Articulatory and Phonological Impairments

A Clinical Focus

Third Edition

Jacqueline Bauman-Waengler

University of Redlands

PEARSON

Boston • New York • San Francisco
Mexico City • Montreal • Toronto • London • Madrid • Munich • Paris
Hong Kong • Singapore • Tokyo • Cape Town • Sydney

Executive Editor and Publisher: Stephen D. Dragin
Editorial Assistant: Katie Heimsoth
Marketing Manager: Kris Ellis-Levy
Production Editor: Paula Carroll
Editorial-Production Service: Omegatype Typography, Inc.
Composition Buyer: Linda Cox
Manufacturing Buyer: Linda Morris
Electronic Composition: Omegatype Typography, Inc.
Cover Administrator: Linda Knowles

For related titles and support materials, visit our online catalog at www.ablongman.com.

Between the time Website information is gathered and then published, it is not unusual for some sites to have closed. Also, the transcription of URLs can result in typographical errors. The publisher would appreciate notification where these errors occur so that they may be corrected in subsequent editions.

ISBN-13: 978-0-205-54925-2
ISBN-10:   0-205-54925-X

Library of Congress Cataloging-in-Publication Data

Bauman-Waengler, Jacqueline Ann.
   Articulatory and phonological impairments : a clinical focus / Jacqueline
Bauman-Waengler.—3rd ed.
      p.   cm.
   Includes bibliographical references and index.
   ISBN-13: 978-0-205-54925-2 (hardcover)
   ISBN-10: 0-205-54925-X (hardcover)
   1.   Articulation disorders. 2.   English language—Phonetics. I.   Title.
   RC424.7.B378 2008
   616.85'5—dc22

                                                            2007025712

Printed in the United States of America

10   9   8   7   6   5   11   10   09

To

Les

and to my mom who always thought my textbook
was "boring" but was still very proud of what I did.
We will all miss her spirit.

About the Author

Jacqueline Bauman-Waengler is a professor in the department of Communicative Disorders at the University of Redlands, California. Her main teaching and clinical emphases are phonetics and phonology, including disorders of articulation and phonology in children and child language disorders. She has published and presented widely in these areas both nationally and internationally. In addition to the third edition of *Articulatory and Phonological Impairments: A Clinical Focus*, Bauman-Waengler adds *Phonetics and Phonology: An Introduction* (published in January, 2008), to her list of publications with Pearson/Allyn & Bacon.

Contents

CHAPTER 8   **Therapy for Phonetic Errors** 245

Preface

The concept for this book grew out of a perceived need to create a bridge between theoretical issues in speech-language pathology and their clinical application. The goal for the third edition has remained the same: to tie strong academic foundations directly to clinical applications. To this end, every chapter contains suggestions for clinical practice as well as marginal notes with so-called clinical applications. This will assist the reader in developing an understanding of how basic concepts and theoretical knowledge form the core for clinical decision making within the assessment and remediation of speech disorders. In addition, the third edition contains learning aids located at the end of every chapter. These include case studies, websites, further readings, critical thinking, and multiple-choice questions that reinforce the presented material from the chapter. One of the strengths of this book has been its strong clinical emphasis. These learning aids support this aspect and add to the diverse foundation of clinical examples.

This third edition has a structure comparable to that of the first two editions. Chapter 1 presents basic concepts that lead to a differentiation between articulation and phonological disorders. This important dichotomy is expanded on in later chapters that address specific phonetic-based assessment and remediation strategies that target articulation disorders, as well as those considered to be more phonologically oriented.

Chapters 2 and 3 include an overview of vowels, consonants, syllable structure, coarticulation, transcription, and diacritics. Chapter 3 reflects the newer transcription systems offered by the International Phonetic Alphabet (IPA) and the Extensions to the IPA (extIPA). The extIPA was specifically developed to address transcription needs of disordered speech. It offers a wide variety of new symbols that can be especially useful for the clinician.

Chapter 4 provides a theoretical foundation that includes the historical development of the conceptual framework surrounding phonetics and phonemics, generative phonology, and nonlinear (multilinear) approaches. This chapter has been changed significantly. The sections on distinctive feature theory and natural phonology have been expanded to include additional analysis procedures that demonstrate the clinical applicability of these theories. The clinical application of natural phonology and phonological processes reappears in later chapters as well.

Normal phonological development is addressed in Chapter 5. New references have been added and a new section relating phonological awareness, emerging literacy, and phonological disorders has been developed. This section provides basic definitions as well as newer literature and research in these areas. Chapters 6 and 7 include diagnostic information, both general and specific, that demonstrates possibilities to differentiate phonetic and phonemic disorders as well as a large array of information, sample worksheets, and clinical applications. Chapter 6 contains a large new section on regional and ethnic dialects as well as English as a second language. The section on regional dialects has been expanded to include information from the Telsur Project at the University of Pennsylvania, and the section on ethnic dialects includes an expanded section on African American Vernacular English. As the number of immigrants to the United States increases, we find a wealth of languages that are being spoken as children learn English as a second language. This chapter examines the vowel and consonant inventories of the five most common foreign languages represented in the United States: Spanish, Vietnamese, Hmong, Cantonese, and Korean. It describes the phonological differences between these languages and American English and provides suggestions as to the pronunciation problems that might occur in speakers of these foreign languages as they learn English as a second language. Chapter 8 is devoted to the traditional phonetic framework for speech sound treatment, and Chapter 9 includes several different phonemic approaches. Maximal oppositions, cycles training, metaphon therapy, and multiple oppositions training are just a few of the concepts treated. Again, clinical applications and examples are provided for all remediation strategies.

The last chapter of the book is devoted to those disorders that are traditionally considered speech disorders. A brief overview is given of the symptom complex and speech characteristics of childhood apraxia of speech, cerebral palsy, cleft palate, mental disabilities, hearing impairment, acquired apraxia of speech, and the dysarthrias. Although a summary of assessment and remediation procedures appears within the text, each section contains updated references, which will lead the reader to additional possibilities.

For instructors, a complimentary *Instructor's Manual and Test Bank* can be ordered from Allyn & Bacon. This manual has been revised to include not only sample test questions but also a large number of additional worksheets and clinical applications. Answers and comments to the learning aids at the end of each chapter are also contained in the Instructor's Manual.

New editions are a constantly evolving process. This third edition has been a serious attempt to leave in place those portions of text that were considered important, but to thoroughly update and add new relevant information that has evolved in the last four years.

$\mathcal{A}$CKNOWLEDGMENTS

The third edition, as with previous editions, starts out appearing as a simple process but ends up being a large time investment supported by a great number of people. First, a special thanks to my companion, Les Beears, who has helped me through all the computer dilemmas and made my life working with computers a whole lot easier. His constant support through all the trials and tribulations of moving and my major and minor crises has been more than a source of strength. I also acknowledge Allyn & Bacon's executive editor and publisher, Steve Dragin, for his friendship and for keeping me moving forward, however difficult that may have been at times. Thanks, too, to my new colleagues at the University of Redlands who have provided a friendly, caring atmosphere that has made my professional life so much happier. Special gratitude goes to my research assistant, Julia Franklin, who provided me with much of the information that is contained at the end of each chapter, and to Angela Benes and Jessica Berger, who were diligent in their search for references, as well as Cassie Hall and Traci Davenport, who helped me with final revisions. I also gratefully acknowledge the following individuals who reviewed and gave suggestions for the third edition: Stephen N. Calculator, University of New Hampshire; Sandra R. Ciocci, Bridgewater State College; Alice M. Dyson, Ball State University; and Audrey M. Glick, University of North Dakota.

1

Clinical Framework

BASIC TERMS AND CONCEPTS

LEARNING OBJECTIVES

When you have finished this chapter, you should be able to:

- Define articulation and articulation disorders.
- Define phonetics and the three branches of phonetics: articulatory, acoustic, and auditory.
- Define and differentiate speech sounds and phonemes.
- Define phonology.
- Differentiate between an articulation and a phonological disorder.
- Explain why articulation impairments are considered to be phonetic disorders, whereas phonological disorders are noted as phonemic problems.

*E*very discipline has a core vocabulary that provides a knowledge base within that particular field of study. Communication sciences and disorders also has such a set of terms. Integral to this discipline, speech and speech disorders represent important constructs. Speech, the exchange of information through speaking or talking, is the most widely used means of communication. One of the main emphases of this book is speech and speech disorders. A speech disorder is a general term that is used to indicate oral, verbal communication that is so deviant from the norm population that it is noticeable or interferes with communication.

Individuals with speech disorders constitute a large percentage of the population with communicative difficulties.

The goal of this beginning chapter is to define and distinguish between certain basic terms. These distinctions will be important when identifying two core concepts within this chapter: articulation and phonological disorders. The term *articulation disorder* is historically older and dates back to the early foundations of what is currently designated as the field of communication disorders. On the other hand, a *phonological disorder* is a more recent label which evidences in part the

1

influence of linguistics on the field of communication disorders. These two different concepts will be important when defining and distinguishing varying types of speech disorders. The following section will define articulation and articulation disorders as well as illustrate their clinical relevance.

ARTICULATION AND ARTICULATION DISORDERS

The term *articulation* and its derivations are often used to describe an individual's speech. They might appear in a referral statement or within a diagnostic report, for example:

> Sandy was referred to the clinic because her parents were concerned about her *articulation* skills.
>
> Bob could *articulate* the sound correctly in isolation, but not in word contexts.
>
> Joe's *articulation* disorder affected his speech intelligibility.

For the purpose at hand, **articulation** refers to the totality of motor processes involved in the planning and execution of sequences of overlapping gestures that result in speech (Fey, 1992). The definition of *articulation* entails, first, that the learning of articulatory skills is a developmental process involving the gradual acquisition of the ability to move the articulators in a precise and rapid manner. Thus, *learning to articulate is a specific kind of motor learning.* Just as children become more adept at certain motor skills as they grow older, their articulation skills develop as well. For example, we do not expect the same level of articulatory abilities from a 2-year-old child as from a 6-year-old. Second, the definition suggests that errors in articulation result from relatively peripheral disturbances of these articulatory processes. Thus, the peripheral motor processes involved in the planning

Articulation is rooted in the Latin word *articulatio,* which stood for the "joining of separate entities." In anatomy, zoology, and biology, this basic definition is preserved, as in "The thyroid cartilage articulates with the cricoid cartilage." Musicians, too, use the word to refer to the joining of separate entities, for example, tone groupings, as in "She played the sonata with feeling and superb articulation." When used by dentists, *articulation* alludes to the joining of teeth, as in "The articulation of the new dentures was better than that of the patient's set of natural teeth." Within communication disorders, the original *articulatio* is exemplified by the joining of the many separate movements needed to establish speech, as in "The child's articulation was characterized by multiple sound errors."

and execution of articulation are impaired; the central language capabilities of the individual remain intact. In summary, articulation is a specific, gradually developing motor skill that involves mainly peripheral motor processes.

If an individual's articulation deviates significantly from the norm, it may be diagnosed as an articulation disorder. An **articulation disorder** refers to difficulties with the motor production aspects of speech, or an inability to produce certain speech sounds (Elbert and Gierut, 1986). Articulation errors are typically classified in light of a child's age, which translates into stages within this developmental process. Younger children are at an earlier stage in this development, whereas older children are at a later stage or may have completed the process. Depending on the age of the child, certain articulation errors may be considered to be typical (age-appropriate errors) or atypical (non–age-appropriate errors).

Articulation and its disorders represent problems with the production of speech sounds. One other basic term relevant to this discussion is *phonetics,* which is the study of speech and speech sounds. Phonetics provides a conceptual foundation for analyzing articulation as well as a clinical framework for assessing and treating articulation disorders. The following section will discuss phonetics and its link to articulation.

PHONETICS AND ITS RELATIONSHIP TO ARTICULATION DISORDERS

The description and classification of speech sounds is the main aim of phonetic science, or phonetics. Sounds may be identified with reference to their production (or "articulation") in the vocal tract, their acoustic transmission, or their auditory reception. The most widely used descriptions are articulatory, because the vocal tract provides a convenient and well-understood reference point. . . . (Crystal, 1987, p. 152)

Generally stated, phonetics is the science of speech (Grunwell, 1987). Such broad definitions delineate speech in its entirety while also effectively indicating the various divisions of phonetics. Thus defined, **phonetics** is the study of speech emphasizing the description and classification of speech sounds according to their production, transmission, and perceptual features. These three branches of phonetics are labeled *articulatory phonetics,* exemplifying speech production, acoustic phonetics, the study of speech transmission, and auditory phonetics.

Articulatory phonetics deals with the production features of speech sounds and their categorization and classification according to specific parameters of their production. Central aspects include how speech sounds are actually articulated, their objective similarities, and their differences. Whereas articulation represents all motor processes resulting in speech in its entirety, articulatory phonetics describes and classifies the specific motor processes responsible for the production of speech sounds. Articulation is typically used

as a more general term to describe the overall speech production of individuals. Articulatory phonetics is a field of study that attempts to document these processes according to specific parameters, such as the manner or voicing of the speech sound. This branch of articulatory phonetics is closely aligned with articulation and its disorders and will be the main emphasis of this text. Definitions and clinical examples are outlined in Table 1.1.

The transmission properties of speech are dealt with in **acoustic phonetics.** Here, the frequency, intensity, and duration of speech sounds, for example, are described and categorized. Within **auditory phonetics,** investigators focus on how we perceive sounds. Our ears are not objective receivers of acoustic data. Rather, many factors influence our perception. Such factors are examined in the area of auditory phonetics.

In the context of this book, we are primarily interested in articulatory phonetics. This specialty area deals with the actualities of how speech sounds are formed. Directly related to this area of phonetics is, of course, articulation.

The description and classification of speech sounds is an integral portion of both the assessment and the treatment of articulation disorders. Knowledge of the production features of speech sounds, information mediated in articulatory phonetics, will guide clinicians when they are evaluating the various misarticulations noted in a clinical evaluation. One important step involves gathering phonetic information on the exact way an individual misarticulates sounds. This type of clinical work involving articulatory phonetics is indispensable in the assessment and treatment of our clients with articulation disorders.

The concept of speech sound is important in our work with articulation and its disorders. However, there is another central term, the *phoneme,* that is connected to phonology and its disorders. The next section will define

Table 1.1   Articulation, Articulation Disorder, and Articulatory Phonetics

Term	Definition	Examples
Articulation	The totality of motor processes involved in the planning and execution of speech.	Describes the speech sound production of individuals, e.g., "He *articulated* the [s] sound correctly." Describes tests that examine speech sound production ability, e.g., "He administered an *articulation* test."
Articulation disorder	Difficulties with the motor production aspects of speech, or an inability to produce certain speech sounds.	A diagnostic category that indicates that an individual's speech sound productions vary widely from the norm, e.g., "He was diagnosed as having an *articulation disorder.*"
Articulatory phonetics	Categorization and classification of speech sounds according to specific production parameters.	How individual sounds are formed, e.g., their place, manner, and voicing characteristics; e.g., clinicians might use their knowledge of articulatory phonetics to determine that the place of articulation, specifically the tongue placement, was deviant from the norm production.

and distinguish between speech sounds and phonemes.

*S*PEECH SOUNDS VERSUS PHONEMES: CLINICAL APPLICATION

Speech sounds are central units in any discussion of disordered speech. Although the human vocal tract is capable of producing a wide array of sounds, including coughing and burping, speech sounds are special sounds because they are associated with speech. **Speech sounds** represent physical sound realities; they are end products of articulatory motor processes. When talking about a child's s-production in the context of an articulation test, for example, we refer to the *speech sound* production of [s].

Speech sounds, then, are real, physical sound entities used in speech. But in addition to their articulatory form, they also have a linguistic function. *Linguistic function* refers to how speech sounds function within a spe-

cific language. For example, which sounds are included in a language and how they are arranged to form meaningful words belong to the linguistic function of speech sounds. Therefore, linguistic function also includes the rules that address how speech sounds can be arranged to produce appropriate words. The term *phoneme* is used in relationship to linguistic function. A **phoneme** is the smallest linguistic unit that is able, when combined with other such units, to establish word meanings and distinguish between them.

If one wants to refer to the physical reality, to the actual production, the term *speech sound* is used. From early to contemporary publications, such phoneme realizations have also been labeled **allophonic variations** (e.g., Shriberg and Kent, 2003; Trubetzkoy, 1939) or **phonetic variations** (Grunwell, 1987). As far as notation is concerned, speech sound productions are usually placed within

> The conceptual nature of the phoneme is more fully developed in Chapter 4.

brackets in phonetic transcription, whereas phoneme values are symbolized by slanted lines, or virgules. For example, [s] indicates that it was a sound someone actually pronounced in a specific manner. On the other hand, /s/ signifies the phoneme "s." Speech sounds or phonetic variations can be examined without reference to a given language system. This is not the case with phonemes. When using the term *phoneme*, we refer exclusively to the function of the sound in question, to its ability to signify differences in word meaning within a *specific* language. Two words that differ in only one phoneme value are called **minimal pairs**. Examples of minimal pairs are *dog* versus *log* and *dog* versus *dot*. See Table 1.2.

How do these terms relate to our clinical decision making? Speech sounds as end products of articulatory motor processes are the units we are describing when we use phonetic transcription to capture an individual's actual productions on an articulation test or spontaneous speech sample. Speech sounds and speech sound errors relate to articulation distortions. However, what if we notice that a child's productions of *swing, sing, ring,* and *wing* all sound the same, for example, that

they all sound like *wing*? The child is not using the necessary phonemic contrasts to signal differences between these words. Both listener and speaker will probably not be able to differentiate between these words because they sound the same. Now we are analyzing the child's phoneme system, the child's ability to use phonemes to establish and distinguish between word meanings. If this occurs consistently throughout the child's speech, we could conclude that the child's phoneme system is limited—that is, restricted when compared to the norm. Phonemes and difficulties in using phonemes contrastively to distinguish meanings relate to *linguistic* abilities, to the individual's language system. This leads us directly into a discussion of phonology, the language-based study of sound systems.

PHONOLOGY AND PHONOLOGICAL DISORDERS

The term *phonology* is basic to the understanding of phonological disorders. **Phonology**, a branch of linguistics, pertains to the description of the systems and patterns of phonemes that occur in a language. It involves determining

Table 1.2 Phoneme versus Speech Sound

Phoneme	Speech Sound
The smallest unit within a language that is able, when combined with other units, to establish word meanings and distinguish between them	Actual realizations of phonemes; referred to as allophonic variations or phonetic variations
Linguistic unit	Concrete, produced, transmitted, and perceived
Used in reference to a particular language system	Can be examined without referring to a specific language system
Basic unit within phonology	Basic unit within phonetics
Notation is within virgules / /, e.g., "the /s/ phoneme"	Notation is within brackets, e.g., "the [f] speech sound"

the language-specific distinctive phonemes and the rule-governed nature of these systems (Mackay, 1987). Phonology is the study of how phonemes are organized and function in communication (Lowe, 1994). Phonology includes the inventory of phonemes of the language in question, thus a list of all the vowels and consonants that function in American English to differentiate meaning. However, phonology also focuses on how these phonemes are *organized* to convey meaning within a language system. Such a description would include how the phonemes can and cannot be arranged to form meaningful words. **Phonotactics** refers to the description of the allowed combinations of phonemes in a particular language.

When an individual's phonology deviates enough from the norm, this could lead to a phonological disorder. A **phonological disorder** refers to an impaired system of phonemes and phoneme patterns within the context of spoken language. The term represents an individual's impairment of the understanding and organization of phonemes within the language system. It is hypothesized that a phonological disorder reflects a language deficiency, specifically a neurolinguistic dysfunction at the phonological level (Grunwell, 1987).

Assessment of a child with a phonological disorder would include gathering information about all the phonemes that the child uses to distinguish meaning—the phonemic inventory. The **phonemic inventory** is the repertoire of phonemes used contrastively by an individual. When compared to the phonemic inventory of General American English, we might find that certain phonemes are not present in the child's speech—that is, the child's phonemic inventory is restricted. In addition, we might analyze the child's phonotactics by examining the position in the word in which these phonemes occur—at the beginning, middle, or end of the word. Children who have difficulties with the organization of their phoneme system might not realize the phonotactics that are typical for American English. Their speech may demonstrate *phonotactic constraints;* in other words, the phoneme use is restricted, the phonemes are not used in all possible word positions.

Phonotactics of General American English include the fact that some phoneme combinations do not occur in American English words. An example would be /ʃ/ + /v/. General American English does have other /ʃ/ combinations, such as /ʃ/ + /r/ (e.g., *shrink*) or /ʃ/ + /t/ (e.g., *wished*). The /ʃ/ + /v/ combination does, however, occur in the phonological system of German. Words such as *Schwester* (/ʃvɛstəʀ/) document this as a *phonotactic* possibility in German.

Phonotactics also includes that some consonant clusters occurring in General American English are restricted in use to certain positions. For example, the clusters "sk" and "ks" cannot occur in the same places. Words or syllables can begin or end with "sk" (e.g., *skate, risk*). This, though, is not the case with "ks." This cluster can occur only at the end of a syllable or word (e.g., *kicks*). This is a *phonotactic* characteristic of the phonological system of General American English.

CLINICAL APPLICATION

Inventory and Phonotactics

Jeff was referred to the school speech-language pathologist by his kindergarten teacher, who was worried about the lack of intelligibility of his speech. The clinician noted that Jeff's phonemic inventory was very restricted. The following phonemes were present in Jeff's speech: /p, b, t, d, k, g, m, n, ŋ, f, v, h, w/. Jeff's phonemic inventory did not include the following phonemes: /s, z, ʃ, ʒ, θ, ð, j, l, r, tʃ, dʒ/. In addition, certain phonotactic constraints were noted. At the beginning of a word, Jeff realized the above noted speech sounds. However, at the end of a word or syllable, only voiced sounds were used. Jeff's phonotactics did not employ voiceless sounds to terminate a word or syllable. Not only was Jeff's phonemic inventory limited, but phonotactic constraints were also discovered.

Phonology is closely related to other constituents of the language system, such as morphology, syntax, semantics, and pragmatics. A child's phonological system, therefore, can never be regarded as functionally separate from other aspects of the child's language growth. Several studies (e.g., Edwards, Fox, and Rogers, 2002; Morrisette and Gierut, 2002; Paul and Jennings, 1992; Ratner, 1994; Rescorla and Ratner, 1996; Roberts, 2005; Scarborough and Dobrich, 1990; Stoel-Gammon, 1989; Storkel, 2001, 2003, 2004; Storkel and Rogers, 2000) have documented that delayed phonological development occurs concurrently with delayed lexical and grammatical development. Although the direct relationship between phonological and grammatical acquisition remains unclear, interdependencies certainly exist between these areas.

PHONETICS VERSUS PHONOLOGY: FORM AND FUNCTION

The speech sounds which are investigated within the area of phonetics have a great many acoustic and articulatory properties which are all important for the phonetician. . . . However, for the phonologist most of them are totally irrelevant as long as they do not function as distinguishing marks between words. Therefore, the speech sound of the phonetician does not coincide with the sound segment of the phonologist. The phonologist considers the sound segment only insofar as it fulfills a certain linguistic function. (Translated from Trubetzkoy, 1939, p. 14)

Any understanding of phonology presupposes its distinction from phonetics. The difference between *form* and *function* has often been used to characterize this distinction. Whereas phonetics emphasizes the form of speech sounds, that is, their concrete actualities, phonology stresses their function as phonemes within the language system. See Table 1.3.

How do we practically differentiate between the form and the function of a specific sound segment in question? When analyzing the speech sound form, a clinician examines all the distinct properties that are associated with its production. It might be noted that [ʃ] is produced without the normal lip rounding or that [s] is produced with the tongue too far forward. The **phonetic inventory** is the repertoire of speech sounds for a particular client, including all the characteristic production features the client utilizes.

On the other hand, if the phoneme function is the goal of the assessment, the clinician would examine the child's phoneme system to determine whether specific phonemes are used contrastively—that is, for the purpose of differentiating between word meanings. A phonemic analysis ignores detailed production characteristics of the sound segment except

Table 1.3 Phonetics versus Phonology

Term	Major Emphasis	Examples
Phonetics	The actualities of speech production	Describes how individual speech sounds are produced, their form
Phonology	The function and organization of phonemes within a given language system	Includes inventory of phonemes within a specific language that functions to differentiate meaning in that language Examines how phonemes can and cannot be arranged to establish meaningful words, i.e., phonotactics

those that distinguish between word meanings in that language. In a phonemic analysis, if a child produces [ʃ] without lip rounding but the sound segment is still perceived as /ʃ/, then the lack of lip rounding would not be relevant. However, if the child's production of [ʃ] is so far off that it is perceived as /s/, this would be important. Its importance lies in the fact that /ʃ/ and /s/ are two separate phonemes in American English; they can be used contrastively to differentiate word meanings, as in *ship* versus *sip*. A phonemic analysis would also examine the phonotactics of a particular client to determine if all sound segments are used in all possible positions.

ARTICULATION DISORDERS VERSUS PHONOLOGICAL DISORDERS

Although the term *phonology* has been a conceptual entity for linguists at least since the beginning of the twentieth century, it is only within the last few decades that it has gained wide usage by speech-language pathologists. For example, describing *phonological processes* when analyzing a child's speech sound error patterns or diagnosing a child as having a *phonological disorder* have their theoretical basis in phonology. In addition, a gradual shift occurred in the 1970s and 1980s away from the label *articulation disorder* to using the term *phonological disorder*. For some, this change was considered necessary as "phonological notions provided a much richer framework for describing normal and disordered speech development" (Kamhi, 1992, p. 262). However, for many, this change in terminology created confusion. One reason for this confusion was the various ways in which the term *phonological disorder* was defined. Another unclear issue related to *how* these new theoretical concepts were to be applied to the assessment and management of children with speech sound/phoneme difficulties. Based on the concep-

tual framework discussed earlier, articulation disorders were defined as disturbances in the relatively peripheral speech motor processes. They result in sounds that are notably different from norm productions. When comparing these characteristics to the previously given definitions, it becomes clear that *articulation disorders are phonetic in nature*.

On the other hand, phonological disorders represent impairments of the understanding and organization of phonemes within a language system. They result in an inadequate phoneme system or in phoneme patterns that are different from those normally noted within a particular language. Phonological disorders are seen as deficiencies in *phoneme function*. For example, the child may demonstrate the ability to produce the sound in question but may be unable to use it appropriately within the phoneme system. *Phonological disorders are phonemic in nature*. See Table 1.4.

Although it does not seem difficult to separate an articulation disorder from a phonological disorder definitionally, opinions vary as to the relationship and interdependencies between the two. The importance in distinguishing between the two terms within the assessment and remediation process is questioned as well as preference among professionals for one term.

For specific speech sound problems, many believe that the term *phonological disorder* is a better label. First, it places speech sound disorders into the broader framework of language. Within this broader framework, attention is focused on the whole system rather than on only one part of the system (Elbert, 1992). This viewpoint also seems more in line with findings that suggest that phonological performance is influenced by pragmatic, morphosyntactic, and semantic levels of organization (e.g., Barlow, 2002; Gierut and Morrisette, 2005; Hoffman, 1990; McCune and Vihman, 2001; Shriberg and Kwiatkowski, 1994; Storkel, 2001; Storkel and Morrisette,

Table 1.4 Articulation Disorders versus Phonological Disorders

Articulation Disorders	Phonological Disorders
Phonetic errors	Phonemic errors
Problems in speech sound production	Problems in the language-specific function of phonemes
Difficulties with speech sound form	Difficulties with phoneme function
Disturbances in relatively peripheral motor processes that result in speech	Disturbances represent an impairment of the understanding of the organization of phonemes within the language system
Speech sound production difficulties do not typically impact other areas of language development such as morphology, syntax, or semantics	Phoneme difficulties may impact other language areas such as morphology, syntax, or semantics

Historically, the term *articulation disorder* has been used as a label for all clients who evidenced speech sound production difficulties. Observed errors were thought to be caused by faulty control of the peripheral articulators. Remediation consisted of increasing precision, speed, and/or mobility of these articulators within the context of speech production. This viewpoint did not emphasize the decisively important fact that speech sounds function within the language system as phonemes. This limited understanding of disordered articulation probably set the stage for embracing a new, more encompassing concept.

2002; Storkel and Rogers, 2000; Velleman and Vihman, 2002). Phonological development is seen as directly linked to the child's developing cognitive and language systems. In addition, it seems clear that some of the sound errors made by children cannot be due to faulty control of the articulators; that is, they cannot be viewed as articulation disorders (Edwards, 1992; Fey, 1992). Although these children may demonstrate adequate production of speech sounds, their rule-governed use in specific contexts or word positions is impaired. For these children, then, the speech sound form is adequate; speech sound function, however, is not.

In an attempt to resolve this labeling issue, Shriberg and Kwiatkowski (1982a) suggested that the term *phonological disorder* be used as a cover term for any problem that involves the speech production process. Thus, both groups of children, those with faulty control of the articulators *and* those with faulty phonemic system organization, would be considered to have a phonological disorder.

Using the term *phonological disorder* in such a broad manner creates several theoretical and practical problems. Definitionally, a phonological disorder represents difficulties with the organization and function of the phoneme system. Does this mean that all children who have speech impairments, even those with so-called simple problems—for example, a distorted [s] or an [r] that is not quite correct—now have problems with the organization and function of their phoneme system? Certainly not. And what about those disorders that have historically been considered as articulation problems, such as the dysarthrias or cerebral palsy? Should these now be considered phonological disorders, too? By labeling all children with speech production problems as "phonologically disordered," more confusion than coherence is gained.

The distinction between articulation and phonological disorders remains decisively important. It keeps definitions clear and is practically applicable to diagnostic and intervention procedures. For the purpose at hand, therefore, a distinction will be made between *phonetic errors,* those in which the peripheral motor processes are disturbed, and *phonemic errors,* those in which the organization and function of the phoneme system is impaired. Although this description of phonetic versus phonemic sound errors is not without problems, the distinction between the two will be applied throughout this text: Phonetic errors result in articulation disorders, whereas phonemic errors represent phonological disorders.

Delineating phonetic from phonemic problems is clinically not an either/or proposition. Often, a child will display characteristics of both phonetic and phonemic errors. Although this division between phonetic and phonemic difficulties may remain at times unclear, a systematic attempt to distinguish between them is one important aspect of clinical decision making.

There is no doubt that the application of phonological principles has added considerably to our understanding of speech errors in children. However, by zealously embrac-

ing these newer concepts, many professionals have started to ignore phonetics due to its alignment with traditional motor-based approaches. The conceptual framework offered by phonetics continues to be a central portion of the assessment and treatment process. "Clearly one cannot employ phonological concepts and techniques without phonetic knowledge, and that knowledge informs clinical assessment and treatment" (Grunwell, 1997, pp. 63–64). Accordingly, after analyzing various treatment perspectives, Shelton (1993) concluded that "both articulatory and phonological concepts contribute to the understanding of children's speech-sound system and related language disorders, but neither is sufficient by itself as a framework for clinical work" (p. 175). For decades, phonetic principles have been the core of assessment and treatment of speech disorders in children and adults. Although phonological principles add to our understanding, they do not replace the valuable knowledge phonetics has to offer.

SUMMARY

This chapter refamiliarized the reader with several terms that are fundamental to the assessment and treatment of articulatory and phonological disorders. Definitions and clinical applications were provided for *articulation, phonetics, speech sound, phonology,* and the *phoneme* as a foundation for this understanding. Form versus function was used to distinguish between phonetics, with its basic unit the speech sound, and phonology, represented by

the phoneme. Phonetics emphasizes the form of speech sounds, whereas phonology stresses the function of phonemes within a language system. Based on these definitions, a differentiation between articulation disorders and phonological disorders was presented. The problems of such a division were discussed in light of the diversity of viewpoints on the subject as well as of the clinical consequences of such a separation.

CASE STUDY

PHONETIC DISORDER
Sandy is a 6-year-old child who was seen in a diagnostic session at the speech and hearing

clinic. Her parents were concerned about her inability to produce an "s" sound. Based on an analysis of a spontaneous speech sample and an articulation test, it was found that Sandy misarticulated "s" and "z" in all transcribed situations. The child was also able to differentiate her mispronunciations from norm productions of [s] and [z]. No other speech sounds were in error, and language skills were found to be within normal limits. Sandy used her distorted realizations in every position in which [s] and [z] should occur. Thus, she seemed to understand the organization of /s/ and /z/ within the language system. The clinician hypothesized that this child was having difficulties with the actual production level only, with the speech sounds [s] and [z], whereas the understanding of their phoneme functions was intact.

PHONEMIC DISORDER

Travis, a 6-year-old first-grader, was referred by his classroom teacher to the speech-language pathologist. The teacher said that although Travis's speech was fairly intelligible, she was concerned about speech and language problems she had noticed in class. Her second concern was that these difficulties might be impacting Travis's emerging literacy skills. According to the teacher, Travis was having difficulty distinguishing between certain sounds and words as the class progressed with elementary reading tasks.

An articulation test and a spontaneous speech sample were analyzed with the following results: Travis had difficulties with s-productions. At the end of a word or syllable, [s] was always deleted. At the beginning of a word or syllable, [s] was produced as [ʃ]. Interestingly enough, when the clinician analyzed other words, she found that Travis could produce [s], but not in its proper context. Thus, several words that contained [f] were articulated with a normal sounding [s] realization. Testing of minimal pairs containing /s/ and /ʃ/ revealed that Travis was having difficulty distinguishing between the phonemic value of the two sounds.

On language tests and in spontaneous conversation, Travis deleted the plural -s and the third person singular -s (e.g., "He, she, it walk"). Comprehension of these grammatical forms was often in error.

The clinician hypothesized that Travis had a phonological disorder—that he had difficulties with the phoneme function and the phonotactics of /s/. This problem was impacting his morphological development. Due to the noted problems in discrimination, this could also have an effect on his beginning reading skills.

THINK CRITICALLY

The following small speech sample is from Tara, age 4;3.

rabbit	[wæbət]	ready	[wɛdi]
feather	[fɛdɚ]	arrow	[ɛwoᵘ]
green	[gwin]	toothbrush	[tutbwəʃ]
this	[ðɪs]	thinking	[θɪŋkɪn]
that	[ðæt]	round	[waᵘnd]
rope	[woᵘp]	bridge	[bwɪdʒ]
rooster	[wustɚ]	street	[stwit]
bathing	[beˈdɪŋ]	thin	[θɪn]
nothing	[nʌtɪŋ]	them	[ðɛm]
bath	[bæt]	breathe	[bwid]

Which speech sound errors are noted in this sample?

Which sounds are substituted for the sounds in error?

Can any phonotactic restraints be noted in the correct productions of "th" and "r"?

Based on this limited information, do you think the child has an articulation disorder or a phonological disorder? Why?

TEST YOURSELF

1. The definition of articulation includes which one of the following?
   a. describes the systems and patterns of phonemes in a particular language
   b. includes phonotactics
   c. refers to the totality of motor processes involved in speech
   d. all of the above

2. The definition of articulation disorder reflects
   a. peripheral motor processes
   b. gradually developing motor skills
   c. mainly peripheral motor processes
   d. all of the above

3. Which one of the following is not included in the definition of phonetics?
   a. the production features of speech sounds
   b. the organizational system of speech sounds
   c. the transmission properties of speech sounds
   d. the perceptual bases of speech sounds

4. Which one of the subdivisions of phonetics would examine the frequency, intensity, and duration of speech sounds?
   a. articulatory phonetics
   b. acoustic phonetics
   c. auditory phonetics

5. If you were studying how foreign students perceive various speech sounds of American English, you would be in which branch of phonetics?
   a. articulatory phonetics
   b. acoustic phonetics
   c. auditory phonetics

6. If you were studying how the production of [s] varies in American English versus Spanish, you would be in which branch of phonetics?

   a. articulatory phonetics
   b. acoustic phonetics
   c. auditory phonetics

7. The definition of phonology includes
   a. the description of the system and patterns of phonemes within a language
   b. the classification and description of how speech sounds are produced
   c. speech sound form
   d. relatively peripheral motor processes involved in speech

8. The allowed combinations of phonemes in a particular language refers to the
   a. phonetic inventory
   b. phonemic inventory
   c. phonotactic constraints
   d. minimal pairs

9. Which one of the following is not included in the definition of phonological disorder?
   a. problems in the language-specific function of phonemes
   b. disturbances in the relatively peripheral motor processes that result in speech
   c. disturbances represent an impairment of the understanding and organization of phonemes
   d. phonemic errors

10. The smallest linguistic unit which is able, when combined with other such units to establish word meanings, is referred to as the
    a. allophonic variation
    b. speech sound
    c. phoneme
    d. phonotactic constraint

WEBSITES

www.phonologicaldisorders.com

This website, created by the author of this textbook, contains basic definitions and characteristics of articulation versus phonological disorders. It also provides references to articles and books which delineate the two. Links are given to other websites and resources.

www.speech-language-therapy.com/phonetic_phonemic.htm

This website distinguishes in an easy-to-read manner between articulation and phonological disorders. Several links are given to areas such as functional speech disorders and a discussion group, which can be accessed from the author's (Carol Bowen) website.

http://scholar.google.com/scholar?q=articulation%20and%20phonological%20disorders&hl=en&lr=&oi=scholart

This website has a list of articles and books that deal with articulation and phonological disorders. Although many references are duplicated and more than ten years old, there are over 5,000 references on this website.

www2.hu-berlin.de/angl/ling_pages/phonology_phonetics.html

This website has some basic definitions of phonetics and phonology. It also lists information on several branches of phonetics (articulatory, acoustic, and auditory phonetics) as well as makes the distinction between segmental and suprasegmental phonology. Several references are also included.

www.unibuc.ro/eBooks/filologie/mateescu/pdf21.pdf

This website, among other things, distinguishes between phonetics and phonology and defines articulatory, auditory, and acoustic phonetics. The definitions appear easy to understand. This appears to be Chapter 2 of a book or manuscript from the University of Bucharest.

www.answers.com/topic/phonology and www.answers.com/topic/phonetics

These websites provide basic definitions and examples of phonology and phonetics. They also provide links to related topics. The website for phonetics gives definitions of articulatory, acoustic, and auditory phonetics.

FURTHER READINGS

Ball, M., & Rahilly, J. (1999). *Phonetics: The science of speech.* London: Arnold.

Catford, J. (2002). *A practical introduction to phonetics* (2nd ed.). Oxford: Oxford University Press.

Handke, J. (2000). *The Mouton interactive introduction to phonetics and phonology.* Berlin, New York: Mouton de Gruyter.

Mackay, I. (1987). *Phonetics: The science of speech production* (2nd ed.). Boston: Allyn & Bacon.

Reid, N. (with H. Fraser). (1996). *Phonetics: An interactive introduction.* Armidale, Australia: The University of New England.

2

Articulatory Phonetics

SPEECH SOUND FORM

LEARNING OBJECTIVES

When you have finished this chapter, you should be able to:

- List the differences in production and function of vowels versus consonants.
- Identify the three descriptive parameters that are used for vowel articulations, and classify the vowels of American English using those three parameters.
- Differentiate between monophthong and diphthong vowels.
- Define centering diphthongs.
- Differentiate between a phonemic and a nonphonemic diphthong.
- Identify the four parameters that are used to describe the articulation of consonants.
- Define the various manners of articulation.
- Classify the consonants of American English according to their organ, place, manner, and voicing characteristics.
- Define coarticulation and assimilation, and describe the different types of assimilatory processes.
- Understand the importance of syllable structure in the assessment process.

*A*rticulatory phonetics deals with the categorization and classification of the production features of speech sounds. A thorough knowledge of how vowels and consonants are generated remains essential for successful assessment and remediation of articulatory and phonological disorders. Although contemporary phonological theories have provided new ways of viewing assessment and treatment of these disorders, knowledge of the speech sounds' production features secures a firm basis for utilizing such procedures. Without this knowledge, phonological process analysis, for example, is impossible.

This chapter discusses articulatory-phonetic aspects of the speech sounds of General American English. The specific goals are

1. to provide a review of the production features of vowels and consonants;
2. to introduce the concepts of coarticulation and assimilation as a means of describing how sounds change within a given articulatory context; and
3. to examine the structure of syllables and their clinical applicability in the assessment and treatment of impaired articulation and phonology.

The production of vowels and consonants, and their subsequent language-specific arrangements into syllables and words, depends on articulatory motor processes. If these processes are impaired, speech sound production will be disordered. Articulatory motor processes depend in turn on many anatomical-physiological prerequisites, which include respiratory, phonatory, or resonatory processes. For example, the speech problems of children with cerebral palsy often originate in abnormal respiratory, resonatory, and/or phonatory prerequisites for articulation. The proper function of such prerequisites, therefore, must first be secured before any articulatory improvement can be expected. Articulatory motor ability is embedded in many different anatomical-physiological prerequisites, which are of fundamental importance to speech-language pathologists.

Basic knowledge in these areas is typically gained from courses and textbooks covering anatomy and physiology of the speech and hearing mechanisms rather than

> For more information about the respiratory, phonatory, resonatory, and articulatory characteristics of cerebral palsy, see Chapter 10.

BOX 2.1 Selected Readings in Anatomy and Physiology of the Speech and Hearing Mechanisms

Culbertson, W. R., Cotton, S. S., & Tanner, D. C. (2006). *Anatomy and physiology study guide for speech and hearing.* San Diego: Plural Publishing.

Kent, R. D. (1997). *The speech sciences.* San Diego: Singular Publishing.

Perkins, W., & Kent, R. (1986). *Functional anatomy of speech, language and hearing: A primer.* Boston: Allyn & Bacon.

Seikel, J. A., King, D. W., & Drumwright, D. G. (2005). *Anatomy and physiology for speech and language* (3rd ed.). Clifton Park, NY: Delmar.

Zemlin, W. R. (1997). *Speech and hearing science: Anatomy and physiology* (4th ed.). Boston: Allyn & Bacon.

from those covering impaired articulation and phonology. This is because the clinical significance of anatomical-physiological knowledge and its application to articulatory and phonological disorders is not always recognized. The anatomical-physiological aspects of such disorders are not within the scope of this chapter. Box 2.1 offers references as an incentive for the reader to rediscover the wealth of information essential to the clinical assessment and remediation of articulatory and phonological impairments.

Vowels VERSUS CONSONANTS

Speech sounds are commonly divided into two groups: vowels and consonants. **Vowels** are produced with a relatively open vocal tract; *no significant constriction* of the oral (and pharyngeal) cavities exists. The airstream from the vocal folds to the lips is relatively unimpeded. Therefore, vowels are considered to be *open sounds*. In contrast, **consonants** are produced with a *significant constriction* in the oral and/or pharyngeal cavities during their production. For consonants, the airstream from the vocal folds to the lips and nostrils encounters some type of articulatory obstacle along the way. Therefore, consonants are considered to be *constricted sounds*. For most consonants this constriction occurs along the sagittal midline of the vocal tract. This constriction for consonants can be exemplified by the first sound in *top*, [t], or *soap*, [s]. For [t] the contact of the front of the tongue with the alveolar ridge occurs along this midline while the characteristic s-quality is made by air flowing along this median plane as the tongue approximates the alveolar ridge. By contrast, during all vowel productions the sagittal midline remains free. In addition, under normal speech conditions, General American English vowels are always produced with vocal fold vibration; they are voiced speech sounds. Only during whispered speech are vowels unvoiced. Consonants, on the other hand, may be generated with or without simultaneous vocal fold vibration; they can be voiced or voiceless. Pairs of sounds such as [t] and [d] exemplify this relevant feature. Pairs of similar sounds, in this case differing only in their voicing feature, are referred to as **cognates.** Voicing features constitute the main linguistically relevant differences that separate the consonant cognates such as [s] from [z] or [f] from [v]. The transcription of various vowels and consonants together with examples of words in which these sounds can be heard are contained in Table 2.1.

Vowels can also be distinguished from consonants according to the patterns of acous-

> The *sagittal midline of the vocal tract* refers to the median plane that divides the vocal tract into right and left halves.

Table 2.1 IPA Symbols (Wise, 1958)

Consonants		Vowels	
Symbol	Commonly Realized In	Symbol	Commonly Realized In
[p]	pay	[i]	eat
[b]	boy	[ɪ]	in
[t]	toy	[eɪ]	ape
[d]	doll	[ɛ]	egg
[k]	coat	[æ]	at
[g]	goat	[a]	father*
[m]	moon	[u]	moon
[n]	not	[ʊ]	wood
[ŋ]	sing	[oʊ]	boat
[θ]	think	[ɔ]	father*
[ð]	those	[ɑ]	hop
[f]	far	[aɪ]	tie
[v]	vase	[aʊ]	mouse
[s]	sun	[ɔɪ]	boy
[z]	zoo	[ɜ]	girl*
[ʃ]	shop	[ɝ]	bird
[ʒ]	beige	[ɚ]	winner
[tʃ]	chop	[ʌ]	cut
[dʒ]	job	[ə]	above
[j]	yes		
[w]	win		
[ʍ]	when*		
[l]	leap		
[r]	red		
[h]	hop		

*May be regional or individual pronunciations.

tic energy they display. Vowels are highly resonant, demonstrating at least two formant areas. Thus, vowels are more intense than consonants; in other words, they are typically louder than consonants. In this respect we can say that vowels have greater sonority than consonants. **Sonority** of a sound is its loudness relative to that of other sounds with the same length, stress, and pitch (Ladefoged, 2006). Due to the greater sonority of vowels over consonants, vowels are also referred to as **sonorants.**

Due to the production features of a special group of consonants and their resulting sonority, certain consonants are also labeled sonorants. **Sonorant consonants** are produced with a relatively open expiratory passageway. When contrasted to other consonants, sonorant consonants demonstrate less obstruction of the airstream during their production. The sonorant consonants include the nasals, the liquids, and the glides. The sonorants are distinguished from the **obstruents,** which are characterized by a complete or narrow constriction between the articulators hindering the expiratory airstream. The obstruents include the stop-plosives, the fricatives, and the affricates.

There are also functional differences between vowels and consonants. In other words, vowels and consonants play different linguistic roles. This has often been referred to as the "phonological difference" between vowels and consonants (Crystal, 1987; Hyman, 1975). The term *consonant* actually indicates this: *con* meaning "together with" and *-sonant* reflecting the tonal qualities that characterize vowels. Thus, consonants are those speech sounds that function linguistically *together with* vowels. As such, vowels serve as the center of syllables, as syllable nuclei. Vowels can constitute syllables all by themselves, for example, in the first syllable of *a-go* or *e-lope.* Vowels can also appear together with one or more consonants, exemplified by *blue, bloom,* or *blooms.* Although there are many types of syllables, the vowel is always the center of the syllable, its nucleus. A small group of consonants can serve as the nuclei of syllables. A consonant that functions as a syllable nucleus is referred to as a **syllabic.** These form and functional differences are summarized in Table 2.2.

> When transcribing, syllabic consonants need a special notation. This is discussed in Chapter 3.

Table 2.2 Features Differentiating Vowels and Consonants

Vowels	Consonants
No significant constriction of the vocal tract	Significant constriction of the vocal tract
Open sounds	Constricted sounds
Sagittal midline of vocal tract remains open	Constriction occurs along sagittal midline of the vocal tract
Voiced	Voiced or unvoiced
Acoustically more intense	Acoustically less intense
Demonstrate more sonority	Demonstrate less sonority
Function as syllable nuclei	Only specific consonants can function as syllable nuclei

American English Vowels

Vowels are commonly described according to certain parameters (Abercrombie, 1967; Crystal, 1987; Heffner, 1975; Kantner and West, 1960; Kent, 1998; Shriberg and Kent, 2003):

1. The portion of the tongue that is involved in the articulation. Example: front versus back vowels.
2. The tongue's position relative to the palate. Example: high versus low vowels.
3. The degree of lip rounding or unrounding.

The four-sided form called a vowel quadrilateral is often used to demonstrate schematically the front–back and high–low positions. The form roughly represents the tongue position in the oral cavity (see Figure 2.1).

The terms *tense/lax* and *open/close* are also used to describe vowels. *Tense* and *lax* refer to

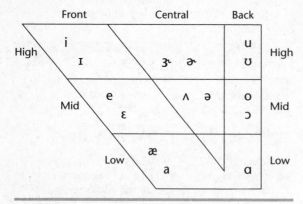

Figure 2.1   Vowel Quadrilateral of General American English Vowels

the degree of muscular activity involved in the articulation and to the length of the vowels in question (Shriberg and Kent, 2003). Therefore, tense vowels are considered to have relatively more muscle activity and are longer in duration than lax vowels. The vowel [i] is considered to be a tense vowel, whereas [ɪ] is lax. When contrasting tense versus lax, one has to keep in mind that these oppositions refer to pairs of vowels that are productionally similar, to vowel cognates. For example, [i] and [ɪ] are considered to be "ee" type vowels, and [u] and [ʊ] are "oo" type vowels.

The terms *close* and *open* refer to the relative closeness of the tongue to the roof of the mouth (Abercrombie, 1967). Again, only vowel cognates are usually characterized with these terms. Using the previous examples, [i] is more close and [ɪ] more open, [u] close and [ʊ] open.

There are two types of vowels: monophthongs and diphthongs. **Monophthongs** remain qualitatively the same throughout their entire production. They are pure vowels (Abercrombie, 1967; Shriberg and Kent, 2003). **Diphthongs** are vowels in which there is a change in quality during their duration (Ladefoged,

"It should be noted that although monophthongs are often referred to as 'pure' vowels, no special virtue attaches to them" (Abercrombie, 1967, p. 60).

2006). The initial segment, the beginning portion of such a diphthong, is phonetically referred to as the **onglide**, its end portion as the **offglide**. Using this notation system, the following descriptions for the most common vowels of General American English are offered.

Front Vowels

[i]   a high-front vowel, unrounded, close and tense.

[ɪ]   a high-front vowel, unrounded, open and lax.

[e]   a mid-front vowel, unrounded, close and tense. In General American English, this vowel is typically produced as a diphthong, especially in stressed syllables or when articulated slowly.

[ɛ]   a mid-front vowel, unrounded, open and lax.

[æ]   a low-front vowel, unrounded, open and lax.

[a]   a low-front vowel, unrounded, close and tense. In General American English, the use of this vowel depends on the particular regional dialect of the speaker. In the New England dialect of the Northeast, one might often hear it.

All front vowels show various degrees of unrounding (lip spreading), with the high-front vowels showing the most. The lip spreading becomes less as one moves from the high-front vowels to the mid-front vowels, finally becoming practically nonexistent in the low-front vowels.

Back Vowels

[u]   a high-back vowel, rounded, close and tense.

[ʊ]   a high-back vowel, rounded, open and lax.

[o]   a mid-back vowel, rounded, close and tense. This vowel is typically produced

There are differences of opinion as to whether certain vowels (specifically [ɔ] and [ɑ]) are tense or lax. This is based partially on definitional differences. Heffner (1975) and Kantner and West (1960) define tense and lax according to the degree of muscular activity. Shriberg and Kent (2003) point out that this has not been verified by experimental studies (e.g., Neary, 1978; Raphael and Bell-Berti, 1975), and they add the dimension of length: Tense vowels are longer in duration than lax ones. Ladefoged (2006) defines tense and lax according to the type of syllable in which the vowel can occur. Only tense vowels can occur in open syllables, that is, in those without a consonant following the vowel (as in the words *bee* and *do*); all other vowels must be considered lax.

as a diphthong, especially in stressed syllables or when articulated slowly.

[ɔ] a low mid-back vowel, rounded, open and lax (Heffner, 1975). The use of this vowel depends on regional pronunciation.

[ɑ] a low-back vowel, unrounded, open and lax (Kantner and West, 1960). There seems to be some confusion in transcribing [ɔ] and [ɑ], although acoustic differences certainly exist. One distinguishing feature: the [ɔ] shows some degree of lip rounding, whereas [ɑ] does not.

Back vowels display different degrees of lip rounding in General American English. The high-back vowels [u] and [ʊ] often show a fairly high degree of lip rounding, whereas the low-back vowel [ɑ] is commonly articulated as an unrounded vowel.

Central Vowels

[ɝ] a central vowel, rounded, tense with r-coloring. Rounding may vary, however, from speaker to speaker. [ɝ] is a stressed vowel. It is typically acousti-

cally more intense, has a higher fundamental frequency, and has a longer duration when it is compared to a similar unstressed vowel such as [ɚ].

[ɚ] a central vowel, rounded, lax with r-coloring. Again, lip rounding may vary from speaker to speaker. This lax vowel is an unstressed vowel.

[ɜ] a central vowel, rounded, tense. [ɜ] is very similar in pronunciation to [ɝ], but it lacks any r-coloring. This vowel is heard in certain dialects. [ɜ] might be found in a Southern dialect pronunciation of *bird* or *worth,* for example. Also, it could be heard in the speech of children having difficulties producing the "r" sound.

[ʌ] a lax, unrounded central vowel. It is a stressed vowel.

[ə] a lax, unrounded central vowel. It is an unstressed vowel.

CLINICAL APPLICATION

Do Children Have Difficulties Producing Vowels?

Vowel errors in children developing phonological skills in a normal manner are relatively uncommon. However, children with phonological disorders may show deviant vowel patterns. Several studies (e.g., Gibbon, Shockey, and Reid, 1992; Penney, Fee, and Dowdle, 1994; Pollock, 2002; Pollock and Keiser, 1990; Reynolds, 1990; Robb, Bleile, and Yee, 1999; Stoel-Gammon and Herrington, 1990) have documented the presence of specific vowel problems in phonologically disordered children. Although certain vowel substitutions seem to be articulatory simplifications that could also occur in normal development, other errors appear to be idiosyncratic. Assessment of vowel qualities should be a portion of every diagnostic protocol. This can easily be achieved with any formal articulation test by transcribing the entire word rather than just the sound being tested.

Diphthongs. As previously defined, a diphthong is a vowel sound that demonstrates articulatory movement during its production. Its initial portion, the onglide, is acoustically more prominent and usually longer than the offglide. Common diphthongs in General American English are **rising diphthongs**. This means that in producing these diphthongs, essential portions of the tongue move from a lower onglide to a higher offglide position; thus, relative to the palate, the tongue moves in a rising motion. This can be demonstrated on the vowel quadrilateral as well (see Figure 2.2).

Certain diphthongs are referred to as **centering diphthongs**. In this case, the offglide, or less prominent element of the diphthong, is a central vowel. In British English, and in some dialects of General American English, this may be a schwa vowel [ə]. Thus, *fear* may be pronounced as [fɪə] or *far* as [faə]. More common in General American English is the use of the central vowel with r-coloring [ɚ] as the offglide. Thus, *fear* is often pronounced as [fɪɚ], *far* as [faɚ], and *bear* as [bɛɚ] (Ball and Rahilly, 1999; Heffner, 1975). Theoretically, any vowel may be combined with [ə] or [ɚ] to form a centering diphthong; however, in General American English certain centering diphthongs are more common than others. Thus, [ɪɚ], [ɛɚ],

and [aɚ], which can be heard in *dear* [dɪɚ], *bear* [bɛɚ], or *farm* [faɚm], are far more prevalent than [iɚ] or [uɚ]. Lowe (1994) refers to the diphthongs which are paired with [ɚ] as **rhotic diphthongs**. Centering diphthongs are also seen transcribed with [r]. Thus, *dear* is transcribed as [dɪr], *bear* as [bɛr], or *farm* as [farm].

There are several different ways to characterize diphthongs as single phonemic units in contrast to two separate vowels. Some transcribers use a bar or bow either above or below the two vowel symbols—[e͞ɪ], [e͡ɪ], or [e͜ɪ], for example. The author has chosen to use the transcription that elevates the offglide portion of the diphthong to indicate its typically lesser intensity and length.

Discrepancies may be noted between the transcriptions of diphthongs offered in this text and the ones in other books. Because phonetic transcription is purely *de*scriptive, never *pre*scriptive, any transcription will, of course, vary according to the actual pronunciation. See Shriberg and Kent (2003) for a thorough discussion of the various ways diphthongs have been transcribed.

[eᴵ] a **nonphonemic diphthong**

It is nonphonemic in the sense that the meaning would *not* change in a particular word if the vowel were to be pronounced as a monophthong [e] versus a diphthong [eᴵ]. Therefore, the meaning would not change if just the onglide was realized. Words pronounced [beᴵk] or [bek], for example, would be recognized as the same word.

[oᵁ] a nonphonemic diphthong

[aᴵ] a **phonemic diphthong**

It is phonemic in the sense that the meaning *would* change in a particular word if only the vowel onglide was produced. Therefore, the vowel was realized as a monophthong. A realization of

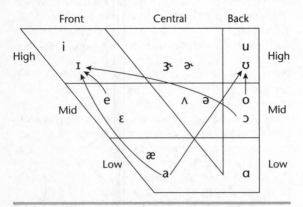

Figure 2.2 Vowel Quadrilateral with Rising Diphthongs

[a] instead of [aɪ] will change the meaning in General American English as the words *sod* [sad] versus *sighed* [saɪd] demonstrate.

[ɔɪ] a phonemic diphthong

The opposition [ʤɔ], *jaw*, versus [ʤɔɪ], *joy*, exemplifies its phonemic value as a

meaning-differentiating sound feature of English.

[aʊ] a phonemic diphthong

Oppositions such as [mas], *moss*, versus [maʊs], *mouse*, exemplify its phonemic value.

CLINICAL APPLICATION

Analyzing the Vowel System of a Child

Occasionally, the vowel system of a client may be restricted or show deviant patterns. In this case, a more in-depth analysis of the vowels produced may be necessary. Vowel systems can be analyzed using the vowel quadrilateral and knowledge of the diphthongs as guiding principles. Front, back, and central vowels as well as diphthongs can be checked in relationship to their accuracy and their occurrence in the appropriate contexts. George, age 5;3, is an example of a child with a deviant vowel system.

George was being seen in the clinic for his phonological disorder. He was a gregarious child who loved to talk and would try to engage anyone in conversation who would listen. The only problem was that George was almost unintelligible. This made dialogue difficult, possibly more so for those who would patiently and diligently try to understand his continuing attempts to interact.

In addition to his many consonant problems, the following vowel deviations were noted:

VOWEL ERRORS

Norm Production	→	Actual Production	Word Examples	Transcriptions		
[eɪ]	→	[ɛ]	grapes	[greɪps]	→	[dɛ]
			table	[teɪbl̩]	→	[tɛboʊ]
[i]	→	[ɪ]	feet	[fit]	→	[fɪ]
			teeth	[tiθ]	→	[tɪ]
			three	[θri]	→	[dɪ]
[ɛ]	→	[æ]	bed	[bɛd]	→	[bæt]
			feather	[fɛðɚ]	→	[fævə]
[u]	correct	[u]	shoe	[ʃu]	→	[tu]
			spoon	[spun]	→	[mun]
[ʊ]	correct	[ʊ]	book	[bʊk]	→	[bʊ]
[oʊ]	correct	[oʊ]	stove	[stoʊv]	→	[doʊ]
			nose	[noʊz]	→	[noʊ]
[ɑ]	correct	[ɑ]	mop	[mɑp]	→	[ma]
			blocks	[blaks]	→	[ba]

George's productions of the back vowels [u], [ʊ], [oᵁ], and [ɑ] are on target. The front vowels do show a deviant pattern, however. Not only is the diphthong [eᴵ] produced as a monophthong, but also the articulatory position of the vowel substitution for [e] is realized lower as [ɛ]. This tendency to lower vowels is also noted in the other productions with front vowels, in which [i] becomes [ɪ] and [ɛ] becomes [æ].

American English Consonants

Four phonetic categories are used to transcribe consonants: (1) organ of articulation, (2) place of articulation, (3) manner of articulation, and (4) voicing features. Most textbooks state that only place, manner, and voicing are used to characterize individual consonants (Edwards, 2003; Lowe, 1994; Shriberg and Kent, 2003). However, they nevertheless often include the organ of articulation. For example, the term *lingual* as in *lingua-dental* or *lingua-palatal*, designates the active organ of articulation. However, when contrasting the lingua-dental sounds [θ] and [ð] to the lingua-palatal sounds [ʃ] and [ʒ], it becomes clear that different portions of the tongue are actively involved in the articulation. The term *lingual* alone does not specify these differences. This text emphasizes the detailed knowledge of production features for specific therapy goals. By adding a category specifically designating the active articulator, the organ of articulation, valuable clarification of consonant articulation is achieved.

Organ of Articulation. Consonants are sounds characterized by the articulators creating a partial or total obstruction of the expiratory airstream. There are active and passive articulators. Active articulators, the so-called **organs of articulation**, are the parts within the vocal tract that actually move to achieve the articulatory result (Crystal, 1987). In describing the consonants of General American English, we are referring specifically to the movements of the lower lip and portions of the tongue. The structures actively involved in the articulation of the consonants of General American English and the resulting phonetic descriptors are contained in Table 2.3. Figure 2.3 displays the divisions of the tongue.

Place of Articulation. The **place of articulation** denotes the area within the vocal tract that remains motionless during consonant articulation, that is, the passive articulator; it is the part that the organ of articulation as active articulator approaches or contacts directly (Crystal, 1987). The upper lip and teeth, the palate, and the velum are the main places of articulation when describing the consonants of General American English. The passive structures of articulation and their resulting phonetic descriptors are contained in Table 2.4. Figure 2.4 displays the structures of the oral cavity as organs and places of articulation.

Manner of Articulation. The **manner of articulation** refers to the type of constriction the organ and place of articulation produce for the realization of a particular consonant. There are various manners of articulation, ranging from complete closure for the production of stop-plosives to a very limited constriction of the vocal tract for the production of glides. The following manners of articulation are used to account phonetically for the consonants of General American English.

Stop-Plosives. During the production of stop-plosives, complete occlusion is secured at specific points in the vocal tract. Simultaneously,

Table 2.3   Phonetic Description: Organ of Articulation

Organ of Articulation	Phonetic Descriptor	Examples
Lower lip	Labial	[p], [b], [m], [f], [v], [w], [ʍ]
Tip of tongue	Apical	[s], [z], [θ], [ð], [r],[1] [l]
Lateral rims of tongue[2]	Coronal	[t], [d], [n], [ʃ], [ʒ]
Surface of tongue	Dorsum	
anterior portion	predorsal	[s], [z]
central portion	mediodorsal	[j], [r]
posterior portion	postdorsal	[k], [g], [ŋ]

1. The transcription used officially by the International Phonetic Association for the American English "r" is [ɹ]. See explanation under rhotics.

2. The term *coronal* designates the apex and the lateral rims of the tongue. While the term *blade* of the tongue also includes its apex, it characterizes an extension into predorsal areas as well. In order to delineate the action of the organ of articulation as closely as possible, the terms *coronal* and *predorsal* will be used instead of *blade*.

the velum is raised so that no air can escape through the nose. The expiratory air pressure builds up naturally behind this closure (stop); compression results, which is then suddenly released (plosive). Examples of stop-plosives are [p] and [b].

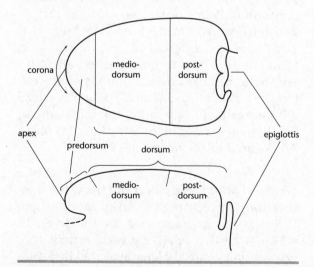

Figure 2.3   Divisions of the Tongue

Fricatives.   Fricatives result when organ and place of articulation approximate each other so closely that the escaping expiratory airstream causes an audible friction. As with the stops, the velum is raised for all fricative sounds. Two examples of fricatives are [f] and [v]. Some fricatives, referred to as **sibilants**, have a sharper sound than others due to the presence of high-frequency components. In General American English [s], [z], [ʃ], and [ʒ] belong to the sibilants.

Nasals.   These consonants are produced with the velum lowered so that the air can pass freely through the nasal cavity. However, there is complete occlusion within the oral cavity between organ and place of articulation. These sounds have been called nasal stops due to the closure in the oral cavity and the ensuing free air passage through the nasal cavity (Ball and Rahilly, 1999). [m], [n], and [ŋ] are the nasal speech sounds of General American English.

Table 2.4   Phonetic Description: Place of Articulation

Place of Articulation	Phonetic Descriptor	Examples
Upper lip	Labial	[p], [b], [m], [w], [ʍ]
Upper teeth	Dental	[f], [v], [θ], [ð]
Alveolar ridge	Alveolar	[t], [d], [n], [s], [z], [l]

Surface of hard palate
    anterior portion
    central portion
    posterior portion
	Palatal
	    prepalatal
	    mediopalatal
	    postpalatal
		
		[ʃ], [ʒ],[1] [r]
		[j], [r]
		(does not normally occur in General American English)

Soft palate	Velar	[k], [g], [ŋ]

1. [ʃ] and [ʒ] are also referred to as postalveolar sounds, indicating a place of articulation just posterior to the highest point of the alveolar ridge. This text will include both of these places of articulation to describe [ʃ] and [ʒ].

Affricates. For affricate sounds, two phases can be noted. First, the velum is raised as a complete closure is formed between organ and place of articulation. As a consequence of these articulatory conditions, expiratory air pressure builds up behind the blockage formed by the organ and place of articulation, the stop phase. Second the stop is then slowly (in comparison to the plosives) released orally, resulting in the friction portion of the speech sound. Affricates should not be viewed as a stop plus fricative combination similar to consonant blends or clusters, such as [ks], in which the stop portion is formed by a different organ and at a different place of articulation than the fricative portion. Rather, affricates are single uniform speech sounds characterized by a slow release of a stopping phase into a homorganic (*hom* = same) friction element. The two most prominent affricates of General American English are [tʃ] and [dʒ].

Glides. For the realization of glides, the constriction between organ and place of articulation is not as narrow as for fricatives. In addition to this relatively wide articulatory posture, glides are also characterized by a gliding movement of the articulators from a rela-

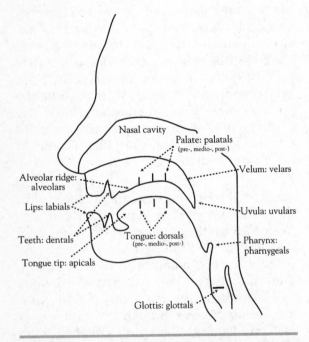

Nasal cavity

Palate: palatals
(pre-, medio-, post-)

Velum: velars

Alveolar ridge:
alveolars

Lips: labials

Uvula: uvulars

Teeth: dentals

Tongue: dorsals
(pre-, medio-, post-)

Pharynx:
pharngeals

Tongue tip: apicals

Glottis: glottals

Figure 2.4 Structures of the Oral Cavity as Organs and Places of Articulation

Stop-plosives are sometimes referred to as stops and sometimes as plosives, depending on the phase of production one wants to draw attention to. Such a division appears at first glance rather academic. There are situations, however, when this distinction becomes important. For example, a client has difficulties realizing a complete occlusion of the lips. This can occur in cases of paralysis of the facial nerve, such as in myasthenia gravis (Thiele, 1980). Such a client has trouble with the stop portion of the production. Other clients—for example, children with developmental verbal dyspraxia—have difficulties with rapid movement patterns of speech. These children can realize the static articulatory postures of the occlusion, but they cannot necessarily release it suddenly enough (Velleman and Strand, 1994). They, therefore, have problems with the plosive phase of the realization and need to be treated quite differently.

Laterals. These sounds are established by a midline closure but lateral openings within the oral cavity. Consequently, the expiratory airstream can pass only around one or both sides of the tongue. [l] is the only lateral consonant of General American English. The laterals together with the rhotics are collectively referred to as **liquids.** According to the classification system of the International Phonetic Alphabet [l] is considered a lateral approximant.

Rhotics. The phonetic characteristics of the rhotics are especially difficult to describe. First, there are at least two types of rhotic productions: *retroflexed* and *bunched* (Shriberg and Kent, 2003). Second, the actual forming of rhotics is highly context dependent. Thus, the production easily changes depending on the features of the surrounding sounds (Kantner and West, 1960). In addition, the positioning of the tongue for individual speakers is highly variable (Shriberg and Kent, 2003). Generally, the *retroflexed* rhotics are produced with the tongue tip in a retroflexed position (*retro* = back, *flex* = turn). The bunched rhotics, on the other hand, show an elevation of the whole corpus of the tongue toward the palate. Perhaps a better classification for [r] is the term *approximant,* which is used within the International Phonetic Alphabet. In this case, [r] is a central approximant. According to the International Phonetic Alphabet, there are two symbols used for the central rhotic approximants. The [ɹ] is a postalveolar approximant in which the tongue tip is raised and points directly upward toward the rear of the alveolar ridge. The [ɻ] is a retroflex production characterized by the tongue tip elevated and bent backward in a more retroflexed position. Officially, there is no IPA symbol for the bunched r-production (Ball and Rahilly, 1999). Table 2.5 contains the various manners

tively constricted into a more open position. The sounds [w] and [j] are considered glides. According to the classification of the International Phonetic Alphabet (IPA), [w] and [j] are considered approximants. **Approximants** are consonants in which there is a much wider passage of air resulting in a smooth (as opposed to turbulent) airflow for these voiced sounds (Ball and Rahilly, 1999).

According to the symbols used by the International Phonetic Association (IPA), the American English rhotics are officially transcribed as [ɹ], an upside down *r*, while the retroflexed is characterized by [ɻ], an upside-down *r* with a retroflexed diacritic. According to the IPA, the [r] symbol is officially reserved for the alveolar trilled "r" sound, which can be heard in Spanish, for example. Because trilled "r" sounds do not exist in General American English, and in order not to complicate matters unnecessarily, it is customary to use the [r] symbol for both the bunched and the retroflexed "r" sounds.

Table 2.5 Phonetic Description: Manner of Articulation

Manner of Articulation	Phonetic Descriptor	Examples
Complete blockage	Stop-plosive	[p], [b], [t], [d], [k], [g]
Partial blockage	Fricative	[f], [v], [s], [z], [ʃ], [ʒ], [θ], [ð]
Nasal emission	Nasal	[m], [n], [ŋ]
Release of stop portion to a homorganic fricative portion	Affricate	[tʃ], [dʒ]
Gliding motion from a more closed to a more open position	Glide	[w], [ʍ], [j]
Lateral airflow	Lateral	[l]
Retroflex blade or bunched dorsum	Rhotic	[r]

of articulation with examples of the consonants of General American English.

Voicing. **Voicing** is the term used to denote the presence or absence of simultaneous vibration of the vocal cords resulting in voiced or voiceless consonants. The voiced and voiceless consonants of General American English are summarized in Table 2.6.

Far more precision may often be necessary to describe how specific consonants are produced. However, this framework of organ of articulation, place of articulation, manner of articulation, and voicing provides a fairly accurate description of General American English consonants.

When Organ, Place, Manner, and Voicing Are Not Enough

In analyzing the articulatory requisites for the realization of [ʃ], we find that it can be described—according to voicing, articulatory organ, place, and manner—as a voiceless coronal-prepalatal fricative. Although that is a generally satisfactory phonetic description, another production characteristic is lip rounding. Describing such an additional feature becomes necessary because some children with "sh" problems do not realize the rounding. In fact, the resulting aberrant production may be due entirely to the absence of this lip-rounding feature.

Table 2.6 Phonetic Description: Voicing

Voicing	Phonetic Descriptor	Examples
With vocal fold vibration	Voiced	[b], [d], [g], [m], [n], [ŋ], [v], [z], [ʒ], [ð], [w], [j], [l], [r]
Without vocal fold vibration	Voiceless	[p], [t], [k], [f], [s], [ʃ], [θ], [ʍ], [h]

The following phonetic descriptions classify the consonants of General American English according to the parameters of voicing, organ, place, and manner.[1]

[p]   voiceless bilabial stop-plosive

(Because both organ and place of articulation are the lower and upper lips, respectively, one should actually say labio-labial. However, the term *bilabial* is usually preferred.)

[b]   voiced bilabial stop-plosive

[t]   voiceless coronal-alveolar stop-plosive

[d]   voiced coronal-alveolar stop-plosive

[k]   voiceless postdorsal-velar stop-plosive

[g]   voiced postdorsal-velar stop-plosive

[f]   voiceless labio-dental fricative

[v]   voiced labio-dental fricative

[s]   voiceless apico-alveolar or predorsal-alveolar fricative

[s] (and [z]) can be produced in one of two ways: with the tongue tip up (i.e., as apico-alveolar fricative [sibilant]) or with the tongue tip resting behind the lower incisors (i.e., predorsal-alveolar fricative [sibilant]).

[z]   voiced apico-alveolar or predorsal-alveolar fricative

[ʃ]   voiceless coronal-prepalatal or coronal-postalveolar fricative with lip rounding

[ʒ]   voiced coronal-prepalatal or coronal-postalveolar fricative with lip rounding

[θ]   voiceless apico-dental or interdental fricative

The [θ] and [ð] are typically produced with either the tongue tip resting behind the upper incisors (i.e., apico-dental) or with the tongue tip between the upper and lower incisors (i.e., interdental).

[ð]   voiced apico-dental or interdental fricative

[m]   voiced bilabial nasal

[n]   voiced coronal-alveolar nasal

[ŋ]   voiced postdorsal-velar nasal

[w]   voiced labial-velar glide or approximant

[ʍ]   voiceless labial-velar fricative (IPA, 1996)

[j]   voiced mediodorsal-mediopalatal glide or approximant

[l]   voiced apico-alveolar lateral or lateral approximant

[r]   voiced mediodorsal-mediopalatal rhotic approximant (bunched) or voiced apico-prepalatal rhotic approximant (retroflexed), officially [ɹ]

Here, the term *apico* refers to the underside of the apex of the tongue.

[h]   voiceless unlocalized open consonant that is, an aspirate

Although this sound is sometimes classified as a laryngeal or glottal fricative, in General American English, there is normally no constriction at the laryngeal, pharyngeal, or oral levels. See Heffner (1975) for a discussion of the [h] production in General American English.

[tʃ]   voiceless coronal-alveolar stop portion followed by a voiceless coronal-prepalatal fricative portion

[dʒ]   voiced coronal-alveolar stop portion followed by a voiced coronal-prepalatal fricative portion

---

1. The organ, place, manner, and voicing features are based on the phonetic descriptions provided by Bronstein (1960) and Kantner and West (1960). These features are seen as descriptive and may, therefore, vary somewhat from speaker to speaker.

CLINICAL APPLICATION

Rhotic Errors versus Central Vowels with R-Coloring

Children with "r" problems, thus, rhotic consonant difficulties, often produce the central vowels with r- coloring ([ɝ] and [ɚ]) in error as well. However, that is not always the case. Note the following patterns seen in Latoria's speech from the Word Articulation Subtest of the Test of Language Development, Primary, Second edition (Newcomer and Hammill, 1988).

Norm Production	→	Actual Production	Word Example	Transcriptions
Rhotics				
[tr]	→	[tw]	tree	[tri] → [twi]
[br]	→	[bw]	bridge	[brɪdʒ] → [bwɪʒ]
[r]	→	[w]	ring	[rɪŋ] → [wɪŋ]
[br]	→	[bw]	zebra	[zibrə] → [zibwə]
[r]	→	[w]	garage	[gəraʒ] → [dʒəwa]
[θr]	→	[θw]	thread	[θrɛd] → [θwɛd]
[tr]	→	[tw]	treasure	[trɛʒɚ] → [twɛʒɚ]
Central Vowels with R-Coloring				
[ɚ]	correct	[ɚ]	feather	[fɛðɚ] → [fɛdɚ]
[ɚ]	correct	[ɚ]	soldier	[soʊldʒɚ] → [soʊʒɚ]
[ɚz]	correct	[ɚz]	scissors	[sɪzɚz] → [sɪzɚz]
[ɝ]	correct	[ɝ]	birthday	[bɝθdeɪ] → [bɝdeɪ]

On the one hand, Latoria has a [w] for [r] substitution ([r] → [w]) for the rhotic consonant [r]. On the other, she can produce the central vowels with r-coloring accurately.

*S*OUNDS IN CONTEXT: COARTICULATION AND ASSIMILATION

Until now, this textbook has discussed articulatory characteristics of General American English speech sounds as discrete units. However, the articulators do not move from sound to sound in a series of separate steps. Speech consists of highly variable and overlapping motor movements. Sounds within a given phonetic context influence one another. For example, if the [s] production in *see* is contrasted to the one in *Sue,* it can be seen that [s] in *see* is produced with some spreading of the lips, whereas there is lip rounding in *Sue.* This difference is due to the influence of the following vowel articulations: [i], a vowel with lip spreading, facilitates this feature in the [s] production in *see,* whereas the lip rounding of [u] influences the production of [s] in *Sue.* These types of modifications are grouped together under the term *coarticulation.* **Coarticulation** describes the concept that the articulators are continually moving into position for other segments over a stretch of speech (Fletcher, 1992). The result of coarticulation is referred to as assimilation. The term **assimilation** refers to adaptive articulatory changes by which one speech sound becomes similar, sometimes identical, to a neighboring sound segment. Such a change may affect one, several, or all of a sound's phonetic constituents; that is, a sound may change its organ, place, manner, and/or voicing properties under the articulatory influence of another sound. Assimilation processes are perfectly natural consequences of normal speech production and are by no means restricted to developing speech in young children. Because the two segments become more alike, assimilatory processes are also referred to as *harmony processes*.

There are different *types* and *degrees* of assimilatory processes. In regard to the different types of assimilatory processes, the following should be noted:

1. Assimilatory processes modifying directly adjacent sounds are called *contact* (or *contiguous*) *assimilations*. If at least one other segment separates the sounds in question, especially when the two sounds are in two different syllables, one speaks of *remote* (or *noncontiguous*) *assimilation* (Heffner, 1975).

The following assimilation processes were noted in the results of children's articulation tests:

Contact
"jumping" [ʤʌmpɪn] → [ʤʌmbɪn]
The voiced [m] impacts the normally voiceless [p].
"skunk" [skʌŋk] → [stʌŋk]
The organ and place of articulation for [s] influence the stop-plosive, changing it from a postdorsal-velar to a coronal-alveolar.

Remote
"yellow" [jɛloʊ] → [lɛloʊ]
Organ, place, and manner of articulation are impacted when the [j] at the beginning of the word becomes identical to the following [l].

"telephone" [tɛləfoʊn] → [tɛdəfoʊn]
Manner of articulation is impacted when the [l] is changed from a lateral to a stop-plosive, similar to the [t] at the beginning of the word.

2. Assimilations can be either *progressive* or *regressive*. In progressive assimilation, a sound segment influences a following sound. This is also referred to as *perseverative assimilation* (Crystal, 1987; Ladefoged, 2006). The previously noted contact assimilations for *jumping* and *skunk* and the remote assimilation for *telephone* are examples of progressive assimilation. A previously articulated sound influenced a following sound.

In regressive assimilation, a sound segment influences a preceding sound. If "is she" [ɪz ʃi] is pronounced [ɪʒ ʃi], changing [s] into [ʒ], regressive assimilation is noted. Regressive assimilations are also known as *anticipatory* assimilations (Crystal, 1987; Ladefoged, 2006).

The following are examples of progressive and regressive assimilation processes:

Progressive
"ice cream" [aɪskrim] → [aɪstrim]
Organ and place of articulation for [s] influence the following stop-plosive, changing it from a postdorsal-velar to a coronal-alveolar stop-plosive production: This is progressive contact assimilation.

"television" [tɛləvɪʒən] → [tɛdəvɪʒən]
Manner of articulation is impacted when the stop-plosive [t] impacts the following [l], changing it from a lateral to a stop-plosive: This is progressive remote assimilation.

Regressive
"pumpkin" [pʌmkɪn] → [pʌŋkɪn]
Organ and place of articulation of [k] influence [m], which is changed from the bilabial to the postdorsal-velar nasal [ŋ]: This is regressive contact assimilation.

"bathtub" [bæθtʌb] → [θæθtʌb]

Organ, place, and manner of articulation are impacted as [θ] influences the previous segment [b]: This is regressive remote assimilation.

In regard to the different degrees of assimilatory influence, one distinguishes between phonemic assimilation and phonetic similitude (Ball and Rahilly, 1999). If an altered segment is perceived to be a different phoneme altogether, this is termed *phonemic assimilation*. *Phonetic similitude* occurs when the change in the segment is such that it is still perceived by speakers of a language as nothing more than a variation or allophone of the original segment. A phonemic assimilation could be exemplified by the change in *ten girls* [tɛn gɚlz] to [tɛŋ gɚlz], the [n] changing to [ŋ] due to the influence of the following postdorsal-velar stop-plosive [g]. An example of a phonetic similitude would be the lip rounding of [s] in *soup* [sʷup] as the [s] is influenced by the lip rounding of the following [u].

Assimilation processes can also be total or partial. Total assimilation occurs when the changed segment and the source of the influence become identical. Partial assimilation exists when the changed segment is close to, but not identical with, the source segment.

The following are examples of total and partial assimilation processes:

Total	"window"	[wɪndoʊ]	→ [wɪnoʊ]
	"Pontiac"	[pɑntiæk]	→ [pɑniæk]
Partial	"handkerchief"	[hæŋkɚtʃɪf]	→ [hæŋkɚtʃɪf]

The term *coalescence* is used when two neighboring segments are merged into a new and different segment. An example of coalescence would be the realization of *sandwich* [sænwɪtʃ] as [sæmɪtʃ]. The bilabial features for the articulation of [w] have impacted the original coronal-alveolar nasal (regressive assimilation), which now is changed to a bilabial nasal [m].

Children at different stages of their speech-language development tend to utilize assimilation processes in systematic ways. This is of obvious interest to clinicians whose task is to separate normal from impaired phonological development. In normally developing children and those with disordered phonology, syllable structure can impact their production possibilities. This will be discussed in the next section.

> Typical assimilation processes and the ages at which these processes occur in children are discussed in Chapter 5.

CLINICAL APPLICATION
Assimilation Processes and Articulation Testing

Assimilatory or harmony processes often occur during an articulation test. It is important to recognize these processes so that the test scoring will not be negatively impacted. The following assimilation processes have been frequently observed by the author:

Word	Expected Response	Child's Response	Impact on Scoring
Santa	[sæntə]	[sænə] total assimilation	Could be scored as an omission of [t]
sandwich	[sænwɪtʃ]	[sæmɪtʃ] total assimilation (coalescence)	Could be scored as an omission of [w] and an [m]/[n] substitution
presents	[prɛzənts]	[prɛzəns] total assimilation	Could be scored as an omission of [t]

Word	Expected Response	Child's Response	Impact on Scoring
A less common example was observed for Danny, age 4;3:			
bath	[bæθ]	[θæθ]	[θ]/[b] substitution
bathtub	[bæθtʌb]	[θæθtʌb]	[θ]/[b] substitution

However, Danny could produce [b] correctly in all other contexts. Note the correct production of [b] at the end of *bathtub*. This was an example of a regressive remote assimilation.

SYLLABLE STRUCTURE

If we are asked to break words down into component parts, syllables seem to be more natural than sounds. For example, speakers of unwritten languages will characteristically use syllable, not sound, divisions. They may even resist the notion that any further breakdown is possible (Ladefoged, 2006). Also, preschool children use syllabification if they try to analyze a word. It is only after children are exposed to letters and writing that they begin to understand the possibility of dividing words into sounds. Thus, syllables appear to be easily recognizable units.

Counting the number of syllables in a word is a relatively simple task. Probably all will agree on the number of syllables in the word *away* or *articulation,* for example. What we might disagree on are the beginning and end points of the syllables in question. To arrive at a consensus, it is first necessary to differentiate between written and spoken syllables.

If one consults a dictionary, written syllabification rules are found. We learn that the word *cutting* is to be divided cut-ting. However, differences may, and often do, exist between written and spoken syllables. The written syllabification rules for *cutting* do not reflect the way we would syllabify the word when speaking. The divisions [kʌ tɪŋ] would be more probable during normal speech. An awareness of existing differences between spo-

ken and written syllable boundaries is important for speech-language specialists.

This is especially critical because a dictionary of rules for the boundaries of *spoken* syllables does not exist. Thus, two competent speakers of a given language may syllabify the same word in different ways. Words such as *hammer* and *window* would probably not cause problems. However, how should one syllabify *telephone,* as [tɛ lə foʊn] or as [tɛl ə foʊn]? That is, does [l] belong to the second or to the first syllable? Variations in the syllabification of spoken words do indeed exist between speakers. To understand this, a look at the syllable structure might be a good way to begin.

Structurally, the syllable can be divided into three parts: *peak, onset,* and *coda* (Sloat, Taylor, and Hoard, 1978). The **peak** is the most prominent, acoustically most intense part of the syllable. Although vowels are clearly more prevalent as syllable peaks, consonants are not strictly excluded. Consonants that serve as the syllable peak are referred to as *syllabics*. A peak may stand alone, as in the first syllable of the word *a-way,* or it can be surrounded by other sounds, as in *tan* or *bring.*

The **onset** of a syllable consists of all the segments prior to the peak, whereas the **coda** is made up of all the sound segments of a syllable following its peak. The segments that compose the onset are also termed *syllable releasing* sounds, and those of the coda are termed *syllable arresting* sounds. Thus, the onset of *meet*

[mit] is [m]; that is, [m] is the syllable releasing sound. The coda, or syllable arresting sound, of *meet* is [t]. This applies also to consonant blends within one syllable. The onset of *scratched* is [skr], its peak is [æ], and the coda [tʃt]. Not all syllables have onsets or codas. Both syllables of *today* [tu deɪ] lack a coda, whereas *off* [ɑf] does not have an onset. The number of segments that an onset or a coda may contain is regulated by rules of the language in question. General American English syllables can have one to three segments in an onset (ray, stay, stray) and one to four segments in a coda (sit, sits, sixth [sɪksθ], sixths [sɪksθs])

The peak and coda together are referred to as the **rhyme** (Carr, 1999). Therefore, in the word *sun*, the onset is "s" and the rhyme is "un." Syllables that do not contain codas are called **open** or **unchecked syllables.** Examples of open, unchecked syllables are *do* [du], *glee* [gli], or the first syllable of *rebound* [ri baʊnd]. Syllables that do have codas are called **closed** or **checked syllables,** such as in *stop* [stɑp] or the first syllable in *window* [wɪn].

The use of specific syllable structures is often neglected when analyzing the speech characteristics of children. However, they do seem to play an important developmental role. A child's first words consist typically of open or unchecked syllables, such as [bɑ] for *ball* or [mɪ] for *milk*. If children start to produce closed syllables, they usually contain only single-segment codas. Similarly, two-syllable words at this stage of development consist usually of open syllables (e.g., Ingram, 1976; Menn, 1971; Velten, 1943; Vihman, Ferguson, and Elbert, 1986). Productions such as [beɪ bi] for *baby* or [ti pɑ] for *teapot* are examples.

Syllable Structure: Clinical Implications

The syllable is also an important unit when assessing and treating children with articulatory or phonological disorders. Sometimes, the syllable unit can give us a more accurate picture of the child's articulatory capabilities than can individual sound productions. The ease of syllable production can be affected by at least three circumstances: (1) the *number of syllables* an utterance contains, (2) the *type of syllable* (open versus closed), and (3) the *degree of syllable stress* (stressed or unstressed) (Fleming, 1971; Kent, 1982). Generally, fewer syllables, open syllables, and stressed syllables usually facilitate accurate productions of specific target sounds.

The designs of most articulation tests document a striking lack of attention to these variables. Most assessment instruments focus on the beginning-initial, the middle-medial, and the end-final sound positions within words. At first glance, it may seem as if initial could be related to the syllable onset, medial to syllable peak, and final to syllable coda. However, this is not the case. For example, the word *window* may be used in an articulation test to assess the production of the word-medial [d] sound, while the word *bathtub* is used to test the word-medial [θ] and [t] sounds. The elicitation of the word *pajamas* tests [dʒ] medially. From these examples, it appears that *medial* indicates anything between the beginning and the end of an utterance.

Is there any comparability between these "medial" positions? Let's examine the syllable structures of these three words:

"window" [wɪn-doʊ]   target [d]

1st syllable	stressed	onset-peak-coda
2nd syllable	unstressed	onset-peak

"bathtub" [bæθ-tʌb]   target [θ] and [t]

1st syllable	stressed	onset-peak-coda
2nd syllable	unstressed	onset-peak-coda

"pajamas" [pədʒæməz]   target [dʒ]

1st syllable	unstressed	onset-peak
2nd syllable	stressed	onset-peak
3rd syllable	unstressed	onset-peak-coda

As one can see, the medial sound [d] in *window* is actually the onset of an unstressed, open syllable. The preceding syllable ends with a coda, thus, two consonants (i.e., [n] + [d]) must be produced in immediate succession. The medial [θ] tested in *bathtub* poses a different problem. It represents the coda of a stressed syllable. Again, there is the complication of two consonants in sequence, [θ] and [t]. The word-medial [t] now appears as a syllable onset in a closed syllable. The third example of medial [dʒ] in *pajamas* exemplifies a quite different articulatory situation again. Here, a three-syllable word is elicited in which the medial [dʒ] is actually an onset of a stressed open syllable.

An analysis of an articulation test according to the syllable structure rather than the word unit would eliminate these problems. If onset, peak, and coda for each syllable are examined, the results also become more accurate and, therefore, clinically more valid. Accuracy of any assessment process is the key to successful treatment. The information attained from examining sound articulation with the syllable as a basic structural unit complements the word-based results and gives additional insight into the child's true articulatory abilities.

SUMMARY

This chapter presented an overview of the form and function of vowels and consonants of General American English. Both vowels and consonants were classified according to their articulatory production features and their linguistic functions. Phonetic descriptors were given to provide the clinician with a detailed account of articulatory action during norm production of vowels and consonants. These features can later be contrasted to those noted in the impaired sound realizations of children and adults with articulatory-phonological impairments.

In the second portion of this chapter, coarticulation, assimilation processes, and syllable structure were defined and examined. Coarticulation and resulting assimilatory processes were described as normal articulatory consequences that regularly occur in the speech of individuals. Assimilatory processes were defined according to the type and degree of sound modification. Examples were given of assimilatory processes in children as well as of the possible impact these processes could have on articulation test results. The last section, on syllable structure, defined the parts of the syllable. Variations in syllable structure do not seem to be accounted for when testing individual sounds within most articulation tests. However, this may be a factor that could affect the articulatory proficiency of children and adults with impaired speech. An analysis of syllable structures would provide the clinician with additional knowledge when evaluating individuals with articulatory-phonological disorders.

CASE STUDY

The following sample is from Tina, age 3;8.

				fan	[vɛn]	ring	[wɪŋ]
				yes	[wɛt]	thumb	[dʌm]
dig	[dɛg]	cat	[tæt]	boat	[bot]	that	[zæt]
house	[haᵘθ]	bath	[bæt]	cup	[tʊp]	zip	[wɪp]
knife	[naf]	red	[led]	lamp	[wæmp]	key	[di]
duck	[dʊt]	ship	[sɪp]	goat	[dot]	win	[jɪn]

Compare the typical vowel productions to those noted in the sample according to (1) the portion of the tongue that is involved in the articulation (front, central, back) and (2) the tongue's position relative to the palate (high, mid, low). For example:

dig	[dɛg]	a high-front vowel changed to a mid-front vowel

Compare the typical consonant productions to those noted in the sample according to voicing, organ, place, and manner characteristics. For example:

house	[ha^{ʊ}θ]	a voiceless apico-alveolar (predorsal-alveolar) fricative is changed to a voiceless interdental (apico-alveolar) fricative

THINK CRITICALLY

1. Some younger children have trouble producing [s] and [z]; they substitute [θ] and [ð] for these sounds. Thus, the word *Sue* would be pronounced [θu] and *zoo* as [ðu]. Both of the target sounds and the substitutions are fricatives. Compare the two articulations and see if you might be able to describe to a child what he or she would have to do to change the articulation from [θ] and [ð] to [s] to [z].
2. Children often have trouble with the lip rounding associated with the sh-sounds ([ʃ] and [ʒ]). Which type of vowel contexts would promote lip rounding? Can you find five words that you could use to assist the lip rounding of [ʃ] or [ʒ]?
3. Identify the following assimilation processes according to the following parameters: contact versus remote, progressive versus regressive, phonemic assimilation, phonetic similitude, or coalescence.

news	[nuz̲]	however	newspaper	[nus̲p̲e^{ɪ}pɚ]
panty	[pænti]	→	[pæni]	
did you	[dɪd ju]	→	[dɪdʒu]	
incubate	[ɪnkjube^{ɪ}t]	→	[ɪŋkjube^{ɪ}t]	
misuse	[mɪsjuz]	→	[mɪʃuz]	

4. Identify the following syllable structures according to (a) onset, peak, and coda and (b) closed or open syllables. For example:

   win.dow → [wɪn.do^{ʊ}]

   1st syllable: onset-peak-coda, closed syllable
   2nd syllable: onset-peak, open syllable

   telephone
   wagon
   shovel
   banana
   pajamas
5. You are testing [k] sounds in the initial, medial, and final positions with a child who is 4 years old with a [t] for [k] substitution. You would like to keep the syllable structure and the stress consistent for all the words used. Therefore, all words should be two syllables in length, stress should be on the same syllable, and syllable structures should be comparable. Find six words that could be used for a 4-year-old child that would test [k] under these conditions.

TEST YOURSELF

1. Vowels are defined as
   a. under normal circumstances having no simultaneous vocal fold vibration
   b. having articulatory constriction along the sagittal midline of the vocal tract
   c. having a relatively unimpeded airstream from the vocal folds to the lips
   d. having relatively less acoustic intensity
2. Which consonants are considered to be sonorant consonants?

a. fricatives and affricates

b. stop-plosives

c. all voiced consonants

d. nasals, liquids, and glides

3. The vowel [i] is described phonetically as a

a. high-front vowel that is unrounded and lax

b. mid-front vowel that is unrounded and tense

c. high-front vowel that is unrounded and tense

d. high-back vowel that is unrounded and tense

4. The consonant [l] is described phonetically as

a. voiced apico-alveolar lateral approximant

b. voiced coronal-alveolar glide

c. voiced predorsal-alveolar lateral approximant

d. none of the above

5. Sibilants are characterized by the presence of high-frequency components. Which one of the following is not a sibilant?

a. [θ]

b. [s]

c. [z]

d. [ʃ]

6. A very young child says [ɡɑɡ] for *dog*. This is which type of assimilation process?

a. regressive phonemic assimilation

b. progressive phonemic assimilation

c. regressive phonetic similitude

d. coalescence

7. A young child says [nɔˈni] for *noisy*. This is which type of assimilation process?

a. progressive contact phonemic assimilation

b. regressive contact phonemic assimilation

c. progressive remote phonemic assimilation

d. progressive remote phonetic similitude

8. Which one of the following words has an unchecked syllable structure?

a. cupcake

b. tomato

c. jumping

d. bathtub

9. What is the rhyme of "reached"?

a. [i]

b. [itʃt]

c. [itʃ]

d. none of the above

10. If you were testing [s] in the medial position, which one of the following words would have the same syllable and stress structure as "cassette"?

a. message

b. receipt

c. basic

d. Lassie

WEBSITES

www.uiowa.edu/~acadtech/phonetics/about.html

This website provides an animated articulatory diagram of each consonant and vowel as well as a description of how the sound is produced. It seems to be very user-friendly. Some of the terminology is a bit different from that used in this text. For example, the term *lingua-*, as organ of articulation, is used for all tongue placements and the terms *tongue blade* and *tongue back* are descriptors for what has been referenced here as *pre-*, *medio-*, and *postdorsal*.

www.everything2.com/index.pl?node_id=441666

This website gives some basic definitions of the various articulators for consonant production, although the tongue as organ of articulation is not mentioned. It does give some basic definitions and examples of manners of articulation and defines vowels according to tongue height, front–back dimensions, and lip rounding. Nasal vowels and the concept of tense versus lax are also a portion of this webpage. Several links are provided, for example, to the International Phonetic Alphabet. Other links are humorous and the webpage is worded in a light style.

en.wikipedia.org/wiki/Vowel and
en.wikipedia.org/wiki/Consonant

These two websites give basic definitions of the vowel and consonant concepts as well as many links to other webpages that are both informative and detailed. These are good reference sources for information.

cla.calpoly.edu/~jrubba/phon/syllables.html

This website, developed by Dr. Johanna Rubba (English Department, Linguistics, Cal Poly State University), deals with syllable structure. Basic definitions are given and several examples are provided. Although the website gives information beyond what this chapter covers, the examples on syllable structure will be helpful.

FURTHER READINGS

Ashby, P. (2005). *Speech sounds*. London: Routledge.

Davenport, M., & Hannahs, J. (2006). *Introducing phonetics and phonology*. London: Arnold.

Garn-Nunn, P., & Lynn, J. (2004). *Calvert's descriptive phonetics* (3rd ed.). New York: Thieme.

Ladefoged, P. (2005). *Vowels and consonants* (2nd ed.). Malden, MA: Blackwell.

Yavaş, M. (2005). *Applied English phonology*. Malden, MA: Blackwell.

3

Phonetic Transcription and Diacritics

LEARNING OBJECTIVES

When you have finished this chapter, you should be able to:

- Define phonetic transcription and explain why it is a notational system.
- Describe how the International Phonetic Alphabet is used.
- Explain the value of transcription for speech-language therapists.
- Define diacritics.
- Identify the diacritics used to delineate consonant sounds.
- Identify the diacritics used to mark vowels.
- Identify the diacritics used to mark stress, duration, and syllable boundaries.

Virtually every book on articulatory-phonological disorders contains a brief discussion of phonetic transcription. In such a section, the symbols and diacritics of the International Phonetic Alphabet are listed together with a comment on the importance of accurate transcription for the assessment procedure. This underplays its importance, however; accurate transcription forms *the* basis for the diagnosis of articulatory-phonological impairments. If clinicians cannot correctly identify and transcribe the productions of their clients, their therapy will not be as goal directed as it should be.

Nevertheless, in training and in clinical practice, phonetic transcription seems to be one of the most neglected areas of study. Although transcription skills are as indispensable as they are difficult to master, the chance to learn them is often limited to one undergraduate course. This meager knowledge base is seldom systematically expanded or revisited in other courses or in most clinical experiences. Many practicing clinicians simply do not feel comfortable with phonetic transcription and therefore, unfortunately, use it as infrequently as possible.

Phonetic transcription is more than just transposing perceived sounds into "strange" symbols; it is above all a process of fine-tuning one's auditory perception for the purpose of successful clinical intervention. Perceptual skills improve with systematic efforts to listen carefully to, and to differentiate accurately between, subtle changes in sound quality. Although this is not a workbook on phonetic transcription (this section does not offer nearly enough information for such a course), phonetic transcription will be emphasized and treated in considerably more detail than is usually the case in textbooks on articulatory-phonological disorders.

The first goal of this chapter is to introduce the International Phonetic Alphabet as the notational system used to document norm productions of vowels and consonants of General American English. However, the transcription of disordered speech requires more than that. It needs additional signs, diacritical marks, that can be added to basic transcription symbols to indicate aberrant sound values. They provide a means of documenting irregular articulatory events. Therefore, this chapter's second goal is to present and discuss some of the more common diacritical markers. Clinical comments are included to exemplify the use of these diacritics. The third goal of this chapter is to examine the clinical implications of phonetic transcription, including the use of diacritics. Examples are provided to demonstrate how phonetic transcription can be used in the assessment process. Familiarity with, and the proper use of, phonetic transcription is seen as an invaluable tool for the diagnosis and treatment of articulatory-phonological impairments.

PHONETIC TRANSCRIPTION AS A NOTATIONAL SYSTEM

Speech is a fleeting event, existing for only the shortest period of time—so short, in fact, that if we don't employ artificial means to preserve speech, we couldn't prove that it had ever ex-

isted, even immediately after the event. Historically, all writing systems were invented to make speech events last longer, to preserve them.

Traditional writing systems do a great job in preserving *what* has been said, but they fall grossly short in indicating *how* it has been said, even though this can be just as important. For example, a speech pathologist needs to document the details of a child's aberrant sound realization. There are no letters in our alphabet for laterally produced s-sounds, for instance. Professionals clearly need more information about *how* a specific speech event has been executed than about *what* has been said. For these special purposes, all traditional writing systems are useless. Special ones had to be invented to serve these needs. *Phonetic transcription* systems were devised in order to document real actualizations of speech events.

Today, the frequently revised International Phonetic Alphabet (IPA) is probably the most widely accepted transcription system in the world (see Figure 3.1). The International Phonetic Association, founded in 1886, published the first IPA in 1888. The International Phonetic Alphabet offers a one-to-one correspondence between phoneme realizations and sound symbols. However, at the same time, many additional signs can be used to identify modifications in the original production. Generally, the IPA serves the professional interests of speech-language pathologists well. Its symbols capture much of what we are interested in. Occasionally, one may be forced to add to the inventory of available symbols in order to characterize an aberrant production. That, though, is to be expected, because phonetic transcription systems are typically designed to transfer standard (but highly impermanent) speech events adequately into (more durable) readable signs. In *aberrant* speech, just about anything can happen, and this may well necessitate additional characters for un-

CONSONANTS (PULMONIC)

	Bilabial	Labiodental	Dental	Alveolar	Postalveolar	Retroflex	Palatal	Velar	Uvular	Pharyngeal	Glottal
Plosive	p b			t d		ʈ ɖ	c ɟ	k ɡ	q ɢ		ʔ
Nasal	m	ɱ		n		ɳ	ɲ	ŋ	N		
Trill	ʙ			r					R		
Tap or Flap				ɾ		ɽ					
Fricative	ɸ β	f v	θ ð	s z	ʃ ʒ	ʂ ʐ	ç ʝ	x ɣ	χ ʁ	ħ ʕ	h ɦ
Lateral fricative				ɬ ɮ							
Approximant		ʋ		ɹ		ɻ	j	ɰ			
Lateral approximant				l		ɭ	ʎ	ʟ			

Where symbols appear in pairs, the one to the right represents a voiced consonant. Shaded areas denote articulations judged impossible.

CONSONANTS (NON-PULMONIC)

Clicks		Voiced implosives		Ejectives	
ʘ	Bilabial	ɓ	Bilabial	ʼ	Examples:
ǀ	Dental	ɗ	Dental/alveolar	pʼ	Bilabial
ǃ	(Post)alveolar	ʄ	Palatal	tʼ	Dental/alveolar
ǂ	Palatoalveolar	ɠ	Velar	kʼ	Velar
ǁ	Alveolar lateral	ʛ	Uvular	sʼ	Alveolar fricative

VOWELS

Where symbols appear in pairs, the one to the right represents a rounded vowel.

OTHER SYMBOLS

ʍ Voiceless labial-velar fricative

w Voiced labial-velar approximant

ɥ Voiced labial-palatal approximant

ʜ Voiceless epiglottal fricative

ʢ Voiced epiglottal fricative

ʡ Epiglottal plosive

ɕ ʑ Alveolo-palatal fricatives

ɺ Alveolar lateral flap

ɧ Simultaneous ʃ and x

Affricates and double articulations can be represented by two symbols joined by a tie bar if necessary.

k͡p t͡s

SUPRASEGMENTALS

ˈ	Primary stress	
ˌ	Secondary stress	ˌfoʊnəˈtɪʃən
ː	Long	eː
ˑ	Half-long	eˑ
˘	Extra-short	ĕ
ǀ	Minor (foot) group	
‖	Major (intonation) group	
.	Syllable break	ɹi.ækt
‿	Linking (absence of a break)	

DIACRITICS

Diacritics may be placed above a symbol with a descender, e.g. ŋ̊

̥	Voiceless	n̥ d̥	̤	Breathy voiced	b̤ a̤	̪	Dental	t̪ d̪
̬	Voiced	s̬ t̬	̰	Creaky voiced	b̰ a̰	̺	Apical	t̺ d̺
ʰ	Aspirated	tʰ dʰ	̼	Linguolabial	t̼ d̼	̻	Laminal	t̻ d̻
̹	More rounded	ɔ̹	ʷ	Labialized	tʷ dʷ	̃	Nasalized	ẽ
̜	Less rounded	ɔ̜	ʲ	Palatalized	tʲ dʲ	ⁿ	Nasal release	dⁿ
̟	Advanced	u̟	ˠ	Velarized	tˠ dˠ	ˡ	Lateral release	dˡ
̠	Retracted	e̠	ˤ	Pharyngealized	tˤ dˤ	̚	No audible release	d̚
̈	Centralized	ë	̴	Velarized or pharyngealized	ɫ			
̽	Mid-centralized	e̽	̝	Raised	e̝	(ɹ̝ = voiced alveolar fricative)		
̩	Syllabic	n̩	̞	Lowered	e̞	(β̞ = voiced bilabial approximant)		
̯	Non-syllabic	e̯	̘	Advanced Tongue Root	e̘			
˞	Rhoticity	ɚ a˞	̙	Retracted Tongue Root	e̙			

TONES AND WORD ACCENTS

LEVEL			CONTOUR		
e̋ or ˥	Extra high		ě or ˩˥	Rising	
é or ˦	High		ê or ˥˩	Falling	
ē or ˧	Mid		e᷄ or ˦˥	High rising	
è or ˨	Low		e᷅ or ˩˨	Low rising	
ȅ or ˩	Extra low		e᷈ or ˧˨˦	Rising-falling	
↓	Downstep		↗	Global rise	
↑	Upstep		↘	Global fall	

Figure 3.1 The International Phonetic Alphabet (revised to 2005). Copyright 2005 by the International Phonetic Association.

usual articulatory events. If such an additional characterization becomes necessary, the specific phonetic value of any added sign must, of course, be described precisely and in detail. If other professionals cannot reliably "read" the transcribed materials, they cannot accurately retransform the symbols into the original phonetic events; that is, they still won't know how the sound was actualized. Under such circumstances, any phonetic transcription becomes pointless.

Phonetic transcription is a purely *descriptive* enterprise. It is nothing but the "spelling out" of an actual speech event by means of special symbols invented to represent the sounds of the utterance in question.

Occasionally, beginning transcription materials consist of lists of orthographically presented words (*book, table, snail,* and so on) that students then have to transfer into phonetic symbols. Such a practice can be misleading. It supports the mistaken notion that there is a *prescriptive* part to phonetic transcription, that it provides some guiding principle about how words are supposed to be pronounced. This is also suggested by dictionaries: Each entry tells the reader how to spell a word correctly, and the following symbols indicate how the word "should be" pronounced. There is, of course, nothing wrong with spelling out how words are commonly pronounced, but any jump from how they *are* pronounced to how they *should be* and are pronounced has nothing to do with the idea behind, and practice of, phonetic transcription.

WHY USE PHONETIC TRANSCRIPTION?

Accurate phonetic transcription is an indispensable clinical tool for speech-language pathologists. That is why it has to be taken so seriously, especially when dealing with the assessment and remediation of impaired articulation and phonology. Without a reliable record of how a child or adult realized a particular speech sound, we simply do not have enough information for goal-directed intervention. Phonetic transcription provides a reasonably accurate written record of what was said and what it sounded like.

Admittedly, phonetic transcription is somewhat troublesome and time consuming. In addition, it certainly has its own problems. Some rules have to be strictly observed in order to overcome these problems. The first thing any aspiring transcriber has to understand is that the human ear is not a microphone. We are unable to *receive* only; we must always *per*ceive; that is, people automatically judge and interpret incoming acoustic signals based on their experience with those signals. In respect to spoken language, this means that when listening to the incoming acoustic signal, the listener unwillingly "distorts" it in the direction of former experiences, including how the listener would have produced it. This "built-in" tendency is the greatest danger to any serious transcription effort. Any higher degree of accuracy achieved while listening to and then describing the *how* of its production is very difficult to attain if perceptual biases rule transcription efforts. To overcome the tendency to "interpret" what was heard requires considerable goodwill, patience, and special training.

There are several other problems that must be considered when using phonetic transcription. For example, many circumstances can affect our transcription, such as the age of the client or an unusual vocal quality. Other factors may produce large variations in the inter- and intra-judge reliability of transcriptions, including the intelligibility of the client

Interjudge reliability denotes the percentage of agreement between two or more people's transcriptions. *Intrajudge reliability* is how well a person agrees with his or her own former transcription.

(Shriberg and Lof, 1991), the position of the sound in the word (Philips and Bzoch, 1969; Shriberg and Lof, 1991), and whether narrow or broad transcription is used (Shriberg and Lof, 1991). Shriberg and Kent (2003) provide an excellent overview of the sources of variation and the factors that affect the reliability of phonetic transcription. These problems are very real, and caution must be exercised when using phonetic transcription. On the other hand, we cannot simply disregard transcription because of its inherent problems or use a private system of noting sound realizations. Instead, the importance of developing good, reliable transcription skills should be stressed. They will prove to be an invaluable resource in the assessment and treatment of articulatory-phonological disorders.

$\mathcal{D}$IACRITICS

Diacritics are marks added to sound transcription symbols in order to give them a particular phonetic value. The set of basic phonetic transcription symbols represents language-specific typical productions. Because speech-language pathologists deal mostly with aberrant articulatory events, it follows that diacritical markers are of special importance when characterizing the speech of their clients. Diacritics are needed to note the clients' deviant sound qualities.

Numerous diacritics are noted in Figure 3.1. Although these diacritics have functioned fairly effectively, extensions to the IPA (extIPA) were diacritics developed specifically to address the transcription of disordered speech. The extIPA symbols, first published in 1990, were revised in 1997. Figure 3.2 is a list of the extIPA symbols. The following discussion on diacritics includes only those frequently used by clinicians. Readers should refer to Figures 3.1 and 3.2 for special transcription needs as they develop.

Diacritics Used with Consonants

Changes in Place of Articulation for Consonants. These symbols describe deviations from normal tongue placement for consonants.

Dentalization. *Dentalization* refers to an articulatory variation in which the tongue approaches the upper incisors. It is marked by [̪] placed under the IPA symbol. For example, the symbol [d] stands for a coronal-alveolar voiced stop. A dentalized realization results when a child places the tip of the tongue not against the alveolar ridge, as the IPA symbol indicates, but against the inside of the upper incisors. A dentalized realization is transcribed as

[d̪] = dentalized [d]

[d̪] occurs quite often as the result of co-articulation. Compare [d]-productions in the words *widow* and *width*. The articulatory influence of the following [θ], an addental or even interdental sound, will probably "dentalize" normally alveolar [d] realizations. Dentalized s-sounds, [s̪] and [z̪], frequently occur in the speech of children (Van Riper, 1978; Weiss, Gordon, and Lillywhite, 1987).

Palatalization. Another modification of consonant articulation is *palatalization*. Only sounds for which the palate is not the place of articulation can be palatalized. Therefore, palatalization can occur with sounds that have a place of articulation anterior or posterior to the hard palate region. If the place of articulation is the alveolar ridge or the upper incisors, palatalization occurs if the anterior portions of the tongue approach prepalatal or mediopalatal portions of the palate, that is, when organ and place of the production are articulated somewhat posteriorly. For velar consonants, palatalization indicates the movement of the place

CONSONANTS (other than those on the IPA Chart)

	bilabial	labiodental	dentolabial	labioalv.	linguolabial	interdental	bidental	alveolar	velar	velophar.
Plosive	p̪ b̪	p͆ ɓ̥	n̪ b̪	t̪ d̪	t̼ d̼					
Nasal		m͆	m̪	n̪	n̼					
Trill				r̪	r̼					
Fricative: central		f͆ v͆	f̪ v̪	θ ð	θ̼ ð̼	ɦ̪ ɦ̪				ʩ
Fricative: lateral+central								ʪ ʫ		
Fricative: nareal	ṁ̥							ṅ̥	ŋ̇	
Percussive	ʬ ʬ						ʭ			
Approximant: lateral				l̪	l̼					

DIACRITICS

↔	labial spreading	θ̢	͈	strong articulation	f͈	ⱷ	denasal	m̃͊
͆	dentolabial	v̼	͉	weak articulation	v̜	ⱷ̇	nasal escape	v̤̇
͆	interdental/bidental	n̪	\	reiterated articulation	p\p\p	͇	velopharyngeal friction	s̰
͇	alveolar	ʃ̠	ͅ	whistled articulation	s̒	↓	ingressive airflow	p↓
͆	linguolabial	d̼	→	sliding articulation	θʃ	↑	egressive airflow	ʃ↑

CONNECTED SPEECH

(.)	short pause
(..)	medium pause
(...)	long pause
f	loud speech [{ꜰ lɑʊd ꜰ}]
ff	louder speech [{ꜰꜰ lɑʊdə‿ ꜰꜰ}]
p	quiet speech [{ᴘ kwaɪət ᴘ}]
pp	quieter speech [{ᴘᴘ kwaɪətə‿ ᴘᴘ}]
allegro	fast speech [{*allegro* fɑːst *allegro*}]
lento	slow speech [{ *lento* sloʊ *lento*}]
crescendo, ralentando, etc. may also be used	

VOICING

˯	pre-voicing	˯z
˳	post-voicing	z˳
₍ₐ₎	partial devoicing	z̬̥
₍ₐ	initial partial devoicing	z̬̥
ₐ₎	final partial devoicing	z̬̥
₍ᵥ₎	partial voicing	s̬
₍ᵥ	initial partial voicing	s̬
ᵥ₎	final partial voicing	s̬
˭	unaspirated	p˭
ʰ	pre-aspiration	ʰp

OTHERS

(‿)	indeterminate sound	(( ))	extraneous noise ((2 sylls))
(V̰), (P̰)	indeterminate vowel, plosive, etc.	¡	sublaminal lower alveolar percussive click
(Pl.vls)	indeterminate voiceless plosive, etc.	ǃ¡	alveolar & sublaminal click ('cluck-click')
( )	silent articulation (ʃ), (m)	*	sound with no available symbol

© 1997 ICPLA

Figure 3.2 ExtIPA Symbols for Disordered Speech (revised to 1997). Copyright 2002 by the International Clinical Phonetics and Linguistics Association. Reprinted with permission.

and organ of articulation in the direction of the palate, to a more anterior articulation. Palatalization causes a typical change in the quality of the sound(s) in question. The diacritical mark for palatalization is a superscript j added to the right of the basic IPA symbol:

[s^j] = palatalized [s]
[t^j] = palatalized [t]

Velarization. *Velarization* refers to the posterior movement of the tongue placement (in the direction of the velum) for palatal sounds. The diacritical mark for velarization is a superscript ɣ placed to the right of the IPA symbol. Thus [t^ɣ] is a velarized [t]. An exception is the so-called dark [l], which in General American English is usually heard in word-final positions, for example in *pull* or *shawl;* also as a syllabic, such as in *little* or *bottle;* preceding a consonant, exemplified by *salt* or *build;* and following high-back vowels [u] (*loop*) or [ʊ] (*look*) (Bronstein, 1960; Carrell and Tiffany, 1960; Small, 2005). The velarization in these cases is often so prominent that even main phonetic characteristics of [l], the articulation of the tongue tip against the alveolar ridge, are sometimes no longer present. In such a case, the velarization actually replaces the typical apico-alveolar l-articulation. The velarized production is an allophonic variation of [l]. Velarized [l]-productions are transcribed [ɫ]:

> The so-called dark and light l-sounds are discussed in more detail in Chapter 8.

[fuɫ] = velarized [l]-sound

Lateralization. [l] is the only lateral in General American English. It cannot be lateralized because it is a lateral already. If during any consonant production other than [l] air is released laterally, we speak of *lateralization.* Not too seldom, [s] becomes lateralized. Articula-

tions of [s] and [z] require a highly accurate placement of frontal parts of the tongue *approximating* the alveolar ridge. This precarious position must be maintained throughout the entire sound duration, a motorically difficult task, especially for young children. To make things easier, children sometimes establish direct contact between the organ and place of articulation. Under these circumstances, the airstream cannot, of course, escape centrally any longer. In an attempt to maintain the fricative effect of [s], the child now releases the air laterally into the cheeks. The result is a conspicuous [s] variation, a lateral lisp. Lateralization is considered a primary articulation; the resulting sound can be categorized as an apico-alveolar lateral fricative. According to the IPA, [ɬ] is the voiceless apico-alveolar fricative, and [ɮ] is its voiced counterpart.

[sɪp] → [ɬɪp] = a lateralized [s]
[zɪp] → [ɮɪp] = a lateralized [z]

The extIPA symbols also provide symbols to distinguish between productions that demonstrate both lateral and central airflow (as opposed to just lateral). The symbols for those are

[su] → [ʪu] = a voiceless alveolar fricative with lateral and central airflow
[zu] → [ʫu] = a voiced alveolar fricative with lateral and central airflow

CLINICAL COMMENTS

Dentalized, palatalized, and lateralized [s] realizations are frequent distortions noted in children. In some children, the dentalized [s̪] may co-occur with a "th" for "s" substitution ([s] → [θ]), as in the following production:

"Santa Claus" [θæn tə klɑs̪] for [sæn tə klɑz]

The too-fronted tongue position of the child's [s]-productions may fluctuate slightly, so that it is perceived at times as [ʂ], at other times as [θ]. It is interesting to note, however, that certain children may also use this dichotomy systematically: [θ] may be realized initiating words or syllables, while [ʂ] is produced terminating words or syllables, for example. Such a possibility should be considered in our assessment.

Differentiating between dentalized, palatalized, and lateralized [s]-productions may seem difficult at first. However, there are clear perceptual qualities that distinguish the three forms of [s] actualization. Dentalized [s]-sounds, [s̪], have a "dull" quality; they lack the sharp, high-frequency characteristic of typical [s]-productions. On the other hand, lateralized [s]-sounds, [ɬ], have a distinct noise component to them that is typically as disagreeable as it is conspicuous. Palatalized [s] variations, [sʲ], approach perceptually a [ʃ] quality. Palatalization of [s] is marked by the anterior portions of the tongue approaching parts of the palate resulting in a somewhat posterior placement of the organ and place of articulation. Comparing the production features of [s] to [ʃ], one notes that [ʃ] realizations also require a more posteriorly placed organ and place of articulation (apico-alveolar [s] versus coronal-prepalatal [ʃ]).

Voice Symbols

Devoicing of Voiced Consonants.   Under normal circumstances, vowels and more than half of our consonants are voiced. If these sounds become devoiced in a speech sample, it needs to be marked. In cases of total devoicing, the IPA symbol for the voiceless counterpart of the voiced sound, its unvoiced cognate, is usually indicated:

[ʃus] for "shoes"

[brɛt] for "bread"

Partial Devoicing.   Often, however, the sound in question is only partially devoiced. The diacritic for partial devoicing is a small circle in parentheses placed under the sound symbol:

[ʃuz̥]

[brɛd̥]

The extIPA also differentiates initial devoicing [˳] and final devoicing [˳].

Voicing of Voiceless Consonants.   Voiceless consonants may also be voiced, especially if they occur between two vowels. A casual pronunciation of *eighteen* might serve as an example. If voiceless consonants become totally voiced, the segment is transcribed with the respective symbol:

[eᶦtin] → [eᶦdin]

Partial Voicing.   If voiceless consonants become partially voiced, the diacritical mark is a lowercase *v* in parentheses under the respective sound symbol:

[eᶦtin] for "eighteen"

Initial and final partial voicing are [ˬ] and [ˬ], respectively.

CLINICAL COMMENTS

Partial voicing and devoicing are difficult to discern and to transcribe correctly. The first impression of transcribers is often some minor qualitative variance—the sound is somehow "off." Such a first impression is usually a good reason to focus subsequently on the voicing–devoicing opposition. This two-step procedure makes it easier to arrive at the difficult judgment: partially voiced or partially devoiced.

Also, in General American English, there is a tendency to devoice (or partially devoice) final consonants. The following are examples from Daniel, age 4;7.

"stove"	[stoᵘv]	→	[stoᵘf]	total devoicing
"slide"	[slaᶦd]	→	[slaᶦd̥]	partial devoicing
"flag"	[flæg]	→	[flæg̥]	partial devoicing
"nose"	[noᵘz]	→	[noᵘs]	total devoicing

The general devoicing tendency in final positions suggests that realizations like these should probably not be considered aberrant productions.

Aspiration and Nonaspiration of Stop-Plosives. Stop-plosives (as well as other consonants) are often described according to two parameters: fortis and lenis. **Fortis** refers to relatively more articulatory effort, whereas **lenis** refers to comparatively less. Most voiceless sounds are realized as fortis consonants, whereas voiced sounds are usually articulated as lenis productions. (One can note the increased articulatory effort on the level of air pressure by contrasting [t] and [d] with a hand in front of the mouth.) The sudden release of the articulatory effort in fortis stop-plosives leads typically to aspiration. This aspiration is noted by using a small superscript *h* following the voiceless stop-plosive sound:

"table"   [tʰeɪbəl]

Stop-plosives, which are normally aspirated, are not marked unless the aspiration is excessive.

Voiceless stop-plosives that are typically aspirated may be produced without this fortis aspiration. In this case, the diacritic for unaspirated stops, [⁼], could be added.

"pie"   [p⁼aɪ]

This example indicates that a normally aspirated [p] has occurred without aspiration.

CLINICAL COMMENTS

Voiceless stop-plosives are usually aspirated at the beginning of words; however, they are not aspirated in consonant clusters. Word-final aspiration is variable (Edwards, 2003).

Unreleased Stop-Plosives.   Stop-plosives can be modified in yet another manner. Unreleased consonants result when the articulatory closure is maintained and not—as usual—released. Although voiceless unreleased stops are more obvious because of their loss of aspiration, voiced stops can be unreleased as well. Unreleased stops typically occur at the end of an utterance or at the end of one-word responses. To indicate an unreleased articulation, the diacritical mark [ˀ] is added:

Boy, was it hot.

[bɔɪ wʌz ɪt hɑtˀ]

CLINICAL COMMENTS

Unreleased consonants should be noted *during* the simultaneous transcription of a client's speech. Just listening to and transcribing from tape recordings can be misleading because, when taped, unreleased consonants can sound similar to consonant omissions. Confusing this production variation with a final consonant deletion could lead to an inaccurate diagnosis. During live transcriptions, we can hear and at least partially see the actual articulation. This provides a much better basis for our judgment: unreleased consonant production or consonant deletion.

The following transcriptions come from an articulation test of Billy, age 4;3:

"cup"	[kʌp]	→	[tʌpˀ]
"music"	[mjuzɪk]	→	[mudɪkˀ]
"book"	[bʊk]	→	[bʊkˀ]
"feet"	[fit]	→	[fitˀ]
"watch"	[watʃ]	→	[watˀ]
"sandwich"	[sænwɪtʃ]	→	[gæmɪtˀ]

Unreleased consonants seldom warrant therapeutic intervention. Billy's case was different. Coming in addition to his many articulation errors, they contributed substantially to a decrease in his intelligibility.

Syllabic Consonants.   Unstressed syllables easily become *reduced syllables*. This means that their vowel nucleus practically disappears. If the vowel nucleus is reduced, the following consonant becomes a syllabic; that is, it becomes the peak of that syllable. This is especially the case in unstressed final syllables when a nasal or the lateral [l] follows the preceding vowel (Heffner, 1975). The proper diacritic mark for such an occurrence is a straight line directly under the syllabic consonant.

$$fɪʃɪŋ → fɪʃən → fɪʃn̩$$

CLINICAL COMMENTS

In spontaneous speech, adults often reduce the unstressed final syllable, as in the following example:

He broke the bottle.

[hi broᵘk ðə batl̩]

In spontaneous speech, and often during an articulation test, children will also demonstrate the use of syllabics. For example:

"little" [lɪtl̩]

"scratching" [skræ tʃn̩]

The boy is fishing; he has a fishing pole.

[ðə̩ bɔɪ ɪz ˈfɪʃn̩ hi hæz ə ˈfɪʃn̩ poᵘl]

While such syllabics, obviously, need to be noted and transcribed, they are considered norm realizations.

Labialization/Nonlabialization of Consonants.
Consonants, with the exception of [ʃ] and [w], are typically unrounded. Lip rounding is a production feature of both of these consonants. If a normally unrounded consonant is produced with lip rounding, this is referred to as labializing the sound in question. When the [ʃ] is produced without lip rounding, this is a nonlabialized production. The diacritic for labialized consonants is a superscript *w* placed to the right of the symbol in question. The diacritic for labial spreading ↔ is placed under the symbol in question to indicate nonlabialization. Labialized consonants can be the result of assimilation processes, as in the following example:

"soup" [sʷup] = labialized [s]

Labialization of normally unrounded consonants due to assimilation is noted, but it is not considered a speech sound problem. On the other hand, [ʃ] is usually produced with at least some degree of lip rounding. The following example indicates [ʃ] without lip rounding:

"ship" [ʃ̪ɪp] = nonlabialized [ʃ]

Unrounded [ʃ] realizations can also be due to assimilation; however, there are children who unround [ʃ] in all contexts. This should be noted and is considered an aberrant production.

CLINICAL COMMENTS

Rounded [s]- and unrounded [ʃ]-sounds are frequent sibilant realizations of children. These may be aberrant productions or context-based assimilation processes. The following is an excerpt from a transcription of Matt, age 4;6:

The boy is swinging really high.

[ðə bɔɪ ɪz sʷwɪŋən rili haɪ]

My mommy made vegetable soup.

[maɪ mami meɪd vɛdʒəbəl sʷup]

In addition to Matt's unorthodox pronunciation of *vegetable*, we note that his [s]-sounds are rounded. In the given context, they may be just assimilation processes regressively influenced by the rounding of the following [w] or [u].

This does not seem to be the case in Chris's transcription, based on an articulation test and a spontaneous speech sample.

"fish"	[fɪʃ]	→	[fɪʃ̪]
"watch"	[watʃ]	→	[waʃ̪]
"chicken"	[tʃɪkən]	→	[ʃ̪ɪkən]
"shovel"	[ʃʌvəl]	→	[ʃ̪ʌvəl]

At lunch I ate a peanut butter sandwich.

[æt lʌnʃ̪ aɪ eɪt ə pinət bʌtɚ ʃ̪ænɪʃ̪]

I wish I had some new tennis shoes,
like Michael Jordan.

[aɪ wɪʃ̪ aɪ hæd sʌm nu tɛnəʃ̪uz laɪk maɪkəl ʃ̪ordən]

Chris, in contrast to Matt, *un*rounds his "sh"-sounds even when they precede a rounded vowel, as in the word *shoes*. He also occasionally uses [ʃ] for [s]- and [tʃ]-sounds.

Derhotacization.   Derhotacization is the loss of r-coloring for the consonant [r] and the central vowels with r-coloring, [ɝ] and [ɚ]. Derhotacized central vowels are transcribed as [ɜ] and [ə]. However, [r], as in *rabbit,* can lose its characteristic r-coloring as well. Children often substitute a [w] for this sound. Another possibility is the [ʋ], which is a voiced labiodental approximant. The [ʋ] sound lacks the high-back tongue position of [w], a labio-velar approximant; however, comparable to the [w], [ʋ] demonstrates a lack of r-coloring.

Diacritics Used with Vowels

Rounding/Unrounding of Vowels.   There are vowels that are normally rounded and others that are normally unrounded—[u] versus [i], for example. The rounding or unrounding of the lips is an important feature of vowel realizations. However, for several reasons, some clients may delete or inappropriately add these characteristics. This results in a distortion of the respective sound quality. The IPA system offers two symbols to indicate rounding and unrounding of vowels. The signs are placed directly under the vowel symbol in question and consist of a small *c*-type notation, which indicates unrounding (or less rounding than is considered normal) when open to the right. When this *c* is inverted, creating an opening to the left, it denotes rounding (or more rounding than is normally the case):

$$[u̜] = \text{unrounded } [u]$$
$$[ɛ̹] = \text{rounded } [ɛ]$$

Changes in Tongue Placement for Vowels.   Deviations in tongue positioning affect vowel

as well as consonant articulations. Different vowel qualities are established essentially by different sizes and forms of the vocal tract. Two main factors determining these sizes and forms pertain to the location of the raised portion of the tongue (front and back dimensions) and to the extent to which the tongue is raised in the direction of the hard or soft palate (high and low dimensions).

Raised/Lowered Tongue Position.   The IPA system offers a set of diacritics that signals the direction of tongue heights on the vertical plane leading to deviations from norm vowel productions. The diacritic [˕] under the vowel symbol marks a lower elevation, whereas the diacritic [˔] under the vowel marks a higher elevation of the tongue than is normally the case for the production of the vowel in question. For example,

$$[s ɪ̞ t]$$

would state that the high-front elevation of the tongue for standard [ɪ] articulation has not been reached in this realization; that is, the tongue articulation was lower than normal, resulting in a perceptible off-quality for [ɪ]. Trying to describe our auditory impression of this sound, we would say that it shifted in the direction of (but not reaching) the sound quality of [e].

Similarly, the transcription

$$[b ɪ̝ t]$$

would indicate a higher-than-normal elevation of the tongue for [ɪ], resulting in a quality that approaches [i] characteristics.

The same principle applies to all vowels. A question that logically follows is whether it makes a difference which symbol we use if the vowel is somewhere in between two qualities. In other words, do a raised [e] ([e̝]), and

> Think of the symbol as a pointer with its base the top of the *T*-type notation. If the pointer projects down [⊤], the tongue has been lowered; if it points up [⊥], the tongue has been raised.

a lowered [ɪ] ([ɪ̞]) signify the same vowel quality? The answer is no. Therefore, in our previous example, one has to make a decision as to whether this vowel realization sounded more like an [e]- or an [ɪ]-type vowel. Based on the transcriber's auditory perception, the basic vowel quality must first be chosen, and then the modifying diacritic mark should be added to it.

Advanced/Retracted Tongue Position. There are also diacritics signaling tongue variations on the horizontal plane that lead to deviations from norm productions. They indicate a tongue position that is too far forward or too far back for a norm production of the vowel in question. The diacritic for vowels produced with a tongue elevation more advanced than usual is [₊]. More retracted protrusions are marked by the diacritic [-]. Both are placed under the vowel symbol: [ɛ̠], for example.

CLINICAL COMMENTS

Changes in the position of the tongue for vowel realizations are often perceptually difficult to target. Although transcribers are aware that the vowel quality is "off," they may not be sure in which direction. If the tongue has been lowered or raised, the vowel quality will sound somehow similar to the neighboring vowel on the vertical plane of the vowel quadrilateral. Thus, a lowered [ɛ] will have a certain [æ] quality, or a raised [ʊ] will approach a [u]. The best reference source in these cases is the vowel quadrilateral. However, this is not as simple if the tongue movements pertain to the horizontal plane—that is, to a tongue position too advanced or retracted. One point of reference is that front vowels that demonstrate a retracted tongue position and back vowels that demonstrate too forward a

tongue position sound somewhat "centralized"—that is, their distinct qualities appear reduced. Therefore, although the vowel can still be identified as the respective front or back vowel, it approaches a [ʌ]-type quality.

Nasality Symbols. During the production of most General American English speech sounds, the velum is elevated to block the escape of the expiratory air through the nasal cavity. There is only one exception to this rule: the nasals. This is what—quite correctly—the textbooks tell us. However, in reality, the conditions are not always so clear-cut. If a nasal follows a vowel, for example, nasality often seeps into the vowel segment; the preceding vowel becomes nasalized:

$$[tæn] \rightarrow [tæ̃n]$$

As long as the nasality doesn't overstep the boundary line of natural assimilatory processes, this nasality remains unmarked. Speakers and listeners perceive these variations as normal. However, if the nasality is perceived as being excessive, or hypernasal, we need to place the "tilde" (which you may have encountered in Spanish language classes) over the respective sound(s). As speech-language specialists, we encounter hypernasality prominently in the speech of clients with dysarthria and cleft palates.

Denasality is also encountered in the speech of our clients. The symbol for denasality is the tilde with a slash through it, placed above the nasal consonant:

$$ni \rightarrow ñi$$

This symbol refers to a reduction of nasal quality. Only nasal consonants can be denasalized. If nasal consonants are perceived as having a total lack of nasal quality (having a completely oral quality), then the symbol for the resulting homorganic voiced stop is used:

$$ni \rightarrow di$$

CLINICAL COMMENTS

One of the characteristics of African American dialect is the total regressive assimilation of postvocalic nasals (e.g., Haynes and Moran, 1989; Wolfram, 1986). The assimilation process is regressive in that the nasal following the vowel changes the characteristic of the preceding vowel into a nasalized vowel. It is considered a *total* assimilation process because the postvocalic nasal consonant is totally gone. The following examples demonstrate this process:

"pen"	[pɛn]	→	[p̃ɛn]	→	[p̃ɛ̃]
"thumb"	[θʌm]	→	[θʌ̃m]	→	[θʌ̃]

These pronunciations were noted on an articulation test from a child, age 4;3, speaking African American dialect:

"broom"	[brum]	→	[brũ]
"airplane"	[ɛɚ pleɪn]	→	[ɛɚ pleɪ̃]
"sandwich"	[sæn wɪtʃ]	→	[sæ̃ wɪtʃ]
"clown"	[klaʊn]	→	[klæ̃ʊ̃]

The total regressive assimilation process ("broom," "airplane," and "sandwich") and the vowel change ("clown") are dialectal in nature. In African American dialect, they represent a regular pronunciation possibility.

Diacritics for Stress, Duration, and Syllable Boundaries

Stress Markers. Every multisyllabic word has its own stress pattern, which may or may not be realized in a regular manner by our clients. The main purpose for all stress realizations is to emphasize certain syllables over others, thus creating a hierarchy of prominence among them.

Primary Stress. The order of prominence is actualized by differences in loudness, pitch, and duration, the loudness differences being the most striking of the three. Generally, two different loudness levels are observed. The loudest syllable is said to have the *primary* stress. It is marked by a superscript short straight line in front of the respective syllable.

"syllable"	[ˈsɪ lə bəl]
"railway"	[ˈreɪl weɪ]
"superior"	[sə ˈpɪr i ɚ]

Secondary Stress. The next loudest syllable bears the *secondary stress.* It is indicated by a subscript short straight line in front of the syllable in question.

"supermarket"	[ˈsu pɚ ˌmɑr kət]
"signify"	[ˈsɪg nə ˌfaɪ]
"phonetic"	[ˌfə ˈnɛ tɪk]

Some people find it difficult to distinguish between subtle loudness differences. For them, it may be of help to know that in General American English, different loudness levels characterizing stress go usually (but not always) hand in hand with changes in pitch. Thus, the louder the syllable, the higher the pitch. To pay attention to pitch differences first, then, may aid in discriminating between differing levels of loudness in stressing. It is also helpful to know that many (but again not all) words in General American English have their primary (or secondary) stress emphasis on the first syllable. A third possibility for those with difficulty in distinguishing stress differences is to vary systematically the loudness in each of the syllables of the word in question, [ˈdʒɛ ˌloʊ] versus [ˌdʒɛ ˈloʊ], for example. Typically, one version of that particular word will sound clearly more acceptable than the other. By a process of elimination, then, one can often ascertain the appropriate stressing pattern.

CLINICAL COMMENTS

Clients with dysarthrias have typical difficulties with stressing. The following transcription exemplifies such a possible displacement of stress.

	"birthday"
Norm speaker:	['bɝθ ˌdeɪ]
Dysarthric speaker:	[ˌbɝθ 'deɪ]

	"umbrella"
Norm speaker:	[ˌəm 'brɛ lə]
Dysarthric speaker:	['ʌm ˌbrə lə]

Duration Symbols. Sounds take up different amounts of time in continuous speech. We are so used to these measurable differences in sound duration that we register changes in these typical lengths automatically as "too short" or "too long." If that is our perceptual impression, we have to indicate it by means of diacritic markers. Normal (i.e., inconspicuous) sound duration remains unmarked.

Lengthening. Longer than normal duration is signaled by either one or two dots following the sound symbol in question. The more dots, the longer the sound.

[fit]   standard vowel duration

[fi·t]   slightly longer than normal vowel duration

[fi:t]   clearly longer than normal vowel duration

Shortening. Shorter than normal speech sound productions also occur. Different degrees of shortening are, as a rule, not indicated.

The diacritic mark for any shortened sounds is [˘] placed above the respective sound symbol.

Shortening of sounds can lead to cutting off a portion of their phonetic properties. Young children with still unstable [s]-sounds sometimes shorten the (normally fairly long) segments to something that may sound like the release portion of [t]. If onset and holding portions of [t] are also identifiable, the obvious transcription would be [t]. However, if that is not the case—that is, if we indeed had an [s]-impression—we would transcribe this as [š].

Syllable Boundaries. Syllable boundaries are indicated by a period placed between the syllables.

"reliable"   [ri.laˈ.ə.bəl]
"attention"   [ə.tɛn.ʃən]

Additional Symbols. The following symbols are not diacritics but are often used when transcribing aberrant speech.

Glottal Stop. The glottal stop ([ʔ]) is produced when a closed glottis is suddenly released after a buildup of subglottal air pressure. The release of air pressure creates a popping noise. The glottal stop is considered an allophonic variation of some stop-plosive productions and can serve to release vowels in stressed syllables (Edwards, 2003) or separate successive vowels between words (Wise, 1958):

"oh"   [ʔoʊ]   releasing a vowel
"Anna asks"   [ænə ʔæsks]   separating successive vowels

Some children with articulatory or phonological impairments use the glottal stop as a sound substitution (Stoel-Gammon and Dunn, 1985).

Bilabial Fricatives. The voiceless ([ɸ]) and voiced ([β]) bilabial fricatives are not phonemes of General American En-glish but can also be used as sound substitutions in ab-errant speech. Both sounds are produced by bringing the lips together so that a horizontally long but ver-tically narrow passageway is left between them for the voiceless or voiced breath stream to pass (Heffner, 1975).

> The bilabial fricatives are phonemes in several languages. For example, [ɸ] is a phoneme of Japanese, whereas [β] has phonemic value in Spanish.

Palatal Fricatives. The voiceless [ç] and voiced [ʝ] mediodorsal-mediopalatal fricatives may be heard as substitutions for [ʃ] and [ʒ]. These sounds are characterized by a more posterior tongue articulation than for [ʃ] or [ʒ]. Thus, both organ and place of articulation are shifted from coronal-postalveolar (or prepalatal) to this mediodorsal-mediopalatal position. The voiceless [ç] sounds similar to a voiceless [j].

Postdorsal-Velar Fricatives. Some children, when attempting to produce the postdorsal-velar stops [k] and [g], may not raise the tongue sufficiently to create a complete clo-sure. In this case, a fricative may result. The symbols for the postdorsal-velar fricatives are [x] for the voiceless sound and [ɣ] for its voiced cognate.

Postdorsal-Uvular Stops. These sounds may again be heard by a child who is attempting to produce [k] or [g]. In this case, the client pro-duces a stop-plosive, but the place of articu-lation is too far back in the mouth, resulting in a sound that might be perceived as having a "guttural" quality. The voiceless postdorsal-uvular stop is transcribed [q], and its voiced counterpart is noted as [ɢ].

Flap, Tap, or One-Tap Trill. The flap, tap, or what is also known as the one-tap trill [ɾ], is a frequent allophonic variation of [t] and [d]. This variation often occurs when stop-plosives are preceded and followed by vowels, as in *city* or *butter.* A single tap of the tongue tip against the alveolar ridge or with a gesture of the tongue tip in that direction character-izes these sounds (Wise, 1958).

"butter"   [bʌɾɚ]
"ladder"   [læɾɚ]

𝒞LINICAL IMPLICATIONS

Phonetic transcription and, especially, its dia-critic marks appear at first glance complicated to handle and difficult to remember. The ob-vious question arises as to how these diacritics could be helpful in our assessment and thera-peutic process. The answer is threefold.

First, accurate phonetic transcription in-volves ear training, a sharpening of our audi-tory discrimination abilities. These skills are indispensable for clinical expertise, some-thing that can never be emphasized enough. Second, phonetic transcription, and especially the use of diacritic markers, provides a gener-ally agreed on, professional way to note certain deviations from norm productions. This sys-tem allows clinicians to communicate freely with other professionals within the field of communication sciences and disorders. Tran-scription symbols can be translated back into actual speech events in the same way that mu-sicians can read notes and translate them back into tunes. Third, by being aware of the many variations that can occur, accurate phonetic transcriptions open up diagnostic possibili-ties that we might not have considered with-out this knowledge. If we don't know what to listen for—unreleased stops or partial devoicing, for example—we might not identify some of the abnormal variations.

CLINICAL APPLICATION

The ExtIPA and Multiple Interdentality

Multiple interdentality, a label dating back to at least the 1930s (Froeschels, 1931, 1937), may often be seen in our clinical population. It is used to describe an immature speech habit in which children produce [t], [d], [l], and [n] with their tongue tip too forward. In other words, the tongue tip is between their teeth—that is, an interdental production. According to the ExtIPA chart (see Figure 3.2), we see that there is a way to transcribe these sounds in the following manner:

$$[t̪], [d̪], [n̪], [l̪]$$

Children with multiple interdentality often have difficulty with [s] and [z] as well. These sounds are also produced interdentally and end up sounding like "th" sounds, thus [θ] and [ð].

---

[s]-sound realizations illustrate well how the use of diacritics can have valuable practical consequences for assessment and intervention. Knowing what to listen for, we find that what once sounded like simply a distorted [s] can now be specified as the actual aberrant form presented: a palatal versus a lateral versus a dentalized [s]-distortion, for example. All these variations can be noted using the respective diacritic markers. In addition, aside from the clarification the notation system provides, detailed knowledge about actual realizations is indispensable for the assessment and successful remediation of [s] errors. By establishing that the [s] appears distorted, we are saying only that its typical production is "off." We have addressed the *acceptability* issue of the sound realization, but not its aberrant *production* features, the most important information

for clinical purposes. However, by comparing the child's actual articulatory features with the known features for regular [s]-productions, we will know precisely which placement characteristics need to be changed therapeutically.

By identifying an [s]-distortion as a palatal [s], for example, detailed information that can be used when planning therapy is given. A palatal [s] is produced with the tongue tip too far back in the direction of the palatal area. Due to this tongue position, the palatal [s] has a [ʃ]-like quality. All other production features are usually in accordance with norm [s]-articulations; the lateral edges of the tongue are raised, and the sagittal grooving necessary for the [s] is present as well. It may be possible, therefore, that the child needs only to move the tongue tip to a more anterior position to produce a regular [s]. Applying this knowledge, therapy becomes not only more goal directed but also much simpler—with the consequence of saving time and possible frustration.

The advantage of knowing how the child actually produces the distorted speech sound becomes even more obvious if we compare two distorted sound productions, one palatal [s] ([sʲ]) and one dentalized [s] ([s̪]), for example. The [s̪] is characterized by a tongue placement too far forward. In this case, the child needs to move the tongue back, posteriorly, to obtain a regular [s]. This would be in direct contrast to the procedure necessary for the [sʲ], in which fronting of organ and place of articulation becomes necessary. Detailed knowledge of the client's production features, then, proves to be an important asset leading to expedient and thorough therapeutic intervention.

Theoretically and practically, the importance of the preceding discussion seems rather obvious. Its essential ingredient is our ability to note and differentiate between changes in sound quality as the basis for our remedial task. By fine-tuning transcription skills, not only are the listener's discrimination and transcription capabilities increased, but also the effectiveness of the whole intervention process improves.

Using Diacritics in the Assessment Process

Andy, age 6;2, was referred to the speech-language specialist by his classroom teacher. According to the teacher, his main problem seemed to be his "speech," which she described as being somewhat difficult to understand and containing many sound errors. After a thorough appraisal, the speech-language specialist was concerned that Andy might have a phonological disorder. When first listening to Andy's spontaneous speech, in addition to his w/r substitutions, she thought that he used [θ] realizations for th-, s-, and sh-sounds. The clinician was worried that Andy was not able to differentiate between these phonemes. She had to admit, though, that there had been some qualitative differences between the productions that she could not quite describe. She decided to continue with her assessment, paying special attention to these sounds. She also used some pictures that pinpointed the th-, s-, and sh-sounds in an elicited speech sample. After carefully listening to Andy's actual productions and later to the recording, the clinician arrived at the following results:

One-Word Articulation Test Results

Norm Production	→	Actual Production	Word Examples	Transcriptions
[s], [z]	→	[s̪], [z̪]	sun	[sʌn] → [s̪ʌn]
			bus	[bʌs] → [bʌs̪]
			zoo	[zu] → [z̪u]
			all consonant clusters with [s]	[s] + consonant → [s̪] + consonant
[ʃ]	→	[sʲ]	shoe	[ʃu] → [sʲu]
			fish	[fɪʃ] → [fɪsʲ]
			dishes	[dɪʃəz] → [dɪsʲəz̪]
[θ]	correct	[θ]	thumb	[θʌm] → [θʌm]
[ð]	correct	[ð]	feather	[fɛðɚ] → [fɛðə]

Selected Spontaneous Speech Sample:

I have a red toothbrush. My mommy tells me every night to brush my teeth.
[aɪ hæv ə wɛd tuθbwəsʲ maɪ mɑmi tɛlz̪ mi ɛvri naɪt tu bwʌsʲ maɪ tiθ]

Today in school we made an art picture.
[tudeɪ ɪn s̪kul wi meɪd ən at pɪksʲə]

We cut out all sorts of things with scissors and pasted them on this sheet of paper.
[wi kʌt aᵘt al s̪oʷəts̪ ʌv θɪŋkz̪ wɪθ s̪ɪz̪əz̪ ænd peɪs̪təd ðɛm an ðɪs̪ sʲit ʌv peɪpə]

Andy did actually differentiate between the th-, s-, and sh-sounds with a dentalized production—[s̪, z̪] for /s/ and /z/, a palatalized [sʲ] for /ʃ/, and correct "th" realizations. In this case, careful transcription made a large difference in the outcome of this assessment.

SUMMARY

Assessment procedures and results should be accurate, professional, and accomplished in an accountable manner. This chapter introduced the International Phonetic Alphabet (IPA) as a widely used system that can provide these requisites for the assessment of articulatory and phonological disorders. The IPA system was developed to document actual phonetic realizations of speech events. It is a means of transferring highly impermanent speech events into more durable graphic representations. Such a system offers the speech-language specialist a way to substantiate assessment results as well as to communicate effectively with other professionals. Transcription should never be considered just an option; accurate transcription is a necessity for professional evaluations.

To increase the effectiveness of the IPA system, certain diacritic markers are used to add production details to the meaning of the basic symbol. These markers are indispensable to the documentation of many of the unusual realizations of our clients. One current diacritic system used for disordered speech, the ExtIPA, was introduced. Such diacritics were itemized, explained, and exemplified in the second section of the chapter. This section also offered clinical comments on many of the diacritics as well as actual phonetic transcriptions utilizing these marks.

The last section of this chapter demonstrated how phonetic transcription and the detailed knowledge acquired through its use in assessment procedures also benefits the intervention process. First, the accuracy needed for the transcription task promotes the fine-tuning of perceptual skills, a clinical proficiency that will, by its very nature, enhance the likelihood of successful intervention. Second, the specificity gained through phonetic transcription, including diacritics, translates into a far more goal-directed treatment approach, which increases clinical efficacy.

CASE STUDY

The following transcription is from Jordan, age 5;6. The first transcription is broad transcription, the second one is narrow transcription.

Broad Transcription

sit	[sɪt]	soap	[soᵘp]
sing	[sɪŋ]	soup	[sup]
sock	[sak]	summer	[sʌmɚ]
sun	[sʌn]	bus	[bʌθ]
miss	[mɪs]	toss	[tas]
goose	[gus]	race	[reˈs]
house	[haᵘs]	pass	[pæs]
zoo	[zu]	zap	[zæp]
bees	[biz]	news	[nuz]
rose	[roᵘz]	trees	[triz]

Narrow Transcription

sit	[s̺ɪt]	soap	[sʲoᵘp]
sing	[s̺ɪŋ]	soup	[sʲup]
sock	[sʲak]	summer	[sʲʌmɚ]
sun	[s̺ʌn]	bus	[bʌθ]
miss	[mɪs̺]	toss	[tasʲ]
goose	[gusʲ]	race	[reˈs̺]
house	[haᵘsʲ]	pass	[pæs̺]
zoo	[zʲu]	zap	[z̺æp]
bees	[biz̺]	news	[nuzʲ]
rose	[roᵘzʲ]	trees	[triz̺]

What additional information do the diacritics provide? Do you see a pattern for the palatalized versus dentalized [s] and [z]?

THINK CRITICALLY

1. What is the difference in production between a dentalized [s], [s̪], and a [θ]? Which articulatory features would you need to change to produce a standard [s]? How would you explain this to a child?
2. What are the production features of [ʃ]? What would you do to change the production to a standard [ʃ]? Are there any vowel contexts you could use to assist in acquiring this standard production?
3. The following transcription is from a child, age 4;2. Label the diacritics and state which ones are context related and which ones would be considered aberrant productions.

[aɪ wʌnt tu goʊ t̪u s̪ʌ bitʃ]

I want to go to the beach.

[sʲæli ɫɛd wi kʊd˺ goʊ]

Sally said we could go.

[dæɾɪ wʌnts̪ tu sʷwɪm]

Daddy wants to swim

[ɪt wɪɫ bi f̬ʌn]

It will be fun.

4. Put in the syllable boundaries and the primary stress markers for the following words:

outspoken

inspiration

national

monumental

October

5. Identify the following symbols. For each, describe when they could be used as sound substitutions.

[x]   [ʔ]   [ɮ]   [ɟ]

TEST YOURSELF

1. IPA stands for which of the following?
   a. International Phonetic Association
   b. International Phonetic Alphabet
   c. both a) and b)
   d. none of the above
2. Which one of the following is not a diacritic used with vowels?
   a. [˕]   c. [ˬ]
   b. [˔]   d. [+]
3. Which one of the following would indicate a nasalized [s]?
   a. [s̩]   c. [s̃]
   b. [s̬]   d. [s̺]
4. Which one of the following would be a standard pronunciation?
   a. [ɮu] zoo   c. [sʲɪŋɚ] singer
   b. [bɛɾi] Betty   d. [kı̝p] keep
5. In the transcription [kætl̩], what does the diacritic under the [l] indicate?
   a. that the [l] is partially devoiced

b. that the [l] is unreleased
c. that the [l] is lateralized
d. that the [l] is the syllable nucleus of the second syllable

6. The voiced labiodental approximant is transcribed as
   a. [β]   c. [ʋ]
   b. [ɣ]   d. [j]
7. The voiced labiodental approximant may be substituted for which sound?
   a. [s]   c. [l]
   b. [r]   d. [ʃ]
8. Which one of the transcriptions would indicate "bird" without the r-coloring on the vowel?
   a. [bɜd]   c. [bɪd]
   b. [bɛd]   d. [bɔd]
9. Which one of the following transcriptions indicates excessive aspiration?
   a. [kʰip]   c. [kı̝p]
   b [kʼip]   d. [kı̈p]

10. The transcription [ʏ̈] would indicate which one of the following?
   a. a vowel position that is too far forward
   b. a vowel position that is too far back
   c. a vowel that is less rounded than is usual
   d. a vowel that is more rounded than is usual

WEBSITES

www.phonologicaldisorders.com

This website, created by the author of this textbook, contains review exercises for phonetic transcription. Examples are also given of additional articulation test results which show how to use phonetic transcription. Links are given to other websites and resources.

www.paulmeier.com/ipa/charts.html

This website was designed by Eric Armstrong of York University, Toronto, Canada, and voiced by Paul Meier of the University of Kansas, United States. It includes the International Phonetic Alphabet and is an interactive website in which you can hear the diphthongs and triphthongs of American English and British English (Received Pronunciation). It is very interesting and user-friendly.

http://web.uvic.ca/ling/resources/phonlab/ipatut/index.html

This is considered a tutorial site for the International Phonetic Alphabet from the University of Victoria, Canada. There are also several other related websites. This one gives the viewer the opportunity to click on the various IPA symbols and hear the vowel sound or the consonant sound. The consonants are imbedded in a vowel-consonant-vowel environment. For beginners using phonetic transcription or for those who would like to familiarize themselves with non–American English sounds, it is a great website.

www.ic.arizona.edu/~lsp/IPA.html

This website is a tutorial from the University of Arizona and it includes vowels, consonants, and examples of several American English dialects. If you go to the homepage, information about American and Canadian dialects is given.

http://www2.arts.gla.ac.uk/IPA/pulmonic.html

This is a webpage from the University of Glasgow, Scotland, United Kingdom, that provides dozens of links to many different topics, including, for example, the International Phonetic Alphabet, movement of the articulators, and online phonetic courses. It is a good resource for several different topic areas in phonetics and phonology.

FURTHER READINGS

Garcia Lecumberri, M., & Maidment, J. (2000). *English transcription course.* London: Arnold.

International Phonetic Association. (1999). *Handbook of the International Phonetic Association: A guide to the use of the International Phonetic Alphabet.* Cambridge, UK: Cambridge University Press.

Pullum, G., & Ladusaw, W. (1996). *Phonetic symbol guide* (2nd ed.). Chicago: University of Chicago Press.

Shriberg, L., & Kent, R. (2003). *Clinical phonetics* (3rd ed.). Boston: Allyn & Bacon.

Small, L. (2005). *Fundamentals of phonetics: A practical guide for students* (2nd ed.). Boston: Allyn & Bacon.

4

Theoretical Considerations and Practical Applications

LEARNING OBJECTIVES

When you have finished this chapter, you should be able to:

- Trace how the development of the speech sound evolved into the phoneme concept.
- Describe the major class features, the cavity features, and the manner of articulation features of the Chomsky and Halle (1968) distinctive feature classification.
- Provide examples of marked and unmarked sounds or sound classes.
- Define natural phonology.
- List examples of the common phonological processes.
- Distinguish the linear from the nonlinear (multilinear) phonologies.
- Describe autosegmental phonology and its use of a tiered representation.
- Explain the metrical trees in relationship to strong and weak stressing.
- Describe the characteristics of feature geometry.
- Understand the importance of optimality theory as a constraint-based approach.

Many students and clinicians are skeptical about theories. They are viewed as unnecessarily difficult to understand, impractical, and not really relevant to diagnostic and therapeutic issues. Some theories may indeed be somewhat difficult to understand because they are attempts to explain highly complex behaviors. For example, Schwartz (1992a) states that a theoretical framework that addresses any aspect of language acquisition requires

1. a theory of abstract knowledge and representation about the subject;
2. the processing of input, how it is represented, and how it is produced; and
3. aspects of developmental change.

It is easy to see why a theoretical framework that attempts to consider all these aspects might be complex.

The second objection to theories is that they are impractical. Actually, theories can be very practical. Theories are based on confirmed observations or systematic experiments. As such, they try to abstract from many practical experiences, attempting to find order and rules amid seemingly entangled details. Theories can also serve as blueprints for practical tasks. For example, phonological theories attempt to explain the structure and function of phonological systems. The structure and function outlined by a specific theory can in turn be used to analyze a particular phonological system. This analysis procedure can then be applied to both normal and disordered phonological systems. Various theories, such as natural phonology generating phonological processes, have resulted in analysis procedures that are used daily to evaluate the phonological systems of children.

The third objection to theories is that they are not relevant to the diagnosis and treatment of individual clients. Because theories guide and direct clinical work, they are fundamentally important and relevant to the diagnostic and therapeutic process. For example, as stated earlier, many students and clinicians are currently using phonological processes to describe patterns of errors and to determine therapeutic goals. The concept of phonological processes evolved from the theory of natural phonology (Donegan and Stampe, 1979; Stampe, 1969, 1972, 1973). The theory of natural phonology applied certain principles of generative grammar, itself another theory that has revolutionized the way professionals view language. Both of these theories have resulted in major changes in diagnostic and therapeutic procedures. Different types of analyses are now employed diagnostically, and a major shift in therapy has occurred due to the impact of these theories. The relevance of theories to our profession should not be underestimated.

Theories also offer a *variety* of clinical possibilities. Each theory provides a somewhat different perspective on the problem to be solved. Therefore, if one theory is used, assessment and treatment will vary from those suggested by a second theory. This gives clinicians several possible directions and approaches from which they can choose. Each theory and its application provide the clinician with unique problem-solving advantages. Without such problem-solving strategies, these features would go unnoticed; valuable diagnostic information would be lost. Thus, theories provide a means of maximizing diagnostic and therapeutic skills. They are significant to the work clinicians do professionally.

Chapters 2 and 3 dealt primarily with production features of articulation—with speech sound forms. The focus in Chapter 4 shifts to phonology—to speech sound function. This shift is a consequence of the fact that contemporary theories in our field are phonological theories; they clearly emphasize the function of the phoneme as a meaning differentiating unit.

The first goal of this chapter is to introduce the reader to some basic terminology and principles underlying many of the contemporary phonological theories. They are contained in the section on phonology. The second goal is to present several phonological theories that have been applied clinically within the discipline. Each phonological theory will be discussed in relationship to its theoretical framework, how it developed, and how it functions. Finally, clinical implications will be suggested for each of the presented theories.

PHONOLOGY

What Is Phonology?

Phonology can be defined as the description of the systems and patterns of phonemes that occur in a language. It involves determining the language-specific distinctive phonemes and the rules that describe the set of changes that take place when these phonemes occur in words (Ladefoged, 2006). Within this system, the smallest entity that can be distinguished by its contrasting function within words is called the *phoneme*. The phoneme is, thus, the central unit of phonology.

Many different theoretical frameworks for phonological investigations exist. However, these various approaches all have one fundamentally important commonality, the differentiation between two levels of sound presentation:

1. the *phonetic level,* with sounds (phones, allophones) as central units, and
2. the *phonemic level,* represented by phonemes.

How Does Phonology Work?

To understand the concept of phonology, it is important to differentiate clearly between speech sounds and phonemes. Speech sounds (phones, allophones) are physical *forms* that are the result of physiological processes and that have objectively verifiable acoustic properties. Phonemes, on the other hand, are defined in terms of their linguistic *function*—that is, in terms of their ability to establish meaningful units in a language.

Phonology as a concept and discipline has undergone considerable changes. The original French and German terms *phonologie* (Baudouin de Courtenay, 1895) and *Phonologie* (Trubetzkoy, 1931) were, under the influence of structuralism, replaced by *functional phonetics* (Jakobson, 1962; Martinet, 1960). The term *functional phonetics* emphasized the functional aspect of speech sounds. Phonology has also been called phonemics (Sapir, 1925), underlining the linguistic function of the phoneme. The term *phonology* is presently preferred and used by most professionals within the field of communication disorders.

How Did the Concept of the Phoneme Develop?

The phoneme as concept and term was born toward the end of the nineteenth century at a point when linguists and phoneticians found it necessary to expand the former single sound concept into a two-dimensional sound concept:

A definition of the phoneme and its relationship to phonology are found in Chapter 1.

1. speech sounds as production realities
2. speech sounds in their meaning-establishing and meaning-distinguishing function, as "phonemes"

In their works, the British phonetician Henry Sweet (1845–1912), the German Eduard Sievers (1850–1932), and the Swiss Jost Winteler (1846–1929) laid the foundation for the understanding of this duality. However, historically, Baudouin de Courtenay deserves the credit for introducing the concept of the phoneme in the year 1870. (The word *phoneme* existed prior to this time, but it was used as another label for speech sound.) N. H. Kruszewski (1881), a student of Baudouin de Courtenay's, further popularized the term in his dissertation. Baudouin de Courtenay interpreted the proposed sound duality as differences between a physiologically concrete sound realization and its mental image. Influenced by the thinking of his time, Baudouin de Courtenay interpreted phonemes as primarily *psychological* sound units, as "psychic equivalents of the sound" (Lepschy, 1970, p. 60), as the sound "intended" by the speaker and "understood" by listeners. This was in contrast to the actually articulated sound, which was seen as a physiological fact. Similarly, the Russian linguist L. V. Ščerba, who succeeded Baudouin de Courtenay, defined the phoneme as "the shortest general sound image of a given language which can be associated with meaning images, and can differentiate words" (Lepschy, 1970, p. 62).

Although still psychologically oriented, the British phonetician Daniel Jones presented a more language-based phoneme concept in the first half of the twentieth century (Jones, 1938, 1950). Jones defined the phoneme as a "family of sounds in a given language which are related in character and are used in such a way that no one member ever occurs in a word in the same phonetic context as any other member" (Jones, 1950, p. 10). According to Jones's definition, as long as speech sounds are understood as belonging to the same category, they constitute a phoneme of that language. For example, as long as [s]-productions, with all their verifiable phonetic differences (different speakers, various circumstances), are evaluated by listeners as being the same, as belonging to the s-category, these allophonic variations represent the single phoneme /s/ in that language.

Today's prevalent phoneme concept is still more functionally oriented. The specific *use* of the phoneme in a language is the primary emphasis. This strictly functional phoneme concept (strongly influenced by Ferdinand de Saussure's [1916/1959] revolutionary new "structuralistic" way to look at language) was introduced by Nikolai S. Trubetzkoy and Roman Jakobson. Trubetzkoy, cofounder of the Prague School of linguistics, wrote that "the phoneme can be defined satisfactorily neither on the basis of its psychological nature nor on the basis of its relation to the phonetic variants, but purely and solely on the basis of its function in the system of language" (Trubetzkoy, 1939/1969, p. 41).

When defining the phoneme, he added that it is "the sum total of the phonologically relevant properties of a sound" (p. 36). "References to psychology must be avoided in defining the phoneme, since the latter is a linguistic and not a psychological concept" (p. 38).

One important aspect of a language's phonological system is its *phonemic inventory.* However, this is not the only variable used in characterizing different phonological systems. Edward Sapir (1921) pointed out that two languages having the same phoneme inventory can, nevertheless, have very different phonologies. Even though inventories may be identical, the way these sound segments can and cannot be arranged to form words may be quite different. Consequently, the *phonotactics,* or "permissible" sound arrangements within a language, is an important aspect of phonemes' "function" and is, therefore, an integral part of the phonology of a given language.

Speech Sound versus Phoneme: Clinical Application

Every utterance has two facets: an audible sequence of speech sounds and their specific meaning conveyed through this sequence. For example, if someone says, "Hey, Joe, over here," there is an audible sequence of sounds [heɪ dʒoʊ oʊvɚ hɪɚ] that conveys a specific meaning. Both the physical form of the speech sound and its language-specific function need to be realized in order for the utterance to be meaningful. If only one aspect is realized, either speech sound form or function, a breakdown in the communicative process will occur. For example, although a child may have the correct speech sound form, in other words, be able to produce [p]–[b], [t]–[d], and [k]–[g], this child might leave out these sounds at the end of a word. Thus, form is accurate but the child's realization of the function is inadequate. In this case, "beet" sounds like "bee" and "keep" becomes "key." A breakdown in communication would probably occur.

Adequate form and function of all segments are basic requirements for meaningful utterances in any language. Form is established by the way the segment in question is produced, by articulatory events. Segment function presupposes the observance of the language-specific rules regarding the arrangement of the speech sound segments. During an utterance, *form* and *function* become combined into meaning-conveying entities.

Segment form and function are also largely dependent on one another. Without acceptable production features, sound segments cannot fulfill their functional task. If, for example, the word *key* is realized as *tea,* a frequent error made by children with t/k substitutions, elements of sound production have interfered with sound function. In this case, the phonological opposition between /t/ and /k/ has been destroyed. Segment function depends on normal segment form.

Also, segment form depends on proper segment function. Without observance of the phonotactic rules governing the language, an acceptable sound production will not transmit the intended message. If, for example, a child produces a correct [s] but does not realize the phonotactic rules combining this [s] with other consonants in clusters, the meaning will be impaired. *Stop* might become *top,* or *hats* is realized as *hat.* For the purpose of effective verbal communication, regular segment form and function are indispensable.

Articulation and Phonological Theories and Therapies: Separation or Unity?

Historically, "correct" single sound realizations were often the central focus of articulation work. The mastering of how sound segments can and cannot be joined together to establish and convey meaning within the respective language was largely neglected. The underlying assumption was that speakers with defective articulation either "know" these rules already or will "learn" them through the various exercises that incorporated the sound in various contexts, for example. Articulation therapies focused on the realization of acceptable speech sound forms.

Today, it is often the other way around. The main orientation is the mastering of the phonological rules that govern the language-specific utilization of the sound segments. Children with phonological disorders do not demonstrate difficulties primarily with the production of the sound segments but instead with their function, with the rule-governed arrangement of these segments. Thus, mastery of the phonological rules, not the speech sound realization, becomes the main goal. Phonological therapies focus on the realization of adequate segment function within a language system.

Both intervention approaches have contributed substantially to the treatment of impaired articulation and phonology. They represent outgrowths of different theoretical viewpoints. However, their high degree of mutual dependency implies that, for successful articulation work, these two approaches are not clinically a matter of "either or" but of "as well as." Of course, based on the specific clinical characteristics of an individual client, one approach may take precedence. If, for example, emphasis on speech sound form were the chosen approach, functional aspects would, nevertheless, also have to be taken into consideration. For example, if a child has just learned the speech sound [ʃ] (i.e., the form is learned), the child will practice this correct production in various syllable shapes according to phonotactic principles. In this example, function follows form. On the other hand, if speech sound function were the main goal, there might be a point in therapy when the clinician would need to consider aspects of speech sound form as well. For example, a child produces a speech sound that appears to be a correctly articulated [f]. However, the child uses this [f] as a substitution for [θ]. The word *bath* is articulated [bæf] and *thing* as [fɪŋ]. In words that normally are articulated with [f], the child uses a [p]; "fan" becomes "pan" and "fig" is articulated as "pig." The child is able to produce the form, but the function of the [f] would need to be taught. Contrasting the phonemes /f/ and /p/ in minimal pairs might help with establishing the function of these two phonemes as meaning differentiating units.

In summary, effective verbal communication always mirrors both aspects of speech sounds, acceptable form and function. Remediation must consider both sides of this duality; they represent two sides of the same coin.

The next section of this chapter will address specific phonological theories. Each section will define, exemplify, and provide clinical examples to demonstrate the application of these theories to clinical assessment and treatment.

CLINICAL APPLICATION

Phonological and Articulation Therapies Working Together

Toby was 5;2 when he was seen by the new speech pathologist. Although he had previously received speech therapy, he was still considered very difficult to understand. A thorough assessment revealed that all fricative sounds were produced as stop-plosives. Thus, [f] and [v] were articulated as [p] and [b], and the voiceless and voiced [s] and [z], [ʃ] and [ʒ], as well as [θ] and [ð] were articulated as [t] and [d]. Toby's phonotactics for these sounds appeared intact. He did produce the noted substitutions consistently in all word positions. Toby often had difficulty discriminating words containing these phonemic oppositions. Thus, if the clinician asked the child to point to the picture of a "pin" versus a "fin" or of a "vase" versus a "base," Toby would often be in error. After completing the evaluation, the clinician decided that Toby had a phonological disorder: Toby did not understand the function of these phonemes in the language system.

The clinician began to work on differentiating and establishing these oppositions in meaningful contexts. Pictures and objects that contained these oppositions were used. The clinician noted that as Toby's discrimination abilities improved, he attempted to produce [f] and [v]; however, these realizations were consistently in error. As Toby struggled to correct the aberrant productions, the clinician realized that he was quickly becoming frustrated. The clinician used her knowledge of speech sound form to show Toby how to produce [f] and [v] in an acceptable manner. Toby was interested, responded quickly to this instruction, and soon could produce regular [f] and [v] sounds. He was very proud of his achievement and responded [naʊ aɪ kæn teɪ ɪt waɪt].

DISTINCTIVE FEATURE THEORIES

Distinctive feature theories are an attempt to determine the specific properties of a sound that serve to signal meaning differences in a language. The task is to determine which features are decisive for the identification of the various phonemes within a given language. Phonetic constituents that distinguish between phonemes are referred to as **distinctive features**.

What Are Distinctive Features?

How does one differentiate between apparent likenesses? For example, how do we distinguish between similar cars, houses, or streets? We look for discernible marks that might set the particular object apart from similar objects. A tree on the corner of a particular street, a brightly colored door on a house, for example, may serve as distinctive features that discriminate between streets or houses. "A distinctive feature is any property that separates a subset of elements from a group" (Blache, 1978, p. 56).

A sound component is said to be distinctive if it serves to distinguish one phoneme from another. These units, which are smaller than sound segments, are considered to be "atomic" constituents of sound segments that cannot be broken down any further (Jakobson, 1949). Theoretically, an inventory of these properties would allow the analysis of phonemes not only of General American English but also of all languages. Thus, distinctive features are considered to be universal properties of speech segments.

How Do Distinctive Features Work?

Distinctive features are the smallest indivisible sound properties that establish phonemes. An inventory of distinctive sound features would demonstrate similarities and dissimilarities between phonemes. These similarities and differences are marked by the presence of certain properties in some phonemes and the absence of these properties in others. The term *binary* is used in most distinctive feature analyses to indicate these similarities and differences. A **binary system** uses a plus (+) and minus (–) system to signal the presence (+) or absence (–) of certain features.

Many different distinctive features must be considered in order to arrive at those that distinguish between phonemes. For example, consonants must be distinguished from vowels, voiced consonants from voiceless consonants, nasals from nonnasals, to mention just a few. If /k/ and /g/ are considered, the following binary oppositions could be established:

/k/	/g/
is a consonant =	is a consonant =
+ consonantal	+ consonantal
is not a vowel = – vocalic	is not a vowel = – vocalic
is not voiced = – voice	is voiced = + voice

In this representation of similarities and dissimilarities, voicing is the only feature that distinguishes /k/ from /g/. Two sound segments are considered distinct and can, therefore, serve as phonemes *if at least one of their features is different.*

The *concept of binarity* goes back to Jakobson's influence on the evolution of distinctive feature theories. Jakobson, Fant, and Halle (1952) formulated that "any minimal distinction carried by the message confronts the listener with a two-choice situation" (paragraph 1.1). It follows that distinctive features are two-valued and require a yes/no decision concerning their presence or absence within sound segments. The concept of binarity has essentially been accepted by later distinctive feature systems. Ladefoged's "Prime Features" (1971) are the clear exception. This system uses multivalued features in its description.

To expand slightly upon this feature system, consider the phonemes /k/, /g/, and /ŋ/. As previously noted, /k/ and /g/ are distinguished from one another by the feature of voicing. How could this feature system be expanded to include the distinctive features that distinguish between /k/, /g/, and /ŋ/?

/k/	/g/	/ŋ/
+ consonantal	+ consonantal	+ consonantal
– vocalic	– vocalic	– vocalic
– voice	+ voice	+ voice
– nasal	– nasal	+ nasal

Although voice distinguishes /k/ from /g/ and /ŋ/, nasality is the feature that differentiates /g/ and /ŋ/, all their other features being the same. In this example, nasality is the distinctive feature that creates an opposition between the phonemes /g/ and /ŋ/.

Presence or absence of the sound segments' distinctive features can be displayed conveniently in a matrix form. Often, the Chomsky–Halle (1968) distinctive feature system is noted in textbooks for speech-language pathologists. However, this is not the only distinctive feature system. Over the years, many different distinctive feature systems have been developed (e.g., Jakobson, 1949; Jakobson, Fant, and Halle, 1952; Jakobson and Halle, 1956; Ladefoged,

1971; Singh and Polen, 1972). Each of these authors had a somewhat different idea about which distinctive features were important when distinguishing between phonemes. Most of the feature systems were binary; however, Peter Ladefoged (1971, 2006) used multivalued features. In addition, most distinctive feature systems used articulatory dimensions to classify the phonemes, although acoustic parameters have been utilized as well (Jakobson, Fant, and Halle, 1952). One distinctive feature system is not necessarily superior to another. They were all developed to address somewhat different aspects of feature distinctions. In addition, many distinctive feature systems originated as a means of analyzing *universal* similarities and differences observed in phoneme systems of many different languages. This goal would of necessity incorporate feature modalities that are not necessary when analyzing General American English speech sounds.

To summarize, distinctive feature systems are an attempt to document specific speech sound constituents that establish phonemes. Distinctive feature theories organize sound constituents according to some productional (or in some cases acoustic) properties that might be utilized in languages to establish meaning differences. The result is a system of contrastive, linguistically relevant sound elements. Historically, many different feature systems exist and many of the newer phonological theories, such as feature geometry, utilize their own somewhat different distinctive features. No one feature system has clear advantages over another. All distinctive feature systems reflect the authors' concept of those characteristics that most aptly define the phoneme.

How Did Distinctive Feature Theories Develop?

The original distinctive feature theories grew out of the phoneme concept, which was developed by the members of the Prague School in the 1930s. Very early in his work, Roman Jakobson, cofounder of the Prague School, hypothesized that the ultimate constituent of language was not the phoneme itself but its smaller components, its distinctive features. Jakobson stressed that these minimal differences serve the function of distinguishing between words that are different in meaning. It is these distinctive features that are functioning to distinguish between *bat* and *pat,* for example.

The Jakobson, Fant, and Halle (1952) system used twelve *acoustic* features based on the sound segments' spectrographic display. Such descriptions soon proved unsatisfactory for linguistic use primarily because similar acoustic representations can be the result of a number of different articulatory gestures. This led to a revision of the original system. In 1956, Jakobson and Halle published a new distinctive feature system that included *articulatory* production features. Many of the later distinctive feature systems (Chomsky and Halle, 1968; Halle, 1962; Ladefoged, 1971, 2006; Miller and Nicely, 1955; Singh, 1968; Singh and Black, 1966; Voiers, 1967; Wickelgren, 1966) were defined primarily according to ar-

---

An example of multivalued features includes using 1, 2, 3, and 4 to distinguish between differences in vowel height. Thus, [æ] is considered [1 height], while [i] is [4 height] (Ladefoged, 2006).

The use of acoustic parameters to specify distinctive features resulted in features such as "compact" and "diffuse." Based on acoustic displays of vowels, (+) compact was defined as a concentration of acoustic energy in the midfrequency region of the spectrum. Low vowels were considered (+) compact. The distinctive feature (+) diffuse was defined by a spread of acoustic energy over a wider frequency range. High vowels and labial, dental, and alveolar consonants were (+) diffuse (Jakobson and Halle, 1956).

ticulatory features (or to a combination of articulatory and acoustic parameters).

Distinctive Feature Theories: Clinical Application

Distinctive feature systems were developed as a means of analyzing phonemes and entire phoneme systems of languages. Each phoneme of the particular system was assessed to determine if the distinctive feature was present (+) or absent (−). Although originally devised to analyze the regular realization of phonemes within and across languages, its analysis potential for disordered speech could not be overlooked. When sound substitution features were compared to target sound features, similarities and differences could be noted.

Distinctive feature systems offered several advantages over the previous analysis systems of classifying errors according to substitutions, deletions, and distortions. First, they provide a more complete analysis. For example, sound substitutions can be broken down into several different feature components, which can then be compared and analyzed. Second, and perhaps more important, distinctive feature systems concentrate on the features that distinguish phonemes within a language. Previous analysis procedures had, at best, focused on phonetic production aspects of speech sounds. With the impact of phonology on the field of communication disorders, this emphasis now shifted to the phoneme and its function within the language system.

Distinctive feature analysis contrasted the features of the target sound to the substitution, resulting in a list of distinctive features that differentiated between the two. This analysis could show whether (1) error and target sounds shared common features and (2) specific error patterns existed.

Therapeutic implications follow logically. If the child can be taught to differentiate between the presence and absence of these differentiating distinctive features, the aberrant sound productions should be easily remediated. However, can children really understand and differentiate between distinctive features? Jakobson's (1942/1968) hypothesis that children acquire features rather than sounds seems to support this assumption. If this is the case, therapy could facilitate this developmental process. In addition, if children acquire features rather than sounds, a certain amount of generalization should occur. Consequently, children should be able to generalize features from sounds they can realize to others they cannot. This could be therapeutically utilized. A child who can produce, for example, + voicing in one phonemic context should be able to generalize this + voicing to other phonemic contexts. Therefore, treatment of one phonemic opposition with specific distinctive features should lead to the norm production of other phonemic oppositions with the same distinctive feature oppositions. This would be a means of treating more than one phoneme in a time-efficient manner.

Over time, several distinctive feature therapy programs were developed (Blache, 1989; Compton, 1970, 1975, 1976; McReynolds and Engmann, 1975; Weiner and Bankson, 1978). However, both the analysis procedures and the clinical applicability of distinctive features for speech-disordered children have been difficult to use and questioned by several authors (Carney, 1979; Foster, Riley, and Parker, 1985; Parker, 1976; Walsh, 1974). Some critical comments have focused on the fact that distinctive feature theory and distinctive features are abstract concepts: Distinctive features are theoretical concepts that were formulated to account for the sound patterns of languages. Carney (1979) further argued that a distinctive feature analysis, based on the phoneme concept, compels the clinician to ignore

Are distinctive features dated? Although distinctive feature therapy does seem to be "out," newer non-linear (multilinear) phonological theories still rely heavily on distinctive features. Markedness is also an important aspect of one of the more contemporary phonological theories—"optimality theory."

phonetic information. This phonetic information, exemplified by [s̪] or [ʃ] , is not classifiable according to distinctive features and may lead to classifying errors inappropriately or not at all. For example, if the child produces a dentalized s-sound, [s̪], how is this classified? There is no distinctive feature for dentalized [s]. The clinician might ignore the distortion, declaring it a norm production, or could perhaps classify it as a [θ]. In both cases, valuable diagnostic and therapeutic information would be lost.

GENERATIVE PHONOLOGY

What Is Generative Phonology?

Generative phonology is an outgrowth of distinctive feature theory, and it represents a substantial departure from previous phonological theories. Pregenerative theories of phonology—that is, those occurring prior to generative phonology (e.g., Jakobson, Fant, and Halle, 1952; Jakobson and Halle, 1956)—distinguished between phonetic and phonemic levels of realization. However, in pregenerative theories, both the phonetic and phonemic levels were analyzed by means of the actual productions, or the concrete realizations, of speech—for example, by using tape recordings of different language samples to assess the systems. Thus, pregenerative theories were developed around the *surface forms*, the actualities of speech production. On the other hand, generative phonologies expanded this concept decisively to include what has been called the underlying form. The **underlying form** is a purely theoretical concept that is thought to represent a mental reality behind the way people use language (Crystal, 1987). Underlying forms exemplify the person's language competency as one aspect of his or her cognitive capacity. The underlying forms also serve as points of orientation to describe regularities of speech reality as they relate to other areas of language, notably morphology and syntax.

Generative phonology, then, assumes two levels of sound representation, an abstract underlying form called *phonological representation* and its modified surface form, the *phonetic representation*. **Phonological rules** are used to demonstrate the relationship between the underlying (phonological) and the surface (phonetic) forms.

How Does Generative Phonology Work?

Distinctive features and phonological rules are central to the concept of generative phonology. *Phonological rules* explain the differences between phonological and phonetic representations. These rules are usually stated in a formalized notation system. This notation system was important, but its practical clinical use was cumbersome and it is no longer used. Although often considered outdated, these features have continued to be utilized in more current phonological therapies, including maximal oppositions (see Chapter 9 for a detailed account of this therapy). This section will introduce the distinctive features system that has been most widely used (Chomsky and Halle, 1968). However, generative phonological rules, specifically their notation, will not be discussed. Grunwell (1987) gives excellent coverage of the notational rules and their application to disordered speech.

Generative Distinctive Features. The first accounts of a generative distinctive feature theory were presented by Noam Chomsky (1957) and

Chomsky and Morris Halle (1968). Chomsky and Halle's (1968) *The Sound Pattern of English* is often cited as the major work in this area. They developed a new set of distinctive features that were different from those proposed by Jakobson and Halle (1956). In *The Sound Pattern of English,* the authors describe five features that are able to establish and distinguish between phonemes: (1) major class features, (2) cavity features, (3) manner of articulation features, (4) source features, and (5) prosodic features.

The *major class features* characterize, and distinguish between, three sound production possibilities that result in different basic sound classes:

1. *Sonorant.* "Open" vocal tract configuration promoting voicing. American English vowels, glides, nasals, and liquids belong to this category.
2. *Consonantal.* Sounds produced with a high degree of oral obstruction, such as stops, fricatives, affricates, liquids, and nasals.
3. *Vocalic.* Sounds produced with a low degree of oral obstruction (not higher than required for the high vowels [i] and [u]), such as vowels and liquids.

Cavity features refer to organ and/or place of articulation:

1. *Coronal.* Sounds produced with the apical/predorsal portion of the tongue ("the blade of the tongue raised from its neutral position," Chomsky and Halle, 1968, p. 304). This cavity feature marks several consonants, for example, [t], [d], [s], [z], [n], and [l]. See Table 4.1 for additional consonants.
2. *Anterior.* Sounds produced in the frontal region of the oral cavity with the alveolar ridge being the posterior border, that is, labial, dental, and alveolar consonants. [m], [n], [b], [p], [d], and [t] are examples.
3. *Distributed.* Sounds with a relatively long oral-sagittal constriction, such as [ʃ], [s], and [z].
4. *Nasal.* Sounds produced with an open nasal passageway—exemplified by the nasals [m], [n], and [ŋ].
5. *Lateral.* Sounds produced with lowered lateral rim portions of the tongue (uni- or bilateral). The only American English example is [l].
6. *High.* Sounds produced with a high tongue position, vowels as well as consonants. Thus, [i], [u], [k], and [ŋ] would be [+ high].
7. *Low.* Vowels produced with a low tongue position—[ɑ], for example. The only consonants qualifying for this category are [h], [ʔ], and pharyngeal sounds. The latter are produced with the root of the tongue as organ of articulation.
8. *Back.* Vowels and consonants produced with a retracted body of the tongue, that is, back vowels and velar and pharyngeal consonants.
9. *Round.* Refers to the rounding of the lips for the production of vowels and consonants. [u] and [w] are [+ round].

Manner of articulation features specify the way organ and place of articulation cooperate to produce sound classes, signaling production differences between stops and fricatives, for example:

1. *Continuant.* "Incessant" sounds produced without hindering the airstream by any blockages within the oral cavity. Vowels, fricatives, glides, and liquids are [+ continuant]; stops, nasals, and affricates are [– continuant].
2. *Delayed release.* Refers to sounds produced with a slow release of a total obstruction within the oral cavity. Affricates such as [tʃ] and [ʤ] are [+ delayed release].

3. *Tense.* Consonants and vowels produced with a relatively greater articulatory effort (muscle tension, expiratory air pressure). [p], [t], [k], [i], and [u], for example, are [+ tense]. [b], [d], [g], [ɪ], and [ʊ], by comparison, are [– tense].

Source features refer to subglottal air pressure, voicing, and stridency:

1. *Heightened subglottal pressure.* American English voiceless aspirated stops ([p], [t], [k]) are [+ HSP] because their production requires an added amount of expiratory airflow that, after freely passing the glottis, accumulates behind the occlusion within the oral cavity.
2. *Voiced.* Produced with simultaneous vocal fold vibration. All American English vowels, glides, liquids, nasals, and voiced stops, fricatives, and affricates are [+ voiced]. [p], [t], [k], [f], [s], and [ʃ], by contrast, are [– voiced].
3. *Strident.* The term *strident* (making a loud or harsh sound) is a feature of American English voiceless and voiced fricatives and affricates. However, the interdental fricatives [θ] and [ð] are [– strident].

Prosodic features are named but not discussed in Chomsky and Halle (1968). To see how several of these distinctive features apply to General American English consonants and vowels, see Tables 4.1 and 4.2.

Generative Naturalness and Markedness. One aspect of distinctive feature theory that seems to have more direct clinical applicability and

Table 4.1 General American English Consonant Matrix According to the Chomsky and Halle (1968) Distinctive Features

	p	b	t	d	k	g	θ	ð	f	v	s	z	ʃ	ʒ	tʃ	dʒ	m	n	ŋ	r	l	w	j	h
Sonorant	–	–	–	–	–	–	–	–	–	–	–	–	–	–	–	–	+	+	+	+	+	+	+	+
Consonantal	+	+	+	+	+	+	+	+	+	+	+	+	+	+	+	+	+	+	+	+	+	–	–	–
Vocalic	–	–	–	–	–	–	–	–	–	–	–	–	–	–	–	–	–	–	–	+	+	–	–	–
Coronal	–	–	+	+	–	–	+	+	–	–	+	+	+	+	+	+	–	+	–	+	+	–	–	–
Anterior	+	+	+	+	–	–	+	+	+	+	+	+	–	–	–	–	+	+	–	–	+	–	–	–
Nasal	–	–	–	–	–	–	–	–	–	–	–	–	–	–	–	–	+	+	+	–	–	–	–	–
Lateral	–	–	–	–	–	–	–	–	–	–	–	–	–	–	–	–	–	–	–	–	+	–	–	–
High	–	–	–	–	+	+	–	–	–	–	–	–	+	+	+	+	–	–	+	–	–	+	+	–
Low	–	–	–	–	–	–	–	–	–	–	–	–	–	–	–	–	–	–	–	–	–	–	–	+
Back	–	–	–	–	+	+	–	–	–	–	–	–	–	–	–	–	–	–	+	–	–	+	–	–
Round	–	–	–	–	–	–	–	–	–	–	–	–	–	–	–	–	–	–	–	–	–	+	–	–
Continuant	–	–	–	–	–	–	+	+	+	+	+	+	+	+	–	–	–	–	–	+	+	+	+	+
Del. Release	–	–	–	–	–	–	–	–	–	–	–	–	–	–	+	+	–	–	–	–	–	–	–	–
Voiced	–	+	–	+	–	+	–	+	–	+	–	+	–	+	–	+	+	+	+	+	+	+	+	–
Strident	–	–	–	–	–	–	–	–	+	+	+	+	+	+	+	+	–	–	–	–	–	–	–	–

Table 4.2   General American English Vowel Matrix According to the Chomsky and Halle (1968) Distinctive Features

	i	ɪ	e	ɛ	æ	ɑ	ɔ	o	ʊ	u	ʌ
Consonantal	−	−	−	−	−	−	−	−	−	−	−
Vocalic	+	+	+	+	+	+	+	+	+	+	+
Coronal	−	−	−	−	−	−	−	−	−	−	−
Anterior	−	−	−	−	−	−	−	−	−	−	−
High	+	+	−	−	−	−	−	−	+	+	−
Low	−	−	−	−	+	+	+	−	−	−	−
Back	−	−	−	−	−	+	+	+	+	+	+
Round	−	−	−	−	−	−	+	+	+	+	−
Tense	+	−	+	−	−	+	−	+	−	+	−

can be found in later theoretical constructs is the concept of *naturalness* and *markedness*. Naturalness and markedness can be seen as two ends of a continuum. The term **naturalness** designates two sound aspects: (1) the relative simplicity of a sound production and (2) its high frequency of occurrence in languages. In other words, more natural sounds are those that are considered easier to produce and occur in many languages. **Markedness**, on the other hand, refers to sounds that are relatively more difficult to produce and are found less frequently in languages (Hyman, 1975). For example, [p] is considered a natural sound (= unmarked). It is easy to produce and occurs in many languages around the world. The affricate [tʃ], though, is a marked sound: It is relatively more difficult to produce and is found infrequently in other languages.

Marked and unmarked features are typically used when referring to cognate pairs, such as /t/ and /d/, and sound classes, such as nasals. Sloat, Taylor, and Hoard (1978) describe the following sounds and sound classes according to markedness parameters:

Voiceless obstruents are more natural (unmarked) than voiced obstruents.

Obstruents are more natural (unmarked) than sonorants.

Stops are more natural (unmarked) than fricatives.

> Obstruents include the stops, fricatives, and affricates. See Chapter 2 for a more complete definition.

Fricatives are more natural (unmarked) than affricates.

Low-front vowels appear to be the most natural (unmarked) vowels.

Close-tense vowels are more natural (unmarked) than open-lax vowels.

Anterior consonants are more natural (unmarked) than nonanterior consonants.

Consonants without secondary articulation are more natural (unmarked) than those with secondary articulation (such as simultaneous lip rounding).

The concept of naturalness versus markedness became a relevant clinical issue when it was observed that children with phonological disorders have a tendency to substitute more unmarked, natural classes of segments for marked ones. For example, children substituted stops for fricatives and deleted the more marked member of a consonant cluster (Ingram, 1989b). Although the results of at least one investigation demonstrated contrary findings (McReynolds, Engmann, and Dimmitt, 1974), most investigations supported the notion that children and adults with speech disorders more frequently showed a change from marked segments to unmarked substitutions (Blumstein, 1973; Klich, Ireland, and Weidner, 1979; Marquardt, Reinhart, and Peterson, 1979; Toombs, Singh, and Hayden, 1981; Williams, Cairns, Cairns, and Blosser, 1970; Wolk, 1986). Markedness is also an important variable in newer theoretical models such as optimality theory (Prince and Smolensky, 1993).

How Did Generative Phonology Develop?

Generative phonology represents the applications of principles of generative (or transformational) grammar to phonology. The concept of generative grammar was first introduced by Noam Chomsky in 1957 in a book titled *Syntactic Structures*. Generative grammar departed radically from structuralistic and behavioristic approaches to grammar, which had dominated linguistic thought during the decades before Chomsky's work. Prior to the introduction of generative grammar, linguists had analyzed the surface forms of sentences into their constituent parts. This type of analysis was found to be inadequate in various respects. An often-used example illustrates this point:

> John is eager to please.
> John is easy to please.

If the two sentences are analyzed according to a structuralistic point of view, the results will indicate that both sentences have exactly the same structure. However, this analysis does not reveal that the two sentences have drastically different meanings. In the first sentence, John wants to please someone else—John is the subject of pleasing. In the second sentence, someone else is involved in pleasing John—John is the object of pleasing.

One aim of generative grammar was to provide a way to analyze sentences that would account for such differences. To do this, a concept was developed that postulated not only a *surface* level of realization but also a *deep* level of representation. *Competence* and *performance* were also terms that distinguished between surface and deep levels of representation. Language competence was viewed as the individual's knowledge of the rules of a language, whereas performance was actual language use in real situations. Structuralists and behaviorists had focused on an individual's performance; generative grammar shifted this focus to include the concept of an individual's language competence. The formulation of rules governing the events between the deep-level competence and surface-level performance was an important goal for generative grammarians.

Distinctive Features and Generative Phonology: Clinical Application

Generative phonology was originally developed to analyze the phonological systems of languages. Its application to phonological development in children has its foundation in Smith's (1973) case study of his son Amahl. Other authors (e.g., Compton, 1975, 1976; Grunwell, 1975; Lorentz, 1976; Oller, 1973) extended these analysis principles to children with disordered phonological systems. Generative phonology, applied in this manner, compares the child's phonological system to the adult's. To do this using the distinctive feature system, the target sound is compared to the child's substitution, noting the distinctive features that are different between the target and substitution.

Distinctive Feature Analysis. A distinctive feature analysis compares the phonetic features of the target sound with the phonetic features of its substitution. Because the distinctive feature system is binary, (+) and (–), similarities and differences between target and substitution can be clearly ascertained. One of the advantages of this analysis is that it allows for a comparison of several sound substitutions to the target phoneme. For example, if a client substitutes [t] for [d], [z], and [ʃ], similarities and differences between all sound features can be compared. In addition, correctly and incorrectly realized features across several phonemes can be examined to see whether patterns exist. A pattern is characterized by frequent use of one or more identical distinctive features when the target sound and the sound substitution are compared.

Most clinical applications use a version of the Chomsky and Halle (1968) distinctive feature system (Elbert and Gierut, 1986; Gierut, 1992; Grunwell, 1987; Lowe, 1994; McReynolds and Engmann, 1975). These distinctive features can be found in Tables 4.1 and 4.2. Any other distinctive feature system could be substituted; the principles of analysis would remain the same. Distinctive feature analysis is also used in feature geometry. (See pages 87–90.)

What to Do?   To describe patterns of errors, the distinctive features of the target phoneme and its substitution(s) are analyzed. Figure 4.1 depicts an example of a worksheet that can be used to identify them.

1. List the target phoneme and the substitution at the top of one of the boxes. If there are several substitutions for one target phoneme, each substitution should be listed in a separate box.

2. List the features that *differ* between the target sound and the substitution in the blank spaces under Feature Differences. Record their (+) or (–) values. These features are taken from the distinctive feature table you are using.

3. Transfer the information from the completed worksheet to the Summary Sheet for Distinctive Feature Analysis (Table 4.3). Table 4.3 provides the number of phonemes affected by each of the specific distinctive features.

In Table 4.4, the results of an articulation test from H. H. are transcribed. A distinctive feature worksheet and summary form are completed for H. H. in Figure 4.2 and Table 4.5. By looking at Table 4.5 we can see that there are four distinctive features that each impact six different phonemes:

– anterior is changed to + anterior (tʃ → t, dʒ → d, k → t, g → d, ʃ → d, ʃ → s),

+ high is changed to – high (tʃ → t, dʒ → d, k → t, g → d, ʃ → d, ʃ → s),

+ continuant is changed to – continuant (f → b, θ → b, ð → d, ʃ → d, s → t, z → t), and

+ strident is changed to – strident (tʃ → t, dʒ → d, f → b, ʃ → d, s → t, z → t).

In summary, distinctive feature systems attempt to capture those phonetic features that distinguish between phonemes of a language. Although these distinctive features are primarily productionally based, they represent an important aspect of a phonemic analysis. Error patterns can clearly be seen when frequently occurring distinctive features are summarized. Distinctive feature analyses cannot account for deletions, assimilations, or changes of the syllable structure.

Natural Phonology

What Is Natural Phonology?

"[Natural phonology] is a natural theory . . . in that it presents language as a natural reflection

Distinctive Feature Worksheet

List all target sounds together with the substitution(s). Use the Chomsky-Halle distinctive feature system to determine which features differ between the target sound and the substitution. List these differences with their "+" and "−" values in the space under the sounds.

Target → Substitution	Target → Substitution	Target → Substitution	Target → Substitution	Target → Substitution
Feature Differences	Feature Differences	Feature Differences	Feature Differences	Feature Differences

Target → Substitution	Target → Substitution	Target → Substitution	Target → Substitution	Target → Substitution
Feature Differences	Feature Differences	Feature Differences	Feature Differences	Feature Differences

Target → Substitution	Target → Substitution	Target → Substitution	Target → Substitution	Target → Substitution
Feature Differences	Feature Differences	Feature Differences	Feature Differences	Feature Differences

Figure 4.1 Worksheet for Distinctive Feature Analysis

Table 4.3 Summary Sheet for Distinctive Feature Analysis Using the Chomsky–Halle Distinctive Feature System

Feature	Feature Change	No. of Phonemes Affected	Feature Change	No. of Phonemes Affected
Sonorant	+ to −	_____	− to +	_____
Consonantal	+ to −	_____	− to +	_____
Vocalic	+ to −	_____	− to +	_____
Coronal	+ to −	_____	− to +	_____
Anterior	+ to −	_____	− to +	_____
Nasal	+ to −	_____	− to +	_____
Lateral	+ to −	_____	− to +	_____
High	+ to −	_____	− to +	_____
Low	+ to −	_____	− to +	_____
Back	+ to −	_____	− to +	_____
Round	+ to −	_____	− to +	_____
Continuant	+ to −	_____	− to +	_____
Delayed Release	+ to −	_____	− to +	_____
Voiced	+ to −	_____	− to +	_____
Strident	+ to −	_____	− to +	_____

Summary: _____

_____

_____

_____

_____

of the needs, capacities, and world of its users, rather than as a merely conventional institution" (Donegan and Stampe, 1979, p. 127). **Natural phonology** incorporates features of naturalness theories and was specifically designed to explain the development of the child's phonological system. The theory of natural phonology postulates that patterns of speech are governed by an innate, universal set of phonological processes. **Phonological processes** are innate and universal; therefore, all children are born with the capacity to use the same system of processes. Phonological processes, as natural processes, are easier for a child to produce and are substituted for sounds, sound classes, or sound sequences when the child's motor capacities do not yet allow their norm realization. These innate, universal natural phonological processes are operating as all children attempt to use and organize their phonological systems. Therefore, all children begin with innate speech patterns but must progress to the language-specific system that characterizes their native language. Phonological processes are used to constantly revise existing differences between the innate patterns and the adult norm production. The theory points out prominent *developmental steps* children go through until the goal of adult phonology is reached in the child's early

Table 4.4   Single-Word Responses to Goldman-Fristoe Test of Articulation for Child H. H.

Target Word	Child's Production	Target Word	Child's Production
1. house	[haʊ]	22. carrot	[tɛwə]
2. telephone	[tɛfoʊ]	orange	[oʊwɪn]
3. cup	[tʌp]	23. bathtub	[bætʌ]
4. gun	[dʌn]	bath	[bæ]
5. knife	[naɪ]	24. thumb	[bʌm]
6. window	[wɪnoʊ]	finger	[bɪnə]
7. wagon	[wædən]	ring	[wɪŋ]
wheel	[wi]	25. jump	[dʌmp]
8. chicken	[tɪtə]	26. pajamas	[dæmi]
9. zipper	[tɪpə]	27. plane	[beɪn]
10. scissors	[tɪtə]	blue	[bu]
11. duck	[dʌt]	28. brush	[bʌs]
yellow	[jɛwoʊ]	29. drum	[dʌm]
12. vacuum	[ætu]	30. flag	[bæ]
13. matches	[mætət]	31. Santa Claus	[tænə dɑ]
14. lamp	[wæmp]	32. Christmas	[tɪtmə]
15. shovel	[dʌvə]	tree	[ti]
16. car	[tɑə]	33. squirrel	[twɜə]
17. rabbit	[wæbɪ]	34. sleeping	[twipɪn]
18. fishing	[bɪdɪn]	bed	[bɛd]
19. church	[tɜ]	35. stove	[doʊ]
20. feather	[bɛdə]		
21. pencils	[pɛntə]		
this	child would not say		

years. Disordered phonology is seen as an inability to realize this "natural" process of goal-oriented adaptive change.

How Does Natural Phonology Work?

The theory of natural phonology assumes that a child's innate phonological system is continuously revised in the direction of the adult phonological system. Stampe (1969) proposed three mechanisms to account for these changes: (1) limitation, (2) ordering, and (3) suppression. These mechanisms reflect properties of the innate phonological system as well as the universal difficulties children display in the acquisition of the adult sound system.

Limitation occurs when differences between the child's and the adult's systems become *limited* to only specific sounds, sound classes, or sound sequences. Limitation can be exemplified by the following: A child might first use a more "natural" sound for a more marked one. For example, all fricatives might be replaced by homorganic stops (e.g., [f] → [p],

Distinctive Feature Worksheet

List all target sounds together with the substitution(s). Use the Chomsky-Halle distinctive feature system to determine which features differ between the target sound and the substitution. List these differences with their "+" and "−" values in the space under the sounds.

Row 1

Target → Substitution
tʃ → t
Feature Differences

−anterior	+anterior
+high	−high
+del. rel.	−del. rel.
+strident	−strident

Target → Substitution
dʒ → d
Feature Differences

−anterior	+anterior
+high	−high
+del. rel.	−del. rel.
+strident	−strident

Target → Substitution
k → t
Feature Differences

−coronal	+coronal
−anterior	+anterior
+high	−high
+back	−back

Target → Substitution
g → d
Feature Differences

−coronal	+coronal
−anterior	+anterior
+high	−high
+back	−back

Target → Substitution
f → b
Feature Differences

+cont.	−cont.
−voice	+voice
+strident	−strident

Row 2

Target → Substitution
θ → b
Feature Differences

+coronal	−coronal
+cont.	−cont.
−voice	+voice

Target → Substitution
ð → d
Feature Differences

+cont.	−cont.

Target → Substitution
ʃ → d
Feature Differences

−anterior	+anterior
+high	−high
+cont.	−cont.
−voice	+voice
+strident	−strident

Target → Substitution
ʃ → s
Feature Differences

−anterior	+anterior
+high	−high

Target → Substitution
s → t
Feature Differences

+cont.	−cont.
+strident	−strident

Row 3

Target → Substitution
z → t
Feature Differences

+cont.	−cont.
+voice	−voice
+strident	−strident

Target → Substitution
r → w
Feature Differences

+conson.	−conson.
+vocalic	−vocalic
+coronal	−coronal
−high	+high
−back	+back
−round	+round

Target → Substitution
l → w
Feature Differences

+conson.	−conson.
+vocalic	−vocalic
+coronal	−coronal
+anterior	−anterior
+lateral	−lateral
−high	+high
−back	+back
−round	+round

Target → Substitution
___ → ___
Feature Differences

Target → Substitution
___ → ___
Feature Differences

Figure 4.2   Distinctive Feature Worksheet for Child H. H.

Table 4.5 Summary Sheet for Distinctive Feature Analysis: Application H. H.

Feature	Feature Change	No. of Phonemes Affected	Feature Change	No. of Phonemes Affected
Sonorant	+ to −	_____	− to +	_____
Consonantal	+ to −	2	− to +	0
Vocalic	+ to −	2	− to +	0
Coronal	+ to −	3	− to +	2
Anterior	+ to −	1	− to +	6
Nasal	+ to −	_____	− to +	_____
Lateral	+ to −	1	− to +	0
High	+ to −	6	− to +	2
Low	+ to −	_____	− to +	_____
Back	+ to −	2	− to +	2
Round	+ to −	0	− to +	2
Continuant	+ to −	6	− to +	0
Delayed Release	+ to −	2	− to +	0
Voiced	+ to −	1	− to +	3
Strident	+ to −	6	− to +	0

Summary: _____

−ant. to +ant: ʧ → t, ʤ → d, k → t, g → d, ʃ → d, ʃ → s

+high to −high: ʧ → t, ʤ → d, g → d, k → t, ʃ → d, ʃ → s

+cont to −cont: f → b, θ → b, ð → d, ʃ → d, s → t, z → t

+strident to −strident: ʧ → t, ʤ → d, f → b, ʃ → d, s → t, z → t

[θ] → [t], [s] → [t]). Later, this global substitution of all fricatives by stops might become *limited* to sibilant fricatives only.

Ordering occurs when substitutions that appeared unordered and random become more organized. Ordering can be exemplified by the following: A child's first revisions may appear unordered. To stay with the stop for fricative example, a child might at first also devoice the voiced stops of the substitution,

thus, ([s] → [t] and [z] → [t]). Thus, *Sue* is pronounced as [tu], but *zoo* is also articulated as [tu]. Later, the child might begin to "order" the revisions by voicing initial voiced stops but still retaining the stop substitution. Now *Sue* is [tu] and *zoo* is [du].

The term **suppression** refers to the abolishment of one or more phonological processes as children move from the innate speech patterns to the adult patterns. Suppression occurs when a previously used phonological process is not used any longer.

According to Stampe (1979), all children embark on the development of their phonological systems from the same beginnings. Stampe sees children as possessing a full understanding of the underlying representation of the adult phoneme system: that is, from the very beginning, the child's perceptual understanding of the phonemic system mirrors the adult's. Children just have difficulties with the peripheral, motor realization of the phonetic surface form. Many authors have questioned the validity of this idea (e.g., Fey, 1992; Oller, Jensen, and Lafayette, 1978; Stoel-Gammon and Dunn, 1985). In addition, Stampe's account of phonological development presents children as passively suppressing these phonological processes. Other contemporary authors, notably Kiparsky and Menn (1977), see children as being far more actively involved in the development of their phonological systems.

In spite of such shortcomings, Edwards (1992) states that "it is not necessary to totally discard the notion of phonological processes just because we may not agree with all aspects of Stampe's theory of Natural Phonology, such as his view that phonological processes are 'innate' and his assumption that children's underlying representations are basically equivalent to the broad adult surface forms" (p. 234). Phonological process analysis has found widespread clinical utilization, although it is used not so much to *explain* developmental speech events, as was the original intent of natural phonologists, as to *describe* the deviations noted in the speech of children.

Because phonological processes are so central to the workings of natural phonology, and to its clinical application, some of the more common processes are listed here with some explanatory remarks.

Phonological Processes

Although many different processes have been identified in the speech of normally developing children and those with phonological disorders, only a few occur with any regularity. Those processes that are common in the speech development of children across languages are called **natural processes.**

Phonological processes are categorized as syllable structure processes, substitution processes, or assimilatory processes. **Syllable structure processes** describe those sound changes that affect the structure of the syllable. **Substitution processes** describe those sound changes in which one sound class is replaced by another. **Assimilatory processes** describe changes in which a sound becomes similar to, or is influenced by, a neighboring sound of an utterance.

Syllable Structure Processes

Cluster reduction. The articulatory simplification of consonant clusters into a single consonant, typically the more "natural" member of the cluster.

Example: [pun] for *spoon.*

Reduplication. This process is considered a syllable structure process because the syllable structure is "simplified"; that is, the second syllable becomes merely a repetition of the first. Total reduplication refers to the exact reduplication of the first syllable. In partial reduplication, the vowel in the second syllable is varied (Ingram, 1976).

Examples:

Total reduplication: [wɑwɑ] for *water.*

Partial reduplication: [babi] for *blanket.*

Weak syllable deletion. The omission of an unstressed syllable.

Example: [nænə] for *baˈnana.*

Final consonant deletion.   The omission of a syllable-arresting consonant.

Example: [hɛ] for *head.*

Substitution Processes

Consonant cluster substitution.   The replacement of one member of a cluster.

Example: [stwit] for *street.*

Note: This is additionally referred to as gliding to indicate the specific type of substitution.

Changes in Organ or Place of Articulation

Fronting.   Sound substitutions in which the organ and/or place of articulation is more anteriorly located than the intended sound. Prominent types include *velar fronting* (t/k substitution) and *palatal fronting* (s/ʃ substitution).

Examples: [ti] for *key;* [su] for *shoe.*

Labialization.   The replacement of a nonlabial sound by a labial one.

Example: [fʌm] for *thumb.*

Alveolarization.   The change of nonalveolar sounds, mostly interdental and labiodental sounds, into alveolar ones.

Example: [sʌm] for *thumb.*

Changes in Manner of Articulation

Stopping.   The substitution of stops for fricatives or the omission of the fricative portion of affricates.

Examples: [tʌn] for *sun;* [dus] for *juice.*

Affrication.   The replacement of fricatives by homorganic affricates.

Example: [tʃu] for *shoe.*

Deaffrication.   The production of affricates as homorganic fricatives.

Example: [ʃiz] for *cheese.*

Denasalization.   The replacement of nasals by homorganic stops.

Example: [dud] for *noon.*

Gliding of liquids/fricatives.   The replacement of liquids or fricatives by glides.

Examples: [wɛd] for *red;* [ju] for *shoe.*

Vowelization (vocalization).   The replacement of syllabic liquids and nasals, foremost [l], [ɚ], and [n], by vowels.

Examples: [teˈbo] for *table;* [lædʊ] for *ladder.*

Derhotacization.   The loss of r-coloring in rhotics [r] and central vowels with r-coloring, [ɝ] and [ɚ].

Examples: [bɜd] for *bird,* [lædə] for *ladder.*

Changes in Voicing

Voicing.   The replacement of a voiced for a voiceless sound.

Example: [du] for *two.*

Devoicing.   The replacement of a voiceless for a voiced sound.

Example: [pit] for *beet.*

Assimilatory Processes (Harmony Processes)

Labial assimilation.   The change of a nonlabial into a labial sound under the influence of a neighboring labial sound.

> Assimilation processes can also be classified according to the type and degree of the assimilatory changes. For definitions and examples, see Sounds in Context: Coarticulation and Assimilation in Chapter 2.

Example: [fwɪŋ] for *swing.*

Velar assimilation.   The change of a nonvelar into a velar sound under the influence of a neighboring velar sound.

Example: [gɑg] for *dog.*

Nasal assimilation.   The influence of a nasal on a nonnasal sound.

Example: [mʌni] for *bunny.*

Note: The place of articulation is retained; only the manner is changed.

Liquid assimilation.   The influence of a liquid on a nonliquid sound.

Example: [lɛloʊ] for *yellow.*

According to natural phonology, phonological processes are recognizable steps in the gradual articulatory adjustment of children's speech to the adult norm. This implies a chronology of phonological processes, specific ages at which the process could be operating and when the process should be suppressed (Grunwell, 1981, 1987; Vihman, 1984). As useful as a chronology of normative data might seem for clinical purposes, tables of established age norms can easily be misleading. Individual variation and contextual conditions may play a large role in the use and suppression of phonological processes.

> Ages of suppression of the various processes are discussed in Chapter 5.

To summarize, natural phonologists assume an innate phonological system that is progressively revised during childhood until it corresponds with the adult phonological output. Limitation, ordering, and suppression are the mechanisms for the revisions that manifest themselves in phonological processes. Phonological processes are developmentally conditioned simplifications in the realization of the phonological system in question. As these simplifications are gradually overcome, the phonological processes become suppressed.

How Did Natural Phonology Develop?

David Stampe introduced natural phonology in 1969. However, several of its basic concepts had been established considerably earlier, most prominent among them being the concepts of naturalness (markedness) and underlying and surface forms, which are important aspects of generative phonology.

Jakobson (1942/1968) extended the concept of naturalness and markedness to *implied universals,* which could be found in different languages, children's acquisition of speech, and the deterioration of speech in aphasics. These universals were even used as a predictive device. Some examples include "fricatives imply stops" and "voiced stops imply voiceless stops." These examples would mean that if a language has fricatives, that language will have stops as well, and if a language has voiced stops in its inventory, the language will also have voiceless stops. Applying these two examples to children's acquisition of speech, children will acquire stops before (homorganic) fricatives. Also, voiceless stops are acquired before their voiced cognates. In an aphasic condition, the breakdown of speech would be characterized by the loss of the later-acquired sounds before the earlier-acquired ones. Thus, aphasics would lose fricatives before (homorganic) stops and voiced stops before voiceless ones. Whether these universal "laws" are generally valid under all of the previously mentioned conditions has been repeatedly questioned. However, they clearly exemplify the concepts of naturalness and markedness as universal phenomena.

Markedness theory also plays a central role in generative phonology and optimality theory (Prince and Smolensky, 1993; McCarthy and Prince, 1995). According to generative phonologists, markedness values are considered to be universal and innate. Thus, Jakobson, with his concept of universal naturalness, and Chomsky and Halle, with their understanding of universal and innate naturalness, set the stage for Stampe's natural phonology. Stampe incorporated the conceptual framework of naturalness into his theory of natural phonology.

At the same time, the meaning and use of the term *underlying form* changed drastically as it was incorporated into natural phonology. Within generative grammar, underlying forms, lexical as well as phonological, are highly abstract entities. They represent *assumed points of reference* that are necessary for the explanation of the many possible surface forms. In contrast, within the context of natural phonology, underlying forms as "models" for surface realizations suddenly gain some concrete reality. The underlying form is *the adult norm* that is the intended goal for children's production efforts.

Natural Phonology: Clinical Application

The concept of phonological processes within natural phonology has impacted both the assessment and the treatment of disordered phonological systems. Assessment procedures using phonological processes consist of contrasting the target word to the child's production. Aberrant productions are identified and labeled according to the phonological process that most closely matches the sound change. Typically, the processes are listed and the frequency of occurrence of individual processes is noted. Frequency of occurrence and the relative age of suppression play a role in targeting a process or processes for therapy. Depending on the age of the child, more frequent processes that should have been suppressed are commonly targeted for therapy. Some authors (Hodson and Paden, 1991; McReynolds and Elbert, 1981) suggest that a process should occur a certain number of times in order for it to be considered a possibility for therapy.

Unlike other analysis procedures, phonological processes can account for changes in syllable or word structures and those due to assimilations. Although phonological processes are not commonly used to identify sound distortions, they could be. For example, [ʂ] could be labeled fronting and [sʲ] backing.

Phonological Process Analysis. A phonological process analysis is a means of identifying substitutions, syllable structure, and assimilatory changes that occur in the speech of clients. Each error is identified and classified as one or more of the phonological processes. Patterns of error are described according to the most frequent phonological processes present and/or to those that affect a class of sounds or sound sequences. The processes utilized to identify substitutions are again primarily productionally based; however, they do account for sound and syllable deletions as well as several assimilation processes.

There are several assessment protocols that analyse phonological processes in articulation tests or in spontaneous speech (Bankson and Bernthal, 1990; Dean, Howell, Hill, and Waters, 1990; Grunwell, 1985a; Hodson, 2004; Ingram, 1981; Khan and Lewis, 2002; Lowe, 1996; Shriberg and Kwiatkowski, 1980). All of them identify each aberrant production according to the phonological process or processes that best represent the changes that have occurred. Most protocols also summarize the phonological processes by counting the total number of specific processes. Table 4.6 represents a protocol for summarizing the established phonological processes from the articulation test and the spontaneous speech sample.

To analyze a speech sample according to phonological processes:

1. Identify the phonological process that best describes the change. More than one phonological process might apply to a given misarticulation. For example, if a child substitutes [d] for [s] ([s] → [d]), this needs to be identified as stopping and voicing.

2. Tally the number of times the child used each process. On the summary form, list the processes and their frequency of occurrence.

The phonological processes and their frequency of occurrence for H. H. are contained in Table 4.7. A word-by-word analyis of his

Table 4.6 Phonological Process Analysis Summary Sheet

Processes	Number of Occurrences
Syllable Structure Changes	
Cluster reduction	_____
Cluster deletion	_____
Reduplication	_____
Weak syllable deletion	_____
Final consonant deletion	_____
Initial consonant deletion	_____
Other _____	_____
Substitution Processes	
Consonant cluster substitution	_____
Fronting	_____
Labialization	_____
Alveolarization	_____
Stopping	_____
Affrication	_____
Deaffrication	_____
Denasalization	_____
Gliding of liquids	_____
Gliding of fricatives	_____
Vowelization	_____
Derhotacization	_____
Voicing	_____
Devoicing	_____
Other _____	_____
_____	_____
_____	_____
Assimilation Processes	
Labial assimilation	_____
Velar assimilation	_____
Nasal assimilation	_____
Liquid assimilation	_____
Other _____	_____
_____	_____
_____	_____

Table 4.7 Summary of Phonological Processes for Child H. H.

Processes	Number of Occurrences
Syllable Structure Changes	
Cluster reduction	16
Cluster deletion	1
Reduplication	0
Weak syllable deletion	2
Final consonant deletion	17
Initial consonant deletion	1
Other _____	_____
Substitution Processes	
Consonant cluster substitution	9
Fronting	15
Labialization	5
Alveolarization	1
Stopping	20
Affrication	0
Deaffrication	0
Denasalization	0
Gliding of liquids	7
Gliding of fricatives	0
Vowelization	0
Derhotacization	7
Voicing	10
Devoicing	3
Other _____	_____
_____	_____
_____	_____
Assimilation Processes	
Labial assimilation	_____
Velar assimilation	_____
Nasal assimilation	_____
Liquid assimilation	_____
Other _____	_____
_____	_____
_____	_____

phonological processes are contained in Appendix 4.1 at the end of this chapter.

As can be seen from Table 4.7, H. H. demonstrates only five different processes 10 or more times: voicing (= 10 times), fronting (= 15 times), cluster reduction (= 16 times), final consonant deletion (= 17 times), and stopping (= 20 times). If the articulation test results are examined (Table 4.4 or Appendix 4.1), one can note that final consonant deletion impacts some of the fricatives, the stop-plosives, the nasals, one of the affricates, and the lateral [l], while stopping affects the fricatives and affricates. On the other hand, fronting is limited to [k], [g], and [ʃ].

Phonological processes can be used to analyze substitutions and deletions, something that distinctive feature analysis was not able to do. In addition, phonological process analysis can generate patterns, by noting the most frequent processes, and allows you to examine the sounds or sound classes that are most frequently included in the various phonological processes.

The next section will introduce the more recent developments in phonological theories, the so-called nonlinear or multilinear phonological theories. They represent a radical departure from the conceptual framework that preceded them.

*L*INEAR VERSUS NONLINEAR PHONOLOGIES

What Are Linear and Nonlinear Phonologies?

Phonological theories, theories of generative phonology included, were based on the understanding that all speech segments are arranged in a sequential order. Consequently, underlying phonological representations and surface phonetic realizations, too, consisted of a string of discrete elements. For example:

Wow, what a test.   [waᵁ wʌt ə tɛst]

The sequence of segments in this phrase begins with [w] and ends with [st]. All segments in between follow each other in a specific order to convey a particular message. Such an assumption that all meaning-distinguishing sound segments are serially arranged characterizes all linear phonologies. Linear phonologies, exemplified by distinctive feature theories and early generative phonology, can be characterized as follows:

1. emphasis on the linear, sequential arrangement of sound segments,
2. assumption that each discrete segment of this string of sound elements consists of a bundle of distinctive features,
3. assumption that a common set of distinctive features is attributable to all sound segments according to a binary + and – system,
4. assumption that all sound segments have equal value and all distinctive features are equal; thus, no one sound segment has control over other units,
5. the phonological rules generated apply only to the segmental level (as opposed to the suprasegmental level) and to those changes that occur in the distinctive features (Dinnsen, 1997).

Linear phonologies with sound segments (and their smaller distinguishing distinctive features) as central analytical units fail to recognize and describe larger linguistic units. Linear phonologies also do not account for the possibility that there could be a hierarchical interaction between segments and other linguistic units. Nonlinear or nonsegmental phonologies attempt to account for these factors.

Hierarchy refers to any system in which elements are ranked one above another.

Nonlinear (or what have been termed **multilinear**) **phonologies** are a group of phonological theories understanding segments as governed by more complex linguistic dimensions. The linear representation of phonemes plays a subordinate role. More complex linguistic dimensions—for example, stress, intonation, and metrical and rhythmical linguistic factors—may control segmental conditions. These theories explore the relationships among units of various sizes, specifically the influence of larger linguistic entities on sound segments. Therefore, rather than a linear view of equal-valued segments (in a left-to-right horizontal sequence), a hierarchy of factors is hypothesized to affect segmental units. Rather than a static sequence of segments of equal value (as in linear phonology), a dynamic system of features, ranked one above the other, is proposed. For example, syllable structure could affect the segmental level. A child may demonstrate the following pattern:

"man"	[mæn]	"window"	[wɪ doʊ]
"dog"	[dɑg]	"jumping"	[dʒʌ pɪ]
"ball"	[bɑl]	"Christmas tree"	[krɪ mə tri]

This child deletes the final consonant of each syllable in a multisyllabic word; however, no final consonant deletion occurs in one-syllable words. In this example, the number of syllables in a word interacts with and affects the segmental level. The number of syllables has priority over the segmental level: It determines segmental features. Nonlinear phonologies would rank syllable structure above the level of sound segments.

Another factor that may affect the segmental level is stress. Children have a tendency to delete segments in unstressed syllables. The following transcriptions demonstrate this:

baˈnana	→	[ˈnænə]
poˈtato	→	[ˈteɪ toʊ]
ˈtelephone	→	[ˈtɛ foʊn]

In these examples, the syllable stress clearly affects segmental realization; word stress has priority over the segmental level. "Instead of a single, linear representation (one unit followed by another with none having any superiority or control over other units), they [nonlinear phonologies] allow a description of underlying relationships that would permit one level of unit to be governed by another" (Schwartz, 1992b, p. 271).

How Do Nonlinear Phonologies Work?

There are many different types of nonlinear/multilinear phonologies. Several new theories have been advanced and others have been modified. All nonlinear phonologies are based on a belief in the overriding importance of larger linguistic units influencing, even controlling, the realization of smaller ones. Nonlinear phonologies also attempt to incorporate this hierarchical order of linguistic elements into analytical procedures, using so-called *tiered representations* of features.

To describe the many different nonlinear phonologies is beyond the scope of this book. *The New Phonologies: Developments in Clinical Linguistics* (Ball and Kent, 1997) is an excellent source of more detailed information on autosegmental phonology, feature geometry, underspecification theory, dependency phonology, government phonology, grounded phonology, optimality theory, and gestural phonology.

This section will be restricted to an introduction to nonlinear phonologies exemplified by autosegmental, metrical, feature geometry, and optimality theories. These theories are in no way superior to other nonlinear phonologies.

Autosegmental Phonology. **Autosegmental phonology** was proposed by John Goldsmith in 1976. Originally, Goldsmith presented this theory to account for tone phenomena in languages in which segmental features interact with varying tones. Parker (1994) illustrates the essential problem in the following manner:

According to the concept of linear (generative) phonology, features extend throughout a segment. Therefore, a segment such as /p/ is considered to be [– voice] throughout its entire segment, while /u/ is [+ voice] throughout its entirety. However, consider the problem posed by affricates. By definition, an affricate begins like a stop and ends like a fricative. The features that differentiate stops and fricatives are + and – continuant. This posed a problem for the linear phonologists because one segment cannot be designated as both + and – one distinctive feature. To solve this problem, the linear phonologists constructed the feature of "delayed release" to designate affricates. However, the feature of delayed release violates the construct of distinctive feature theory in that this property does not extend throughout the entire segment.

Autosegmental phonology proposed that changes within the boundary of a segment could be factored out and put onto another "tier." Thus + and – continuant could be placed on another level to indicate the change within the segment boundary. A diagram of an affricate such as /tʃ/ would look accordingly:

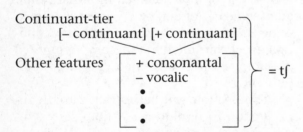

As can be seen, a single segment on one tier can be associated with more than one segment on another tier. Using the example of /tʃ/, the + consonantal segment can be associated with + and – continuant on another tier. In fact, the term *autosegmental* refers to the concept that certain segments are autonomous—they do not have a one-for-one match on another level.

As mentioned earlier, Goldsmith's (1976) dissertation addressed tone phenomena in so-called tone languages. This concept was used to

> Tone languages, which represent a large number of the languages of the world, are distinguished by changes in the meaning of a word simply by changing the pitch level at which it is spoken. Thus, phonemic differences can be signaled by distinctive pitch levels known as tones or tonemes (Crystal, 1987). For example, in Mandarin Chinese, four different tones with the identical sound segments [ma] result in words that mean "mother," "hemp," "horse," and "scold." Autosegmental phonology placed these tones on a tier above the sound segments, demonstrating the overriding importance of these tones for the meaning of the word.

explain *one-to-many mappings* (one tone associated with more than one segment) and *many-to-one mappings* (more than one tone associated with one segment). However, this "tiered" organization can demonstrate many characteristics of children's speech as well—relationships between certain syllable types and production of sound segments, for example.

For an understanding of autosegmental phonology, specific terms need to be defined:

Tiers	Separable and independent levels that represent a sequence of gestures or a unified set of acoustic features.
Association lines	Indicators for connections between autosegments on different tiers. Association lines cannot cross.
Linkage condition	Any condition governing the association of units on each tier. A linkage condition states, for instance, that if a segment is not linked to a position on another tier, it will not be phonetically realized.
Skeletal (or CV) tier	A representation of a syllable and its hierarchically related components' onset and rhyme.
Onset	Onset of a syllable. Includes all segments before the nucleus.

Rhyme   Cover term for nucleus (vowel) and coda (the arrest of the syllable).

The following diagram depicts the skeletal tier of a CVC syllable:

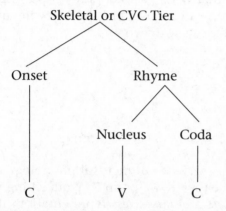

Skeletal or CVC Tier

The following is an example of a child who deleted final consonants in two-syllable words. The following diagram illustrates this relationship:

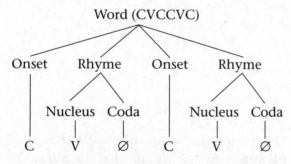

Word (CVCCVC)

Autosegmental phonology also accounted for *feature spreading*. Certain features such as + and – rounding, for example, can spread to other vowels and consonants. There are two rules for spreading. First, + and – round spreads from a vowel to adjacent consonants. Second, + and – round spreads from a consonant to an adjacent consonant up to a vowel. The following examples demonstrate the two types of feature spreading. The solid line is an inherent feature, while the dotted line represents a spread feature specification:

1. [+ round] spreads from a vowel to adjacent consonant.

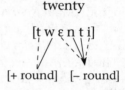

soy sauce

[s ɔɪ s ɑ s]

[+ round]   [– round]

2. [+ round] spreads from a consonant to an adjacent consonant up to a vowel.

twenty

[t w ɛ n t i]

[+ round]   [– round]

Feature spreading also occurs with such features as [+ voice] and [+ nasal].

To summarize, autosegmental phonology was originally conceived to account for cases in which a single segment is associated with two mutually exclusive features. It has since been expanded to demonstrate relationships between certain syllable types and consonant realizations. Feature spreading accounts for examples in which the feature or property of one segment spreads to adjacent segments.

CLINICAL APPLICATION

Using Autosegmental Phonology to Analyze an Error Pattern

The following autosegmental chart is for a child who produces all initial consonant clusters (two- and three-sound clusters) as [d]:

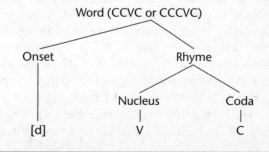

Word (CCVC or CCCVC)

Metrical Phonology. **Metrical phonology** (Liberman, 1975; Liberman and Prince, 1977) extended a hierarchical-based analysis to stress. In linear phonology, for example, stress was not handled in a binary + and – way; rather, there were an infinite number of prominence values that could be assigned to stress. The stress assignment rules of linear phonology produced a relative ordering within any given string of sound segments. This relative ordering can be used (1) to analyze the relative stressing of individual *words* within a sentence (sentence stress) as well as (2) to analyze the relative stressing of *syllables* within a word (word stress). The following example demonstrates the linear phonology stress assignment of individual words (word stress) and when these words are placed within a sentence. The numeral 1 indicates the primary stress:

Word stress

   a. customer

     1   3 2

   b. services

     1 3 2

Sentence stress

   c. customer services

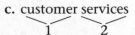

       1   2

   d. He is the supervisor of customer services.

     4 6 5   1   7   2   3

This system of assigning stress to words within phrases appeared inadequate to Liberman and Prince. For example, the words *customer services* are assigned two different values in examples c and d even though the same words are used. Stress assignment rules in linear (generative) phonology were relational and changed depending on the prominence given to the words within a phrase (Hogg and McCully, 1989).

Metrical phonologists proposed another concept for understanding and analyzing stress. "Metrical trees" are used to reflect the syntactic structure of an utterance. To show the relative prominence of each constituent in an utterance, stress patterns are represented by a binary branching of these metrical trees. One branch is labeled S for "stronger" stress and the other W for "weaker" stress. Applying this principle to an example, the following metrical tree can be drawn:

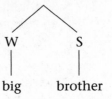

Thus, every tree in metrical phonology must have either a W S or an S W branching. This renders a binary stress representation. If the phrase is expanded, the following stress pattern emerges:

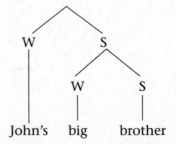

This pattern indicates that *brother* has more prominence than *big* and that the phrase *big brother* is more stressed than *John's*. The same relationship, then, is maintained between *big* and *brother* in both metrical representations.

The second basic concept in metrical phonology pertains to the syllable.

Although word boundaries are indicated in generative phonology, the syllable structure was not considered. Metrical phonologists indicate not only the number of syllables within a word but also which consonants belong (or are hypothesized to belong) to each syllable.

The notation uses the Greek letter sigma (σ) to indicate the individual syllables:

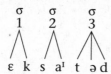

This hierarchical arrangement can also be used to include the morphological representation of the word together with its syllabic divisions. The Greek symbol mu (μ) denotes the morphemes within this word:

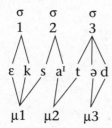

Such an analysis clearly indicates the difference between syllabic and morphological boundaries.

To summarize, metrical phonology is a theoretical construct that extends hierarchical analysis procedures to stress and syllable boundaries. Stress is analyzed according to a binary "strong" and "weak" system rather than to a relational numbering system that was used by earlier phonologists, including the linear (generative) phonologists. This hierarchical analysis has also been used when dividing words into syllables. Syllabic analyses allow for comparisons between syllable and morpheme boundaries.

CLINICAL APPLICATION

Using Metrical Phonology to Analyze an Error Pattern

The following metrical tree demonstrates a child's deletion of unstressed syllables in the two-syllable word *above* and the three-syllable word *umbrella*:

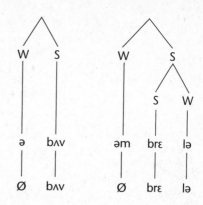

Feature Geometry. **Feature geometry** represents a group of theories that have adopted the tiered representation of features used in autosegmental phonology. However, feature geometry theories have added a number of other hierarchically ordered feature tiers. Feature geometry attempts to explain why some features (and not others) are affected by assimilation processes (known as *spreading* or *linking* of features) while others are affected by neutralization or deletion processes (known as *delinking*) (Dinnsen, 1997). There are several different tier representations in feature geometry. Figure 4.3 is a feature geometry representation that was provided by Bernhardt and Stemberger (1998) based on the proposals of Bernhardt (1992a, 1992b), Clements (1985), McCarthy (1988), and Sagey (1986).

In accordance with principles of nonlinear phonologies, feature geometry also utilizes hierarchically organized levels of representation, so-called tiers. These tiers interact with one another. Some features are designated as nodes, which means that they may dominate more than one other feature and serve as a link between the dominated feature and

> Note that distinctive features also play a central role in the newer nonlinear/multilinear phonologies. According to Bernhardt and Stemberger (1998), the distinctive features for feature geometry are based on those of Chomsky and Halle (1968), except for the features for place of articulation, which follow Sagey (1986).

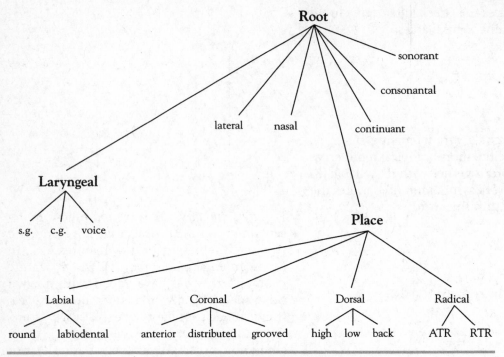

Figure 4.3   Feature Geometry of the English Consonant System

Source: From *Handbook of Phonological Development from the Perspective of Constraint-Based Nonlinear Phonology* (p. 92), by B. H. Bernhardt and J. P. Stemberger, 1998, San Diego, CA: Academic Press. Copyright 1998, reprinted with permission from Elsevier Science.

higher levels of representation. For example, in Figure 4.3, the Place node serves as a link between the Labial, Coronal, Dorsal, and Radical nodes and the Root node. Features at a higher level of representation are said to dominate other features. The Place node, for example, dominates the different places of articulation (Labial, Coronal, and Dorsal nodes). The Place node must be activated, so to speak, before a specific place of articulation can be chosen. Or, the Laryngeal node as a higher level of representation must be functioning before [+ voice] can be designated. Features that are dominated are considered to be subordinate or at a lower level of representation.

The following is a brief explanation of the different nodes and features, summarized from Bernhardt and Stemberger (1998).

Laryngeal features

1. [+ voiced] sounds produced with vocal fold vibration (e.g., [d], [i]).
2. [+ spread glottis] the vocal cords are spread wide, leading to low-amplitude voice at the glottis (e.g., voiceless aspirated stops [t^him] are + s.g. [h], as well as [f], [θ], [s], and [ʃ]).
3. [+ constricted glottis] the vocal cords are pulled together tightly, so that regular periodic vibration is impossible (e.g., all + c.g. segments are – voiced, glottal stops are + c.g.).

Manner features

1. [+ sonorant] sounds in which the pressure above the larynx allows the vocal cords to vibrate continuously, without any rise

in pressure above the larynx (e.g., voiced vowels, glides, liquids [r] and [l], [h], and nasals are + sonorant).

2. [+ consonantal] sounds with a narrow constriction in the oral and/or pharyngeal cavities that significantly impede the flow of air (e.g., stops, affricates, nasals, fricatives, laterals, taps, and trills are + consonantal).

3. [+ continuant] sounds in which air continues to move through the oral cavity (e.g., vowels, glides, liquids, and fricatives).

4. [+ nasal] sounds with the velum lowered so that air moves through the nasal cavity (e.g., nasals).

5. [+ lateral] sounds in which central airflow is blocked in the oral cavity, but in which air is directed over at least one side of the tongue (e.g., laterals).

6. [+ tense] sounds produced with relatively greater "muscular tension" (e.g., tense vowels, voiceless obstruents).

Place features

Lips

1. [Labial] sounds made with more involvement of one or both lips (e.g., bilabials [p, b, m], labiodentals [f, v], and [r], [w] are + labial).

2. [+ round] sounds involving protrusion of the lips with narrowing at the corners of the mouth (e.g., all rounded vowels and labialized consonant [kʷ], [r], and [w] are + round. Bilabials and labiodentals are – round).

3. [+ labiodental] labial sounds that are made with only one lip (e.g., [f] and [v]).

The tip of the tongue

1. [Coronal] sounds made with raising of the tip or blade of the tongue (e.g., [t, d, s, z, ʃ, ʒ, θ, ð, n, r, l, and j] plus high-front vowels are included).

2. [+ anterior] coronal sounds made at the alveolar ridge or further forward (e.g., [t, d,

θ, ð, n, l] are + anterior, – anterior includes [ʃ, ʒ, tʃ, dʒ, r, and j], and front vowels).

3. [+ distributed] coronal sounds made with a wide area of contact between the tip/blade of the tongue and the roof of the mouth or teeth (e.g., [tʃ, dʒ, f, v, ʃ, ʒ, r, and j] are + distributed, – distributed sounds include [t, d, s, z, n, and l]).

4. [+ grooved] coronal sounds made with a grooved tongue, a narrow channel at or near the midline (e.g., alveolar fricatives [s, z, ʃ, ʒ] and affricates).

The tongue body

1. [Dorsal] sounds made with the back of the tongue (e.g., [k, g, ŋ], back vowels, [w], and [j] also dark [l]).

2. [+ back] sounds with the back of the tongue body raised or lowered (e.g., velar sounds [k, g, ŋ, w], including the dark [l], back and central vowels).

3. [+ high] sounds where the tongue body is raised (e.g., high vowels, [k, g, ŋ, w, and j].

4. [+ low] sounds where the tongue body is lowered (e.g., low vowels).

The tongue root

1. [Radical] sounds in which the root of the tongue is advanced or retracted (e.g., pharyngeal and pharyngealized consonants, not typical for American English speech sounds).

2. [Advanced Tongue Root (ATR)] sounds in which the tongue root is advanced (e.g., high vowels, [i], [e], [u], and [o] are + ATR, consonants are blank for this feature).

As can be seen from the preceding explanation, the use of features and the definition of certain features are different from those proposed by Chomsky and Halle (1968).

Another nonlinear theory, the *theory of radical underspecification* (Archangeli, 1988; Archangeli and Pulleyblank, 1994; Bernhardt, 1992b; Kiparsky, 1982; Pulleyblank, 1986), suggests that underlying representations contain only "unpredictable" features. A predictable feature is one that would be commonly associated with that particular segment or class of sounds. For example, nasals are typically voiced (although there are unvoiced nasals in some African languages). Voicing for nasals is, then, predictable and would not be contained in the underlying representation. Or, because all sonorants are voiced, this is again a predictable feature and is not contained in the underlying representation. On the other hand, obstruents can be [+ voice] or [– voice]; therefore, the unpredictable nature of this feature is contained in the underlying representation.

Rules in nonlinear analysis are restricted to two basic operations: *spreading* (known as *linking*) and *deletion* (known as *delinking*) of phonological information from one tier to another. Spreading of features could be exemplified by the production of [gʌk] for *duck*. The coronal place node for /d/ is subject to linking or assimilation from the dorsal place node feature of /k/. Thus, the dorsal place node of the final [k] in *duck* affects the initial [d]. The end result is that the initial [d] is produced as [g]. The place of articulation is moved from coronal [d] to dorsal [g]. Delinking could be exemplified by the production of [dʌ] for *duck*. Under the assumption that the underlying representation is intact, the final consonant slot for that production is delinked from the representation along with the actual features of /k/. Linking and delinking result from, and are constrained by, principles of association between tiers. These principles are outlined in Bernhardt and Stemberger (1998) and could be used as a reference for more detailed analysis procedures.

To summarize, one nonlinear phonology, feature geometry, theorizes that segments are composed of multitiered hierarchically organized features. Specific nodes that can dominate other features and link various levels of representation are designated. According to this theory, features can link (assimilate) or delink, causing neutralization or deletion. Principles of association are used to explain occurrences between tiers.

Optimality Theory. **Optimality theory**, first formalized by Prince and Smolensky (1993) and McCarthy and Prince (1995), is considered a constraint-based approach. Constraints are a limit to what constitutes a possible pronunciation of a word (Stemberger and Bernhardt, 1997). When constraints are applied linguistically, a set of grammatical universals is said to exist that includes the fact that all languages have syllables and that certain syllable patterns seem to be more (or less) common. For example, in General American English, there are words that begin with three consonants, such as *street*, but not any that begin with four consonants in a row. Therefore, we could say that American English has a constraint on how many consonants can occur at the beginning of a word; three consonants are acceptable, but four are not. Languages will demonstrate certain constraints if compared to one another. For example, Hawaiian allows no more than one consonant in a row, resulting in words such as *kanaka* for "man." When comparing this to English, which allows several consonants in a row, in such words as *street* and *sixths,* we could say that Hawaiian has a constraint against more than one consonant as an onset or as a syllable coda. Constraints characterize patterns that are and are not possible within or across languages. Applying this principle generally to children with articulatory-phonological disorders, it could be stated that a child who does not produce syllable codas, thus evidences final-consonant deletion, has a constraint against producing final codas.

Constraints are based on principles of markedness. Thus, each constraint violation indicates markedness in that respect. Constraints are a means of (1) characterizing universal patterns that occur across languages, (2) demonstrating variations of patterns that occur between languages, and (3) determining markedness indicated by constraint violations (Archangeli and Langendoen, 1997).

Markedness is discussed on pages 69–70 and 74 of this chapter.

Optimality theory, as a constraint-based approach, was originally developed to explain the differences that occur between languages. Optimality theory presupposes a Universal Grammar and states that constraints characterize universals; however, constraints can be violated. Some constraints are very important (within and across languages) and are rarely violated, whereas others are not as important and can be violated. In this sense, constraints are *violable*. If we examine constraints in this manner, we will find that the following universal trends are considered typical (unmarked) properties of syllables. To the right of the constraint is the name given to it according to Archangeli and Langendoen (1997):

Syllables begin with a consonant.	ONSET
Syllables have one vowel.	PEAK
Syllables end with a vowel.	NOCODA
Syllables have at most one consonant at an edge.	*COMPLEX

In examining this list, we can see whether there are constraint violations in American English.

1. *Syllables begin with a consonant: ONSET.* Not all syllables begin with a consonant, as demonstrated by words such as *away* and *eat*. Probably in General American English most syllables do, however, begin with a consonant. This is a violable constraint (although it is maintained most of the time) in American English.

2. *Syllables have one vowel: PEAK.* In American English this seems to be the case all the time. Some syllables consist of syllabic consonants such as [bi.tl̩] or [fɪʃ.n̩]; however, no syllables contain two vowels. In American English this is a constraint that is *rarely*, if at all, violated.

3. *Syllables end with a vowel: NOCODA.* Not all syllables in American English end with a vowel. Many syllables end with a consonant in words such as *hat, clock,* and *antique.* This constraint is violated in American English.

4. *Syllables have at most one consonant at an edge: *COMPLEX.* This is also violated in American English. Words such as *clocks* and *streets* demonstrate a violation of this constraint.

In summarizing, we could state that some of the previously mentioned constraints are violated while others are not. This could lead to a rank ordering of constraints from those constraints that are never or rarely violated → to those that are sometimes violated → to those that are often violated. Those constraints that are *rarely* violated are considered higher-order constraints and are separated from others by a double arrow >>. Those violable constraints are separated from each other by a comma. Based on the previous discussion, the following rank ordering could be made:

PEAK>>ONSET, NOCODA, *COMPLEX

Thus, in American English the constraint PEAK (syllables have one vowel) is not violated. Therefore, it is separated from the others ONSET, NOCODA, *COMPLEX by >>. The others, which can be violated, are separated by commas. Therefore, one important concept within optimality theory is the rank ordering of the constraints.

Optimality theory, like other linguistic theories, proposes an input (an underlying representation), an output (the surface representation), and a relation between the two. The only specification of the input is that it is linguistically well formed; it does not contain variables that are not grammatical. The output is the actual production. Optimality theory does not account for differences between the input and output in terms of rules (as in generative grammar) or processes (as in natural phonology), but in terms of constraints. In optimality theory the relation between the input and output is mediated by two formal mechanisms: the generator (GEN) and the evaluator (EVAL). The generator links the input with potential outputs. It can add, delete, or rearrange, for example. The evaluator judges the outputs to determine which one is the *optimal* output. For any given input, such as [pɪg], which is the mental representation of the word *pig,* the GEN can generate an infinite number of possible phonetic outputs for that form. All these output forms compete with one another, but one output must be chosen as the optimal one. The EVAL evaluates all these different outputs and chooses the output that is the optimal response for that particular language. These output forms are evaluated through the constraints and their ranking within that language. The constraints and their relative rankings, thus, restrict the possible output forms (Ball, 2002; Barlow, 2001).

There are two types of constraints functioning within this mechanism: faithfulness and markedness. Faithfulness constraints require that input and output forms be identical to one another. If segments between the input and output are deleted, inserted, or rearranged, the faithfulness constraint is violated. If a child produces the word *skip* as [sɪp], then the faithfulness constraint has been violated. Markedness constraints require outputs to be unmarked or simplified in structure. *Unmarked features* are those that are easier to perceive or produce or those that occur frequently across languages. Consonant clusters are considered to be marked (see *COMPLEX mentioned previously). Thus, the child who produces *skip* as [skɪp] violates the markedness constraint. However, a child who says the word *skip* as [sɪp] has not violated this constraint; the output is unmarked or simplified.

As can be seen, faithfulness and markedness constraints are conflicting; there is an antagonistic relationship between the two. The conflict between faithfulness and markedness leads to violation of constraints, or what is termed *constraint violability.* Every utterance violates some constraint; if faithfulness is maintained, then markedness is violated. (The most unmarked syllable would be something like [bɑ], so any more complex syllable structure would be in some violation of markedness.)

So how does the EVAL judge which one is the most optimal form? At this point the theory postulates that the rank ordering of the constraints becomes the deciding factor. Lower-ranked constraints can be violated to satisfy higher-ranking constraints. In our previous example, ONSET, NOCODA, or *COMPLEX could be violated to satisfy PEAK.

If this theory is applied to phonological development, the hypothesis is that children acquire the correct ranking of the constraints as they develop. Immature patterns demonstrate that this ranking, according to the language in question, has not yet been mastered. Individual patterns of normal development are seen as products of the individual's idiosyncratic constraint rankings. Applying this to children with phonological disorders, these children also have their own unique constraint rankings. Our job is to find out the rankings that would then account for their error patterns. The next step is to try to rerank the constraints so that they are more in line with the input. It is assumed that markedness constraints (thus, the typical simplification that occurs in relationship to the production features) must be demoted. Demotion is a process where higher-ranking constraints that do not match the adult rankings become lower—that is, they become more easily violated. If they are more easily violated, then the rankings will eventually match the adult ones.

The names of constraints and how they are abbreviated from text to text varies. Table 4.8 is a list of possible constraints that is summarized from Barlow (2001).

Optimality theory uses tableaus to demonstrate the rank order of constraints. Tableaus are boxes with the word listed on the far left followed by the rank-ordered constraints.

Higher-ranking constraints are to the left. The following tableau demonstrates the ranking of constraints if a child were to say [pɪ] for *pig*.

/pɪg/ pig	*CODA	MAX
a. [pɪg]	*!	
b. ☞ [pɪ]		*

☞ = optimal output, optimal candidate, or the one with the fewest, lowest violations; * = constraint violation; *! = fatal violation (a violation that eliminates a candidate completely).

Here, the optimal output refers to the child's output, not the adult form. As can be seen from this tableau, the markedness constraint CODA (no final consonants, no coda) is ranked higher than the faithfulness constraint

Table 4.8 Markedness and Faithfulness Constraints, with Examples of Violations and Nonviolations

Constraint	Definition	Violation	Nonviolation
Markedness			
*COMPLEX	No clusters	*sweep* → [swip]	*sweep* → [sip]
*CODA	No final consonants (no codas)	*cat* → [kæt]	*cat* → [kæ]
*FRICATIVES	No fricatives	*sun* → [sʌn]	*sun* → [tʌn]
*LIQUIDS	No liquids	*lake* → [lek]	*lake* → [wek]
		rain → [ren]	*rain* → [wen]
*LIQUID-[l]	No liquid [l]	*lake* → [lek]	*lake* → [wek]
*LIQUID-[r]	No liquid [r]	*rain* → [ren]	*rain* → [wen]
Faithfulness			
MAX	No deletion	*cat* → [kæ]	*cat* → [kæt]
		sweep → [sip]	*sweep* → [swip]
DEP	No insertion	*sweep* → [səwip]	*sweep* → [swip]
IDENT-FEATURE	Don't change features	*lake* → [wek]	*lake* → [lek]
		sun → [tʌn]	*sun* → [sʌn]
IDENT-[cons]	Don't change [consonantal]	*lake* → [wek]	*lake* → [lek]
IDENT-[cont]	Don't change [continuant]	*sun* → [tʌn]	*sun* → [sʌn]

Source: From "Case Study: Optimality Theory and the Assessment and Treatment of Phonological Disorders," by J. Barlow, 2001, *Language, Speech, and Hearing Services in Schools, 32,* p. 245. Copyright © 2001 by the American Speech-Language-Hearing Association. Reprinted by permission.

of MAX (no deletions) as the child has violated the faithfulness constraint MAX. On the other hand, if one examines the norm adult pattern, MAX would be ranked higher than CODA. In this rather simplified example, the CODA constraint must be demoted to obtain final consonants.

Optimality theory offers a new way of viewing both the acquisition of phonological patterns and the categorizing of disordered phonological systems. The concept of constraints and demoting constraints reminds one of phonological process suppression. However, the theoretical model and the information gained are far more detailed and give the clinician valuable information about what the child can do and not just what the child is incapable of doing.

How Did Nonlinear Phonology Develop?

John Firth, professor of general linguistics at the University of London, was a key figure in the development of modern linguistics in the United Kingdom. In a way, nonlinear phonology, too, can be traced back to Firth's (1948) so-called prosodic analysis. For the first time, Firth challenged the one-sided linguistic importance of the phonemic units in their consecutive linearity. He advocated the necessity for additional nonsegmental analyses, "prosodies," which represent larger linguistic entities, such as syllables, words, and phrases. He postulated that speech is a manifestation of consecutively ordered units *as well as* a manifestation of larger prosodic units that bind phonemes together into linguistically more comprehensive units. Different analytical systems may need to be set up in order to explain the range of contrasts involved. With this approach, known as *polysystemicism,* the concept of nonlinear phonology was born.

Contemporary nonlinear/multilinear phonologies are an outgrowth of generative pho-nology. Chomsky and Halle's (1968) major contribution, *The Sound Pattern of English,* was innovative in its description of two levels of representation, a surface phonetic representation and an underlying phonemic representation. Although the idea of distinctive features was taken from the Prague School of linguistics, Chomsky and Halle understood the distinctive feature concept in a different way and modified it accordingly. Nonlinear phonologies adopt the generative concepts of distinctive features and surface-level and underlying representation. However, these new phonologies understand the surface-level representation in a very different way.

Chomsky and Halle's generative phonology described speech components in a linear manner: It was segment based. The components of any utterance were arranged in a sequence, with one discrete segment following the next. A common set of distinctive features is attributed to all segments, and each feature is specified by the assignment of a binary value. This limited the generation of phonological rules in several respects. First, only whole segments could be deleted or added. The only other modifications that could occur in the segment were achieved by changing the + or – values of one or more distinctive features. (Thus, this system analyzes only additions, deletions, or substitutions; analysis of non-phonemic distortions is not possible.) Second, because all segments are equally complex and all distinctive features are equal within this system, there is no reason to expect that any one segment, or any one distinctive feature, might be affected by any given phonological rule. However, many observations and investigations have reported, for example, that certain sounds and sound classes appear to be especially vulnerable to assimilation, whereas others cause assimilation (Dinnsen, 1997). Third, early generative phonology adopted the division between the segmentals and the suprasegmentals that the structural linguists had used to describe and analyze speech events. However, such a division does not allow a vertical, hierarchical understanding of the interaction between segmental units and prosodic features. The nonlinear phonologies represent a challenge to the earlier segment-based approaches. "Nonlinear phonological theory is another step in the evolution of our understanding of phonological systems" (Bernhardt and Stoel-Gammon, 1994, p. 126).

Nonlinear Phonologies: Clinical Implications

Although contemporary nonlinear phonologies began with Goldsmith's (1976) dissertation on autosegmental phonology, many different nonlinear phonological theories have since been proposed. This section has attempted to briefly introduce four nonlinear approaches: autosegmental phonology, metrical phonology, feature geometry, and optimality theory. However, it should be kept in mind that many other nonlinear phonologies exist.

Several of these nonlinear approaches have been applied to the analysis of disordered phonological systems. In the 1980s, Leonard and Brown (1984) and Pollock and Schwartz (1988) demonstrated how disordered phonological systems could be analyzed utilizing autosegmental principles. Bernhardt and Stoel-Gammon (1994) applied principles of grounded phonology (Archangeli and Pulleyblank, 1994) to the analysis of phonologically disordered speech. Stemberger and Bernhardt (1997) used optimality theory (McCarthy and Prince, 1993; Prince and Smolensky, 1993) to develop an intervention plan in a case study of a child. Dinnsen (1997) examined how underspecification theory, more specifically radical underspecification theory (Archangeli, 1988; Kiparsky, 1982; Pulleyblank, 1986), can explain both the normal acquisition of phonological systems and disordered phonology.

More recently, many different articles have featured application of principles of optimality theory to the assessment process and to the selection of treatment targets. Based on a case study, Barlow (2001) and Dinnsen and O'Connor (2001) demonstrated how optimality theory could be utilized to analyze a child's speech and to arrive at treatment targets. Bernhardt and Holdgrafer (2001a, 2000b) have outlined in detail how an in-depth phonological analysis can be generated that incorporates several nonlinear principles.

Feature geometry has been widely applied to the analysis of phonological disorders in children (Bernhardt, 1990, 1992a, 1992b, 1994; Bernhardt and Gilbert, 1992; Bernhardt and Stemberger, 1998; Bernhardt and Stoel-Gammon, 1994; Chin and Dinnsen, 1991; Von Bremen, 1990).

CLINICAL APPLICATION

More Information—Feature Geometry versus Phonological Processes

Let's look at the difference between how feature geometry versus phonological processes would explain an example of a child who says [gʌ] for *duck* and [dʌ] for *dumb.* If phonological processes are assigned to these substitutions and deletions, the following results are noted:

| "duck" | [dʌk] | → | [gʌ] | backing [d] → [g]
 final consonant deletion [k] → Ø |
| "dumb" | [dʌm] | → | [dʌ] | final consonant deletion [m] → Ø |

Although these phonological processes are easily identifiable, they give no information about the child's underlying representation. Where to begin in therapy would be a relatively arbitrary choice that would be based on the number of times the processes were observed and the age at which they should be suppressed. Feature geometry demonstrates that the underlying representation for this child includes information about the dorsal place node, that is, about /k/ and /g/. This is evidenced by the dorsal production of [g] in [gʌ] for *duck*. Articulatory constraints, however, prevent realization of final consonants. If this was just a case of final consonant deletion, both *duck* and *dumb* should have been realized as [dʌ]. In the underlying representation, the child might be trying to differentiate between *duck* and *dumb*. This suggests that if the articulatory constraints could be eliminated, the child's g/d substitution (backing) might also be eliminated. The concept of feature geometry and underlying representation provides us with more insight into reasons for the child's output patterns.

Autosegmental and metrical phonologies have not received as much application as other nonlinear theories. Autosegmental phonology was conceived to account for cases in which a single segment is associated with two mutually exclusive features. Although it was originally applied to tone languages, it might also offer some applicability to disordered phonological systems. One important factor that is absent from many phonological theories is the child's production of nonphonemic distortions, for example, a dentalized s-production ([s̪] for /s/). According to generative phonology, this distortion must be classified either as /s/, therefore [+ strident], or as /θ/, [– strident]. It is possible, however, that this single segment [s̪] could share these two seemingly mutually exclusive features of [+ strident] and [– strident]. If so, autosegmental phonology may offer a means of analyzing these types of distortions. Feature spreading within autosegmental phonology is structured to analyze assimilation processes but also offers a means of specifying coarticulatory conditions that might be useful in therapy.

Although not used extensively in clinical application, metrical phonology, which extends hierarchical analysis procedures to stress and syllable boundaries, suggests several possibilities in its application to disordered phonological systems. Kehoe (2001) has documented how a metrical approach can form the basis for an analysis of multisyllabic word productions, and Velleman and Shriberg (1999) have used metrical phonology to analyze the speech of children with suspected developmental apraxia of speech. Stress, both within a word and within a sentence, often plays a decisive role in the production of segments. Metrical phonology offers analysis procedures that emphasize the interrelationships that might exist between stress and segment production. The comparison of syllable and morphological boundaries within metrical phonology provides the potential to link phonological segmental production to other language areas.

To summarize, many different nonlinear phonologies have been developed within the last decade or so. Some of them have been applied to case studies of children with disordered phonological systems. The results seem to indicate that these phonologies promise new insights into, and a deeper understanding of, the phonological system. Future research should document which of these theories can provide the clinician with new possibilities for the assessment and treatment of individuals with impaired phonological systems.

SUMMARY

This chapter first introduced some of the basic terminology and principles underlying contemporary phonological theories. The relationship between the sound form and the sound function (as phoneme) was established as a basis for the understanding of phonological theories. The development of the phoneme concept was traced historically to provide a foundation for the understanding of how phonological theories could evolve from this "new" concept. Clinical application of these basic principles stressed the interrelationship between sound–form and sound–function.

The remainder of this chapter was a summary of several different phonological theories that impact the assessment and treatment of phonological disorders. These theories were enumerated in a historical sequence. The linear phonologies were represented by distinctive feature theory, generative phonology, and natural phonology. The nonlinear phonologies included autosegmental, metrical, feature geometry, and optimality theory. Each phonological theory was discussed in respect to what the theoretical framework stands for, how it developed, how it functions, and its clinical implications.

The field of phonology is constantly evolving. Current phonological theories are an attempt to describe the phonological system with all its complexity in a different manner. Although some of the newer models have yet to stand the test of time and research, all offer new insights into the intricate nature of normal and impaired phonological systems.

CASE STUDY

The distinctive feature analysis procedure can be demonstrated using a slightly modified clinical example from Chapter 2, pages 33–34. The following sample is from Tina, age 3;8.

dig	[dɛg]	boat	[bot]
house	[haʊθ]	cup	[tʊp]
knife	[nɑf]	lamp	[wæmp]
duck	[dʊt]	goat	[dot]
cat	[tæt]	ring	[wɪŋ]
bath	[bæt]	thumb	[tʌm]
red	[wed]	that	[dæt]
ship	[sɪp]	zip	[ðɪp]
fan	[fɛn]	key	[ti]
yes	[jɛθ]	win	[wɪn]

The following errors are noted:

[s] → [θ]	house, yes
[k] → [t]	duck, cat, cup, key
[θ] → [t]	bath, thumb
[r] → [w]	red, ring
[ʃ] → [s]	ship
[l] → [w]	lamp
[g] → [d]	goat
[ð] → [d]	that
[z] → [ð]	zip

These target sounds and substitutions can be inventoried using the Distinctive Feature Worksheet. The following patterns emerge: The most frequent distinctive features include high (5 times), anterior (4 times), coronal (4 times), and back (4 times).

A phonological process analysis procedure can be demonstrated using the same child, Tina, age 3;8.

Target→Error		Phonological Process
[s]→[θ]	house, yes	fronting
[k]→[t]	duck, cat, cup, key	velar fronting
[θ]→[t]	bath, thumb	stopping + backing*
[r]→[w]	red, ring	gliding
[ʃ]→[s]	ship	palatal fronting
[l]→[w]	lamp	gliding
[g]→[d]	goat	velar fronting
[ð]→[d]	that	stopping + backing*
[z]→[ð]	zip	fronting

Summarizing the phonological processes, we see that fronting (including both velar and palatal fronting) affected five sounds (s → θ, k → t, ʃ → s, g → d, and z → ð). Both stopping + backing (θ → t and ð → d) and gliding (l, r → w) were noted on two different sounds.

---

*Although *backing* was not covered, it is considered to be an idiosyncratic process that can be found in the speech of children with phonological disorders. **Backing** refers to a substitution in which the organ and/or place of articulation is more posteriorly located than the intended sound.

THINK CRITICALLY

The following are the results of an articulation test from Ryan, age 6;6:

horse	[hoᵘɚθ]	pig	[pɪk]	chair	[ʃɛɚ]
wagon	[wægən]	cup	[kʌp]	watch	[waʃ]
monkey	[mʌŋki]	swinging	[s̪wɪŋɪŋ]	thumb	[fʌm]
comb	[koᵘm]	table	[teˈbəl]	mouth	[maᵘf]
fork	[foɚk]	cat	[kæt]	shoe	[su]
knife	[naˈf]	ladder	[læɾɚ]	fish	[fɪs]
cow	[kaᵘ]	ball	[bɑl]	zipper	[ðɪpɚ]
cake	[keˈk]	plane	[pweˈn]	nose	[noᵘθ]
baby	[beˈbi]	cold	[koᵘd]	sun	[θʌn]
bathtub	[bæftəb]	jumping	[dʌmpən]	house	[haᵘθ]
nine	[naˈn]	TV	[tivi]	steps	[stɛp]
train	[tweˈn]	stove	[θtoᵘv]	nest	[nɛt]
gun	[gʌn]	ring	[wɪŋ]	books	[bʊkθ]
dog	[dɑg]	tree	[twi]	bird	[bɝd]
yellow	[wɛloᵘ]	green	[gwin]	whistle	[wɪθəl]
doll	[dɑl]	this	[dɪθ]	carrots	[kɛɚət]

1. Summarize the substitutions according to distinctive features. Which distinctive features occur most frequently?

2. Summarize the errors according to phonological processes. Which phonological processes occur most frequently?

TEST YOURSELF

1. Which one of the following does not belong to the phoneme/phonology concept?
   a. meaning-establishing and meaning-differentiating function of sound units
   b. underlying form or representation
   c. production realities
   d. sound unit function within a particular language system
2. Which one of the following is a major class feature that distinguishes sounds produced with a high degree of oral obstruction?
   a. sonorant   c. vocalic
   b. consonantal   d. coronal
3. Which one of the following statements concerning phonological processes is *not* true?
   a. they are innate
   b. they are universal
   c. children with different language backgrounds begin with different sets of phonological processes
   d. they are used to simplify productions for the child in the developmental period
4. If a child says [waʃ] for *watch,* this is an example of which phonological process?
   a. stopping   c. deaffrication
   b. affrication   d. labialization
5. Which one of the following is true about nonlinear/multilinear phonologies?
   a. segments are governed by more complex linguistic dimensions such as stress
   b. emphasis is on the sequential arrangement of sound segments
   c. all sound segments have equal value
   d. no one sound segment has control over the other units
6. Which one of the following terms is not representative of autosegmental phonology?
   a. tiers are separable and independent levels
   b. certain segments are autonomous and do not have a one-for-one match on another level
   c. strong and weak stress are emphasized
   d. feature spreading is also a portion of this concept
7. According to metrical phonology, the word *potato* has which one of the following stress patterns?
   a. weak branching to "po," strong branching to "tato"; further divided into strong branching on "ta," weak branching on "to"
   b. strong branching on "po," weak branching to "tato"; further divided into strong branching on "ta," weak branching on "to"
   c. weak branching to "po," strong branching to "tato"; further divided into weak branching on "ta," strong branching on "to"
8. Which one of the following terms is not associated with feature geometry?
   a. spreading
   b. distinctive features
   c. faithfulness
   d. delinking
9. In optimality theory, the constraint "markedness" requires outputs to be
   a. the same as the input
   b. simplified in structure
   c. marked
   d. demoted
10. If a child produces [ta] for *stop*, then which one of the following constraints is violated?
    a. *COMPLEX   c. *FRICATIVES
    b. *CODA   d. MAX

WEBSITES

www.phonologicaldisorders.com

This website, created by the author of this textbook, contains basic definitions and examples of phonological processes. It also gives examples of articulation test results that are analyzed according to phonological processes. Links are given to other websites and resources.

www.speech-language-therapy.com/Table2.htm

This website from Caroline Bowen summarizes some more common phonological processes and gives examples of each process. For a beginning review, this website could be helpful.

www.essex.ac.uk/speech/teaching-01/documents/df-theory.html

This website from Mark Tatham (1999 copyright) gives a brief discussion of distinctive feature theory. It provides references and a discussion on redundancy. It also has "clips" scattered throughout the website, which give you a more in-depth discussion of the various terms.

www.chass.utoronto.ca/~contrast/#Summary

This website reports on a research project on markedness that was conducted by Elan Dresher and Keren Rice (funded by the Social Science and Humanities Research Council of Canada). It outlines the goals of the project and provides an overview of markedness and how the topic could be extended to other areas such as second language acquisition.

http://egg.auf.net/99/docs/abstracts/polgardi.html

This relatively compact website, created by Krisztina Polgardi, discusses government phonology and optimality theory. There is a link to the Plovdiv website, which gives more broad-based information about phonology.

http://camba.ucsd.edu/phonoloblog/index.php/2006/12/04/review-phonological-development-and-disorders-in-children/

This website provides a book review of *Phonological Development and Disorders in Children* (Hua and Dodd, 2006, published by Multilingual Matters). It is a good read and gives a lot of interesting information on the multilingual perspective, which is the focus of the book.

FURTHER READINGS

Archangeli, D., & Langendoen, T. (1998). *Optimality theory: An overview.* Malden, MA: Blackwell.

Ball, M., & Kent, R. (1997). *The new phonologies: Developments in clinical linguistics.* San Diego: Singular.

Bernhardt, B., & Stemberger, J. (1998). *Handbook of phonological development: From the perspective of constrain-based nonlinear phonology.* San Diego: Academic Press.

Bernhardt, B., & Stemberger, J. (2000). *Workbook in nonlinear phonology for clinical application.* Austin, TX: ProEd.

Lombardi, L. (2001). *Segmental phonology in optimality theory: Constraints and representations.* New York: Cambridge University Press.

APPENDIX 4.1

1. Transcription of H. H. According to Pre-, Inter-, and Postvocalic Positions

Target Word	Child's Production	Position	Description
1. house	[haʊ]	postvocalic	[s] deletion
2. telephone	[tɛfoʊ]	[unstressed syllable deletion—noted but not counted on matrices]	
		postvocalic	[n] deletion
3. cup	[tʌp]	prevocalic	[k] → [t]
4. gun	[dʌn]	prevocalic	[g] → [d]

Target Word	Child's Production	Position	Description
5. knife	[nɑɪ]	postvocalic	[f] deletion
6. window	[wɪnoʊ]	intervocalic	[nd] → [n]
7. wagon	[wædən]	intervocalic	[g] → [d]
wheel	[wi]	postvocalic	[l] deletion
8. chicken	[tɪtə]	prevocalic	[tʃ] → [t]
		intervocalic	[k] → [t]
		postvocalic	[n] deletion
9. zipper	[tɪpə]	prevocalic	[z] → [t]
		vowel nucleus	[ɚ] → [ə]
10. scissors	[tɪtə]	prevocalic	[s] → [t]
		intervocalic	[z] → [t]
		nucleus + postvocalic	[ɚz] → [ə]
11. duck	[dʌt]	postvocalic	[k] → [t]
yellow	[jɛwoʊ]	intervocalic	[l] → [w]
12. vacuum	[ætu]	prevocalic	[v] deletion
		intervocalic	[kj] → [t]
		postvocalic	[m] deletion
13. matches	[mætət]	intervocalic	[tʃ] → [t]
		postvocalic	[z] → [t]
14. lamp	[wæmp]	prevocalic	[l] → [w]
15. shovel	[dʌvə]	prevocalic	[ʃ] → [d]
		postvocalic	[l] deletion
16. car	[tɑə]	prevocalic	[k] → [t]
		vowel nucleus	[ɚ] → [ə]*
17. rabbit	[wæbɪ]	prevocalic	[r] → [w]
		postvocalic	[t] deletion
18. fishing	[bɪdɪn]	prevocalic	[f] → [b]
		intervocalic	[ʃ] → [d]
		postvocalic	[ŋ] → [n], this is considered a variation in regular pronunciation and not an error, not counted

---

* [ɑɚ] is considered to be a centering diphthong; therefore, it is the nucleus of the syllable.

Target Word	Child's Production	Position	Description		
19. church	[tɜ]	prevocalic	[tʃ]	→	[t]
		vowel nucleus	[ɝ]	→	[ɜ]
		postvocalic	[tʃ] deletion		
20. feather	[bɛdə]	prevocalic	[f]	→	[b]
		intervocalic	[ð]	→	[d]
		vowel nucleus	[ɚ]	→	[ə]
21. pencils	[pɛntə]	intervocalic	[ns]	→	[nt]
			[lz] deletion		
this	child would not say	postvocalic			
22. carrot	[tɛwə]	prevocalic	[k]	→	[t]
		intervocalic	[r]	→	[w]
		postvocalic	[t] deletion		
orange	[oᵘwɪn]	intervocalic	[r]	→	[w]
		postvocalic	[ndʒ]	→	[n]
23. bathtub	[bætʌ]	intervocalic	[θt]	→	[t]
		postvocalic	[b] deletion		
bath	[bæ]	postvocalic	[θ] deletion		
24. thumb	[bʌm]	prevocalic	[θ]	→	[b]
finger	[bɪnə]	prevocalic	[f]	→	[b]
		intervocalic	[ŋg]	→	[n]
		vowel nucleus	[ɚ]	→	[ə]
ring	[wɪŋ]	prevocalic	[r]	→	[w]
25. jump	[dʌmp]	prevocalic	[dʒ]	→	[d]
26. pajamas	[dæmi]	[unstressed syllable deletion—noted but not counted in matrices]			
		prevocalic	[dʒ]	→	[d]
		[i] in end noted as a diminutive, final consonant deletion not counted in matrices			
27. plane	[beⁱn]	prevocalic	[pl]	→	[b]
blue	[bu]	prevocalic	[bl]	→	[b]
28. brush	[bʌs]	prevocalic	[br]	→	[b]
		postvocalic	[ʃ]	→	[s]
29. drum	[dʌm]	prevocalic	[dr]	→	[d]
30. flag	[bæ]	prevocalic	[fl]	→	[b]
		postvocalic	[g] deletion		

Target Word	Child's Production	Position	Description
31. Santa Claus	[tænə dɑ]	prevocalic	[s] → [t]
		intervocalic	[nt] → [n], considered a normal assimilation, counted as correct
		intervocalic	[kl] → [d]
		postvocalic	[z] deletion
32. Christmas tree	[tɪtmə ti]	prevocalic	[kr] → [t]
		intervocalic	[sm] → [tm]
		intervocalic	[str] → [t]
33. squirrel	[twɜə]	prevocalic	[skw] → [tw]
		vowel nucleus	[ɝ] → [ɜ]
		postvocalic	[l] deletion
34. sleeping	[twipɪn]	prevocalic	[sl] → [tw]
		postvocalic	[ŋ] → [n] this is considered a variation in regular pronunciation and not an error, not counted
bed	[bɛd]		
35. stove	[doʊ]	prevocalic	[st] → [d]
		postvocalic	[v] deletion

2. Phonological Processes for H. H.

Target Word	Child's Production	Position	Description
1. house	[haʊ]	postvocalic	final consonant deletion
2. telephone	[tɛfoʊ]		weak syllable deletion
		postvocalic	final consonant deletion
3. cup	[tʌp]	prevocalic	velar fronting
4. gun	[dʌn]	prevocalic	velar fronting
5. knife	[naɪ]	postvocalic	final consonant deletion
6. window	[wɪnoʊ]	intervocalic	cluster reduction
7. wagon	[wædən]	intervocalic	velar fronting
wheel	[wi]	postvocalic	final consonant deletion
8. chicken	[tɪtə]	prevocalic	stopping
		intervocalic	velar fronting
		postvocalic	final consonant deletion

Target Word	Child's Production	Position	Description
9. zipper	[tɪpə]	prevocalic vowel nucleus	stopping + devoicing derhotacization
10. scissors	[tɪtə]	prevocalic intervocalic nucleus postvocalic	stopping stopping + devoicing derhotacization final consonant deletion
11. duck yellow	[dʌt] [jɛwoʊ]	postvocalic intervocalic	velar fronting gliding
12. vacuum	[ætu]	prevocalic intervocalic postvocalic	initial consonant deletion cluster reduction + cluster substitution (velar fronting) final consonant deletion
13. matches	[mætət]	intervocalic postvocalic	stopping stopping + devoicing
14. lamp	[wæmp]	prevocalic	gliding
15. shovel	[dʌvə]	prevocalic postvocalic	stopping + fronting + voicing final consonant deletion
16. car	[tɑə]	prevocalic nucleus	velar fronting derhotacization
17. rabbit	[wæbɪ]	prevocalic postvocalic	gliding final consonant deletion
18. fishing	[bɪdɪn]	prevocalic intervocalic postvocalic	stopping + labialization + voicing stopping + fronting + voicing not counted, normal variation
19. church	[tɜ]	prevocalic nucleus postvocalic	stopping derhotacization final consonant deletion
20. feather	[bɛdə]	prevocalic intervocalic nucleus	stopping + labialization + voicing alveolarization + stopping derhotacization
21. pencils	[pɛntə]	intervocalic postvocalic	cluster substitution (stopping) cluster deletion
22. carrot	[tɛwə]	prevocalic intervocalic postvocalic	velar fronting gliding final consonant deletion
orange	[oʊwɪn]	intervocalic postvocalic	gliding cluster reduction

Target Word	Child's Production	Position	Description
23. bathtub	[bætʌ]	intervocalic	cluster reduction
		postvocalic	final consonant deletion
bath	[bæ]	postvocalic	final consonant deletion
24. thumb	[bʌm]	prevocalic	stopping + labialization + voicing
finger	[bɪnə]	prevocalic	stopping + labialization + voicing
		intervocalic	cluster reduction + velar fronting
		nucleus	derhotacization
ring	[wɪŋ]	prevocalic	gliding
25. jump	[dʌmp]	prevocalic	stopping
26. pajamas	[dæmi]		weak syllable deletion
		prevocalic	stopping
		postvocalic	diminutive—use of [i]
27. plane	[beɪn]	prevocalic	cluster reduction + voicing
blue	[bu]	prevocalic	cluster reduction
28. brush	[bʌs]	prevocalic	cluster reduction
		postvocalic	palatal fronting
29. drum	[dʌm]	prevocalic	cluster reduction
30. flag	[bæ]	prevocalic	cluster reduction, cluster substitution (stopping + labialization + voicing)
		postvocalic	final consonant deletion
31. Santa Claus	[tænə dɑ]	prevocalic	stopping
		intervocalic	[nt] → [n] considered normal assimilation, not counted
		intervocalic	cluster reduction, cluster substitution (velar fronting + voicing)
		postvocalic	final consonant deletion
32. Christmas tree	[tɪtmə ti]	prevocalic	cluster reduction, cluster substitution (velar fronting)
		intervocalic	[sm] → [t] cluster reduction, cluster substitution (stopping)
		intervocalic	[str] → [t] cluster reduction
33. squirrel	[twɜə]	prevocalic	cluster reduction, cluster substitution (velar fronting)
		nucleus	derhotacization
		postvocalic	final consonant deletion

Target Word	Child's Production	Position	Description
34. sleeping	[twipɪn]	prevocalic	cluster substitution (stopping, gliding)
		postvocalic	not counted, normal variation
bed	[bɛd]		
35. stove	[doʊ]	prevocalic	cluster reduction, cluster substitution (voicing)
		postvocalic	final consonant deletion

3. Spontaneous Speech Sample for H. H.

Looking at pictures:

[dæ ə pɪtə əv ə tɑ]
That a picture of a dog.

[hi ə bɪ dɑ]
He a big dog.

[hi baʊ ən hæ ə tawə]
He brown and has a collar.

[oʊ dæ ɪt ə tɪti]
Oh, that is a kitty.

[wi hæf ə tɪti]
We have a kitty.

[wi dɑt aʊ tɪti ə waːŋ taˈm]
We got our kitty a long time.

Conversation with Mom:

[tæn wi do tu mədanoʊ]
Can we go to McDonald?

[aˈ wʌ ə tibɜdə]
I want a cheeseburger.

[aˈ wʌ fɛnfaˈθ]
I want french fries.

[wɛ ɪt bɪwi]
Where is Billy?

[hi tʌm tu mədanə wɪt ʌt]
He come to McDonald with us?

[xxxxx maˈ haʊ]
xxxx My house.

[mɑmi lɛ do]
Mommy let go.

[lɛ do naʊ]
Let go now.

Talking about summer vacation:

[wi doʊf tu dæmɑt]
We drove to Grandma.

[si wɪf ɪn oʊ +haˈo]
She live in Ohio.

[si hæt ə fɑm]
She has a farm.

[si hæt watə taʊt]
She has lot'a cows.

[taʊt ju noʊ mu taʊ]
Cows, you know, moo cow.

[deˈ it ə ho wɑt]
They eat a whole lot.

Normal Phonological Development

5

LEARNING OBJECTIVES

When you have finished this chapter, you should be able to:

- Describe the primary function of the infant's respiratory, phonatory, resonatory, and articulatory systems at birth, and explain the general changes that occur before babbling begins.
- Identify the types of auditory perceptual skills that infants demonstrate prior to their first words.
- List characteristics of each of the prelinguistic stages.
- Explain the role of individual variability during the early period of speech sound development.
- Define and provide examples of the various syllable structure, substitution, and assimilation processes noted in this chapter.
- Describe the relationship between phonological development, metaphonology, and learning to read.

*T*his chapter outlines the prelinguistic behavior and phonological development of children from birth to their school years. **Prelinguistic behavior** refers to all vocalizations prior to the first actual words. **Phonological development** refers to the acquisition of speech sound form and function within the language system. In accordance with current terminology, this is now referred to as phonological development rather than as speech sound development, as it was in the past. To some, this may signal only a difference in wording; however, the concept has actually undergone a fundamental change. **Speech sound development** refers primarily to the gradual articulatory mastery of speech sound forms within a given language. Thus, the proficiency of a child to produce standard patterns speech sounds is measured. *Phonological development,* on the other hand, implies the acquisition of a functional sound system intricately connected to the child's overall growth in language. Learning to produce a variety of sounds is not the same as learning the contrasts between sounds that convey differences in meaning.

The first goal of this chapter is to explore briefly certain aspects of the structural and functional development that must occur prior to speech sound production in the infant. In addition, the development of specific perceptual skills will be discussed.

The second goal is to examine some of the available information on articulatory and phonological development. Organized according to segmental form as well as prosodic development, this survey ranges from the prelinguistic stages to the near completion of the phonological system during the early school years. In reviewing the literature, an attempt will be made to discuss the various studies so that the reader will become aware of differences in design and purpose, which have often resulted in contrasting outcomes. In addition, it should be noted that much of the literature focuses on the child's acquisition of speech sounds. Little information is available on the child's gradual development of the phonemic function and phonotactic constraints of these segments within a language. When possible, these studies will also be included.

The third goal of this chapter is to highlight interdependencies between language acquisition, phonological development, and emerging literacy. Developing phonology cannot be meaningfully separated from other aspects of emerging language; it represents an integral part of the child's total language acquisition process. Although cognitive and motor abilities certainly play important roles in the unfolding of phonology, the child's acquisition of semantic, morphosyntactic, and pragmatic skills influences it as well.

Various studies have provided guidelines for determining if a child demonstrates normal versus impaired phonological development. These "mastery" studies are typically based on the results of testing a large number of children, setting a percentage for each age group for normal articulation of the speech sound in question, and, finally, establishing age levels that are considered to be the time frame for acquisition of each sound. As important as these studies are, the role of individual variation, especially in a child's younger years, should not be underestimated. The development of speech sounds and the acquisition of a child's phonological system remains an individual process. Although certain trends can be noted when comparing these studies containing large numbers of children, individual variation continues to play a large role in the total acquisition process. Both factors—general trends noted in large scale studies and the child's individual growth and development—are important factors to consider when evaluating whether a child has an articulatory/phonological disorder.

Aspects of Structural and Functional Development

As the infant begins its journey from primarily crying behavior to babbling and words, important anatomical structures that are prerequisites for sound production need to be taken into consideration. Both the structure and the function of respiratory, phonatory, resonatory, and articulatory mechanisms must advance decisively before any regular articulatory processes can occur. These necessary changes, which continue through infancy and early childhood, are directly reflected in the transformation from prelinguistic to linguistic sound productions. The following summary from Bosma (1975), Kent (1997), and Kent and Murray (1982) presents a broad outline of the development of the respiratory, phonatory, resonatory, and articulatory systems during this time span.

The shape, size, and composition of the respiratory system are dramatically modified from infancy to adulthood. Newborns and infants are, of course, perfectly able to accumulate enough air pressure against a closed glottis to "phonate" quite impressively. Although small, compared to those of adults, babies' lungs are proportionally large for their body structure. Their subglottal pressure is considerable and continues to be so throughout childhood. For example, when comparable loudness levels are contrasted, children demonstrate higher subglottal pressure values than do adults (Stathopoulos and Sapienza, 1993). In addition, compared to the adult, only approximately one-third to one-half of the alveoli are present in the lungs of the newborn (Hislop, Wigglesworth, and Desai, 1986). It is not until the child is approximately 7 to 8 years old that the number of alveoli approaches the adult value (Hislop, Wigglesworth, and Desai, 1986; Kent, 1997). It is also around this age that children's respiratory function demonstrates adult patterns. Developmental milestones in the respiratory system are summarized in Table 5.1.

The changes in the phonatory and resonatory systems from infancy to childhood are especially impressive. This anatomical–physiological development leads directly to their future secondary physiological function for articulatory purposes. However, in newborns, the larynx and vocal tract reflect exclusively primary functions; that is, they are at this time unable to fulfill any articulatory tasks. For example, the oral cavity (with tongue and lips) and the pharyngeal cavity are utilized primarily for sucking and swallowing

Table 5.1   Milestones in the Development of the Respiratory System of the Child

Age	Typical Patterns
Birth	Rest breathing is approximately 30 to 80 breaths per minute. Frequent paradoxical breathing occurs exemplified by the rib cage making an expiratory movement as the abdomen performs an inspiratory movement. Only between one-third to one-half of the number of alveoli are present at birth.
1.5 to 3 years	Rest breathing rate decreases to approximately 20 to 30 breaths per minute at age 3. Respiratory control increasingly supports the production of longer utterances during this time frame. The number of alveoli increases rapidly, beginning to approximate adultlike values at the end of this period. Small conducting airways surrounding the alveoli increase their dimensions in a similar fashion.
7 to 8 years	Rest breathing is approximately 20 breaths per minute. Adultlike breathing patterns are now beginning to be achieved. Number of alveoli reaches adult values at age 8.

Sources: Hislop, Wigglesworth, and Desai (1986); Kent (1997); Thurlbeck (1982); and Zeltner, Caduff, Gehr, Pfenninger, and Burri (1987).

actions. The tongue, which in young infants fills out the oral cavity completely, leaves practically no space for the buccal area, the space between the outside of the gums and the inside of the cheeks. In addition, a prenatally acquired "sucking pad," an encapsulated structure of the cheek supporting the lateral rims of the tongue for more effective sucking action, helps to fill out this space entirely. The production of sounds is under these conditions severely restricted. The ability to produce speech sounds is a highly complex process that depends primarily on many anatomical–physiological changes that occur as a product of growth and maturation. Figure 5.1 shows the tongue displacement and the size of several anatomical structures of the newborn infant.

The larynx, too, has to develop structurally before it can effectively contribute to the speech process. In newborns, for example, the artytenoid cartilages and the large posterior portion of the cricoid cartilage are disproportionately large when compared to an adult larynx (see Figure 5.2). The vocal processes where the vocal folds attach are also large in relation-

ship to the other structures. This means that they reach deeply into the vocal folds, thus stifling their vibratory action. In addition, the infant's larynx sits closely under the angle between neck and chin. This high, semifixated position of the larynx does not allow the vocal tract to be effectively elongated in a downward direction. This elongation is indispensable for some resonating effects during vowel articulation, for example.

Stabilization of the pharyngeal airway (necessary for an upright position) is another significant postnatal development. Anatomical changes include the downward displacement of the hyoid bone and larynx, away from the base of the skull and the mandi-

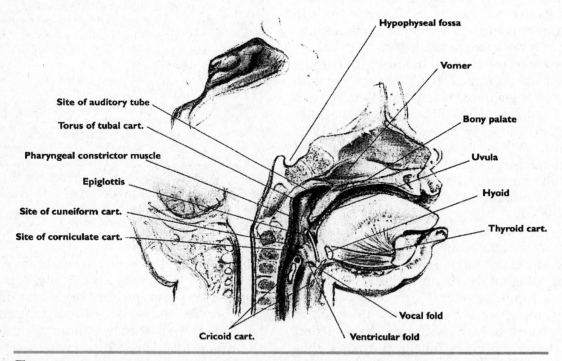

Figure 5.1 Paramedian Section of the Pharyngeal, Oral, and Nasal Area of the Newborn Infant
The tongue is displaced slightly downward, away from the palate, and forward.

Source: From "Anatomic Physiologic Development of the Speech Apparatus," by J. F. Bosma, in *The Nervous System, Vol. III: Human Communication and Its Disorders* (p. 470), edited by D. B. Tower, 1975, New York: Lippincott-Raven Publishers. Copyright 1975 by Lippincott-Raven Publishers. Reprinted with permission.

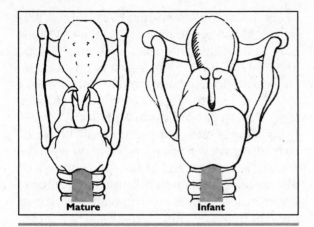

Figure 5.2 Posterior View of Skeletons of Larynx of Mature Man and of Infant
The infant's larynx is, of course, much smaller than the adult's. The sketches are intended to indicate proportional differences of some laryngeal structures only.

Source: From "Anatomic Physiologic Development of the Speech Apparatus," by J. F. Bosma, in *The Nervous System, Vol. III: Human Communication and Its Disorders* (p. 477), edited by D. B. Tower, 1975, New York: Lippincott-Raven Publishers. Copyright 1975 by Lippincott-Raven Publishers. Reprinted with permission.

ble, and the loss of the aforementioned sucking pad. All of these changes must occur as prerequisites for the articulation of speech sounds.

After the child's first words, around the child's first birthday, the speech mechanism undergoes further enlargement and changes in form. Expansions of the laryngeal and pharyngeal cavities are prominent

> To verify the decisive importance of movements of the larynx for normal vowel production, place your index finger lightly on the V-shaped notch of the thyroid cartilage of the larynx with the middle finger and thumb on either side of the lamina. In this position, articulate [i] versus [u]. The downward movement during [u] can easily be felt.

examples. These expansions co-occur with changes in the form and mobility of the arytenoid cartilages, soft palate, and tongue. The following changes characterize this development:

1. The thyroid cartilage enlarges more than the cricoid cartilage.
2. The epiglottis becomes larger and more firm.
3. The arytenoid cartilages, which were relatively large in the early stages of this development, now change little in size; they adapt structurally and functionally to the other laryngeal structures.
4. The vocal and ventricular folds—that is, the "true" and "false" vocal folds—lengthen. This has the effect that more of the vocal folds' muscular portion is now freed for normal vocal cord vibration.

Skeletal enlargement of the skull and laryngeal areas during childhood occurs mostly in posterior and vertical directions. This allows the velum more room and thus more mobility. However, the oral area is the site of the greatest changes in available space and resulting mobility of the anatomical structures. Due to these skeletal changes, the tongue no longer completely fills the mouth. In addition, the tongue and lips become elongated and acquire further mobility. The fine-tuning and coordination of the lip, mandible, tongue, and velar movements for regular voice and speech production are now increasingly acquired.

To summarize, during infancy, we see enormously complex developmental changes. The infant's larynx, mouth, and pharyngeal areas evolve from a mechanism able to serve only respiratory and feeding purposes to a vocal tract that is structurally and functionally ready for the production of speech sounds.

In the study by Birnholtz and Benacerraf (1983), auditory stimulation was provided by an electrolarynx placed several inches from the mothers' abdomens. Using ultrasound, the researchers observed that fetuses aged between 24 and 28 weeks after conception demonstrated notable eye blink behavior approximately half a second after the beginning of the electrolarynx buzz. In this study, 680 fetuses were tested. Only 8 of the 680 did not evidence this eye blink behavior. After birth, it was found that 2 of the 8 infants were deaf and that the remaining 6 had a variety of central nervous system disorders.

ASPECTS OF PERCEPTUAL DEVELOPMENT

Although it has often been documented that infants are able to discriminate minimal differences in speech sounds within the first months after their births (Best and McRoberts, 2003; Best, McRoberts, and Goodell, 2001; Eilers, 1980; Houston and Jusczyk, 2000; Kuhl, Stevens, Hayashi, Deguchi, Kiritani, and Iverson, 2006), their auditory experiences actually begin even before birth. Using ultrasound technology, researchers have been able to detect fetal eye blink responses to a loud noise between 24 and 28 weeks after conception (Birnholtz and Benacerraf, 1983). Using loudspeakers close to the mothers' abdomens, Lecanuet, Granier-Deferre, and Bushnel (1989) presented the syllables [babi] or [biba] to nineteen women in their last trimester of pregnancy. Changes in fetal heart rate demonstrated that almost all of the fetuses reacted when the syllable stimulation varied—for example, when stimulation changed from [babi] to [biba]. Also, within the first days after birth, infants demonstrate a preference for their own mothers' voices and will actively change their sucking rate to hear her voice more often than another female's voice (DeCasper and Fifer, 1980). And at 4 days

of age, babies of French-speaking mothers prefer the sound of French over Russian (Bertoncini, Morais, Bijeljac-Babic, McAdams, Peretz, and Mehler, 1989; Mehler, Jusczyk, Lambertz, Halsted, Bertoncini, and Amiel-Tison, 1988).

These results support the notion that infants start to pay attention and "learn" something about voice and speech probably prior to birth. However, what evidence do we have about the infant's and child's perception and discrimination of speech sounds and phonemic contrasts? The following is an overview of these perceptual skills.

- *Categorical perception.* **Categorical perception** refers to the tendency of listeners to perceive speech sounds varied along a continuum according to the phonemic categories of their native language. Thus, variations in voice onset time will produce a clear listener distinction between [ba] or [pa], as if an actual boundary divided the two. Based on changes in measured sucking rates, categorical perception for /b/ and /p/ in the syllables [ba] and [pa] has been demonstrated in infants as young as one month of age (Eimas, Siqueland, Jusczyk, and Vigorito, 1971). Infants under 3 months of age can detect differences in place and manner of articulation for consonants (Jusczyk, 1992). Other studies related to the perception of phonemic contrasts in infants include Cohen and Cashon (2003), Houston and Jusczyk (2000), Jusczyk and Luce (2002), Kuhl (1980), Mareschal and French (2000), Maye and Weiss (2003), and Maye, Werker, and Gerken (2002), for example.

Peter W. Jusczyk (1948–2001) was involved in the first studies of infant speech perception and over the next thirty years became one of the most influential contributors to research in infant perception and language acquisition. A review of his many contributions can be found in Gerken (2005).

- *Discrimination of non-native sounds in infants.* If children demonstrate categorical perception at such an early age, it was hypothesized that they might have an inborn ability to make these distinctions. In order to test this hypothesis, a task was devised in which the discrimination skills of young infants were tested with unknown phonemes of nonnative languages—that is, languages to which they had not been exposed. Although adult nonnative speakers could not discriminate these pairs, results demonstrated that up to approximately 6 to 8 months of age, infants could indeed discriminate between two nonnative sounds that were very similar in their production characteristics (Best and McRoberts, 2003; Trehub, 1976; Werker and Tees, 1983). By 10 to 12 months, this discrimination ability had disappeared and the infants' performance was as poor as that of English-speaking adults (Werker and Tees, 1983). The conclusion drawn was that language experience may result in the loss of this discrimination ability. We do not discriminate between categories that are nonfunctional in our own native language.

- *Perceptual constancy.* The ability to identify the same sound across different speakers, pitches, and other changing environmental conditions is known as **perceptual constancy.** Perceptual constancy for vowels and consonants within different vowel contexts has been noted in children from 5½ to 10 months of age (Kuhl, 1980; Maye and Gerken, 2000; Werker and Fennell, 2004).

- *Perception of phonemic contrasts.* Shvachkin (1973) and Garnica (1973) examined the ability of toddlers from 10 to 22 months to associate minimally paired nonsense syllables to different objects. Could the child learn to differentiate between phonemes that signal word meaning differences? These studies found that in all children there was a developmental progression in the ability to make these distinctions; that is, some distinctions appear easier

to detect than others. However, considerable variability was noted between the children as to which features were discriminated earlier and which later.

- *Early perceptual abilities related to language development and disorders.* Recent studies (Kuhl, Conboy, Padden, Nelson, and Pruitt, 2005; Tsao, Liu, and Kuhl, 2004; Werker and Tees, 2005) document that early perceptual abilities appear to be related to later language development in children. Tsao, Liu, and Kuhl (2004) measured speech discrimination in 6-month-old infants using a conditioned head-turn task. At 13, 16, and 24 months of age, language development was assessed in these same children using the MacArthur Communicative Development Inventory. Results demonstrated significant correlations between speech perception at 6 months of age and later language (word understanding, word production, and phrase understanding). The finding that speech perception performance at age 6 months predicts language at age 2 years supports the idea that phonetic perception may play an important role in language acquisition. Early perceptual studies may also show evidence of later difficulties, such as dyslexia (Bogliotti, 2003; Richardson, Leppaenen, Leiwo, and Lyytinen, 2003). For example, Lyytinen and colleagues (2001) investigated 107 children with a familial risk of dyslexia, comparing them to 93 children without familial risk. The earliest significant differences between groups were found using brain potential responses to speech sounds at only a few days old and head turning at 6 months old, which were conditioned to reflect categorical perception of speech sounds. No differences were found between the groups in other measures, such as parental reports of vocalization, motor behavior, or growth of vocabulary (using the MacArthur Communicative Development) before age 2. Similarly, no group differences were found in cognitive and language development assessed by the Bayley Scales of Infant Development and the Reynell Developmental Language Scales before age 2.5.

An infant's early perceptual abilities include a wide range of competencies. Many of these abilities develop prior to the actual production of first words. It appears that the infant's early perceptual abilities may also impact later language development, while lack of specific skills may be a portion of the symptom complex of disordered language learning.

The next section examines another aspect of the infant's behavior: the prelinguistic stage. This stage describes those vocalizations prior to the first real words. We will also see that specific competencies in this behavior will also impact later language development.

PRELINGUISTIC STAGES: BEFORE THE FIRST WORDS

Child language development is commonly divided into *prelinguistic behavior,* vocalizations prior to the first true words, and *linguistic development,* which starts with the appearance of these first words. This division is exemplified by the use of early nonmeaningful versus later meaningful sound productions. Jakobson's *discontinuity hypothesis* (1942/1968) clearly emphasized a sharp separation between these two phases. According to his theoretical notion, babbling is a random series of vocalizations in which many different sounds are produced with no apparent order or consistency. Such behavior is seen as clearly separated from the following systematic sound productions evidenced by the first words. The division between prelinguistic and linguistic phases of sound production, according to

Jakobson, is often so complete that the child might actually undergo a period of silence between the end of the babbling period and the first real words.

Research since that time (e.g., de Boysson-Bardies, 2001; Nathani, Ertmer, and Stark, 2006; Oller, 1980; Oller, Wieman, Doyle, and Ross, 1976; Stark, 1980, 1986) has repeatedly documented (1) that babbling behavior is not random but rather that the child's productions develop in a systematic manner, (2) that the consonantlike sounds that are babbled are restricted to a small set of segments, and (3) that the transition between babbling and first words is not abrupt but continuous; late babbling behavior and the first words are very similar in respect to the sounds used and the way they are combined. It also appears that the child's perceptual abilities are quite developed before the first meaningful utterances. For example, some word comprehension is evident at approximately 7 to 9 months of age (Owens, 2008). The presence of phonemic contrasts in very young children has also been previously documented. Although this acquisition is gradual, more general contrasts begin at approximately 1 year of age. Findings like these suggest that the child's language system starts to develop prior to the first spoken meaningful words, during the prelinguistic period.

The following is an overview of the *prelinguistic stages* of production described by Stark (1986). Although these are referred to as stages, there is overlap from one period of development to the next. In addition, individual variation between children necessitates that the ages given are approximates.

Stage 1: Reflexive crying and vegetative sounds (birth to 2 months). This stage is characterized by a large proportion of reflexive vocalizations. *Reflexive vocalizations* include cries, coughs, grunts, and burps that

NORMAL PHONOLOGICAL DEVELOPMENT

seem to be automatic responses reflecting the physical state of the infant. *Vegetative sounds* may be divided into grunts and sighs associated with activity and clicks and other noises, for example, which are associated with feeding.

Stage 2: Cooing and laughter (2 to 4 months). During this stage, *cooing* or *gooing* sounds are produced during comfortable states. Although these sounds are sometimes referred to as vowel-like, they also contain brief periods of consonantal elements that are produced at the back of the mouth. Early comfort sounds have quasi-resonant nuclei; they are produced as a syllabic nasal consonant or as a nasalized vowel (Nakazima, 1962; Oller, 1980). From 12 weeks onward, a decrease in the frequency of crying is noted, and most infants' primitive vegetative sounds start to disappear. At 16 weeks, sustained laughter emerges (Gesell and Thompson, 1934).

Stage 3: Vocal play (4 to 6 months). Although there is some overlap between Stages 2 and 3, the distinguishing characteristics of Stage 3 include longer series of segments and the production of prolonged vowel- or consonantlike steady states. It is during this stage that the infant often produces extreme variations in loudness and pitch. Transitions between the segments are much slower and incomplete when compared to older children. In contrast to vowels in Stage 2, those in Stage 3 demonstrate more variation in tongue height and position.

Stage 4: Canonical babbling (6 months and older). Although **canonical babbling**—the collective term for the reduplicated and nonreduplicated babbling stages—usually begins around 6 months of age, most children continue to babble into the

time when they say their first words. Stark (1986) describes reduplicated and nonreduplicated, or variegated, babbling as follows: **Reduplicated babbling** is marked by similar strings of consonant–vowel productions. There might be slight quality variations in the vowel sounds of these strings of babbles, but the consonants will stay the same from syllable to syllable. An example of this is [əmama]. **Nonreduplicated** or **variegated babbling** demonstrates variation of both consonants and vowels from syllable to syllable. An example of this is [batə]. A major characteristic of this babbling stage is smooth transitions between vowel and consonant productions.

From the previous description, one might conclude that these babbling stages are sequential in nature, a child first going through reduplicated babbling and then later nonreduplicated babbling. This has indeed been documented by Elbers (1982), Oller (1980), and Stark (1986), to mention a few. However, more recent investigators have questioned this developmental pattern. For example, Mitchell and Kent (1990) assessed the phonetic variation of multisyllabic babbling in eight infants at 7, 9, and 11 months of age. Their findings showed that (1) nonreduplicated babbling was present from the time the infant began to produce multisyllabic babbling, not evolving out of an earlier period of reduplicated babbling; and (2) no significant difference existed between the amount of phonetic variation for the vocalizations when the infants were 7, 9, and 11 months old. These and other findings (Holmgren, Lindblom, Aurelius, Jalling, and Zetterstrom, 1986; Smith, Brown-Sweeney, and Stoel-Gammon, 1989) suggest that both reduplicated and variegated forms extend throughout the entire babbling period.

At the beginning of this stage, babbling is used in a self-stimulatory manner; it is not used to communicate to adults. Toward the end of this stage, babbling may be used in ritual imitation games with adults (Stark, 1986).

Stage 5: Jargon stage (10 months and older). This babbling stage overlaps with the first meaningful words. The **jargon stage** is characterized by strings of babbled utterances that are modulated primarily by intonation, rhythm, and pausing (Crystal, 1986). It sounds as if the child is actually attempting sentences but without actual words. Because many jargon vocalizations are delivered with eye contact, gestures, and intonation patterns that resemble statements or questions, parents are convinced that the child is indeed trying to communicate something to which they often feel compelled to respond (Stoel-Gammon and Menn, 1997).

The following section examines the child's segmental productions toward the end of the canonical babbling stage. Because the productions cannot yet be said to be true vowels and consonants of a particular language system, they will be referred to as **vocoids** and **contoids**, respectively. These terms were introduced by Pike (1943) to indicate nonphonemic speech sound productions.

Vocoids

Several early investigations with a large number of children were those carried out by Irwin and colleagues in the 1940s and 1950s (e.g., Chen and Irwin, 1946; Irwin, 1945, 1946, 1947a, 1947b, 1948, 1951; Irwin and Chen, 1946; Winitz and Irwin, 1958). According to the data on fifty-seven children from 13 to 14 months of age, there was a continued predominance of the [ɛ], [ɪ], and [ʌ] vocoids. Thus, front and central vocoids were found to be favored over high and back vocoids. Later investigations (Davis and MacNeilage, 1990; Kent and Bauer, 1985) generated similar results.

Contoids

Several authors have investigated the contoids, which predominate in the late babbling stage. Locke (1983) provides an excellent overview of the results from three major investigations (see Table 5.2). The agreement between these studies is far more striking than the differences. As can be seen from Table 5.2, the most frequent contoids were [h], [d], [b], [m], [t], [g], and [w]. The twelve most frequently produced contoids represent about 95 percent of all the segments transcribed in the three studies (Locke, 1983). These results stand in contrast to earlier statements that babbling consists of a great multitude of random vocalizations. On the contrary, these and other investigations (Locke, 1990; Vihman, Macken, Miller, Simmons, and Miller, 1985) suggest that only a rather limited set of phones is babbled.

Looking at Table 5.2, it appears that there were not any non-English sound segments utilized by the infants studied. However, this is partially conditioned by the investigative methods employed and by the perceptual limitations inherent in phonetic transcription. As to the investigative methodology, in the Irwin studies, only three non-English sounds were transcribed; the rest were ignored. The Fisichelli study considered exclusively English sounds. The Pierce and Hanna investigation, on the other hand, did document that the infants produced several non-English sounds with some frequency. Other investigations (e.g., Stockman, Woods, and Tishman, 1981) have confirmed the occurrence of non-English

Table 5.2   Relative Frequency of English Consonantlike Sounds in the Babbling of 11- to 12-Month-Old American Infants[1]

More Frequent Consonants				Less Frequent Consonants			
Sound	*A*[2]	*B*	*C*	*Sound*	*A*[2]	*B*	*C*
h	31.77	21.0	18.3	v	1.03	1.0	0
d	20.58	30.0	13.5	l	.96	1.0	1.6
b	9.79	5.0	10.0	θ	.85	0	0.4
m	6.69	1.0	7.2	z	.56	0	0
t	4.34	0	3.6	f	.37	0	0.4
g	4.15	12.0	8.4	ʃ	.37	0	0
s	3.45	0	0.4	ð	.34	0	0.8
w	3.39	17.0	8.4	ŋ	.33	1.0	3.2
n	2.65	1.0	4.4	ʒ	.10	0	0
k	2.12	1.0	6.3	r	.10	0	0
j	1.77	9.0	11.6	tʃ	0	0	0
p	1.63	0	1.6	dʒ	0	0	0
Totals	92.33	97.0	93.7		5.01	3.0	6.4

1. The three investigations represented are *A:* Irwin (1947a); *B:* Fisichelli (1950); *C:* Pierce and Hanna (1974).

2. The *A* columns total less than 100% because the difference (2.66%) represents several sounds in Irwin's original tabulations that have no phonemic equivalent in American English phonology (e.g., [ʔ ç χ]).

Source: From *Phonological Acquisition and Change* (p. 4), by J. L. Locke, 1983, Orlando, FL: Academic Press. Copyright 1983 by Academic Press. Reprinted with permission.

sounds in this late babbling period, although not to any high degree.

The phrase *perceptual limitations inherent in phonetic transcription* refers to the difficulty encountered when trying to transcribe non-native speech sounds. Someone not trained in listening for and transcribing non-English sounds certainly will encounter grave problems recognizing and categorizing them. Locke (1983) summarizes this difficulty appropriately by stating that "there might have been more [non-English sounds] if the listeners were themselves non-English [speakers], or more effectively oriented to non-English sounds and modes of symbolization" (p. 5).

Syllable Shapes

During the later babbling periods, open syllables are still the most frequent type of syllables. In Kent and Bauer (1985), for example, V, CV, VCV, and CVCV structures accounted for approximately 94 percent of all syllables produced. Although closed syllables were present, they were found to be very limited in the repertoires of these infants.

Babbling and Its Relationship to Later Language Development

Jakobson's discontinuity hypothesis denounced any link between babbling and later language development. However, babbling behavior is one aspect of early communication that is emerging as a predictor of later language ability. Several researchers have suggested that both the quantity and the diversity of vocalizations do indeed play a role in later language development.

Attempts have been made to correlate the quantity of vocalizations at a certain babbling age to later language performance (e.g., Brady, Marquis, Fleming, and McLean, 2004; Camp, Burgess, Morgan, and Zerbe, 1987; Kagan, 1971; McCune and Vihman, 2001; Paavola, Kunnari, and Moilanen, 2005; Roe, 1975, 1977; Rothgaenger, 2003). Here, quantity was defined as the number of vocalizations during a specific time period. Although somewhat different criteria were used in the various studies, the results showed that the amount of prelinguistic vocalizations was positively related to later language measures.

Diversity of vocalizations was measured by (1) the number of different consonant-like sounds heard in the babbling of infants, (2) the number of structured CV syllables, (3) the proportion of vocalizations containing a true consonant, and (4) the ratio of consonantlike sounds to vowel-like sounds (Bauer, 1988; Bauer and Robb, 1989; de Boysson-Bardies, 2001; McCarthren, Warren, and Yoder, 1996; Munson, Edwards, and Beckman, 2005; Nathani, Ertmer, and Stark, 2006; Oller, Eilers, Neal, and Schwartz, 1999: Paul, 1991; Paul and Jennings, 1992; Reed, 2005; Rescorla and Ratner, 1996; Stoel-Gammon and Otomo, 1986; Whitehurst, Smith, Fischel, Arnold, and Lonigan, 1991). Summarizing the results of these methodologically varying studies, it appears that (1) less language growth is seen in children with more vocoid-babble compared to those with more contoid-babble, (2) greater language growth is related to greater babble complexity, and (3) greater language growth is related to the increased diversity of contoid productions.

Knowledge of Babbling Stages and Diagnostics

Speech-language pathologists, especially those in early intervention services, are often confronted with children who are still within the babbling stages of development. Knowledge of the babbling stages, which includes characteristics and approximate ages of occurrence, can be very helpful in our assessment process. Consider the following information from the parents of Megan, who is 16 months old.

The early intervention program was contacted by Megan's parents, who had been referred by the child's pediatrician. Megan was born four weeks premature and had been followed very closely by both the parents and the pediatrician. She had started to walk around 11 months of age and the parents reported that all developmental milestones up to that point had been within normal limits. The parents were concerned because Megan did not have any real words. Children of acquaintances had begun to talk when they were 10 to 12 months old.

The speech-language pathologist visited the family home and noted that Megan was a very active toddler who was busy with her toys and enjoyed attention. Occasionally, Megan produced utterances that consisted of single vowels, for example, [a]; CV structures ([ba], [da], [ma]); and CVCV syllables ([mama], [babi], [dada], [dati]). According to the parents, repeated attempts at getting Megan to imitate these babbles had not met with success. It was observed (and the parents verified) that Megan did not use strings of babbles with any intonational patterns, that is, Megan did not produce jargon speech.

Based on these results, we could deduce that Megan is within the canonical babbling stage. However, she has not reached the point at which she is imitating these babbles in ritualized games with her parents, nor is she using jargon speech. According to the approximate ages presented, jargon speech begins around 10 months of age. Megan is now 16 months old. This information gives us a general idea of where Megan stands at the moment within the period of prelinguistic development.

Prosodic Feature Development

Vowels and consonants are combined to produce syllables, words, and sentences. At the same time that we articulate these sound segments, pronunciation varies in other respects. For example, as adults a wide range of pitch and loudness variables are utilized that can change the meaning of what is said in a number of ways. Consider the sentence: "You want that.↘" said with a falling tone at the end compared to "You want that?↗" said with a rising tone at the end. (One can even imagine that if *that* is stressed and the vowel prolonged with an excessive rising tone in the second sentence, something incredible is being desired.) The sound segments in these two sentences [ju wʌnt ðæt] relate to *what* we say; *prosodic features* refer to *how* we say it. **Prosodic features** are larger linguistic units, elements occurring across segments, that are used to influence what we say. The linguistically most relevant prosodic features we realize in speech are pitch, loudness, and tempo variations (which include sound duration). They have specific functions and may be analyzed separately. If combined, they constitute the *rhythm* of a particular language or utterance.

The development of prosodic features in infants has gained considerable importance in research in the last years. Current research begins to document their development and supports the hypothesis positing a close interaction between prosodic features, early child-directed speech (motherese), and early language development (Bonvillian, Raeburn, and Horan, 1979; Delack and Fowlow, 1978;

Fernald et al., 1989; Hallé, de Boysson-Bardies, and Vihman, 1991; Hsu and Fogel, 2001; Jacobson, Boersma, Fields, and Olson, 1983; Kent and Murray, 1982; Robb and Saxman, 1990; Stern and Wasserman 1979; Turk, Jusczyk, and Gerken, 1995; Whalen, Levitt, and Wang, 1991). Clearly, far more information is available in the area of sound segment development. However, a better understanding of prosodic features and their development may offer us valuable insights into the transition from babbling to the first words and the close interconnection of segmental and prosodic feature acquisition.

Coinciding with the canonical babbling stage, or starting at approximately 6 months of age, the infant utilizes patterns of prosodic behavior. Certain features are now employed consistently, primarily intonation, rhythm, and pausing (Crystal, 1986). Acoustic analysis shows that falling pitch is the most common intonation contour for the first year of life (Delack and Fowlow, 1978; Kent and Murray, 1982; Snow, 1998a, 1998b, 2000). Prosodic patterns continue to diversify toward the end of the babbling period to such a degree that names such as *expressive jargon* (Gesell and Thompson, 1934) and *prelinguistic jargon* (Dore, Franklin, Miller, and Ramer, 1976) have been applied to them. These strings of babbles typically end in a manner that is characteristic of adult General American English intonation patterns, giving the impression of sentences without words.

TRANSITION FROM BABBLING TO FIRST WORDS

Several studies suggest that babbling and early words have much in common (e.g., de Boysson-Bardies and Vihman, 1991; Davis and MacNeilage, 1990; Ferguson and Farwell,

1975; Kent and Bauer, 1985; Oller, Wieman, Doyle, and Ross, 1976; Stark, 1980; Vihman, Ferguson, and Elbert, 1986). In fact, they are often so similar that difficulties arise in differentiating between the two. The main characteristics of the transition from babbling to first words include:

1. primarily monosyllabic utterances
2. frequent use of stop consonants, followed by nasals and fricatives
3. bilabial and apical productions
4. rare use of consonant clusters
5. frequent use of central, mid-front, and low-front vowels ([ʌ, ɛ, æ])

In spite of the similarities, data from Vihman and colleagues (1986) and Davis and MacNeilage (1990) revealed the following distinctions between babbling and first words:

1. A large diversity existed between the children's productions in each of the areas investigated (phonetic tendencies, consonant and vowel inventories, and word selection). The more words the children acquired, the more this diversity seemed to diminish (Vihman, Ferguson, and Elbert, 1986).
2. Frequent use of [l] in one child's speech (Davis and MacNeilage, 1990), although other studies noted that this consonant was not used to any significant degree.
3. The majority of the children utilized voiced stops in babbling but not in words; [g] was the most prominent example of this (Vihman, Ferguson, and Elbert, 1986).
4. Vowels produced during babbling were used as substitutes for other vowel productions in words. The high-front vowel [i] was a frequent substitute (Davis and MacNeilage, 1990).
5. Productions were context dependent. For example, high-front vowels occurred more

frequently following alveolars; high-back vowels following velars; and central vowels after labial consonants (Vihman, 1992). However, little evidence of these context dependencies was found in the Tyler and Langsdale (1996) study. The wide range of individual variability could in part explain the differences they encountered.

𝒯HE FIRST FIFTY WORDS

Around a child's first birthday, a new developmental era begins: the *linguistic phase*. It starts the moment the first meaningful word is produced. That sounds plain enough, but there are some problems defining the first meaningful word. Must it be understood and produced by the child in all applicable situations and contexts? Must it have an adultlike meaning to the child? How do you categorize utterances that do not resemble our adult representation but are, nevertheless, used as words by the child in a consistent manner?

Most define the **first word** as an entity of relatively stable phonetic form that is produced consistently by the child in a particular context and is recognizably related to the adultlike word form of a particular language (Owens, 2008). Thus, if the child says [ba] consistently in the context of being shown a ball, this form would qualify as a word. If, however, the child says [dodo] when being shown the ball, then this would not be accepted as a word because it does not approximate the adult form.

Children frequently use "invented words" (Locke, 1983) in a consistent manner, thereby demonstrating that they seem to have meaning for the child. These vocalizations—used consistently but without a recognizable adult model—have been called **proto-words** (Menn, 1978), **phonetically consistent forms** (Dore et al., 1976), **vocables** (Ferguson, 1976), and **quasi-words** (Stoel-Gammon and Cooper, 1984).

The time of the initial productions of words is usually called the *first-fifty-word stage.* This stage encompasses the time from the first meaningful utterance at approximately 1 year of age to the time when the child begins to put two "words" together at approximately 18 to 24 months. Whether this stage is actually a separate developmental entity may be questioned. The first word may be a plausible starting point, but the strict fifty-word cut-off point is, according to several studies, purely arbitrary (Ferguson and Farwell, 1975; Nelson, 1973). Nevertheless, it appears that the child produces approximately fifty meaningful words before the next generally recognized stage of development, the *two-word stage,* begins.

During the first-fifty-word stage, there seems to be a large difference between the production and the perceptual capabilities of the child. For example, at the end of this stage, when children can produce approximately fifty words, they are typically capable of understanding around 200 words (Ingram, 1989a). This fact must have an effect on the development of semantic meaning as well as on the phonological system. It must be clearly understood that by analyzing the child's verbal productions during this stage, we are looking at only one aspect of language development. The child's perceptual, motor, and cognitive growth, as well as the influence of the environment, all play indispensable roles in this stage of language acquisition.

In examining the course of phonological development during this period, we see that it is heavily influenced by the individual words the child is acquiring. Children are not just learning sounds, which are then used to make up words, but, rather, they seem to learn word units that happen to contain particular sets of sounds. Ingram (1976) called this a *presystematic stage* in which contrastive words rather than contrastive phones (i.e., as phonemes)

are acquired. The presystematic stage can be related to Cruttenden's (1981) *item learning* and *system learning* stages of early phonological development. In **item learning**, the child first acquires word forms as unanalyzed units, as productional wholes. Only later, characteristically after the first-fifty-word stage, does **system learning** occur, during which the child acquires the phonemic principles that apply to the phonological system in question.

The early portion of the item learning stage is known as the *holophrastic period,* the span of time during which the child uses one word to indicate a complete idea. In addition, the link between the object, its meaning, and the discrete sound segments used to represent the object is not yet firmly established. For example, a child might produce [da] to indicate a dog. The next day, the production might change somewhat to, perhaps, [do]. This time, the production may not refer to a dog alone but also to a cow or horse. According to Piaget (1952), the child is still within the sensorimotor period of development and so has not yet achieved full imitative ability or object permanence. Sounds and meanings drift and change.

Segmental Form Development

Several authors (e.g., Ferguson and Farwell, 1975; Ingram, 1989b) have noted *phonetic variability* and a *limitation of syllable structures* and *sound segments* during the first-fifty-word stage. **Phonetic variability** refers to the unstable pronunciations of the child's first fifty words. Although this has been well documented (Farwell, 1976; Kiparsky and Menn, 1977; Stoel-Gammon and Cooper, 1984), it appears that some productions are more stable than others. Ferguson and Farwell (1975) call this category of words stable forms. However, the authors do not provide a measure for this stability, and, from their examples, it is often not clear why certain words are considered more stable than others. To complicate matters, it seems that some children have a tendency to produce more stable articulations from the beginning of this stage. Stoel-Gammon and Cooper (1984) and French (1989) provide data on children whose phonetic realizations were stable from the first real word.

The second characteristic of this stage is the limitation of syllable structures and segmental productions utilized. From their relatively small repertoire of words, it would seem logical to conclude that children do not produce a large array of syllable structures and sound segments. However, what are the actual limitations during the first-fifty-word stage?

First, certain syllable types clearly predominate. These are CV, VC, and CVC syllables. When CVCV syllables are present, they are full or partial syllable reduplications. This, of course, does not mean that other syllable types do not occur. Looking, for example, at the data from Ferguson and Farwell (1975), French (1989), Ingram (1974), Leopold (1947), Menn (1971), Stoel-Gammon and Cooper (1984), and Velten (1943), these syllables are indeed the most frequently occurring. However, the children produced other syllables as well. Menn's Daniel, for instance, produced CCVC [njaj], Leopold's Hildegard a CCVCV [prɪti], and Ferguson and Farwell's T a CVCVVC [wakuak]. If the individual children are examined to see if patterns emerge, differences can be found. Certain children seem to favor specific types of syllables. For example, some children evidence CVC structures to a moderate degree from the very beginning of this stage. With others, CVC syllables appear only later and do not constitute any major part of the child's phonology until after the first-fifty-word stage (Ingram, 1976).

Second, what are the speech sound limitations that can be observed during the first-fifty-word stage? More specifically, which

vowels and consonants are present, and which ones are not? Two studies that have had a large impact on this question are those presented by Jakobson (1942/1968) and Jakobson and Halle (1956). After studying several diary reports of children from various linguistic backgrounds, they concluded that the first consonants are labials, most commonly [p] or [m]; these first consonants are followed by [t] and later [k]; fricatives are present only after the respective homorganic stops have been acquired; and the first vowel is [a] or [ɑ], followed by [u] and/or [i].

Over the years, Jakobson's postulated universals have undergone a good deal of scrutiny. Although most of the investigators (e.g., Oller et al., 1976; Stoel-Gammon and Cooper, 1984; Vihman et al., 1986) have concentrated on consonant inventories, Ingram (1976) has attempted to grapple with the acquisition of vowels. Using the data from four case studies (Ingram, 1974; Leopold, 1947; Menn, 1971; Velten, 1943), he compared the vowels in the first fifty words. General trends could be noted, and most children seemed to follow the acquisitional pattern of [a] preceding [i] and [u].

Consonant inventories follow the same pattern. Although certain similarities have been verified, several investigations have pointed out the wide range of variability between individual subjects (e.g., Ferguson and Farwell, 1975; Stoel-Gammon and Cooper, 1984; Vihman, 1992; Vihman et al., 1986). If one wants to generalize, then the marked use of voiced labial and dental stops and nasals has to be underlined. Ferguson and Garnica (1975) make the point that [h] and [w] are also among the first consonants acquired. Findings substantiating these generalizations drawn from five different investigations are summarized in Table 5.3. Table 5.3 compares the consonant inventory of seven children labeled "Stanford" (Vihman et al., 1986) to nineteen other children from research studies noted in the table.

Comparing Jakobson's Results to the First Words of Two Children

The following are the first words of Joan Velten (Velten, 1943) and Jennika Ingram (Ingram, 1974).

	Joan			Jennika	
Age	Words	Actual Production	Age	Words	Actual Production
;10	up	[ap]	1;3	blanket	[ba], [babi]
	bottle	[ba]		byebye	[ba], [baba]
;11	bus	[bas]		daddy	[da], [dada], [dadi]
	put on	[baza]		dot	[dat], [dati]
	that	[za]		hi	[haⁱ]
1;0	down	[da]		mommy	[ma], [mami], [mama]
	out	[at]		no	[no]
	away	['ba ba]		see	[si]
	pocket	[bat]		see that	[siæt]
1;1	fuff	[af], [faf]		that	[da]
	put on	[ba'da]	1;4	hot	[hat]
1;2	push	[bus]		hi	[haⁱ], [haⁱdi]
	dog	[uf]		up	[ap], [api]
	pie	[ba]		no	[nodi], [dodi], [noni]
1;3	duck	[dat]			
	lamb	[bap]			
1;4	M	[am]			
	N	[an]			
	in	[n̩]			

If the month increments are seen as later phases of development, the following order occurs in the first words for Joan and Jennika:

	Joan	Jennika
Vowels	[a] → [u]	[a], [i], [o], [æ], [aⁱ]
Consonants	[p], [b] → [s], [z] → [t], [d] → [f] → [m], [n]	[b], [d], [t], [h], [m], [n], [s] → [p]
Syllable shapes	VC, CV → CVC, CVCV	CV, CVCV, CVC → VC, VCV
	CVCVs are not reduplications	Most CVCVs are reduplications
Phonetic variability	More stable forms	More variability

Both Joan's and Jennika's vowel development follows Jakobson's findings: [a] is followed by, or co-occurs with, [i] and/or [u]. Joan's order of consonant development, though, shows clear differences from the order described by Jakobson. For example, she does seem to use the fricatives [s] and [z] before the homorganic stops [t] and [d]. Both children demonstrate rather late development of specific bilabial sounds that, according to Jakobson, are the earliest consonants: for Joan [m] and for Jennika [p] are later than fricatives.

Table 5.3 Initial Consonant Productions within the First-Fifty-Word Vocabularies of Seven Stanford Subjects and Nineteen Other English-Speaking Children

	Stanford	Others		Stanford	Others[1]
p	×	+	ʃ	+	+
b	×	×	ʒ	0	0
t	×	+	tʃ	–	–
d	×	+	dʒ	–	–
k	×	+	m	×	×
g	+	+	n	×	+
f	+	–	ŋ	–	–
v	–	0	l	–	–
θ	+	–	r	+	–
ð	+	–	w	+	+
s	–	–	j	+	–
z	–	–	h	+	+

Note: × = all children in study; + = over half but not all children in study; – = more than one but less than half children in study; 0 = none of the children.

1. Data derived from Ferguson and Farwell (1975); Shibamoto and Olmsted (1978); Leonard, Newhoff, and Mesalam (1980); and Stoel-Gammon and Cooper (1984).

Source: From "Phonological Development from Babbling to Speech: Common Tendencies and Individual Differences," by M. M. Vihman, C. A. Ferguson, and M. Elbert, 1986, *Applied Psycholinguistics, 7,* p. 28. Copyright 1986 by Cambridge University Press. Reprinted with permission.

As can be seen, all the children have words containing [b] and [m]. More than half of the children in the studies produced [p], [t], [d], [k], [g], [ʃ], [n], [w], and [h] consonants as well.

Longitudinal Findings. Longitudinal research follows a child or a group of children over a specific time frame. It has the advantage of observing the acquisition process of individual children. However, longitudinal research is often limited in that only one child or a small group of subjects is evaluated. Stoel-Gammon (1985) presented a longitudinal investigation that not only utilized spontaneous speech but also looked at a sizable number of children.

Thirty-four children between 15 and 24 months of age participated in this study. The investigation was constructed to look at mean-ingful speech only; therefore, the subjects were grouped according to the age when they actually began to say at least ten identifiable words within a recording session. This resulted in three groups of children: Group A children, who had ten words at 15 months; Group B, who had ten words at 18 months; and Group C, who had ten words at 21 months. The

It should be noted that the Vihman, Ferguson, and Elbert (1986) data in Table 5.3 reduce the individual variation among children considerably. For example, if child A produces two words with word-initial [n] while child B produces forty-three words with [n], both of those children are counted for [n] use in this table. However, the use of this particular sound in the two children's inventories is hardly comparable.

resulting data provide information about early consonant development and can be summarized as follows:

1. A larger inventory of sounds was found in the word-initial than in the word-final position.
2. Word-initial inventories contained voiced stops prior to voiceless ones; the reverse was true for word-final productions.
3. The following phones appeared in at least 50 percent of all the subjects by 24 months of age:

   [h, w, b, t, d, m, n, k, g, f, and s] word-initially
   [p, t, k, n, r, and s] word-finally

4. The liquid [r] nearly always appeared first in a word-final position.
5. If the mean percentage of norm consonant productions was calculated (Shriberg and Kwiatkowski, 1982b), 70 percent accuracy was achieved. Because there is obviously a large difference between the inventory produced by 2-year-olds and that produced by adults, the author states that this accuracy level suggests that children are primarily attempting words that contain sounds within their articulatory abilities.
6. The order of appearance of initial and final phones was relatively constant across the three groups of children tested. Individual differences in the appearance of phones related to the classes of fricatives/affricates and liquids.

Although individual variability was observed in this investigation, the ability to follow the children in a longitudinal manner from the same point (ten identifiable words in a recording session) regardless of their age seemed to reduce the extreme variability noted in other cross-sectional research. Although this study did not contain a large number of subjects, it certainly suggests some clinical implications.

CLINICAL APPLICATION

Developmental Research and Therapeutic Implications

It is often stated that speech-language pathologists follow a developmental model in therapy; that is, sounds or processes that are developmentally earlier are targeted before those that are later. Stoel-Gammon's (1985) data support techniques utilized in therapy:

1. *Sounds first appear in the word-initial position.* In therapy, a newly acquired sound is typically placed in the word-initial position. Developmental data give evidence that this is indeed easier for the child.
2. *Anterior stops and nasals are acquired earlier.* In therapy, this is often used as a guiding principle. These sounds are very early and should, therefore, be in the speech of children. Even most children with phonological disorders have them in their consonant inventories.

There are also some interesting results from this study that are not often employed in therapy:

1. *The liquid [r] nearly always appeared in word-final position.* Based on this finding, words such as *more* and *bear* might be easier than *red* or *rope* for the child with [r] difficulties (assuming that the child has difficulty with the central vowels with r-coloring *and* the approximant [r]).
2. *Word-initial inventories contained voiced stops first; word-final inventories contained voiceless stops first.* According to this finding, the child with [k] and [g] problems might benefit from first working on [g] in the word-initial position before [k] in the word-final position. (This is based on the earlier result that sounds appear first in the word-initial position followed by later use in the word-final position.)

Due to the limited number of subjects, this application of Stoel-Gammon's (1985) results to therapeutic practice is probably premature. The intent here is to demonstrate how research findings can directly impact therapy.

Individual Acquisition Patterns. Throughout this discussion, individual variability has been stressed. The next question follows automatically: Do children show individual acquisition patterns or strategies? In other words, do children build their phonological inventory around certain sounds? If so, do these sounds represent a child's preference for a particular sound or set of sounds? Ferguson and Farwell (1975) referred to *salience* and *avoidance* factors. *Salience* implies that children will acquire words that contain sounds within their phonological inventories. The **salience factor** is defined as a child's active selection in early word productions of words containing sounds that are important or remarkable (salient) to the child. The **avoidance factor** is defined as the avoidance of words that do not contain sounds within a child's inventory. (This principle seems to apply only to the production of words; investigations relative to comprehension have not produced similar results. See Hoek, Ingram, and Gibson, 1986.) Production selection and avoidance have often been observed; for example, Schwartz and Leonard (1982) add experimental support to this claim.

Individual strategies employed may include preferences for certain sounds, certain syllable structures, and/or sound classes or sound features. Individual preference can also refer to those objects and contexts that the child enjoys more than others. The child's preference and environment will most certainly have an effect on which words are acquired and which phonetic inventory is established during the production of the first fifty words.

Prosodic Feature Development

As the child moves from the end of the babbling period to first words, the previously noted intonational contours continue. The falling intonation contour still predominates, although both a rise–fall and a simple rising contour have also been observed (Kent and Bauer, 1985).

An important aspect of communication during the first-fifty-word stage is *prosodic variation*. Examples of children's speech during this time have included pitch variations to indicate differences in meaning. For example, a falling pitch on the first syllable, [da↓ da], as daddy entered the room versus [da↑ da], a rising pitch on the first syllable, was realized when a noise was heard outside when daddy was expected (Crystal, 1986). Prosodic features are also used to indicate differences in syntactical function. Bruner (1975) labels these prosodic units *place-holders*. A demand or question, for example, is often signaled first by prosody; words are added later. For example, a child aged 1;2 first used the phrase "all gone" after dinner by humming the intonation. Approximately a month passed before the child's segmental productions were somewhat accurate (Crystal, 1986). One widely held view is that these prosodic units fulfill a social function. They are seen as a means of signaling joint participation in an activity shared by the child and the caregiver. Several authors suggest that prosodic features are evidence of developing speech acts (Dore, 1975; Halliday, 1975; Menn, 1976). A word with a specific intonation pattern might indicate requesting, calling, or demanding, for example. The following prosodic features associated with intentional communication have been observed (Marcos, 1987):

10 to 12 Months

First words, naming, labeling

> Begin with a falling contour only. Flat or level contour, usually accompanied by variations such as falsettos or variations in duration or loudness. Example: At 10 and 11 months, Hildegard (Leopold, 1947) lengthened the vowels of words such as [de:] for *there*.

13 to 15 Months

Requesting, attention getting, curiosity, surprise, recognition, insistence, greeting

Rising contour. High falling contour that begins with a high pitch and drops to a lower one. This is noted in the previous example of [da↑ da].

Prior to 18 Months

Playful anticipation, emphatic stress

High rising and high rising–falling contour. Example: A child might use a high rising intonation pattern on *ball* to indicate that the game is about to begin.

Around 18 Months

Warnings, playfulness

Falling–rising contour. Rising–falling contour. Example: A child might use a falling–rising contour on *no* to indicate that he or she has been warned not to do that, that is, to repeat this warning. The same *no* with a rising–falling contour could be used during a game to indicate that daddy is not going to get the ball.

As can be noted, intonational changes seem to develop prior to stress. Although various pitch contours appear earlier than the first meaningful words, contrastive stress is first evidenced only at the beginning of the two-word stage or at the age of approximately 1;6. During the first-fifty-word stage, the observed pitch variations can be said to represent directional sequences (rising versus falling, for example) or range patterns (high versus low within the child's pitch range). For a more detailed analysis of early intonational development, see Crystal (1986) and Snow, (1998a, 1998b, 2000).

THE PRESCHOOL CHILD

This section stresses information on the developing phonology of the child from approximately 18 to 24 months, the end of the first-fifty-word stage, to the beginning of the sixth year. It is during this time that the largest growth within the phonological system takes place. However, not only is the child's phonological system expanding but also large gains are seen in other language areas. From 18 to 24–30 months of age, the child's expressive vocabulary has at least tripled from 50 to 150–300 words (Lipsitt, 1966; Mehrabian, 1970), while the receptive vocabulary has grown from 200 to 1,200 words (Weiss and Lillywhite, 1981). The transition from one-word utterances to two-word sentences, a large linguistic step, is typically occurring at this time. With the production of two-word sentences, the child has entered the period of expressing specific semantic relationships: the beginning of syntactical development.

Around the child's fifth birthday, the expressive vocabulary has expanded to approximately 2,200 words, and about 9,600 words are in the child's receptive vocabulary (Weiss and Lillywhite, 1981). Almost all of the basic grammatical forms of the language—such as questions, negative statements, dependent clauses, and compound sentences—are now present as well (Owens, 2008). More important, the child knows now how to use language to communicate in an effective manner. Five-year-olds talk differently to babies than they do to their friends, for example. They also know how to tell jokes and riddles, and they are quite able to handle the linguistic subtleties of being polite and rude.

A child's phonological development at 18 to 24 months still demonstrates a rather limited inventory of speech sounds and phonotactic possibilities. At this time, perception seems to somewhat precede production. By the end of the preschool period, around the child's fifth birthday, an almost complete phonological system has emerged.

All these changes occur in less than four years. Although this section focuses on phonological development, such a discussion must always be seen within the context of the equally large expansions in morphosyntax, semantics, and pragmatics that occur during this time.

Segmental Form Development: Vowels

One area of sound acquisition that has been widely neglected in most discussions of phonological development is the acquisition of vowels. This neglect has been at least partially justified with the statement that children have acquired all vowels within the English sound inventory by the age of 3 (Templin, 1957). Little information is available on the development of vowels. This section on vowel development in preschool children will utilize the data presented by Irwin and Wong (1983) and Velten (1943). Although several methodological problems with Irwin and Wong's (1983) investigation have been pointed out (see Smit, 1986), it nevertheless examines the vowel productions in spontaneous conversations of children from 18 to 72 months of age. The Velten (1943) data come from a diary study of Joan Velten.

By examining the Irwin and Wong data, it can be seen that the children show the acquisition of [ɑ], [ʊ], [i], [ɪ], and [ʌ] at 18 months if the criterion is set at 70 percent accuracy. For the individual subjects at this age level, the correct production of vowels ranged from 23 percent to 71 percent. By 24 months, the only vowels that did not reach 70 percent group accuracy were [ɝ] and [ɚ]. By the age of 3, all the vowels were accounted for with virtually no production errors. Interestingly enough, at

age 4, the accuracy for [ɚ], [u], and [ə] dropped again to less than 90 percent.

These findings generally support Templin's claim that vowels are mastered at age 3. The drop in accuracy at age 4 might indicate that some younger children simply avoided those vowels before.

Another view of vowel acquisition is offered by diary studies. Velten's (1943) data show that prior to the age of 21 months, her daughter utilized the [a] vowel. After a surge in vocabulary at 21 months, the vowel [u] was added. When this child is compared to Irwin and Wong's (1983) data, large discrepancies between the two become obvious. Again, the previously discussed concepts of salience and avoidance may apply to the described differences. Some children possibly select, for the most part, words that consist of sounds within their repertoire, avoiding those words and sounds that are not. Salience and avoidance in conjunction with individual phonetic preference could account for the noted differences.

Far more information is needed in the area of vowel acquisition. From the limited amount of data presently available, it appears that vowels are indeed generally mastered by the age of 3. Whether individual variation plays a large role in this acquisition process still needs to be documented. This is an interesting area of research, especially in light of the deviant vowel systems that are often noted in children with phonological disorders.

Segmental Form Development: Consonants

Cross-Sectional Results. It appears that no chapter on phonological development can be complete without looking at the large sample studies that began in the 1930s (Wellman, Case, Mengert, and Bradbury, 1931) and have continued periodically since that time. However, it seems appropriate to preface such a discussion with the problems inherent in these studies.

Large sample studies were initiated to look at a large number of children in order to examine which sounds were mastered at which age levels. To this end, they evaluated most of the speech sounds within a given native language. With a few exceptions (Irwin and Wong, 1983; Olmsted, 1971; Stoel-Gammon, 1985, 1987), these studies have used methods similar to articulation tests to collect their data; that is, the children were asked to name pictures and certain sounds were then judged productionally "correct" or "incorrect."

In this type of procedure, general as well as specific problems arise. First, the fact that the child produces the sound "correctly" as a one-word response does not mean that the sound can also be produced "correctly" in natural speech conditions. Practitioners have always been aware of the often large articulatory discrepancies between one-word responses and the same sounds used in conversation. Second, the choice of pictures/words will certainly affect the production of the individual sounds within the word. Not only does the child's familiarity with the word play a role but also factors such as the length of the word, its structure, the stressed or unstressed position of the sound within the word, and the phonetic context in which the sound occurs. These factors help or hinder production. Therefore, strictly speaking, the only conclusion that can be drawn from cross-sectional studies is that the children could or could not produce that particular sound in that specific word.

The third point is a theoretical issue. As stated repeatedly in this textbook, there has been an adoption of certain newer concepts and terminology within the field of speech-language pathology. This chapter, for example, is called phonological development, not speech sound development. With the inclusion of the terms *phonology* and *phonological*

development, certain conceptual changes have been accepted. These cross-sectional studies are perhaps indicative of the inventory of speech sounds children typically possess at certain ages, but they are not a documentation of a particular child's phonological system.

Specific methodological differences between various cross-sectional studies are also important factors when interpreting the results. These include the criteria used to determine whether the child has "mastered" a particular sound. Although this has been elaborated on in several articles and books (e.g., Smit, 1986; Vihman, 2004), it is worth mentioning again. Table 5.4 provides a comparison of several of the larger cross-sectional studies.

Looking at age comparisons in Table 5.4, a difference in reported mastery of three or more years can be observed for some sounds. For example, note the difference between the ages of mastery for the [s] in the more recent Prather, Hedrick, and Kern (1975) and in the older Poole (1934) study. The Poole investigation has a mastery age of 7½ years, whereas the Prather and associates investigation shows an age level of 3 years. A three-year difference can be found for [z] acquisition when the Prather and associates data are compared to the Templin (1957) results. Again, Prather, Hedrick, and Kern assign a much earlier level of mastery. One question that is often asked in this context is: Does this mean that children are now producing sounds "correctly" at an earlier age? The answer is no; many of these differences are a consequence of the way *mastery* was defined. Poole, for instance, stated that 100 percent of the children must use the sound correctly in each of the positions tested. Prather and associates and Templin, on the other hand, set this level at 75 percent. In addition, rather than using the 75 percent cut-off level for all three positions (initial, medial, and final) as Templin had done, Prather,

Table 5.4 Age Levels for Speech Sound Development According to Six Studies

	Wellman (1931)	Poole (1934)	Templin (1957)	Sander (1972)	Prather (1975)	Arlt (1976)
m	3	3½	3	before 2	2	3
n	3	4½	3	before 2	2	3
h	3	3½	3	before 2	2	3
p	4	3½	3	before 2	2	3
f	3	5½	3	3	2–4	3
w	3	3½	3	before 2	2–8	3
b	3	3½	4	before 2	2–8	3
ŋ		4½	3	2	2	3
j	4	4½	3½	3	2–4	
k	4	4½	4	2	2–4	3
g	4	4½	4	2	2–4	3
l	4	6½	6	3	3–4	4
d	5	4½	4	2	2–4	3
t	5	4½	6	2	2–8	3
s	5	7½	4½	3	3	4
r	5	7½	4	3	3–4	5
ʧ	5		4½	4	3–8	4
v	5	6½	6	4	4	3½
z	5	7½	7	4	4	4
ʒ	6	6½	7	6	4	4
θ		7½	6	5	4	5
ʤ			7	4	4	4
ʃ		6½	4½	4	3–8	4½
ð		6½	7	5	4	5

Source: From *Assessment and Remediation of Articulatory and Phonological Disorders* (p. 47), by N. A. Creaghead, P. W. Newman, and W. A. Secord, 1989, Boston: Allyn & Bacon. Copyright © 1989 by Allyn & Bacon. Reprinted by permission.

Hendrick, and Kern used only two positions (initial and final) for their calculations. This clearly changes the ages to which mastery can be assigned. A shift to earlier acquisition noted in the Prather, Hendrick, and Kern study could be accounted for by these methodological changes. Also, as Smit (1986) points out, the Prather and associates results are based on incomplete data sets, especially at the younger age groupings. Although Prather, Hendrick, and Kern began with twenty-one subjects in each age group, several of these children did not respond to many of the words. Thus, at times, only eight to twelve children were used to calculate the norms. The children who did not respond to some words may have been avoiding them because they felt that they could not pronounce them "correctly."

> The lack of response from the younger children could reflect the aforementioned avoidance factor: Words that contain sounds not in the child's inventory will be avoided.

Ingram (1989a) points out problems related to the Templin study summing them up as follows:

> Templin's study provides a useful descriptive overview of English phonological acquisition. . . . Here, however, we will conclude with a caution about using large sample data such as these for anything more than the most general of purposes, setting out a series of problems with Templin's study in particular and large sample studies in general. The limitations of such studies need to be emphasized since their results may be inappropriately used both for theoretical and practical purposes, the latter including cases where a child might be misidentified as being speech-delayed because of his performance on a Templin-style articulation test. (p. 366)

What, then, is the alternative? Several investigators (e.g., Irwin and Wong, 1983; Stoel-Gammon, 1985) have attempted to improve the situation by using spontaneous speech and/or longitudinal investigations. Although spontaneous speech samples are in some respects better than the picture-naming tasks, several problems remain. Their use can also give us a biased picture. We actually probe into only a small portion of the child's conversational abilities and then generalize, assuming that this is representative of the child's overall performance. Also, factors outside our control might determine which words and sounds the child does produce and which ones he or she does not. As a result, the sample obtained will probably not contain all the sounds in that particular child's phonetic inventory.

> The avoidance factor may also influence spontaneous speech. Words might be avoided that contain sounds that the child cannot say.

Longitudinal data, on the other hand, can give us a real insight into the individual acquisition process, an important aspect missing in cross-sectional studies. The following discussion examines data from longitudinal studies on consonant development in children.

Longitudinal Results. Several longitudinal studies of consonant development exist, but they report on either a single child or a small group of children (e.g., Leopold, 1947; Menn, 1971; Vihman et al., 1985). Therefore, the data cannot be readily generalized. However, Vihman and Greenlee (1987) used a longitudinal methodology to examine the phonological development of ten 3-year-old children with the following results:

1. Stops and other fricatives were substituted for [ð] and [θ] by all children.
2. Over half of the children also substituted [r] and [l] sounds (gliding) and employed palatal fronting, in which a palatal sound is replaced by an alveolar ([ʃ] becomes [s]).
3. Two of the ten children demonstrated their own particular "style" of phonological acquisition.
4. On the average, 73 percent of the children's utterances were judged intelligible by three raters unfamiliar with the children. However, the range of intelligibility was broad, extending from 54 percent to 80 percent. As expected, children with fewer errors were more intelligible than those with multiple errors. Another factor also played a role: The children who

used more complex sentences tended to be more difficult to understand.

This last finding is significant. It documents the complex interaction between phonological development and the acquisition of the language system as a whole. The simultaneous acquisition of complex morphosyntactic and semantic relationships could well have an impact on the growth of the phonological system. It has been hypothesized that **phonological idioms** (Moskowitz, 1971) or **regression** (Leopold, 1947) occurs as the child attempts to master other complexities of language. Both terms refer to accurate sound productions that are later replaced by inaccurate ones. When trying to deal with more complex morphosyntactic or semantic structures, the child's previously correct articulations appear to be lost, replaced by inaccurate sound productions.

CLINICAL APPLICATION

Using Cross-Sectional Mastery Level Charts: Yes or No?

This textbook has pointed out some of the problems inherent in large cross-sectional studies that provide ages of sound mastery. Should these charts then be discarded? Probably not. Sound mastery charts give useful information about the general ages and order in which speech sounds develop. They can provide a broad framework for comparison, especially for beginning clinicians.

Clinicians should remember, however, that varying methodologies and criteria for sound mastery across investigations have produced a wide range of acquisition ages. Differences in ages of mastery for some sounds are often 3 to 4½ years apart. Based on the results of the Sander (1972) study, a clinician could justify doing [s] therapy with a 3-year-old, but according to the Poole (1934) investigation, a clinician should wait until the child is 7½ years old to work on [s]. These sound mastery charts should never be the single deciding factor for intervention. A colleague once remarked,

"When I worked in the public schools, we first decided if the child should be in therapy or not. Then we used the specific sound mastery chart that documented our decision." Clinical decision making involves much more than comparing a child to the mastery ages provided by cross-sectional research.

Phonological Processes

Within the last decade, the study of phonological development has shifted from examining the mastery of individual sounds to the acquisition and ordering of the phonological system. According to natural phonology, there seems to be a time frame during which normally developing children do suppress certain processes. This approximate age of suppression is helpful when determining normal versus disordered phonological systems and can be used as a guideline when targeting remediation goals.

> Definitions and examples of phonological processes are given in the Natural Phonology section of Chapter 4.

The following section will address some developmental aspects of syllable structure, substitution, and assimilation processes.

Syllable Structure Processes. Syllable structure processes are manifestations of the general tendency of young children to reduce words to basic CV structures. They become evident between the ages of 1;6 and 4;0, when there is a rapid growth in vocabulary and the onset of two-word utterances (Ingram, 1989b).

<u>Reduplication</u> is an early syllable structure process. Ingram (1989b) notes that it is a common process during the child's first-fifty-word stage. There was no evidence of this process in the youngest group of children (1;6 to 1;9) in the Preisser, Hodson, and Paden (1988) study.

<u>Final consonant deletion</u> is a relatively early process. Preisser and associates (1988) state that it was extremely rare in the utterances of

the children in the 2;2 to 2;5 age group. Ingram (1989b) and Grunwell (1987) note the disappearance of this process around age 3.

Unstressed syllable deletion, sometimes called *weak syllable deletion,* lasts longer than final consonant deletion, to approximately 4 years of age (Ingram, 1989b). This is also confirmed by Grunwell's (1987) data. However, Preisser, Hodson, and Paden (1988) noted that most of the children in their sample appeared to have suppressed this process by around their second birthday. (Only 3 percent of the twenty children over age 2;2 demonstrated unstressed syllable deletion.)

Cluster reduction is a syllable structure process that lasts for a relatively long time. Haelsig and Madison (1986) noted cluster reductions that still occurred in 5-year-old children, while Roberts, Burchinal, and Footo (1990) evidenced rare instances of this process in their 8-year-old children. In the Smit (1993a) study, there was some evidence of cluster reduction in the 8;0- to 9;0-year-old children for specific initial consonant clusters (approximately 1 to 4 percent of the 247 children for primarily three-consonant clusters). Greenlee (1974) describes four developmental stages of consonant reduction: (1) deletion of the entire cluster: [it] for *treat;* (2) reduction to one cluster member: [tit] for *treat;* (3) cluster is realized but one member is substituted: [twit] for *treat;* (4) norm articulation: [trit]. The Smit (1993a) and McLeod, van Doorn, and Reed (2001) data support Stages 2 through 4, whereas Stage 1, complete deletion of a cluster, was very rare or not seen at all even in the 2-year-old subjects.

Epenthesis refers to the insertion of a sound segment into a word, thereby changing its syllable structure. The intrusive sound can be a vowel as well as a consonant, but most often it is restricted to a schwa insertion between two consonants. This schwa insertion—for example, [pəliz] for *please*—is used to simplify the production difficulty of consonant clusters. Smit (1993a) and Smit, Hand, Freilinger, Bernthal, and Bird (1990) report that between the ages of 2;6 and 8;0, schwa insertion in clusters is a common process.

Substitution Processes. *Stopping* refers most frequently to the replacement of stops for fricatives and affricates. Due to the fact that fricatives and affricates are acquired at different ages, stopping is not a unified process but should be broken down into the individual sounds for which this process is employed. Table 5.5 summarizes the ages at which stopping is suppressed for the different fricative sounds.

Fronting denotes the tendency of young children to replace palatals and velars with alveolar consonants. Frequently occurring fronting processes consist of [ʃ] → [s], palatal fronting, and [k] → [t], velar fronting. Palatal fronting may also occur in affricate productions, [tʃ] → [ts] and [dʒ] → [dz]. Lowe, Knutson, and Monson (1985) found velar fronting to be more prevalent than palatal fronting. They also found that fronting rarely occurred after the age of 3;6. Based on the Smit (1993b) data, both velar fronting and palatal fronting were still noted until approximately age 5;0, although the frequency of occurrence is very limited (less than 5 percent of the 186 children).

Gliding of [r] and [l] seems to extend beyond 5;0 years of age (Grunwell, 1987; Smit, 1993b) and can be infrequently found even in the speech of children as old as age 7 (Roberts et al., 1990; Smit, 1993b). The suppression of these and other common processes are summarized in Tables 5.5 and 5.6.

Assimilation Processes. There are many different assimilation processes that occur in the speech of children. Children at different

Table 5.5   Age of Suppression of Stopping

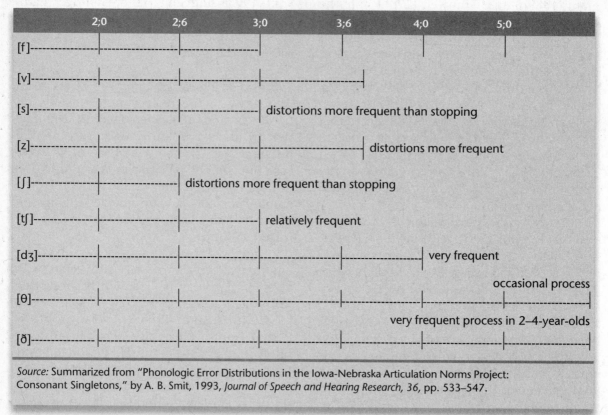

	2;0	2;6	3;0	3;6	4;0	5;0
[f]						
[v]						
[s]		distortions more frequent than stopping				
[z]		distortions more frequent				
[ʃ]	distortions more frequent than stopping					
[tʃ]	relatively frequent					
[dʒ]		very frequent				
[θ]	occasional process					
[ð]	very frequent process in 2–4-year-olds					

Source: Summarized from "Phonologic Error Distributions in the Iowa-Nebraska Articulation Norms Project: Consonant Singletons," by A. B. Smit, 1993, *Journal of Speech and Hearing Research, 36,* pp. 533–547.

> Assimilation is discussed in some detail in Chapters 2 and 4.

stages of their speech development tend to utilize assimilation processes in systematic ways. One of the most frequently occurring assimilatory processes is *velar harmony* (Smith, 1973). Prominent examples are:

[gɔk]   for "dog"
[keɪk]   for "take"
[kɑk]   for "talk"

However, regressive assimilation processes are not limited to velar consonants. Smith (1973) reported similar regressive assimila-

tions in which bilabials influenced preceding nonlabial consonants and consonant clusters. Among his examples:

[bebu]   for "table"
[bɔp]   for "stop"
[mibu]   for "nipple"

Although not all children display these types of assimilation processes, they may be part of the normal speech development in 1;6- to 2-year-olds. If they persist beyond age 3;0, they begin to constitute a danger sign for a disordered phonological system (Grunwell, 1987).

Table 5.6 Age of Suppression for Several Processes

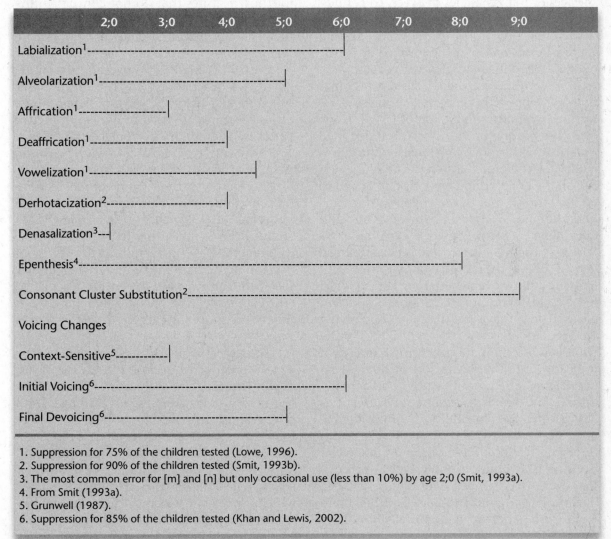

	2;0	3;0	4;0	5;0	6;0	7;0	8;0	9;0
Labialization[1]								
Alveolarization[1]								
Affrication[1]								
Deaffrication[1]								
Vowelization[1]								
Derhotacization[2]								
Denasalization[3]								
Epenthesis[4]								
Consonant Cluster Substitution[2]								
Voicing Changes								
Context-Sensitive[5]								
Initial Voicing[6]								
Final Devoicing[6]								

1. Suppression for 75% of the children tested (Lowe, 1996).
2. Suppression for 90% of the children tested (Smit, 1993b).
3. The most common error for [m] and [n] but only occasional use (less than 10%) by age 2;0 (Smit, 1993a).
4. From Smit (1993a).
5. Grunwell (1987).
6. Suppression for 85% of the children tested (Khan and Lewis, 2002).

Developmental Issues: Natural Phonology versus Nonlinear Phonology

Nonlinear phonologies, exemplified by autosegmental theory, metrical phonology, feature geometry, and optimality theories, are discussed in the previous chapter. Developmental implications for optimality theory are noted in Chapter 4. This discussion will concentrate on how feature geometry theory explains the acquisition of children's phonological systems.

First, let's compare the acquisition process when feature geometry is contrasted to Stampe's (1979) generative model of natural phonology. Phonological processes represent surface-level mismatches between the child's and the adult's norm productions. Therefore, if the child says [to$^{\upsilon}$p] for *soap*, we say that there is a mismatch in the form; that is, the child has used the natural process of stopping. As the child's phonological system becomes more developed, this process is suppressed, resulting in a norm production of [so$^{\upsilon}$p]. However, as a portion of this theory, it is assumed that the child's underlying representation was adultlike. Therefore, although the child says [to$^{\upsilon}$p], the child's underlying system is said to be fully intact; that is, the child has the same understanding of the /s/ phoneme as an adult does. One problem with this explanation is that it is highly abstract and lacks empirical data to support the claims about the child's underlying adultlike representation. For example, if the child always produces [t] for [s], what indication do we have that the child's underlying representation matches the adult's? Even if the child can discriminate between [t] and [s], it indicates only that some sort of differentiation has occurred, not that the child actually utilizes the same discrimination categories that adults use. In addition, phonological processes do not explain why certain substitution processes occur and others do not. Velar fronting is a common phonological process. However, why are velar consonants replaced by alveolars and not bilabials? For this, there is no explanation in the natural phonology construct.

Feature geometries account for the developmental process in a different manner. First, the child is viewed as coming to the language-learning process with a "set of universally determined templates with regard to segmental properties" (Yavaş, 1998, p. 277). In feature geometry, concrete underlying representations can be formulated that match the child's production but do not contradict properties of the adult target system. This is done by stating that

the underlying representation is *underspecified* for those features that do not contrast in the child's system. If a child replaces [k] with [t], the place features of coronal versus dorsal are underspecified. In the absence of phonemic contrasts in the child's system and the subsequent lack of an underlying specification, so-called default features are formulated. These default features are used to explain the error patterns. The child who replaces all [k]-productions with [t] demonstrates that there is no place of articulation contrast between nonlabial stop-plosives. Dorsal and coronal features have no underlying representation: They are underspecified. However, [t] is seen as the default feature. When either [t] or [k] is needed, [t] is supplied as the default. In the course of development, the child's underlying underspecified features give way to more specified representations that create a match between the child's phonological system and the target system.

The feature geometry tiers also represent the general order of acquisition of features (Yavaş, 1998). Thus, higher-level features, those closer to the root node, such as supralaryngeal and laryngeal features, are developmentally earlier than those that are lower or more deeply embedded on the tier, such as coronal, labial, and dorsal place features. As children develop, their phonological mismatches are typically related to features that are lower on the feature geometry tiers. Laryngeal and supralaryngeal features are dominated by the root node. Therefore, according to this framework, early distinctions should develop between nasal versus nonnasal and voiced versus voiceless contrasts. Looking at the developmental patterns of children, we see that these are indeed some of the earliest contrasts—[p], [b], and [m], for example.

In addition, common processes—that is, those that typically occur in the development of children's phonological systems versus idiosyncratic or unusual processes—can be accounted for by using feature geometry's tiered representation. Velar fronting ([k] → [t]) is a common process that involves changes in the place node. On the other hand, an idiosyncratic or unusual process, such as liquid stopping ([r] → [d]), affects a major class feature (sonorant) at the root node. According to the implications of feature geometry, these two "substitutions" would indicate something quite different in the development of the child's phonological system.

Feature geometry is an innovative way to look at phonological development. Although certain hierarchical features and specific theories are still being debated, it has much to offer within the framework of a developing phonological system. For more information on phonological development and nonlinear phonology, the reader is advised to turn to the *Handbook of Phonological Development from the Perspective of Constraint-Based Nonlinear Phonology* by Bernhardt and Stemberger (1998).

Prosodic Feature Development

At the time when children begin to use two-word utterances, a further development in the usage of suprasegmentals occurs: *contrastive stress*. This term indicates that one syllable within a two-word utterance becomes prominent. The acquisition process seems to proceed in the following order.

First, within the child's two-word utterance, a single prosodic pattern is maintained; the two words have a pause between them that becomes shorter and shorter. The next step appears to be the prosodic integration of the two words into one tone-unit. A **tone-unit**, or what is often called a sense-group, is an organizational unit imposed on prosodic data (Crystal, 1986). Such a tone-unit conveys meaning beyond that implied by only the verbal production. When the two words become one tone-unit (i.e., without the pause between them and with one intona-

tional contour), one of these words becomes more prominent, usually louder and associated with an identifiable pitch movement (Crystal, 1986). At the end of this process, there exists a unifying rhythmic relationship between the two items; thus, pauses become less likely. The following developmental pattern could be observed:

> Daddy (pause) eat
> Daddy (pause shortens) eat
> 'Daddy 'eat (no pause, both stressed)
> 'Daddy eat (first word stressed)

The use of contrastive stress in the two-word stage may be used to establish *contrastive meaning* (Brown, 1973). It is assumed that the meaning of the combined one-tone utterance is different from the meaning of the two words in sequence. Later, we see that this contrastive stress is used to signal differences in meaning with similar words. Thus, " 'Daddy eat" could indicate that "Daddy is eating," while "Daddy 'eat" could indicate, perhaps, that "Daddy should sit down and eat."

The existing studies of prosodic feature development agree that the acquisition of intonation and stress begins at an early age. Adultlike intonational patterns are noted prior to the appearance of the first word, while the onset of stress patterns seems to occur clearly before the age of 2. However, true mastery of the whole prosodic feature system does not seem to take place until children are at least 12 years old (Atkinson-King, 1973; Malikouti-Drachman and Drachman, 1975).

THE SCHOOL-AGE CHILD

By the time children enter school, their phonological development has progressed considerably. At age 5;0, most of them can converse freely with everyone and make themselves understood clearly to peers and adults alike. However, their pronunciation is still recognizably different from the adult norm. Phonologically, they still have a lot to learn. Although their phonological inventory is nearly complete, this system must now be adapted to many more and different contexts, words, and situations. Other phonological features are obviously not mastered at all at this time. Certain sounds are still frequently misarticulated and some aspects of prosodic feature development are only beginning to be incorporated.

Most of the research in child phonology has centered on the development of phonological skills in the first five years of life. However, recent interest in later phonological acquisition has evolved in part due to the established relationship between learning to speak and learning to read.

Segmental Form Development

The development of a child's phonological system includes both perceptual and productional maturation. Although the focus of this chapter is on production, it should be emphasized that the school-age child's perceptual skills are still very much in the process of growing. The gradual establishment of phonemic categorization skills, for example, continues well beyond 5 years of age, and it may not be until 14 years of age that children can reliably give categorical responses to certain types of synthetic stimuli (Fourcin, 1978). Tallal, Stark, Kallman, and Mellits (1980) reported that the perceptual constancy of children's phonemic categorizations still changes between 5 and 9 years of age. Also, the recognition of isolated words under quiet and noisy environmental conditions demonstrates improvement until at least age 10 (Elliott et al., 1979). The processing ability of specific continuous speech samples is still measurably slower for fifth-graders than for

adults (Cole and Perfetti, 1980), and the ability to understand specifically structured sentences under difficult listening conditions continues to develop until the age of 15 (Elliott, 1979). Perceptually, children are still fine-tuning, certainly during the beginning school years, and in some respects far beyond.

Information on the productional development of the phonological system comes from quite different methodological backgrounds. Most of the information available is based on the results of articulation tests, that is, based on responses to picture naming. If we look at these investigations (e.g., Lowe, 1986, 1996; Templin, 1957), we find that acceptable pronunciation of certain sounds is not achieved until between age 4;6 and 6;0. The most common later sounds are [θ, ð, ʒ] (Sander, 1972). Other findings (Ingram, Christensen, Veach, and Webster, 1980) include one or more of these consonants: [r, z, v]. Based on single-item pronunciation, most investigators agree that children complete their phonemic inventory by the age of 6;0 or, at the latest, 7;0. However, data from the Iowa-Nebraska Articulation Norms (Smit, 1993b) found dentalized [s] productions in 10 percent of the 9-year-old children tested. Table 5.7 indicates the later developing sounds found in large cross-sectional studies.

One must keep in mind that most of these results are responses to single-word tasks. To assume, based on this type of task, that these sounds are now "learned" does not take into account the complexity of their use in naturalistic contexts, in new words, and in conversational situations.

Consonant clusters also prove difficult for the school-age child. The acquisition of clusters usually takes place anywhere from about age 3;6 to age 5;6. During this time, the child may demonstrate consonant cluster reduction, lengthening of certain elements of the cluster, for example [s:no], or epenthesis. In

Table 5.7 Later-Developing Sounds with Approximate Ages of Mastery

Sound	Age of Mastery	Source
[s]	7½ , 9	Poole (1934), Smit (1993b)[1]
[z]	7½ , 9	Poole (1934), Smit (1993b)
[r]	7½ , 8	Poole (1934), Smit (1993b)
[v]	6½ , 6, 5½	Poole (1934), Templin (1957), Smit (1993b)
[ʃ]	6½ , 5½	Poole (1934), Smit (1993b)
[ʒ]	6, 6½ , 7	Wellman et al. (1931), Poole (1934), Templin (1957)
[θ]	7½ , 6, 6	Poole (1934), Templin (1957), Smit (1993b)
[ð]	6½ , 7, 7	Poole (1934), Templin (1957), Smit (1993b)
[tʃ]	5, 5½	Wellman et al. (1931), Smit (1993b)
[dʒ]	7, 5½	Templin (1957), Smit (1993b)

1. For the Smit (1993b) data, mastery levels were not determined. For the purpose of this table, a sound has been considered mastered if the estimated percentage of acceptable use is approximately 90 percent.

epenthesis, the child inserts a schwa vowel between two consonantal elements of a cluster, as in [səno], for example. The Iowa-Nebraska data submitted by Smit (1993a) offer interesting insight into twenty-seven different initial clusters. In this study, 1,049 children between the ages of 2;0 and 9;0 were screened using an articulation test format. The data can be summarized as follows:

1. On fourteen of the twenty-seven initial clusters tested, a small percentage of children in the 8;0- to 9;0-year-old group (N = 247, frequency of occurrence = approximately 2 percent) reduced two consonant clusters to a single element. These clusters included [pl], [kl], [gl], [sl], [tw], [kw], [tr], [dr], [fr], [sw], [sm], [sn], [st], [sk].
2. The consonant clusters [br] and [θr] demonstrated a higher frequency of consonant cluster reduction (5 to 15 percent) for children from ages 5 to 9.
3. For the 5;6- to 7;0-year-olds, the consonant clusters that fell at 75 percent or below group accuracy included [sl], [br], [θr], [skw], [spr], [str], and [skr].
4. Epenthesis, or schwa insertion in consonant clusters, occurs frequently up to age 8;0. The 9-year-olds exhibited schwa insertion rarely.

These data demonstrate that consonant cluster realizations are not adultlike for all children even at age 9.

In addition, the timing of the sounds within consonant clusters is also not yet comparable to adult performance in school-age children (Gilbert and Purves, 1977; Hawkins, 1979). When the temporal relationships between the elements of a cluster were compared for children and adults, it was found that differences, particularly in voice onset time, were still present at 8;0 years of age.

Although this information indicates that phonological development extends past the age of 7, most of the available research has focused on the development of the phonological inventory. Unfortunately, other features of the phonological system are still relatively uncharted territory. For example, the development of allophonic variations in older children should also be addressed. How do children learn the acceptable range of phonetic variation in different contexts within their speech community? Local (1983) exemplified this process by tracing the acquisition of one vowel produced by a boy between the ages of 4;5 and 5;6. The variability of sound production and the learning of its acceptable allophonic limitations are decisively important tasks for the developing school-age child.

The intricate interrelation of normal phonological development with other areas of language growth, which has been previously emphasized, demands attention at this point in the child's development as well. The acquisition of vocabulary, for example, is a monumental task to be accomplished in a relatively short time. When children begin kindergarten, they are said to have an expressive vocabulary of approximately 2,200 words (Weiss and Lillywhite, 1981). New sound sequences occurring in words that will now be attained require not only increased oral-motor control and improved timing skills but also the internalization of new phonological rules. For instance, the conditions under which voiceless stops in English need to be aspirated might now become a new achievement.

The acquisition of morphology is also related to phonological growth. The learning of specific morphological structures implies the learning of phonological rules. The child has to understand under which conditions the plural suffix -s is voiced or voiceless, for example. This interconnection between morphology and phonology has been termed **morphophonology**, which refers to the study of the different allomorphs of the morpheme and the rules governing their use. For example, the child's production of [əz] to indicate the plural form for *glass* versus [s] as the plural of *boat* falls within the study of morphophonology as do the rules governing the productional changes from *divide* to *division* and from *explode* to *explosion*. Research findings in this area (e.g., Atkinson-King, 1973; Ivimey, 1975; Myerson, 1978) substantiate that children as old as 17 are still acquiring certain morphophonological patterns. The complex interrelationship between the phonological system and other components of language continues into the child's later school years.

Phonological Awareness, Emerging Literacy, and Phonological Disorders

One other important aspect that needs to be addressed in this section pertains to the interconnections between learning to speak and learning to read. Although a general concensus has not been reached as to which variables are indispensable for acquiring reading, there does seem to be a close relationship between early speech and emerging literacy. Thus, a strong correlation between the phonological development, especially segmentation skills, and later reading achievement has been found (e.g., Clarke-Klein and Hodson, 1995; Lundberg, Olofsson, and Wall, 1980). Moreover, early language development, specifically the perceptual processing of sounds, has been found to be one of the strongest predictors of later reading acquisition (Lundberg, 1988). Some of these skills develop during the early school years.

Metaphonological skills are also related to reading. A subcategory of metalinguistics, **metaphonology** involves the child's conscious awareness of the sounds within that particular language. It includes how those sounds are combined to form words. Therefore, metaphonological skills pertain to the child's ability to discern how many sounds are in a word or which sound constitutes its beginning or end. Phonological awareness abilities are one important metaphonological skill. There is a growing body of knowledge that documents the relationship between phonological awareness and emerging literacy. The following section will briefly summarize these results.

Research over at least two decades has affirmed the importance of phonological awareness and its relationship to reading acquisition (e.g., Chaney, 1992; Lonigan, Burgess, and Anthony, 2000; Olofsson and Neidersoe, 1999; Stanovich, 2000). Reviews of the literature have noted that strong phonological awareness skills are characteristics of good readers, whereas children with poor phonological awareness skills in kindergarten and early school years are far more likely to become poor readers (e.g., Catts, Fey, and Zhang, 2001; Leafstedt, Richards, and Gerber, 2004; Marcel, 1980; Torgesen, 2000). This section will define phonological awareness, discuss the various levels of phonological awareness, and examine the impact articulation/phonological disorders have on developing phonological awareness skills and early literacy.

Phonological awareness is an individual's awareness of the sound structure or phonological structure of a spoken word in contrast to written words (Gillon, 2004). It is the child's conscious ability to detect and manipulate sound segments, such as moving sounds around in a word, combining certain sounds together, or deleting sounds (Smith, Simmons, and Kameenui, 1995). Phonological awareness should be examined in the broader scope of phonology, as we find that long before children become aware of the phonological structure of words, they have specialized phonological knowledge. This knowledge allows them to make a judgment about whether a word is part of their native language, to self-correct any speech errors or mispronunciations, and to discriminate between acceptable and unacceptable variations of a spoken word (Yavaş, 1998).

Phonological awareness uses a single modality—the auditory one. It is the ability to hear sounds in spoken words in contrast to recognizing sounds in written words, which accesses the child's coding abilities. **Coding** is translating stimuli from one form to another—for example, from auditory to written form or from written to auditory. Phonological awareness should also be separated from phonemic awareness. Phonological awareness is a more general term that refers to all sizes of sound units, such as words (e.g., How many words are in the sentence *He hit the ball*?); syllables (e.g., How many syllables does *banana* have?); onset-rimes (e.g., Which one of these words rhymes with *bed: man, lock*, or *head*?); and phonemes (e.g., What is the first sound in *dog*?). **Phonemic awareness**, however, refers only to the phoneme level and necessitates an understanding that words are comprised of individual sounds. Examples would include the child's ability to segment and match sounds (e.g., What is a word that starts with the same sound as *Cathy*?) and the ability to manipulate sounds (e.g., What would *mean* be without the final *n* sound?). The concepts of phonological and phonemic awareness should also be separated from phonological processing.

Phonological processing is the use of sounds of a language to process verbal information in oral or written form that requires working- and long-term memory (Wagner and Torgesen, 1987). Research provides strong support that phonological processing includes two broad dimensions: coding and awareness (Hurford et al., 1993; Liberman and Shankweiler, 1985; Smith, Simmons, and Kameenui,

1995). Coding, which contains two dimensions, phonetic and phonological, includes multiple processes that require memory and coding from one form of representation to another. An example might be that the child learns that the letters *sh* sound a certain way. This knowledge is stored in memory, which the child must access when trying to sound out a new word, *shelf*. The distinction between the two coding dimensions is the type of memory that is accessed. In other words, phonetic coding takes place in working memory for such processes as sounding out unfamiliar words.

In contrast, phonological coding is related to the semantic lexical abilities in long-term memory. This seems to involve a three-step process. First, written symbols are matched to the pronunciation of the written word. Second, the pronunciation of the written word is matched with the pronunciation of words in memory. Third, pronunciations of words in memory are linked with meaning for retrieval of meaning and pronunciation (Wagner and Torgesen, 1987; Wesseling and Reitsma, 2000). At least four types of phonological processing skills demonstrate differences between normal readers and poor readers: memory span (retention of new strings of verbal items), recall of verbal information (in contrast to recall of nonverbal items), articulation rate, and rapid naming (Cornwall, 1992, Torgesen, 2000, Torgesen, Wagner, Simmons, and Laughon, 1990).

Thus, phonological awareness is a subdivision of phonological processing; however, phonological awareness is less complex than coding in the demands it puts on memory and processing of information. Phonological awareness is a multilevel skill of breaking down words into smaller units and it can be described in terms of syllable awareness, onset-rime awareness, and phoneme awareness (Gillon, 2004). A variety of measures can be used to evaluate a child's knowledge of these three levels.

Syllable Awareness. Awareness at the syllable level requires that the child understands that words can be divided into syllables. For example, the word *baby* has two syllables: "ba" and "by." Tasks used to evaluate syllable awareness include (1) syllable segmentation (How many syllables, or beats, are in *banana*?); (2) syllable completion (Here is a picture of a rainbow. I'll say the first part of the word and you can complete it. Here is a rain___); (3) syllable identity (Which part of "rainbow" and "raincoat" sound the same?); and (4) syllable deletion (Say "rabbit." Now say it again without the "ra").

Onset-Rime Awareness. This awareness involves recognition of the onset of the syllable (all sounds prior to the vowel nucleus) and the rime, or the rest of the syllable, which includes the syllable peak and coda. (See Chapter 2 for a review of syllable structure.) Onset-rime awareness is typically measured by using some type of rhyming tasks. To be able to rhyme, the child must be able to separate the onset from the rime of the word. Thus, the child knows that *cat, bat,* and *hat* rhyme as the onset changes in each; however, the rime stays the same: "at." Tasks that measure onset-rime awareness include (1) spoken rhyme recognition (Do these words rhyme: *hop* and *top*?); (2) which one does not rhyme (Which word does not rhyme: *cat, sat, car*?); (3) spoken rhyme production (Tell me a word that rhymes with *dog*); and (4) onset-rime blending ("c" "at" is blended to "cat").

Phonemic Awareness. This skill can be measured in a number of ways. For each of the tasks the child's ability to manipulate sounds is tested. Examples include (1) phoneme detection (Which one of the following words has a different first sound: *rose, red, bike, rabbit*?); (2) phoneme matching (Which word begins with same sound as "rose"?); (3) phoneme isolation (Which sound do you hear at the beginning of "toad"?); (4) phoneme completion (Here is a picture of a ball. Can you finish the word for me? "ba__"); (5) phoneme blending (I am going to say a word in a funny way. Can you tell me what the word is? *b—i—g*); (6) phoneme deletion (Can you say "toad" without the "d" sound?); (7) phoneme segmentation (How many sounds are in "jeep"?); (8) phoneme reversal (Say "ball." Now say "ball" backwards: "lab"); (9) phoneme manipulation (Say "meat." Now say it again but this time change the "m" and the "t" around: "team"); and (10) spoonerisms (for example, *hot dog* becomes *dot hog*).

There seems to be a developmental progression in the acquisition of phonological awareness skills. First, an awareness of larger units, such as words and syllables, precedes awareness of smaller units, such as individual sounds. In a comprehensive study by Lonigan, Burgess, Anthony, and Barker (1998), which tested several different levels of phonological/phonemic awareness in 356 children between the ages of 2 and 5, the following results emerged. First, age influenced the performance on all tasks. Although accelerated growth was evident between the ages of 3 and 4 years, it was not until around age 5 that children were able to consistently perform phoneme detection tasks. Second, the linguistic complexity of the task influenced performance. Children across age groups showed stronger performance on blending and deleting at the word level (*dog + house = doghouse*), followed by success at the syllable level (*win + dow = window*), and the weakest performance at the phoneme level (*d + o + g = dog*). Third, performance on the phonological awareness tasks was moderately correlated to scores on receptive and expressive language

tasks at the 4- and 5-year-old level, but not at the younger ages.

Although stable performance of phonological awareness tasks may not be evident until 4 years of age, some 2- and 3-year-old children can demonstrate phonological awareness knowledge. Maclean, Bryant, and Bradley (1987) appear to be one of the earliest investigators who found that a moderate percentage of 3-year-old children can perform competently on a rhyme detection task. When Lonigan and colleagues (1998) reduced the load on memory by having the child look at three pictures and point to the picture that did not rhyme, then close to 25 percent of the 2½-year-old children scored above chance on the task.

It must be noted that some researchers have questioned the progressive nature of phonological development. In other words, the seemingly noted fact that syllable awareness emerges before rhyme awareness, and rhyme awareness before phoneme awareness, was not evidenced in all children. For example, individual reports of older poor readers document children who performed better on phoneme manipulation tasks as opposed to performance on rhyme tasks (Duncan and Johnston, 1999). These findings are contrary to the trends noted in most other children. Further research will be necessary before we will be able to say whether there is a smooth progression from larger units of awareness (syllable and rhyme awareness) to smaller units, such as phonemic awareness.

The next question that arises is whether phonological awareness abilities are predictive of later reading and spelling competencies. In a large number of studies that attempted to control for variables such as memory, intellectual ability, and home and preschool environments (e.g., Lundberg, Olofsson, and Wall, 1980; Share, Jorm, Maclean, and Matthews, 1984; Torgesen, Wagner, and Rashotte, 1994;

Torneus, 1984), the following findings are suggested:

1. There is a positive relationship between phonological awareness and reading. Children with phonological awareness skills learn to read more easily than children who do not have these skills (Snow, Burns, and Griffin, 1998).
2. Performance on phonological awareness tasks in kindergarten and first grade is a strong predictor of later reading achievement (Hecht, Burgess, Torgesen, Wagner, and Rashotte, 2000; Torgesen, Wagner, Rashotte, Burgess, and Hecht, 1997).
3. Direct training of phonological awareness and sound-letter correspondence with children who are not yet reading improves their reading and spelling skills (Adams, Foorman, Lundberg, and Beeler, 1997; Swank, 1997).
4. Phonological awareness teaching works best when combined with instruction in sound-letter correspondence (Bradley and Bryant, 1983).

Finally, the relationship between phonological awareness, developing literacy, and speech disorders is relevant to this discussion. Approximately 4 percent of 6-year-old children will approach reading with a speech impairment (Shriberg, Tomblin, and McSweeney, 1999). Are these children's phonological awareness skills impacted by their speech problems? If so, will these children be at a greater risk for developing reading and spelling difficulties? It appears that children with articulation disorders—and therefore motor-based problems that affect the mechanics of actually producing the sound—are not at high risk for literacy problems (e.g., Bishop and Adams, 1990; Catts, 1993; Dodd, 1995). However, those children who have a phonological disorder, impacting the processing of phonological information, which might include semantic, syntactic, and/or morphological levels, are potentially at risk for written language difficulties. The extent of this problem is probably determined by their patterns of linguistic strengths and weaknesses (Gillon, 2004). Therefore, the specific findings from children with expressive phonological difficulties and their phonological awareness skills may be summarized as follows:

1. As a group, children with phonological difficulties show deficits on a variety of phonological awareness tasks (e.g., Bird and Bishop, 1992; Bird, Bishop, and Freeman, 1995; Gillon, 2000; Marion, Sussman, and Marquardt, 1993; Webster and Plante, 1992).
2. Without intervention, these difficulties with phonological awareness persist over time. Difficulties have been especially noted in acquiring phonemic level skills (e.g., Gillon, 2002; Snowling, Bishop, and Stothard, 2000).
3. Children with additional spoken language impairments generally experience poorer long-term outcomes in reading and writing when compared to children with isolated phonological production difficulties (Bishop and Adams, 1990; Catts and Kamhi, 1999; Goswami and Bryant, 1990; Hodson, 1994; Hulme and Snowling, 1992; Lewis, Freebairn, and Taylor, 2000; Snowling, Goulandris, and Stackhouse, 1994; Stackhouse, 1993, 1997; Wells, Stackhouse, and Vance, 1996).
4. In addition to phonological awareness difficulties, children with expressive phonological problems display weaknesses in other areas that appear to be important for literacy development, including letter-name knowledge and verbal working memory (e.g., Webster, Plante, and Couvillion, 1997).

5. The type of phonological disorder is relevant to predicting reading outcomes. Thus, children who show consistent use of unusual or idiosyncratic errors (as opposed to normal developmental processes) may evidence more severe difficulties in acquiring literacy skills (e.g., Dodd et al., 1995; Leitao, Hogben, and Fletcher, 1997).

6. The severity of a child's phonological disorder influences literacy outcomes. Children with severe phonological disorders, significant phonological processing difficulties, and other language impairments are very likely to have persistent reading and spelling difficulties (e.g., Bird et al., 1995; Bishop and Robson, 1989; Larrivee and Catts, 1999; Stackhouse, 1982, 1997). However, for the most part, these children respond positively to phonological awareness instruction, which can prevent the long-term effects (Gillon, 2000).

To summarize, phonological awareness is a subcategory of phonological processing. It contains many different levels of skills and seems to demonstrate a systematic developmental sequence. It is highly correlated to later reading and spelling abilities. Children with phonological difficulties demonstrate more problems with phonological awareness, and consequently difficulties with reading acquisition. These reading and spelling deficits may persist, especially in children with idiosyncratic errors and those with severe phonological problems.

Prosodic Feature Development

Prosodic features assume grammatical function. For example, specific intonation patterns are employed to differentiate between statements and certain questions in English ("He is coming."↘ versus "He is coming?"↗). Contrasting stress realizations signal different word classes ('*construct* versus con 'struct). On the sentence level, the combined effects of higher pitch and increased loudness usually convey communicatively important modifications of basic meaning ("This is a 'pen" versus "'This is a pen"). This section examines the grammatical function of prosodic features in school-age children and their relationship to phonological development.

As previously noted, the child begins to use intonational patterns toward the end of the first year of life. As the child's grammatical abilities develop, new uses of intonation emerge. For example, the contrast between rising and falling pitch differentiates the two grammatical functions of a tag question in English ("asking" as in "We're ready, aren't we?"↗ and "telling" as in "We're ready, aren't we!" ↘). Differences in intonation patterns like these appear to be learned during the child's third year (Crystal, 1987). However, the learning of intonation goes on for a long time. Studies report that children as old as 12 years were still acquiring some of the fundamental functions of English intonation, especially those for signaling grammatical contrasts (Cruttenden, 1985; Ianucci and Dodd, 1980; Wells, Peppé, and Goulandris, 2004). As reported by Crystal (1987), even teenagers have been shown to have difficulty understanding sentences in which intonation and pausing are used to differentiate meanings. His example: "She dressed, and fed the baby" (indicating she dressed herself and then fed the baby) versus "She dressed and fed the baby" (indicating she dressed as well as fed the baby). Thus, while certain intonational features seem to be among the earliest phonological acquisitions, others may be some of the last.

Several studies have examined the use of contrastive stress both on the word level ('*record* versus re'*cord*) and on the sentence level (determining whom Mary hit in the following sentences: "John hit Bill and then *Mary* hit him" versus "John hit Bill and then Mary hit *him*") (e.g., Atkinson-King, 1973; Chomsky, 1971; Hornby and Hass, 1970; Myers and Myers, 1983). Although the ages differ depending on the type and design of the research, results suggest that children are still learning certain aspects of contrastive stress up until the age of 13.

The acquisition of prosodic features is a gradual process that in some respects extends into the teens. It is closely connected to the new phonological, morphosyntactic, semantic, and pragmatic demands placed on the developing child. As the complexity of the linguistic environment and the child's interaction with that environment increase, so do the subtle intricacies of each of these language levels.

SUMMARY

First, this chapter provided an overview of structural and functional development in infancy and early childhood. At birth, the infant's respiratory, phonatory, resonatory, and articulatory systems are not fully developed. Many changes must occur before the systems are ready to support regular sound and voice production. In addition, the child's perceptual abilities are developing. The second portion of this chapter summarized early perceptual skills, including categorical perception and phonemic awareness. The third section of this chapter traced the segmental form and prosodic feature development of children from vocalizations prior to babbling to the time when their speech sound inventory has reached an adultlike form. The prevalence of certain sounds and syllable shapes was traced from babbling to the first words. As the number of words in children's vocabularies increases, inventory and complexity of syllables grow as well. During this early stage of expansion, the prosodic feature intonation begins to be used to signal different intentions.

The preschool child's development is characterized by a large growth in all aspects of language; the acquisition of new phonological features is a portion of this quickly maturing system. Although cross-sectional studies have attempted to provide so-called mastery ages for sounds, these results cannot be easily generalized. Longitudinal data that document individual variability in sound acquisition among children as well as the influence of other language areas on phonological skills were then summarized. The suppression of many phonological processes is occurring within this time interval as well. Based on research findings, approximate ages were given for the suppression of several common phonological processes. The differences between natural phonology (the suppression of phonological processes) and the phonological development hypothesized by nonlinear/multilinear phonologies were addressed.

Both segmental form and prosodic features continue to mature during the school years. Although the sound inventory is approaching adultlike form, many aspects of the phonological system are still maturing. The child needs to learn morphophonemic variations as well as metaphonological skills. Metaphonological skills were briefly discussed in relationship to the emerging literacy of children. During the school years, phonological development often impacts the child's abilities to learn to read and write. The close interdependencies between phonology, language development, and literacy learning point to the importance of normal phonological development in children.

CASE STUDY

DIAGNOSTIC IMPLICATIONS OF PHONOLOGICAL PROCESS SUPPRESSION

Approximate ages of suppression have been provided for several common phonological processes. This information can be helpful during our diagnostic assessment. The following phonological processes were identified in Clint, age 3;6.

Word	Production	Phonological Process
house	[haʊ]	final consonant deletion
cup	[kʌ]	final consonant deletion
gun	[gʌ]	final consonant deletion
shovel	[ʃʌbəl]	stopping of [v]
vacuum	[bækju]	stopping of [v], final consonant deletion
vase	[beɪ]	stopping of [v], final consonant deletion
scratching	[krætʃɪŋ]	consonant cluster reduction
skunk	[kʌŋk]	consonant cluster reduction
star	[tɑɚ]	consonant cluster reduction
jumping	[dʌmpɪŋ]	stopping of [dʒ]
jelly	[dɛli]	stopping of [dʒ]
jeep	[dip]	stopping of [dʒ]
that	[dæt]	stopping of [ð]
bath	[bæt]	stopping of [θ]
feather	[fɛdɚ]	stopping of [ð]

Similar processes were also noted in conversational speech.

Which of the noted processes should be suppressed by age 3;6? Final consonant deletion is usually suppressed by around age 3;0, while stopping of [v], [θ], [ð], and [dʒ] extends to age 3;6 or beyond. Consonant cluster reduction is also a process that is suppressed at a relatively late age. Based on these results, the only process that might cause concern at this age would be final consonant deletion. Again, discretion must be exercised when using these approximate ages of suppression as the sole criterion for determining the necessity for intervention.

THINK CRITICALLY

1. Lori is a 20-month-old toddler who is brought to your clinic by her parents who are concerned that Lori has not begun to say real words. Although she babbles strings of babbles, such as [baba], [maba], [toto], and [dada], she does not evidence true words nor does she impose intonation or rhythmic patterns on the babbles. The parents report that just recently (within the last two to three weeks) Lori will occasionally imitate a babble that she has just produced if the parents have her attention and immediately say her babble back to her. What prelinguistic stage is Lori in? She is 20 months old. Approximately how delayed is she in respect to speech development?

2. The following results of an articulation test are from Ryan, age 6;6. We noted distinctive features and phonological processes for Ryan in Chapter 4.

horse	[hoᵁɚθ]	pig	[pɪk]	chair	[ʃɛɚ]
wagon	[wægən]	cup	[kʌp]	watch	[waʃ]
monkey	[mʌŋki]	swinging	[s̬wɪŋɪŋ]	thumb	[fʌm]
comb	[koᵁm]	table	[teˡbəl]	mouth	[maᵁf]
fork	[foɚk]	cat	[kæt]	shoe	[su]
knife	[naˡf]	ladder	[læɾɚ]	fish	[fɪs]
cow	[kaᵁ]	ball	[bɑl]	zipper	[ðɪpɚ]
cake	[keˡk]	plane	[pweˡn]	nose	[noᵁθ]
baby	[beˡbi]	cold	[koᵁd]	sun	[θʌn]
bathtub	[bæftəb]	jumping	[dʌmpən]	house	[haᵁθ]
nine	[naˡn]	TV	[tivi]	steps	[stɛp]
train	[tweˡn]	stove	[θtoᵁv]	nest	[nɛt]
gun	[gʌn]	ring	[wɪŋ]	books	[bʊkθ]
dog	[dɑg]	tree	[twi]		
yellow	[wɛloᵁ]	green	[gwin]		
doll	[dɑl]	this	[dɪθ]		
bird	[bɝd]	whistle	[wɪθəl]		
carrots	[kɛɚət]				

Based on Ryan's age, compare which sounds might be considered in *error* if the ages of speech sound development from the Poole (1934) versus the Templin (1957) investigations are used (p. 130). (Actually any two studies could be used for comparison.) Discuss the problems when using these sound mastery age levels.

3. Use the results generated in Chapter 4 that identified the phonological processes noted for this elicitation task (p. 98). Based on the age of the child (6 years, 6 months), identify which phonological processes are age appropriate, which ones might be considered borderline, and which ones should be suppressed at his age.

TEST YOURSELF

1. Prelinguistic behavior refers to
   a. the development of an infant's vocal tract
   b. the ability to perceive speech sounds prior to birth
   c. all vocalizations prior to a child's first words
   d. prosodic feature development

2. Infants begin to learn about voice and speech
   a. prior to birth (in the womb)
   b. at birth when others begin talking to them
   c. when they start babbling
   d. when they say their first word
3. Canonical babbling includes
   a. reduplicated babbling

b. nonreduplicated babbling
c. reflexive babbling
d. a and b
e. none of the above

4. Which prosodic feature seems to be the first to develop?
   a. contrastive stress
   b. intonation
   c. syllable stress
   d. durational variations

5. Which stage typically is the beginning of the lingustic phase of language development?
   a. canonical babbling
   b. nonreduplicated babbling
   c. first fifty words
   d. two-word stage
   e. holophrastic period

6. What syllable shapes predominate the first 50-word stage of language development?
   a. CV, VC, and CVC
   b. CVCC
   c. CCVC
   d. CVCVCC

7. Which one of the following is among the later-developing sounds?
   a. [f]   c. [s]
   b. [j]   d. [k]

8. Which of the following is *not* a syllable structure process?
   a. cluster reduction
   b. final consonant deletion
   c. gliding
   d. reduplication

9. If a child says [tip] for *keep,* this is an example of which type of process?
   a. stopping
   b. gliding
   c. fronting
   d. epenthesis

10. Which one of the following refers to the child's conscious awareness of sounds within his or her native language?
   a. morphophonology
   b. metaphonology
   c. phonetic coding
   d. phonotactics

WEBSITES

www.phonologicaldisorders.com

This website, created by the author of this textbook, provides references to articles and books which describe several different aspects of phonological development. Links are given to other websites and resources.

www.speech-language-therapy.com/acquisition .html

This website by Caroline Bowen contains information on phonological development and phonological process suppression. There are helpful charts and downloadable pdf files on developmental norms and ages of speech sound acquisition. References are included at the end of the website.

www.waisman.wisc.edu:8000/vocal/index.html

For anyone who would like more information on vocal tract development, this website, from the Waisman Center at the University of Wisconsin-Madison, cites recent research on vocal tract development from infancy through adolescence. Additional links and resources are also provided.

www.personal.psu.edu/mam1034/csd300 .phonologicalprocesses.html

This website was developed by Meredith Massucci at Penn State University. It offers definitions and examples of normal phonological processes and idiosyncratic or atypical processes. The explanations are from "Fundamentals of Phonetics" (Small, 2005) and are presented in a clear manner for the beginning student.

http://home.cogeco.ca/~monicafitz/stages.htm

This website offers an explanation of the prelinguistic stages of development. It provides a reference page as well as a section on theories. The theories do not include nonlinear-based approaches. The site is simple to use and understand and easy to navigate.

www.asha.org/public/speech/development/
child_hear_talk.htm

This website, by the American Speech-Language-Hearing Association (ASHA), provides an easy-to-read chart on developmental milestones of hearing/understanding and talking. The chart only includes up to 5 years of age.

FURTHER READINGS

Ferguson, C., Menn, L., & Stoel-Gammon, C. (1992). *Phonological development: Models, research, implications.* Timonium, MD: York Press.

Gillon, G. (2004). *Phonological awareness: From research to practice.* New York: Guilford Press.

Hua, Z., & Dodd, B. (Eds.). (2006). *Phonological development and disorders: A multilingual perspective.* North Somerset, UK: Multilingual Matters.

Lowe, R. (2002). *Workbook for the identification of phonological processes and distinctive features.* Austin, TX: Pro-Ed.

McGuinness, D. (2005). *Language development and learning to read: The scientific study of how language development affects reading skill.* Cambridge, MA: MIT Press.

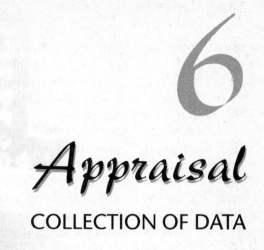

6
Appraisal
COLLECTION OF DATA

LEARNING OBJECTIVES

When you have finished this chapter, you should be able to:

- Compare and contrast "screening" and a "comprehensive assessment."
- Identify the advantages and disadvantages of articulation tests.
- Explain the importance of stimulability testing.
- Determine the areas of assessment when evaluating the speech mechanism.
- Define emerging phonology.
- Identify the specific procedures that can be used to aid in the evaluation of an unintelligible child.
- Differentiate between standard English and vernacular English.
- Differentiate between a regional and a cultural dialect.
- Describe the features of African American English.
- Evaluate the role that the speech-language therapist might play when assessing a child with limited English proficiency.
- Describe the speech sound characteristics of Spanish English, Vietnamese English, Hmong English, Cantonese English, and Korean English.
- Identify the procedures that should be considered when evaluating a dialect speaker.

$\mathcal{T}$he last chapters have provided a foundation that can now be applied to the diagnosis and treatment of impaired articulation and phonology. Before our diagnosis begins, two questions should be asked: (1) What information do we actually need? and (2) How should we gather that information? Consider a child coming to us whose parents are concerned because the child's speech is virtually unintelligible. On the other hand, consider an adolescent who seeks therapy because of a somewhat conspicuous [s]-production. These two individuals present completely different situations, different ages, different degrees of impairment, and differences in the information we would need to effectively evaluate the situation. How, then, do we assess these diverse situations? Let's begin by looking at the various parts of an assessment.

Assessment is one of the most important tasks a clinician will perform; it is the basis for treatment decisions. **Assessment**, the clinical evaluation of a client's disorder, can be divided into two phases: appraisal and diagnosis (Darley, 1991). **Appraisal** refers to the collection of data, whereas **diagnosis** represents the end result of studying and interpreting these data. Therefore, the appraisal portion of our assessment would answer the two questions previously stated concerning what information we actually need and how we gather that information. Appraisal is a very important aspect of our assessment. The collection of too little or unspecific information will not provide enough data for an adequate diagnosis. At the other extreme, collecting too much or unnecessary data is wasting the client's and clinician's valuable time. Therefore, professional assessment demands qualified (and verifiable) decisions throughout the appraisal process.

This chapter deals with the appraisal portion of assessment. Its first goal is to identify the constituent parts of an appraisal—that is, the different types of data needed for a comprehensive diagnosis. These parts will be identified and procedures outlined for each of the appraisal methods. The second goal is to emphasize the clinician's role in choosing among available measures—that is, the clinical decision-making process leading to the selection of instruments serving each individual client maximally. Because the selection of appraisal instruments will necessarily influence the interpretation of the collected data, every appropriate choice will lead to a more complete diagnosis. Effective assessments are essential for clinical procedures; they lead us through the entire diagnostic and therapeutic process.

BOX 6.1   Interviewing and Obtaining Case History Information: Bibliographical Sources

Crowe, T. (Ed.). (1997). *Applications of counseling in speech-language pathology and audiology.* Baltimore: Lippincott Williams and Wilkins.

Haynes, W. O., & Pindzola, R. H. (2004). *Diagnosis and evaluation in speech pathology* (6th ed.). Boston: Allyn & Bacon.

Rollin, W. (2000). *Counseling individuals with communication disorders* (2nd ed.). Boston: Butterworth-Heineman.

Ruscello, D. M. (2000). *Tests and measurements in speech language pathology.* Woburn, MA: Butterworth-Heinemann.

Shipley, K. G., & McAfee, J. G. (2004). *Assessment in speech-language pathology: A resource manual* (3rd ed.). San Diego, CA: Singular Thomson Learning.

Shipley, K. G., & Roseberry-McKibbin, C. (2006). *Interviewing and counseling in communicative disorders: Principles and procedures.* Austin, TX: Pro-Ed.

Tomblin, J. B., Morris, H. L., & Spriestersbach, D. C. (2000). *Diagnosis in speech-language pathology* (2nd ed.). San Diego, CA: Singular Thomson Learning.

The collection of data pertains to at least four different areas: (1) the case history, (2) interviews with parents and other professionals, (3) school and medical records, and (4) the evaluation by the clinician. Procedures and information important for the first three areas are covered in many texts. Selected sources are given in Box 6.1. This chapter will cover only the fourth and most specific task, the evaluation by the clinician.

EVALUATION BY THE CLINICIAN

Clinicians collect data in two different ways: through a procedure known as screening or through a more comprehensive evaluation.

A **screening** consists of activities or tests that identify individuals who merit further evaluation. A screening procedure does not collect nearly enough data to establish a diagnosis; it only demonstrates the need for further testing. Screening measures can be formal or informal. Formal measures include elicitation procedures, which often have normative data and cutoff scores. Informal measures are typically devised by the examiner and may be directed toward a particular population or age level. Screenings are typically used to give the clinician an initial impression of a large group of children. For example, public schools may screen all kindergarten and first-grade children. Screenings are beneficial for those individuals who "fail" the procedure and are later more comprehensively evaluated. Screenings are not always reliable in that some individuals may "pass" the procedure but still demonstrate impairments. Screenings were not devised to serve as a database for a diagnosis; they are too limited in their scope. In contrast, a **comprehensive evaluation** is a series of activities and tests that allows a more detailed and complete collection of data. A *comprehensive phonetic-phonemic evaluation* is the core of the appraisal for articulatory/phonological impairments. It includes data from the following sources:

- an articulation test and stimulability measures
- conversational speech assessment in varying contexts
- hearing testing
- speech mechanism examination
- the possible selection of additional measures such as language testing, perceptual performance, contextual testing, and/or cognitive assessment (Bernthal and Bankson, 2004; Lowe, 1994)

The following section will examine each of these portions of the appraisal process, begin-

ning with an initial impression and its usefulness in the collection of data.

INITIAL IMPRESSION

Clinicians can start collecting data even before the formal appraisal actually begins—for example, by closely observing the conversation between the caregiver and the child, the teacher and the child in a classroom situation, or the child communicating with his or her peers. This initial contact will provide an important first impression. The task is to notice certain features of the conversation and put them onto a simple form like the one in Figure 6.1. Although more and other variables have to be considered later, this record of the initial impression is meant to aid in planning and organizing the remainder of the assessment.

If the initial impression is that the child is partly or totally intelligible, then the next step, the collection of data from an articulation test, could be initiated. If, on the other hand, the initial impression yields an unintelligible child, additional procedures for data collection may need to be considered, especially for the spontaneous speech sample. Very young children, dialect speakers, and individuals with English as a second language will all require additional considerations. Guidelines for these populations are found later in this chapter.

ARTICULATION TESTS

Some Advantages and Disadvantages of Articulation Tests

Articulation tests are typically designed to elicit spontaneous naming based on the presentation of pictures. Most consonants of General American English are tested in

Figure 6.1   Sample Form for the Initial Impression

Name _____   Age _____

Conversational partner _____   Date _____

Intelligibility

Good _____   Partly intelligible _____   Unintelligible _____

Single-word responses and continuous speech show comparable intelligibility _____

Single-word responses are more intelligible than continuous speech _____

General overview of misarticulations

Affects consonants _____

Affects consonants and vowels _____

Noted misarticulations _____

_____

_____

Other factors affecting intelligibility (for example, hyper- or denasality, vocal loudness or quality, rate of speech)

_____

Caregiver's/teacher's/peer's response to misarticulations

No response _____   Asks for repetition _____   Tries to correct _____

Child's response to parent's/caregiver's intervention _____

_____

_____

the initial, medial, and final positions of words.

There are several advantages to using an articulation test. First, these tests are relatively easy to give and score; the necessary time expenditure is usually minimal. This is an attractive feature for those who feel limited in the time they can spend with appraisal procedures. Second, the results provide the clinician with a quantifiable list of "incorrect" sound productions in different word positions. This is clearly relevant to further assessment and planning of therapy. Third, several of the tests provide standardized scores. These scores allow the clinician to compare the individual client's performance with the performance of other children of a similar age. In addition, these scores could be used to document the client's need for, and progress in, therapy.

There are, however, also several problems inherent in articulation tests. Many of them have already been discussed (see Chapter 2 and Chapter 5) and can be summarized as follows:

1. An articulation test examines sound artic-ulation in selected isolated words. How-ever, eliciting sounds based on single-word responses can never give adequate infor-mation on the client's production realities in connected speech. Sound articulation within selected words may not be repre-sentative of the child's ability to produce a particular sound under natural speech conditions.

2. Articulation tests do not give enough in-formation about the client's phonological system. Articulation tests are measures of speech sound production; they are pho-netic tests. As such, they were never meant to provide enough assessment data for a phonological analysis. Although some spontaneous naming measures analyze sounds in error according to phonological processes, the information they provide is not enough for a comprehensive phono-logical analysis.

3. Articulation tests do not test all sounds in all the contexts in which they occur in General American English. Although this would admittedly be a rather large task, some articulation tests do not even test all of the speech sounds of General American English. If scored according to the direc-tions provided, most articulation tests do not test vowels, for example, and very few consonant clusters are sampled.

4. The sounds actually tested do not occur in comparable phonetic contexts; that is, they are not context controlled. For exam-ple, the sounds before and after the tested consonants are different from word to word. The words used are also of varying lengths and complexities. This presents the child with a task that changes in its production difficulty from word to word.

5. Articulation tests, like all standardized tests, are selected probes into rather limited aspects of an individual's total articulatory behavior and/or abilities. An articulation test examines only a very small portion of that child's articulatory behavior—it explores the child's speech performance with particular test items, on a certain day, in a unique testing situation. It would not be realistic to generalize that such limited results represent a reliable measure of the client's articulatory abilities, let alone the client's phonological system.

Factors to Consider When Selecting a Measure of Articulation

When selecting a measure of speech sound competency, several factors are important. In addition to the test's construct and its tech-nical characteristics, the following should be considered: (1) the test's appropriateness for the age or developmental level of the client, (2) the test's ability to supply a standardized score, (3) the test's analysis of the sound errors, and (4) the test's inclusion of an adequate sam-ple of the sound(s) relevant to the individual client at hand.

Appropriateness for the Age or Developmental Level of the Client. Although the age ranges vary, most tests can be administered to chil-dren from approximately 3 years to school age. Selection becomes a troublesome issue for very young and for older adolescent or adult clients. Younger clients, and this may include 2-year-olds or delayed 3- and 4-year-olds, may not re-spond well to a formal articulation test. Some younger children might react better to those tests that contain large colored pictures. For other children, the naming of actual objects or spontaneous speech may be the only way to assess sound production skills. For the evaluation of adolescent or adult clients, two problems exist. First, many of the tests are not standardized for children beyond the ages of 12 or 13. In addition, most articulation tests are oriented toward a much younger population. This may prove demeaning for older adolescents and adults and therefore is inappropriate. Certain articulation tests contain printed sentences that can be read by clients. Although the sentence content and the reading level are designed for early school-age children, articulation tests that provide sentences to be read might prove less of a problem for older clients.

> Later in this chapter, the section on Special Considerations will examine alternative ways to assess younger clients with emerging phonological systems.

Ability to Provide a Standardized Score. Some articulation tests are not standardized; that is, standardized scores are not available as outcome measures. Therefore, the results obtained from a client cannot be compared to the performance of other children of a similar age. If it is important that the results of an articulation test yield standardized scores, tests should be selected correspondingly.

Analysis of the Sound Errors. There are many different tests to choose from. Some are labeled articulation tests, whereas others purport to be tests of *phonology*. Articulation tests and tests of phonology do not differ in their examination format (both use the same format: spontaneous picture naming) but in their analysis of the results. Typically, tests of phonology categorize misarticulations according to phonological processes. Although the clinician could go through any articulation test noting the number and type of phonological processes used, those tests that already contain such a procedure will probably allow the clinician a more expedient assessment.

CLINICAL APPLICATION

Using Articulation Tests to Examine Phonological Processes

The evaluation of phonological processes is a portion of several articulation tests (e.g., Assessment Link between Phonology and Articulation [ALPHA], Lowe, 1996; Bankson-Bernthal Test of Phonology, Bankson and Bernthal, 1990; and Khan-Lewis Phonological Analysis, which uses the responses from the Goldman-Fristoe Test of Articulation, Khan and Lewis, 2002). Phonological processes can be determined from the results of any articulation test. The clinician examines the results of the articulation test and notes the phonological processes employed. The following is an example from the PAT-3: Photo Articulation Test (Lippke, Dickey, Selmar, and Soder, 1997):

Word	Child's Response	Phonological Process
saw	[tɑ]	stopping [s] → [t]
pencil	[pɛnθəl]	consonant cluster substitution [ns] → [nθ], fronting [s] → [θ]
house	[haʊ]	final consonant deletion [s] → ø
spoon	[pun]	consonant cluster reduction [sp] → [p]
skates	[keɪtθ]	consonant cluster reduction [sk] → [k]
		consonant cluster substitution [ts] → [tθ], fronting
stars	[tɑɚ]	consonant cluster reduction [st] → [t]
		final consonant deletion [z] → ø*
zipper	[dɪpɚ]	stopping [z] → [d]

*In this example, the production is characterized as a final consonant deletion because [ɑɚ] is considered a centering diphthong.

Which phonological processes are operating and how often they occurred could then be analyzed.

Test's Inclusion of an Adequate Sample of the Sound or Sounds Relevant for the Individual Client. Articulation tests typically contain words that sample the sound inventory of General American English. Thus, most of the consonants of General American English are tested within the test. However, most articulation tests do not sample the most frequently misarticulated sounds in a large number of different contexts. For example, the [s] may be tested in only two or three different words. An adequate number of words containing the sound in various word positions is often not available. Supplemental testing with additional words can always be achieved later, but a test that provides adequate goal-directed material for individual clients uses our diagnostic time more efficiently.

Assessment Procedures to Supplement Articulation Tests

Which assessment strategies, then, can be employed to minimize the previously mentioned shortcomings of articulation tests?

1. *If a word contains any aberrant vowel or consonant productions, transcribe the entire word.* This gives valuable additional information about the client's sound production skills. For example, assume that the tested word is *yellow*, that the initial [j] is being evaluated, and that the child says [jɛwoᵘ]. According to the scoring instructions, the initial [j] would be noted as being "correct" and the clinician would

> Articulation tests are often referred to as citation-form testing. The *citation form* refers to the spoken form of a word produced in isolation, as distinguished from the form it would have when produced in conversational speech. Both citation-form testing and spontaneous speech sampling should be used to collect data for a comprehensive evaluation.

continue on to the next item. However, if the entire word has been transcribed, the clinician can later evaluate the [l] production and compare it to the other words on the test that contain [l]. (In addition, some articulation measures test only sounds in the initial and final word positions; however, some clients demonstrate difficulties with medial productions.) Transcribing the entire word complements the test information considerably and supplies insights into vowels and consonant cluster productions as well.

2. *Supplement the articulation test with additional utterances that address the noted problems of the client.* The target sound(s) should be sampled in various vowel contexts and word positions, for example. There are several ways to do this. One is to develop a list of words containing the needed sound(s). This has the advantage of tailoring the supplemental materials to exactly fit the client's needs. One could also use commercially prepared materials. Two examples are McDonald's Deep Test of Articulation (McDonald, 1964) and Secord's Clinical Probes of Articulation Consistency (C-PAC) (Secord, 1981a). McDonald's deep test uses pictures to elicit a compound word, such as *hot + dog = hotdog*. The words formed are not typical compound words of General American English; however, a variety of phonetic contexts can be sampled this way. The C-PAC assesses the targeted consonant before and after various vowels (in one-syllable words, consonants initiating and terminating the word), in consonant clusters, in sentences, and during storytelling. For children who cannot read, the elicitation mode is imitative. These commercially available protocols have the advantage of assessing a sound in a variety of contexts without any preparation on the part of the clinician.

3. *Always sample and record continuous speech.* Although it has been well documented that production differences exist in children between single-word tasks (citing) and spontaneous speech (talking) (e.g., Andrews and Fey, 1986; DuBois and Bernthal, 1978; Faircloth and Faircloth, 1970; Morrison and Shriberg, 1992; Shriberg and Kwiatkowski, 1985; Stoel-Gammon and Dunn, 1985), many practitioners continue to use articulation tests as the sole basis for their analysis procedures. Morrison and Shriberg (1992) state that "citation-form testing yields neither typical nor optimal measures of speech performance" (p. 271). An articulation test is not good enough for the appraisal and diagnosis of clients with phonetic and/or phonemic disorders. See the section on spontaneous speech sampling for further information.

4. *Determine the stimulability of the error sounds.* This task can be easily and relatively quickly accomplished at the end of an articulation test. See the following section on stimulability testing.

Organizing Articulation Test Results: Describing the Error

Most articulation tests include a form that can be used to record the client's responses. By completing this form, the clinician obtains information about the accuracy of the sound articulation and the position of this sound within the test word. Each articulation test gives directions on how to record accurate and inaccurate sound realizations. To describe sound errors, there are at least three different scoring systems (Shriberg and Kent, 2003). The following scoring systems are available:

Two-Way Scoring.   A choice is made between a production that is "right" (accurate articulation of the sound in question) and "wrong" (inaccurate articulation). Two-way scoring can be used effectively to give feedback to the client and to document therapy progress. It can also be used in a screening protocol. However,

because of its limitations and its inability to render any usable information about the kind of aberrant articulation taking place, the two-way scoring system is inappropriate for the scoring of articulation tests.

Five-Way Scoring.   This system uses a classification based on the type of error. "Correct," or norm productions, constitute one category. The other four categories are (1) deletion or omission—that is, a sound is deleted completely; (2) substitution—a sound is replaced by another sound; (3) distortion—the target sound is approximated but not closely enough to be considered a norm realization; and (4) addition—a sound or sounds are added to the intended sound. The five-way scoring system is commonly suggested in the manuals of articulation tests. However, this system has several inherent problems.

First, articulation tests often do not define, or give examples of, which articulatory patterns are considered within normal limits. There are many dialectal and contextual variations that could result in a somewhat different but entirely acceptable pronunciation. For example, the alveolar flap [ɾ] is a common pronunciation for [d] in *ladder*. Should this variation be considered "correct" if the medial d-sound is being tested? Clinicians should be aware of these common variations and how they may impact their scoring. Second, the category of deletion or omission may include the presence, rather than the absence, of a sound. Normally, deletion implies that a sound segment has been eliminated, as in [mu] for *moon,* for example. However, Van Riper and Irwin (1958) include glottal stops, unvoiced articulatory placements, and short exhalations under omissions as well. If the production of [wæʔən] for *wagon* is considered, according to these authors, the [g] would be classified as a deletion. Actually, it would be more accurate to label this as a substitution of a glottal stop for

[g]. This ambiguous definition of deletion can detract from the accuracy of the results when sound realizations are later analyzed. Third, the terms *substitution* and *distortion* have a long history of definitional unclarity. Some authors (Van Riper, 1978; Van Riper and Irwin, 1958; Winitz, 1975) state that a more precise way of considering distortions is to regard them as substitutions of non-English sounds. For example, a child produces [ʃ] in which the organ and place of articulation is too far back; that is, rather than prepalatal, it has a palatal placement. There is a palatal fricative, transcribed as [ç], that is a regular speech sound in many languages. Therefore, this palatal [ʃ] production could be designated either as a distortion of [ʃ] or as a substitution of [ç] for [ʃ]. Such vagueness in regard to what constitutes a distortion versus a substitution can also impact the scoring of many articulation tests.

Phonetic Transcription. Transcription systems describe speech behavior. The goal of any phonetic transcription is to represent spoken language by written symbols. Of the three scoring systems mentioned, phonetic transcription requires the highest degree of clinical skill. The goal is not to *judge* specific misarticulations but to *describe* them as accurately as possible. Phonetic transcription has several advantages over the other two systems: (1) it is far more precise; (2) it gives more information about the misarticulation, which is helpful for both assessment and intervention; and (3) among professionals, it is the most universally accepted way to communicate information about articulatory features. Phonetic transcription uses broad transcription of the speech sounds of General American English and narrow transcription, diacritics that further delineate the characteristics of the sounds produced. Both broad and narrow transcription are indispensable for a comprehensive evaluation. This scoring system will be used for the following analyses of citation articulation tests as well as spontaneous speech sampling.

Stimulability Testing

Another assessment procedure often used by clinicians during the appraisal process is stimulability testing. **Stimulability testing** refers to testing the client's ability to produce a misarticulated sound in an appropriate manner when "stimulated" by the clinician to do so. Many variations in this procedure exist, but commonly, the clinician asks the client to "watch and listen to what I am going to say, and then you say it" (Bernthal and Bankson, 2004). Although there is no standardized procedure for stimulability testing, an isolated sound is usually first attempted. If a norm articulation is achieved, the sound is placed within a syllable and subsequently in a word context. The number of models provided by the clinician typically varies from one to five attempts (Diedrich, 1983).

For many clinicians, stimulability testing is a standard procedure concluding the administration of an articulation test. It gives a measure of the consistency of a client's performance on two different tasks: the spontaneous naming of a picture and the imitation of a speech model provided by the clinician. Such information is very helpful in appraising the articulatory capabilities of a client. (See Bleile, 2002; Hodson, Scherz, and Strattman, 2002; Khan, 2002; Lof, 2002; Miccio, 2002; and Tyler and Tolbert, 2002.)

Children's articulatory stimulability has been used to determine therapy goals and to predict which children might benefit more from therapy. It has been suggested that sounds that were more stimulable would be easier to work on in therapy; therefore, highly stimulable sounds would be targeted first (Rvachew and Nowak, 2001). When used as a means of predicting which children might benefit from therapy, high stimulability was correlated with more rapid therapeutic success (Miccio, Elbert, and Forrest, 1999). It was also proposed that high stimulability might mean that children were on the verge of acquiring the sounds and would not even need therapeutic intervention (Khan, 2002). Although stimulability testing seems to be one type of data collected by most clinicians, its effect on treatment targets is still questionable. In her article on treatment efficacy, Gierut (1998) points out that two studies (Klein, Lederer, and Cortese, 1991; Powell, Elbert, and Dinnsen, 1991) have documented that targeting nonstimulable sounds prompted change in those sounds *and* other untreated stimulable sounds. In comparison, treatment of a stimulable sound did not necessarily lead to changes in untreated stimulable or nonstimulable sounds. Gierut concludes that treatment of nonstimulable sounds may be more efficient than treatment of stimulable sounds due to the widespread change that seems to occur. However, another study (Rvachew, Rafaat, and Martin, 1999) noted lack of treatment progress on nonstimulable sounds when compared to stimulable ones.

As a portion of the data collected in a client's appraisal, stimulability testing gives useful information. However, stimulability testing should not be the only source when deciding whether a client receives services or which therapy sequence to choose.

$\mathcal{S}$PONTANEOUS SPEECH SAMPLE

Over the years, numerous authors have documented the differences that exist in children's speech when single-word citing responses are compared to spontaneous speech (e.g., Andrews and Fey, 1986; Campbell and Shriberg, 1982; DuBois and Bernthal, 1978; Healy

and Madison, 1987; Hoffman, Schuckers, and Daniloff, 1989; Klein, 1984; Masterson, Bernhardt, and Hofheinz, 2005; Menyuk, 1980; Morrison and Shriberg, 1992; Wolk and Meisler, 1998). However, assessment and treatment protocols continue to be based primarily on the results of citation articulation tests. Some clinicians may argue that they don't have time to complete the transcription and analysis of a spontaneous speech sample. However, these samples can serve many different functions. For example, conversational speech samples can supply additional information about the language, voice, and prosodic capabilities of the client. Specific semantic, morphosyntactical, and pragmatic analyses could supplement additional language testing when required. The conversational speech sample is not optional, but rather a basic necessity for every professional appraisal.

Although any conversational speech sample is more representative of a client's production capabilities than a one-word citation-form test, the type of sampling situation also plays a role. Several authors have found an increase or decrease in errors depending on the production task required. First, more complex linguistic contents generally cause an increase in misarticulations (Panagos and Prelock, 1982; Panagos, Quine, and Klich, 1979; Schmauch, Panagos, and Klich, 1978). Second, different communicative needs can also influence production accuracy. For example, Menyuk (1980) reported the improvement of speech patterns in five children when they were trying to relate information that was important to them.

Organizing the Continuous Speech Sample

A continuous speech sample should be planned and executed in a systematic manner in order to minimize the time investment and maximize the results. Here are some suggestions.

Begin with the Articulation Test. One goal of a continuous speech sample in a comprehensive assessment is to compare the child's productions on a single-word citation task to those in continuous speech. Errors that have been noted in single words can be helpful in planning the continuous speech sample. For example, if the child demonstrates error productions for [s], [ʃ], [tʃ], [dʒ], and [l] on the articulation test, or if the articulation test does not sample particular sounds, these could be targeted.

Provide Objects or Pictures that May Elicit Targeted Sounds. Objects and pictures containing the targeted sounds can then become a portion of the spontaneous speech procedure. Comparability between citing and talking tasks could be increased by attempting to trigger some of the same words that were on the articulation test.

Plan the Length of the Sample. There has been a lot of discussion about which sample length furnishes adequate information for a comprehensive assessment. Grunwell (1987) states that "100 different words is the minimum size of an adequate sample; 200–250 words is preferable" (p. 55). On the other hand, Crary (1983) found that 50-word samples for process analysis provided as much information as 100-word speech samples. Unfortunately, this problem does not have an easy solution. Although 50 words seems more palatable, a sample of that size might not give the needed information.

It should be kept in mind that in normal conversation, children articulate between 100 and 200 syllables per minute (Culatta, Page, and Wilson, 1987). Therefore, three minutes of conversational speech should render approximately 450 syllables or, depending on the length of each word, about 200 words. In most cases this will probably constitute an adequate sample. If allowances are made for nonspeech events, interaction with the clinician, and deletion of certain portions due to lack of intelligibility, a 200- to 250-word sample should take no more than ten to fifteen minutes to record. With most children, much of the transcription can be attained spontaneously. Assuming that another ten to fifteen minutes is required later to transcribe portions of the sample from tape, the total recording and transcribing time amounts to around thirty minutes. In light of the acquisition of needed information for goal-directed therapy, this is not a large time investment. Perhaps a lack of the necessary transcription skills deters clinicians more than the actual time involvement.

Plan Diversity into the Sample. Various communicative situations should be a portion of the recorded speech sample. A variety of situations will ensure that the sample adequately represents the phonetic and phonemic skills of the client. This may include several different talking situations, such as picture description, storytelling, describing the function of objects, or problem solving. Communicative diversity could also include the client talking with caregivers or siblings. The recording time for each different sample needs to be only two to three minutes. Varying communicative situations will also allow for articulatory differences that occur between pragmatically and linguistically diverse samples.

Monitor Your Recording and Gloss Any Utterances that Might Later Be Difficult or Impossible to Understand from the Taped Recording. Diligent monitoring will ensure that the quality of the recording remains constant. This can mean anything from readjusting the microphone if the client moves to asking the client to repeat an utterance if it is not completely intelligible. It is helpful and often necessary to gloss the word or phrase, especially if later transcription difficulties are anticipated. **Glossing** means repeating with normal pronunciation what the client has just said for easier identification later. This can be done quite naturally so that it will not interfere with the structured situation.

Transcribe As Much of the Spontaneous Speech Sample As Possible during the Recording.   Live transcriptions have the advantage of capturing phonetic detail that may be lost with a tape recording. They also decrease the subsequent transcription time. In addition, listening to one or two minutes of conversation before transcribing may dramatically increase transcription effectiveness due to the clinician's adjustment to the client's pronunciation patterns. Unintelligible utterances should be clearly marked (language sampling techniques use a series of *X*s to note unintelligibility). It is not necessary to spend a considerable amount of time trying to decipher these responses. Instead, it is better to gloss the utterance whenever the intelligibility of the response might be later questioned.

$\mathcal{E}$VALUATION OF THE SPEECH MECHANISM

An evaluation of both the structure and the function of the client's speech mechanism is a prerequisite for any comprehensive appraisal. Its intent is to assess whether the system appears adequate for regular speech sound production. At first glance, the examination of the speech-motor system looks like a relatively simple procedure that has often been described. However, the interpretation of the results is not necessarily as straightforward as it would seem.

It might be beneficial to view the results of the evaluation of the speech mechanism along a continuum in which one end indicates nor-

mal structure and function while the other end indicates grossly deviant structural and/or functional inadequacies. At the normal end of the continuum, assume that the client has passed all required procedures. This is commonly the case, and no further speech-motor testing appears to be necessary—the client has passed the oral-speech assessment.

At the other end of the continuum, results could show such a pronounced structural or functional aberration from norm that an organic cause of the speech difficulties needs to be concluded. If organicity is noted, further testing by the clinician and/or referral to a medical expert are warranted.

Between the endpoints of this continuum exists a broad range of structural and functional deviations that may or may not directly impact the adequate production of speech sounds. Often, clinicians will find minor structural and/or functional inadequacies that don't appear severe enough to be considered "organic," yet certainly do not qualify as "passing." Interpreting such results is often difficult. Our evaluation of the speech mechanism is actually just a screening measure requiring more testing and possible referral when any functional and/or structural inadequacies are found. One possible screening form for the evaluation of the speech-motor system is summarized in Appendix 6.1.

What to Look for When Evaluating the Speech Mechanism

Examining the Head and Facial Structures.   One of the first impressions is provided by simply observing the client's face and head. Sitting opposite the client, first evaluate the size and the shape of the head. Relative to the body size, the head should appear normal—not too large and not too small. In addition, the shape should be considered. The relationship between the cranium (the upper portion of the skull containing the brain) and the facial skeleton (the lower portion of the skull containing, among other structures, the articulators) should be evaluated. The cranial portion should not appear too large nor the facial area too small or vice versa. Micrognathia, for example, is marked by an unusually small jaw. Next, the symmetry of the facial features should be inspected. Do the right and left sides of the face appear fairly similar both in proportion and in overall appearance? *Proportion* refers to the structures on both sides being on corresponding planes and their dimensions being similar on both sides. For example, right and left eyes are level and both appear to be about the same size. *Appearance* refers to the overall shape of the structures in question and to the normal state of resting muscle—that is, to the muscular tone. Oddly shaped eyes, nose, or mouth would be a deviancy within this category. In addition, any drooping of the structures or lack of muscle tone on one side of the face should be noted. At rest, the right and left sides of the lips should be even, the red of the lips, or vermilion, forming a smooth curve. Appearance and proportions of the nares (the nostrils), the nasal septum (the structural division of the nose, dividing the nasal cavity into right and left halves), the philtrum (the vertical groove between the upper lip and the nasal septum), and the columella (the vertical ridges on either side of the philtrum) should be evaluated. In short, any striking features of the head and face should be noted. This would include a fairly common syndrome called adenoid facies. Adenoid facies is the result of chronic or repeated infections that lead to enlarged adenoids, mouth breathing, a shortening of the upper lip, and an elongated face (Zemlin, 1998).

Examining Breathing. Respiration can be indirectly observed by examining breathing patterns. The clinician should observe and evaluate the client's breathing patterns at rest (silent breathing) and during speech. During silent breathing, the client's mouth should be closed with no noticeable clavicular breathing (excursions in the clavicular area that cause the shoulders to move up and down during breathing). In addition, during silent breathing, the amount of time between the inspiratory and expiratory phases should be fairly equal. Therefore, an approximately one-to-one relationship exists between the time for inspiration and for expiration. During speech production, the normal time relationship between inspiratory and expiratory phases is somewhere between one and two+; that is, depending on the length of the utterance, the expiratory phase should be at least twice as long as the inspiratory. Any irregularities in breathing patterns should be noted. This includes irregular breathing patterns, muscular jerks or spasms during breathing, forced inhalations or exhalations, or any other (especially recurrent) conspicuous respiratory movements.

Examining the Oral and Pharyngeal Cavity Structures. The structures involved in this area of the speech mechanism examination include the teeth, the tongue, the palate, and pharyngeal areas.

The Teeth. First, the occlusion of the teeth is important. Normal occlusion (Class I) is characterized by the lower molars being one-half of a tooth ahead of the upper molars. There are several different types of malocclusions, including Class II malocclusion (overbite), Class III malocclusion (underbite), open bite, and cross bite. (Definitions of these malocclusions are given in Appendix 6.1.) Next, the clinician should check to see if all teeth are present and whether the spacing and their axial orientation appear adequate. The *axial orientation* of the teeth refers to the positioning of the individual teeth. Abnormalities in this respect would pertain to irregularly "tipped" or rotated teeth. Malocclusions of the teeth and missing teeth may affect the production of specific speech sounds.

The Tongue. First, examine the size of the tongue in its relationship to the size of the oral cavity. Does it appear too large, overfilling the oral cavity (macroglossia), or does it seem too small for the cavity size (microglossia)? Both of these conditions would signal a deviancy. In addition, the tongue's appearance is examined to see if the color appears normal and if the muscular dorsum of the tongue demonstrates a healthy muscle tone. Any "shriveled" tongue appearance might signal a paralytic condition. Next, the surface of the tongue needs to be observed. It should be relatively smooth. Any fissures (grooves or cracks in the dorsum of the tongue), lesions (wounds or abrasion), and fasciculations (any visible "bundling" of muscles) would indicate a deviancy. Finally, the tongue needs to be examined in its resting position. It should look symmetrical without any muscular twitching or movements.

The Hard and Soft Palate. Up until this point, the clinician has observed just structures. Examination of the hard and soft palate goes beyond observation. It necessitates feeling structures with your finger and evaluating structures within the pharyngeal cavity. Therefore, it is necessary that the clinician wear examining gloves and be equipped with a small penlight to carry out the task. The hard palate's color, the size and shape of the palatal vault, and the presence or absence of clefts, fissures, and fistulas (openings or holes in the palate) are determined. The midline of the hard and soft palates is usually a pink and whitish color; a blue tint may suggest a submucous cleft. To exclude this possibility, the clinician should feel along the midline of the hard palate to ensure that the underlying bony structure is intact. The uvula should be examined and its length and any structural abnormalities noted. A bifid uvula (a uvula that is split into two portions), for example, may indicate a submucous cleft. Finally, the fauces (the passage between the oral and the pharyngeal cavities) and the pharyngeal area itself need to be assessed. Excessive redness or a swollen appearance of the tonsils and/or adenoids might indicate an inflammation and warrants medical referral.

Functionally Assessing the Speech Mechanism. The functional integrity of the speech mechanism is as important as adequate structures. In this portion of the assessment, the movement patterns of the lips, mandible, tongue, and velum are examined. For the purpose at hand, proper function means not only that the client can move the structures on command but also that the range, smoothness, and speed of the movements are adequate. As the client is performing the various tasks, the clinician should pay attention to the following:

1. Can the client adequately perform the task?
2. Is the range of movements adequate?
3. Are the movements integrated and smooth?
4. Given the age of the client, is the speed of movement within normal limits?

If the client cannot move individual structures on command but movements are noted during involuntary tasks—for example, the client cannot stick out the tongue when asked to do so but can stick out the tongue to lick a postage stamp—this could in-

> The sections on childhood apraxia of speech and apraxia of speech in adults in Chapter 10 will offer further suggestions in this area.

dicate an apraxic condition. Further testing becomes necessary. The major goal of this portion of the assessment is to determine whether the functional integrity of the articulators appears adequate. Isolated functional deviancies do not necessarily translate into an inability to articulate certain speech sounds. They only suggest motor problems. Such functional difficulties should be evaluated in light of the client's articulatory performance, articulatory limitations, and intelligibility. Several different functional tasks for lips, mandible, tongue, and velum are indicated in Appendix 6.1.

SELECTION OF ADDITIONAL ASSESSMENT MEASURES

Approximately 80 percent of the clinical population with "delayed speech" have associated language problems (Keating, Turrell, and Ozanne, 2001; Shriberg, 1991; Shriberg, Kwiatkowski, Best, Hengst, and Terselic-Weber, 1986; Shriberg, Kwiatkowski, and Rasmussen, 1990; Toppelberg, Shapiro, and Theodore, 2000). Therefore, language testing is recommended for every child who has a phonetic and/or phonemic disorder. In addition, a hearing screening is essential. Other measures may include the testing of specific auditory discrimination skills and an appraisal of the cognitive abilities of the client. Selection of additional tests will largely depend on an evaluation of the background information, medical and/or school records, and the clinical impression of the individual client.

Hearing Screening

A hearing screening is a portion of every assessment procedure. According to the revised set of "Guidelines for Identification Audiometry" (American Speech-Language-Hearing Association [ASHA], 1985) and the "Guidelines for Audiologic Screening" (ASHA, 1997), the following procedures should be a portion of the audiologic screening:

1. taking a history, which includes noting recent episodes of ear pain (otalgia) and/or ear discharge (otorrhea)
2. visual inspection to determine the presence of structural defects, and ear-canal and eardrum abnormalities
3. identification audiometry
4. acoustic immittance measurements

Referral criteria for each are included in Table 6.1.

Especially with children, the clinician should have knowledge of any developmental history that could affect the child's hearing status. This would include a history of episodes of otitis media, "earaches," or the placement of tubes. Shriberg and Kwiatkowski (1982a) verified that one-third of children enrolled in speech or language intervention had histories of recurrent middle-ear disease. Although controversy exists surrounding the exact role chronic otitis media plays in the acquisition of phonology, it may at least interact with other risk factors in some children. This interaction could easily lead to a greater risk of delayed or impaired communication skills.

Language Testing

Due to the high percentage of language problems in children with speech disorders, language screening belongs to the evaluation process. This can be done using formal, standardized assessment measures or informal evaluations. For example, the previously recorded speech sample could be analyzed to determine if morphosyntactic and semantic skills are age-appropriate. As with any screening tool, if the client does not pass the procedure, further testing becomes necessary.

Table 6.1 Referral Criteria for Audiologic Screening

History Information		
Recent history of earaches, ear pain (otalgia)	⟶	Refer
Recent history of ear discharge (otorrhea)	⟶	Refer
Visual Inspection of the Ear		
Structural defect of the ear, head, or neck	⟶	Refer
Ear-canal abnormalities, including blood or effusion, occlusion, inflammation, excessive cerumen, tumor, and/or foreign material	⟶	Refer
Eardrum abnormalities, including abnormal color, bulging eardrum, fluid line or bubbles, perforation, retraction	⟶	Refer
Identification Audiometry		
Procedure: Air conduction screening at 20 dB HL at 1,000, 2,000, and 4,000 Hz*		
Failure to respond at one frequency in either ear	⟶	Refer
Tympanometry		
Procedure: Static admittance, equivalent ear-canal volume, and tympanometric width are used in the screening protocol.		
Flat tympanogram and equivalent ear-canal volume (V_{ec}) outside normal range	⟶	Refer
Low static admittance (Peak Y) on two successive occurrences in a 4–6 week interval	⟶	Refer
Abnormally wide tympanometric width (TW) on two successive occurrences in a 4–6 week interval	⟶	Refer

*According to ASHA (1985, 1997), these criteria may require alteration for various clinical settings and populations.

Source: Summarized from *Guidelines for Screening for Hearing Impairments and Middle Ear Disorders,* 1990. Copyright 1990 by the American Speech-Language-Hearing Association.

Several language screening measures are available for children of all ages. Box 6.2 gives a few examples of standardized and nonstandarized language screening measures for preschool and school-age children.

Specific Auditory Perceptual Testing

For many years, the appraisal of auditory perceptual skills, specifically speech sound discrimination testing, was a standard procedure for all clients with speech sound difficulties.

The reasoning was that faulty speech sound perception often caused, or was linked to, the production problems. This was promoted by earlier works such as Van Riper's (1939b) *Speech Correction,* in which discrimination training was seen as a necessary portion of every therapy sequence.

Investigations into the relationship between auditory discrimination abilities and the production of speech sounds have extended over half a century (e.g., Anderson, 1941; Aungst and Frick, 1964; Cohen and

BOX 6.2 Selected Language Screening Measures for Preschool and School-Age Children

Birth to 3 Years Screening Measures

Brigance, A. (2004). *Brigance inventory of early development—II*. N. Billerica, MA: Curriculum Associates.

Fankenburg, W., Archer, P., Bresnick, B., Dodds, J., Edelman, N., Maschka, P., & Shapiro, H. (1992). *Denver II*. Denver, CO: Denver Developmental Materials Publishing Co.

Glover, M., Preminger, J., & Sanford, A. (2002). *The early learning accomplishment profile for developmentally young children birth to 36 months (E-LAP)*. Lewisville, NC: Kaplan Press.

LeBuffe, P., & Naglieri, J. (2003). *Devereux early childhood assessment*. Lewisville, NC: Kaplan Early Learning Company.

Linder, T. (1993). *Transdisciplinary play-based assessment: A functional approach to working with young children*. Baltimore, MD: Paul H. Brookes.

Newborg, J., Stock, J., Wnek, L., Guibaldi, J., & Suinicki, J. (1984). *Battelle developmental inventory (screening scale)*. Allen, TX: DLM Teaching Resources.

Preschool, School-Age Screening Measures

Blank, M., Rose, S., & Berlin, L. (1978). *Preschool language assessment instrument* (2nd ed.). Austin, TX: PRO-ED.

Gauthier, S., & Madison, C. (1998). *Kindergarten language screening test (KIST-2)* (2nd ed.). Austin, TX: PRO-ED.

Hresko, W., Reid, D., & Hammill, D. (1999). *Test of early language development (TELD-3)* (3rd ed.). Austin, TX: PRO-ED.

Morgan, D., & Guilford, A. (1989). *Adolescent language screening test (ALST)* (3rd ed.). Austin, TX: PRO-ED.

Semel, E., Wiig, E., & Secord, W. (1995). *CELF-3 screening test*. New York: The Psychological Corporation.

Speech-Ease Associates. (1985). *Speech-Ease screening inventory (K–1)*. Austin, TX: PRO-ED.

Diehl, 1963; Hall, 1938; Kronvall and Diehl, 1954; Lapko and Bankson, 1975; Locke, 1980b, 1980c; Mase, 1946; Monnin and Huntington, 1974; Prins, 1963; Travis and Rasmus, 1931; Williams and McReynolds, 1975; Winitz, 1969; Winitz, Sanders, and Kort, 1981). The results of these and many other studies were inconclusive: Some investigators found a positive relationship between auditory discrimination and articulation skills but others did not. Several reasons for the variation of these results have been suggested (Schwartz and Goldman, 1974; Sherman and Geith, 1967; Weiner, 1967; Winitz, 1984). These different outcomes, however, did not support the cause–effect relationship earlier hypothesized. As a result of these findings, auditory discrimination testing seemed to lose much of its value as a standard assessment procedure.

Currently, speech sound discrimination testing is typically done only with those clients who demonstrate a collapse of two or more phonemic contrasts into a single sound (Bernthal and Bankson, 2004). If a child substitutes [w] for [r] and [l], this would exemplify the collapse of three phonemic contrasts into a single sound: /w/, /r/, and /l/ would all be represented by the phoneme /w/. Auditory discrimination testing is a means of ascertaining whether clients who do not utilize phonemic contrasts might also not perceive the difference between these contrasts.

Within the last few years, auditory discrimination testing has departed from the testing of general discrimination skills. General tests of auditory discrimination would include measures such as the Auditory Discrimination Test (Wepman, 1973) and the Goldman-Fristoe-Woodcock Diagnostic Auditory Discrimination Test (Goldman, Fristoe, and Woodcock, 1970). Although these tests are designed to measure general auditory deficiencies, they do not give enough information about the discrimination skills of specific phonemic collapses noted in individual clients. Both Locke (1980c) and Winitz (1984) advocate the use of specific auditory discrimination testing that (1) is tailored to the individual client, (2) considers the client's speech sound difficulties or the collapse of the particular phonemic contrasts, and (3) includes the productionally problematic phonetic environment in words and in more meaningful sentence contexts.

Speech Production Perception Task (Locke, 1980c). This task utilizes selected stimuli based on the child's aberrant productions. The clinician first identifies these productions. For example, the child says [wæmp] for *lamp*. The norm production [læmp] and the child's production [wæmp] are now used to construct the perception task. The norm production is identified as the *stimulus production* (SP) and the child's aberrant production as the *response production* (RP). A perceptually similar third phoneme, the *control production* (CP), is also used when constructing the task. In this case, [ræmp] could be selected. Next, the clinician presents a picture of the stimulus production, in this example a picture of a lamp. The child is then asked "Is this a _____?" The three stimuli—stimulus production, response production, and control production—are presented in a random order. Figure 6.2 exemplifies this perception task.

Discrimination Testing and the Phonological Performance Analysis (Winitz, 1984). Winitz offers additional suggestions that could be incorporated into the assessment of auditory discrimination skills of clients:

1. *The test items should be relevant and client oriented.* General auditory discrimination tests are not a good measure of the client's difficulties. If a child produces [r] incorrectly, for example, tasks should concentrate on the child's discrimination of [r] and not of [l] or [t].
2. *The specific aberrant productions of the client should be targeted.* The client's production should be contrasted to the norm production of the sound in question. If a child lateralizes [s], the child's abilities to discriminate between a lateral [s] and a regular [s] should be examined. Therefore, the clinician must be able to replicate any of the client's distortions.
3. *The phonetic context in which the incorrect productions occur must be considered.* The clinician must know whether the client's production occurs in the word-initial, -medial, or -final position; in singletons or in consonant clusters; or with specific vowels, for example. If a child evidences deletion of [z] at the end of a word, the discrimination testing should emphasize the presence versus the absence of [z] in this position—for example, *toe* versus *toes.* Similarly, a child who produces an unrounded [ʃ] preceding front vowels should be tested with words with front vowels— for example, *ship, sheep,* and *sheet.*

Winitz (1984) also proposes that a phonological performance analysis supplement the aforementioned auditory discrimination tasks. The purpose of such an analysis is to determine whether children perceive the distinction between contrastive sounds that they misarticulate. Although the previous suggestions are guidelines for appraising all clients with speech sound difficulties, the phonological performance analysis is appropriate for those who demonstrate the collapse of two (or more) phonemic contrasts. Minimal pairs containing the respective phoneme contrasts are embedded in sets of three identical sentences with a somewhat connected topic. Each set of sentences has an appro-

Figure 6.2 Speech Production Perception Task

| Child's Name _____ | Sex: M F | Birthdate: _____ |
| | | Age: _____ |

Date _____		Date _____		Date _____	
Production Task					
Stimulus	Response*	Stimulus	Response	Stimulus	Response
[læmp]	[wæmp]	[ ]	[ ]	[ ]	[ ]
SP /l/ RP /w/	CP /r/	SP / / RP / /	CP / /	SP / / RP / /	CP / /
Stimulus	Response	Stimulus	Response	Stimulus	Response
1. [ræmp]	yes NO	1.	1.		
2. [wæmp]	yes NO	2.	2.		
3. [læmp]	YES no	3.	3.		
4. [læmp]	YES no	4.	4.		
5. [wæmp]	yes NO	5.	5.		
6. [ræmp]	yes NO	6.	6.		
7. [ræmp]	yes NO	7.	7.		
8. [læmp]	YES no	8.	8.		
9. [wæmp]	yes NO	9.	9.		
10. [læmp]	YES no	10.	10.		
11. [wæmp]	yes NO	11.	11.		
12. [ræmp]	yes NO	12.	12.		
13. [wæmp]	yes NO	13.	13.		
14. [læmp]	YES no	14.	14.		
15. [ræmp]	yes NO	15.	15.		
16. [wæmp]	yes NO	16.	16.		
17. [læmp]	YES no	17.	17.		
18. [ræmp]	yes NO	18.	18.		
RP____ CP____ SP____		RP____ CP____ SP____		RP____ CP____ SP____	

*The correct response is in uppercase letters.

Source: From "The Inference of Speech Perception in the Phonologically Disordered Child, Part II: Some Clinically Novel Procedures, Their Use, Some Findings," by J. L. Locke, 1980, *Journal of Speech and Hearing Disorders, 45,* p. 447. Copyright 1980 by the American Speech-Language-Hearing Association. Reprinted by permission.

priate illustrative picture. After reading one set of sentences, the clinician tells the child to select the picture that best represents the meaning of the sentences. At a later point in the assessment process, the child is read the second set of sentences and again asked to pick the appropriate picture. Although the phonological performance analysis attempts to test minimal pairs in connected sentences rather than in isolated word productions, the development of such a battery for each child not only would be time consuming but also would probably tax a clinician's artistic and creative skills. To aid in this task, several examples of sentences contrasting commonly substituted sounds in minimal pairs are contained in Chapter 8.

Cognitive Appraisal

Speech-language pathologists are not qualified to perform formal IQ testing. However, the results of a cognitive appraisal may be important when developing further assessment and treatment goals. IQ testing might then be initiated by referring the client to appropriate professionals. Often, such test results may be obtained through medical, school, or client records.

Caution should be exercised, though, when interpreting the results of IQ measures of children demonstrating phonetic-phonemic disorders. First, a large percentage of children with speech disorders also demonstrate language difficulties. Some cognitive assessment tools use tasks very similar to those used to assess language. Therefore, IQ scores may be affected by the child's language incompetencies. This is particularly a problem with full-scale IQ scores (Nelson, 1998). For this reason, some authors have suggested using nonverbal cognitive measures (Paul, 2007), although tests designed to evaluate nonverbal cognitive skills may appraise only a limited aspect of cognition (Johnston, 1982; Kamhi, Minor, and Mauer, 1990). Second, intelligibility may play a role in the assessment of children with moderate to severe phonemic difficulties, particularly if verbal IQ measures are used. Nonverbal measures would be helpful with the unintelligible child; however, as previously noted, these tests appear restricted. Third, cognitive measures, similar to other standardized tests, do not adequately reflect the abilities of children from culturally and linguistically diverse backgrounds. Although the sample used to norm a particular test typically contains a percentage of children from culturally and linguistically diverse backgrounds (usually the same percentage as these minorities are represented within the U.S. population), this percentage is so small that the inherent test bias for these populations is not eliminated. The presence of language and/or phonetic-phonemic impairments may further compound the interpretation of IQ scores of children from culturally or linguistically diverse backgrounds.

Although the results of a cognitive appraisal may give helpful guidelines for planning subsequent assessment and remediation strategies, the interpretation of the results is not without its problems. Clinicians should be aware of the type of cognitive assessment instrument used to appraise the individual (e.g., verbal versus nonverbal) and the limitations of each measure. *Extreme care should be exercised when interpreting the scores of children from linguistically and culturally diverse backgrounds.*

CLINICAL APPLICATION

How Much Time Does a Comprehensive Appraisal Require?

A comprehensive phonetic-phonemic appraisal seems to involve a considerable amount of time. However, gathering data could be distributed over several therapy sessions. The following sequence is possible if a clinician is limited to twenty minutes of data collection per setting.

Time #1	Impression of intelligibility.
	Hearing screening.
	Speech-motor screening.
Time #2	Articulation test + stimulability measures.
Interim planning	Analyze articulation test and plan spontaneous speech sample.

Time #3   Spontaneous speech sample in at least two different settings.

Could include sample with family, siblings, classmates.

Time #4   Supplemental testing, if necessary. This could include additional word lists to supplement articulation test, specific auditory discrimination testing, language screening, etc.

$\mathcal{S}$PECIAL CONSIDERATIONS

The Child with Emerging Phonology

The period of **emerging phonology** is the time span during childhood in which conventional words begin to appear as a means of communication. Although this level of development usually occurs when children are toddlers, it may also occur in older children with more severe deficits in language learning. Within the assessment process, special consideration must be given to the child with an emerging phonological system. Both the diagnostic procedures themselves and the analysis of the results will be different for this population.

Characteristics of Children with Emerging Phonological Systems. Children with emerging phonology are referred for speech-language services for several reasons. First, some may have been born with known risk factors. Identifiable developmental disorders include Down syndrome and other genetic disorders, known hearing impairments, and cerebral palsy. Second, some children will have early acquired disorders secondary to diseases or trauma such as encephalitis, closed head injury, or abuse. Third, children will be brought by parents who are concerned about the child's development: Parents might have observed differences in the expressive communication abilities and/ or intelligibility of their child compared to other children of a similar age. Fourth, chil-

dren will be referred through various sources because they are "late talkers" and their expressive language is slow to emerge.

The group of children with developmentally delayed emerging phonology is typically characterized by small expressive vocabularies showing a reduced repertoire of consonants and syllable shapes (Nathani, Ertmer, and Stark, 2006; Paul and Jennings, 1992; Pharr, Ratner, and Rescorla, 2000; Rescorla, Mirak, and Singh, 2000). Often, their words are unintelligible. The limited phonological system may also impact further semantic and morphosyntactic development. Therefore, it is important to appraise the phonological system within the broader framework of the child's developing language system. In addition to hearing screening, assessment procedures should always include language testing for this group of children.

Procedural Difficulties with These Children. Previously noted assessment procedures encompass several different tasks that provide useful and necessary information. However, for children at this level of development, several of these tasks may be difficult to complete.

1. *Articulation tests and stimulability measures.* Depending on the client's developmental level, the administration of standardized articulation tests and stimulability measures might not be possible because these children are not yet skilled at following directions or at imitating. An alternative method might include the naming of objects. However, due to the limited expressive vocabulary of most of these children, this adaptation may have severe limitations.

What to Do? With the caregivers' help, one can usually procure a fairly complete sample of words the child is using. Based on the production of these words, the child's consonant and vowel inventory as well as syllable shapes can be established. Such words can be obtained in a number of ways. The following possibilities are given as suggestions:

1. Have the family tape-record the child saying specific spontaneous and elicited words at home.
2. Have the caregiver bring from home a few objects that the child can name.
3. Have the caregiver keep a log of the intended words that the child can produce as well as the approximate way in which each word was pronounced.

Although a tape recording is a good idea, the quality must be secured so that the productions can be accurately evaluated. Based on personal clinical experience, asking the caregiver to bring familiar objects from home and keeping a log of utterances usually provide more diagnostic information than tape recordings. Bringing in familiar objects from the home environment is especially productive in the initial session. For a young child in an unfamiliar setting, this might provide a small comfort zone that will open communication doors. Caregiver logs of the child's spoken words become a necessity when attempting to appraise the shy child who does not communicate at the first or even second meeting. Clinicians need to keep in mind that caregivers are not skilled in phonetic transcription, so they will be limited in their abilities to write down how the child pronounced a certain word. Explanations and examples should be given to the caregiver on how to proceed with this task.

2. *Spontaneous speech sample.* Children with emerging phonological systems who are being evaluated for a possible communication disorder probably do not talk a lot. When they talk, utterances may contain only one or two

words and what they say may be partially unintelligible. Collecting a spontaneous speech sample may, therefore, be a challenge. However, spontaneous samples not only provide data for establishing sound and syllable inventories but also establish communicative situations that elicit spontaneous utterances. If the child is using primarily single words, a one-word utterance analysis such as Bloom's (1973) or Nelson's (1973) will quantify the types of words the child is using. As mentioned earlier, a child's emerging phonological system should be examined and evaluated within the broader parameters of the child's emerging language as a whole.

What to Do? Techniques described in the previous section on articulation testing can also be used to obtain a conversational speech sample. With the shy child who does not respond in an unfamiliar setting, observations of the child's communicative interaction with the caregivers before or after the session may give valuable information.

3. *Examination of the oral-facial structures and the speech-motor system.* Important diagnostic information will be gained if a relationship can be verified between the speech-motor abilities and the slow speech development of these children. However, the assessment of the structure and function of the speech-motor system is often very difficult to obtain from younger children. This is in part due to their intolerance of the procedures needed to complete an oral examination as well as to their limitations in imitating sounds and movements on command.

What to Do? Several fun situations can be initiated to assist in this process. Paul (2007) suggests pretending to make clown or fish faces together, letting the child first look inside your mouth with a small flashlight, and then pretending to look for a dinosaur or elephant in the child's mouth. However, even with the best ideas, clinicians will often fail to get the cooperation of a young child. One possibility would be to wait until the child becomes better acquainted with the clinician and then attempt the procedure again. A second possibility is to gather information about the child's feeding and babbling behaviors. Questions about the child's feeding behavior might help discover related developmental disorders. Box 6.3 contains some sample questions about feeding that could be used to gather information about the speech-motor system of the child indirectly. Babbling history could attempt to establish the quantity and diversity of the child's babbling. Both quantity and diversity of babbling behaviors have been correlated to measures of language.

> The relationship between babbling and language development was discussed in Chapter 5.

4. *Hearing screening.* A hearing screening is indispensable for children with emerging phonological systems for a number of reasons (the high prevalence of otitis media and its impact on hearing is only one). Speech-language specialists equipped with a portable audiometer typically use a screening procedure that has the client signaling, by raising a hand, for example, when a tone is heard. This type of screening procedure may not be possible with children at this age. However, conditioned response audiometric screening may yield results.

What to Do? If screening attempts have failed, the child needs to be referred for a comprehensive audiological evaluation.

5. *Additional tests.* It is well documented that children with phonological disorders often have language problems as well (e.g., Keating, Turrell, and Ozanne, 2001; Shriberg, 1991;

BOX 6.3 Questions to Assess the Feeding Behavior in the Child with an Emerging Phonological System

During sucking of liquids, did any of the following occur?

- Tongue thrusting (abnormally forceful protrusion of the tongue from the mouth)
- Lip retraction (drawing back of the lips so that they form a tight line over the mouth)
- Jaw thrusting (abnormally forceful and tense downward extension of the mandible)
- Lip pursing (a tight purse-string movement of the lips)
- Jaw clenching (abnormally tight closure of the mouth)
- Tonic bite reflex (abnormally strong jaw closure when the teeth or gums are stimulated)

During swallowing, did/do any of the following occur?

- Drooling
- Excessive mucus present
- Coughing, choking, gagging
- Hyperextension of head or neck

During biting and chewing, do any of the following occur?

- Abnormal movements of the jaws, lips, and tongue with solid foods of different consistencies
- Munching versus chewing motions (munching is the earliest form of chewing and involves a flattening and spreading of the tongue combined with up-and-down jaw movement, whereas chewing is characterized by spreading and rolling movements of the tongue and rotary jaw movements)
- Abnormal patterns

Source: Summarized from "Feeding At-Risk Infants and Toddlers," by M. Jaffe, 1989, *Topics in Language Disorders, 10*(1), pp. 13–25.

Shriberg et al., 1986; Shriberg, Kwiatkowski, and Rasmussen, 1990; Webster, Majnemer, Platt, and Shevell, 2005). Therefore, the language abilities of these children need to be assessed. For younger children between 2 and 3

The reader is referred to Language Testing in this chapter for selected language measures that can be used for the birth to 3 population.

years of age, the language assessment instrument must be selected with care. Because of these children's limited attention spans, difficulties in following directions, and their relatively poor imitation skills, even some standardized language tests normed for these ages may not be successfully administered.

What to Do? There are numerous developmental tests that rely partially or totally on the information supplied by the caregiver about the child's level of functioning. The analysis of language in naturalistic contexts can also be used to assess the child's pragmatic, morphological, syntactical, and semantic competencies. See, for example, Lund and Duchan (1993).

Analyzing the Child's Emerging Phonological System. Several authors suggest that an independent analysis be used with children who are at this level of phonological development (Bernthal and Bankson, 2004; Paul and Jennings, 1992; Stoel-Gammon and Dunn, 1985). An **independent analysis** takes only the client's productions into account; they are not compared to the adult norm model. Because only a relatively limited number of consonants and vowels are typically present in the child's inventory, a comparison to the adult norm model would not be helpful for later assessment and intervention. At this stage of the child's development, more information can be gained by seeing which sounds and syllable shapes *are* present. The child's inventory must first be expanded before comparisons to the adult model can be made.

Three kinds of data are collected for the independent analysis: the inventory of speech sounds, the syllable shapes the child uses, and any constraints noted on sound sequences.

The inventory of speech sounds includes all vowels and consonants found in the accumulated word productions of the child. Data on syllable shapes would pertain to single sound productions to signify a word (V, C) and to the use of both open and closed syllable forms (CV, CVCV, CVC). Sound production constraints would include any sound or sound combinations that are used only in certain word or context positions. Examples of this category would include [p] used only word-initially or [d] used only in CVCV structures.

CLINICAL APPLICATION
Inventory of Speech Sounds, Syllable Shapes, and Constraints

Ted is a 1;8-year-old Down syndrome child who is being followed in the early intervention program. These twelve words have been recorded by his mother and the speech-language pathologist.

"yes"	[jɛ]	"pig"	[pɪ]
"mom"	[mʌm]	"hug"	[hʌk]
"daddy"	[dædi]	"bike"	[baɪ]
"hello"	[hoʊ]	"duck"	[dʌk]
"grandpa"	[dapa]	"truck"	[tʌk]
"bye"	[baɪ]	"cow"	[daʊ]

Vowel inventory: [i, ɪ, ɛ, æ, a, oʊ, aɪ, aʊ, ʌ]

Consonant inventory: [m, p, b, t, d, k, j, h]

Syllable shapes: CV, CVC, CVCV

Constraints: [k] is used only in a postvocalic position after the central vowel [ʌ].

An Index of Severity. For children with emerging language skills, Paul and Jennings (1992) suggest a procedure used to obtain an index of severity of phonological delay. This index is based on the number of different consonants and the syllable shapes represented in the child's productions. For both indices, data from normally developing children were compared to those of children with small expressive vocabularies. Table 6.2 describes the procedures and subsequent results that can be used to examine the severity of phonological delay.

Table **6.2** An Index of Severity of Phonological Delay (Paul and Jennings, 1992)

Total Number of Consonants		
Procedure:	The gathering of words for the analysis is based on a ten-minute communications sample. The total number of different consonants are counted.	

Results:	Children	Age	Average Number of Consonants
	Norm	18–24 mos.	14
	Small expr. vocab.	18–24 mos.	6
	Norm	24–36 mos.	18
	Small expr. vocab.	24–36 mos.	10

The child's average number of different consonants can be compared to see if they are closer to the number produced by the norm children or to those with small expressive vocabularies.

Syllable Structure Level (SSL)	
Procedure:	This analysis is based on 20–50 vocalizations.
	It examines intelligible words and nonconventional vocalizations.
	Based on the syllable shape, each utterance is assigned a certain level.
	The ratings given to each vocalization are added together and divided by the total number of vocalizations rated.

Levels:

Level 1: vocalization is composed of only a voiced vowel (V syllable shape [ɑ], [u]), a voiced syllabic consonant (C syllable shape [l̩], [m̩]), or CV syllable in which the consonant is a glottal stop, glide, or [h] ([wi], [hɑ]). The following are examples of Level 1 vocalizations: [i], [oʊ], [l̩], [m̩], [n̩], [hɑ], [wa], [ʔa], [ja], [ju].

Level 2: vocalization is composed of a VC ([ʌp], [ɪk]), CVC with a single consonant ([bab], [mɑm]), or a CV shape that contains consonants other than those noted at Level 1 ([tu], [mu]). Voicing differences are disregarded; therefore, [bip] or [toʊd] would be considered Level 2. The following are examples of Level 2 vocalizations: [ʌk], [um], [ab], [papa], [baba], [noʊ], [tɛdi], [kaka], [lala].

Level 3: vocalization is composed of syllables with two or more different consonant types ([dɑli], [kɪti]). Voicing differences only would be considered Level 2. The following are examples of Level 3 vocalizations: [bati], [boʊmo], [dʌk], [hɛlo], [jʌki], [hat], [koʊt].

Results:	Norm children at 24 months of age	SSL = 2.2
	Children with small expressive vocabularies at 24 months of age	SSL = 1.7

The child's SSL average can be compared to see whether it is closer to the average for children in the norm group or to the average for children with small expressive vocabularies.

CLINICAL APPLICATION

Index of Severity

Further utterances were gathered from Ted, who was presented in the previous Clinical Application. The syllable structure level is noted for each vocalization.

"yes"	[jɛ]	Level 1	"pig"	[pɪ]	Level 2
"mom"	[mʌm]	Level 2	"hug"	[hʌk]	Level 3
"daddy"	[dædi]	Level 2	"bike"	[baɪ]	Level 2
"hello"	[hoʊ]	Level 1	"duck"	[dʌk]	Level 3
"grandpa"	[dapa]	Level 3	"truck"	[tʌk]	Level 3
"bye"	[baɪ]	Level 2	"cow"	[daʊ]	Level 2

Additional nonconventional vocalizations:

[ha]	Level 1	[oʊ]	Level 1
[dɪdɪ]	Level 2	[bubu]	Level 2
[pu]	Level 2	[i]	Level 1
[bæbæ]	Level 2	[pabi]	Level 2
[bʌpi]	Level 2	[ja]	Level 1
[m̩]	Level 1	[ʌ]	Level 1

- Total Number of Consonants: 8
  Syllable Structure Level: 1.83

Ted is 20 months of age. His total number of consonants is much closer to the average found for the children with small expressive vocabularies. Although Ted's syllable structure is higher than those found in children with small expressive vocabularies, it is still closer to the average for that group when compared to the norm children at 24 months of age.

The Unintelligible Child

The speech of unintelligible children is so disordered that the speaker's message cannot be understood. Unintelligible children are not limited to any specific age group. For example, Hodson and Paden (1981) report children who at 8 years of age were considered unintelligible.

Characteristics of Unintelligible Children. Hodson and Paden (1981) evaluated the speech of sixty unintelligible children ranging from 3 to 8 years of age. All of these highly unintelligible children evidenced varying degrees of difficulty with the production of liquids, stridents, and consonant clusters. Prevalent phonological processes in the speech of these children were cluster reduction, stridency deletion, stopping, gliding and vocalizations of liquids, and labial and nasal assimilations. Hodson (1984) notes that the least intelligible children were those who omitted entire classes of sounds. A few of the children produced no obstruents, either before or after the vowel nucleus (*bed* was realized as [ɛ] or [wɛ]), and a small number of the children did not produce sonorant consonants (*run* was pronounced [ʌ]).

Procedural Difficulties with Unintelligible Children. Children 3 years and older will usually not have difficulties completing an articulation test, stimulability testing, or the speech-motor assessment. Even with reduced intelligibility, a single-word articulation test will probably render transcribable results that can be used for a phonetic/phonemic analysis. The major difficulty for the clinician when evaluating unintelligible children is being able to understand and transcribe a spontaneous speech sample. With careful structuring, an understandable spontaneous speech sample may be possible even with unintelligible children.

What to Do?

1. *Choose the topic and attempt to structure the situation as much as possible.* If the context is unknown—that is, if the unintelligible child is talking about a self-generated topic—the clinician will have even more difficulty understanding the sample. Scripts of action events, routine events, and scripted events (Lund and

Duchan, 1993) will give structure and predictability to the conversation. Scripts of action events depict everyday occurrences with predictable elements. Therefore, if children are asked to explain what they do at McDonald's to get a hamburger, the predictability of the events should aid comprehension. *Routine events* begin, progress, and end in essentially the same way each time they occur. If the topic is baseball and the child should explain what the person coming up to bat must do, the known progression of events will again help the clinician understand the conversation. *Scripted events* are activities that have been performed previously and, therefore, all participants have expectations of how they will progress. For example, a child and clinician could fix the wheel on a broken toy truck. The clinician would then ask the child to explain what they had just done. If the clinician models sentences, for example, "First, we saw that the truck had a missing wheel. Next, we looked for the wheel," the child might use similar sentence patterns. Again, the predictability of the utterances should increase the clinician's ability to understand what the child is attempting to say.

2. *Gloss the utterances the child says as much as possible.* Any utterances that may later be difficult to understand from the tape recording should be glossed by the clinician. Glossing means repeating the child's utterance according to norm pronunciation. If the child says [aᴵoᵛoᵛm] for "I go home," the clinician repeats the utterance in a regular manner so that it is recorded together with the sample.

The Dialect Speaker

Dialect is a neutral label that refers to any variety of a language that is shared by a group of speakers. Although this section focuses on the variations in speech sounds represented by a dialect, it should be kept in mind that dialects also encompass specific use of vocabulary, word forms (such as plural endings), sentence structure, and melody patterns.

The technical use of *dialect*, as a neutral term, implies no particular social or attitudinal evaluations of the term; that is, there are no "good" or "bad" dialects. Dialects are simply those language variations that typify a group of speakers within a language. The factors that may correlate with a particular dialect usage may be as simple as geographical status or as complex as a notion of cultural identity. It is important to keep in mind that socially acceptable or so-called "standard" versions of a language constitute dialects as much as those varieties that are considered socially isolated or stigmatized language differences. In American English there is also a dialect referred to as Standard English.

There appear to be two sets of representations of Standard English: a formal and an informal version (Wolfram and Schilling-Estes, 2006). **Formal Standard English**, which is applied primarily to written language and the most formal spoken language situations, tends to be based on the written language and is exemplified in guides of usage or grammar texts. When there is a question as to whether a form is considered Standard English, then these grammar texts are consulted. An informal definition of Standard English is more difficult to define. **Informal Standard English** takes into account the assessment of the members of the American English–speaking community as they judge the "standardness" of other speakers. This notion exists on a continuum ranging from standard to nonstandard speakers of American English and relies far more heavily on grammatical structure than pronunciation patterns (Wolfram and Schilling-Estes, 2006). In other words, listeners will accept a range of regional variations in pronunciation but will not accept the use of socially stigmatized grammatical structures. For example, a rather pronounced Boston or New York regional dialect is accepted, but structures such as "double negatives" would not be considered Standard English. On the other hand, **vernacular dialects** refer to those varieties of spoken American English that are considered outside the continuum of Informal Standard English (Wolfram and Schilling-Estes, 2006). Vernacular dialects are signaled by the presence of certain structures. Therefore, a set of nonstandard English structures mark them as being vernacular. For example, the presence of double negation, lack of subject-verb agreement, and using variations from standard verb forms would constitute features that would label the speaker as utilizing a vernacular dialect. Although there may be a core of features that exemplify a particular vernacular dialect, not all speakers display the entire set of structures described. Therefore, differing patterns of usage exist among speakers of one particular vernacular dialect.

Dialects may vary along several parameters. First, one can describe a dialect according to its hypothesized causative agent. In this way, two main categories are formed: (1) those dialects corresponding to various geographical locations, which are considered **regional dialects;** and (2) those dialects that are generally related to socioeconomic status and/or ethnic background, labeled as **social** or **ethnic dialects.** In addition, dialects are classified according to their linguistic features. This would include the phonological, morphosyntactical, semantic, and pragmatic differences that are distinctive when the speakers representing that dialect are compared to informal Standard English. It appears that regional dialects typically at least demonstrate phonological and semantic features that are unique. On the other hand, social and ethnic dialects may vary along *all* of the previously stated linguistic features.

Regional Dialects. Traditionally, individuals who have studied dialect (dialectologists) have listed three main dialect groups in the United States: northern, midland, and southern. More recent scholars prefer a simple north–south distinction, although there are still significant differences in the boundaries of each proposed area. Many researchers believe that there are no discrete dialect boundaries and no clear-cut dialect divisions within American English. However, data from the Telsur Project show clear and distinct dialect boundaries with a high degree of similarity within each dialect. The Telsur Project of the Linguistics Laboratory of the University of Pennsylvania is one of the largest and most extensive ongoing collections of data related to the dialect regions of the United States. The data consist of phonetic transcriptions and acoustic analyses of vowel systems of informants. These data have been recently compiled in the Atlas of North American English (Labov, Ash, and Boberg, 2005) and represent the active processes of change and diversification that the authors have been tracing since 1968 (Labov 1991, 1994, 1996; Labov, Yaeger, and Steiner, 1972). Their results document four major dialect regions: the North, the South, the West, and the Midland. The first three demonstrate a relatively uniform development of the sound shifts of American English, each moving in somewhat different directions. The fourth region, the Midland, has considerably more diversity and most of the individual cities have developed dialect patterns of their own. The following is given as a brief summary of these four major dialect regions.

North. The area referred to as North is divided into the North Central region, the Inland North, Eastern New England, New York City, and Western New England. For the short vowels [ɪ], [ɛ], [æ], [ʊ], [ʌ], and [ɑ-a-ɔ], these areas all evidence a specific vowel shift (the

Northern Cities Vowel Shift, which is discussed in Labov, 1991, for example). For the long vowels, which include the diphthongs, the North Central and the Inland North regions maintain a long high position, which is typical of the vowel quadrilateral that has been presented in this text. The r-coloring of postvocalic r-productions, such as in *farm* [fɑɚm], is also maintained in these areas.

On the other hand, the Eastern New England area demonstrates r-lessness in which (1) rhotic diphthongs such as those noted in *farm* [fɑɚm] and *porch* [poᵊɚtʃ], (2) stressed central vowels with r-coloring such as in *bird* [bɝd] and *shirt* [ʃɝt], and (3) unstressed central vowels with r-coloring such as in *mother* [mʌðɚ] and *over* [oᵘvɚ] will lose the r-coloring, resulting in possible pronunciations such as [fɑəm] or [fɑm] for *farm*, [poᵘətʃ] or [poᵘtʃ] for *porch*, [bɜd] for *bird*, [ʃɜt] for *shirt*, [mʌðə] for *mother,* and [oᵘvə] for *over.*

In addition, the two vowels [ɑ] and [ɔ] are merged into an intermediate vowel, typically [ɑ] or more frequently [a]. Thus, distinct pronunciations for words such as *caught* [kɔt] and *cot* [kɑt] are not realized. Instead, one similar vowel is used for both words. The exception to this is the city of Providence (Rhode Island), which has the characteristic r-lessness but does not merge the [ɑ] and [ɔ] vowels.

New York City has a unique dialect that is not reproduced further west and therefore cannot fit neatly into any larger regional groupings. The long vowels maintain a high position, similar to that noted for the North Central and Inland North areas. There is consistent r-lessness of postvocalic "r" except for the central vowel with r-coloring [ɚ] (the vowel sound heard in *bird*) and when a final "r" is followed by a vowel in the next word, such as *The car is here*. In addition, the [æ] vowel splits into a lax and tense form and the production differences between [ɑ] and [ɔ] are maximal, the [ɔ] vowel being raised to a mid-high posi-

tion. No clear patterns of sound change seem to be occurring in Western New England.

South. The South demonstrates a vowel shift referred to as the Southern Shift (see Labov, 1991). However, a small area of the Southeast is distinct from the rest of the South: the two cities of Charleston (South Carolina) and Savannah (Georgia). In these cities there is a small degree of vowel change. Another characteristic of the southern region is the [ɑ]–[ɔ] distinction. With the exception of the margins of the South—western Texas, Kentucky, Virginia, and the city of Charleston—this distinction is marked not by a change in the vowel quality but by a back upglide for [ɔ]. Thus, acoustically the nuclei of the vowels are very similar; however, [ɔ] is productionally signaled by a back upgliding movement of the tongue.

Midland. Speakers in the Midland area do not seem to participate in the vowel shifts that are noted in the South and North. Labov, Ash, and Boberg (2005) divide the Midland into two sections: South and North. The consistently noted feature of the South Midland is the fronting of [oᵘ], resulting in a [ʌ]-like quality. Exceptions are Louisville (Kentucky) and Savannah (Georgia). Using this criterion, Philadelphia is a member of the South Midland, and Pittsburgh and St. Louis are considered North Midland.

West. The diversity of dialects declines steadily as one moves westward, resulting in a diffusion of northern, midland, and southern characteristics. Although there are exceptions, characteristics of the West are aligned with those of the Midland. The most prominent feature of western phonology is the merger of [ɑ] and [ɔ]; however, as noted previously, this is not unique to the West. The second feature that emerges is the fronting of the vowel [u] as in *two* or *do*, which is produced with a tongue position that is more anterior than typical, for example. Although these two characteristics are also noted in the South Midland, there appears to be a much higher frequency of their occurrence in the West.

Regional dialects are related to geographical regions within the United States. These regional boundaries have shifted over the years and different researchers have described the regions somewhat differently. Table 6.3 is a somewhat different view of regional dialects evidenced within the United States. It includes two of the minor regional dialects, Ozark English and Appalachian English, as well as the geographic areas where these dialects can be heard (Carver, 1987; Christian, Wolfram, and Nube, 1988). Certain phonological changes are associated with each of these dialects. However, they are not mutually exclusive but rather demonstrate considerable overlap of several features. Table 6.4 itemizes some of the overlap in the regional dialects as well as in African American English.

Other important variables of dialect have also been recognized in the study of American English. Two of these are the social and ethnic dimensions of dialect. This next section will examine these two aspects as they relate to phonological variations within the United States.

Ethnicity. Often, the terms *race, culture,* and *ethnicity* are used interchangeably within professional literature and informal conversations. However, there are distinctions between each of these terms. **Race** is a biological label that is defined in terms of observable physical features (such as skin color, hair type and color, head shape and size) and biological characteristics (such as genetic composition). **Culture** is a way of life developed by a group of individuals to meet psychosocial needs. It consists of values, norms, beliefs, attitudes, behavioral styles, and traditions. **Ethnicity** refers to commonalities such as religion, nationality, and region. Although race is a biological distinction, it can take on ethnic meaning if members of a biological group have evolved specific ways of living as a subculture (Battle, 1993).

Several different kinds of relationships may exist between ethnicity and language variation. For ethnic groups that maintain a language other then English, there is the

Table 6.3 Additional Regional Dialects with Notable Changes in Pronunciation

Dialect	Geographical Area
New York	Metropolitan New York
New England	Upper Maine, the Narragansett Bay region, and metropolitan Boston
Southern	Coastal plains from Virginia to eastern Texas; includes most of North Carolina, South Carolina, Georgia, Alabama, Mississippi, and Louisiana
Ozark English	Northern Arkansas, southern Missouri, and northwestern Oklahoma
Appalachian English	Areas of Kentucky, Tennessee, Virginia, North Carolina, and West Virginia (southern Appalachians, Ozarks, Bluegrass area of Kentucky, and Nashville basin area)

Sources: Carver (1987); Christian, Wolfram, and Nube (1988).

Table 6.4 Specific Phonological Features of Regional and Cultural Dialects

Phonological Feature	Example		Dialects
Changes in r-Sounds			
Loss of r-coloring on central vowels	*bird* *father*	= [bɜd] = [faðə]	New York, New England, Southern, African American English
Neutralization of [r] in postvocalic clusters	*farm*	= [fɑm]	New York, New England, Southern
Neutralization of [r] in an intervocalic word position	*Carol*	= [kɛəl]	African American English, Appalachian English, Ozark English
Neutralization of [r] after a consonant	*throw*	= [θoʊ]	Appalachian English, Ozark English
Changes in Individual Consonants			
Initial [w] reduction	*will*	= [ɪl]	Appalachian English, Ozark English
Substitution of t/θ and d/ð initiating a word	*that* *think*	= [dæt] = [tɪŋk]	Appalachian English, Ozark English, African American English
Substitution of f/θ and v/ð intervocalic and in final word position	*bathtub* *mouth*	= [bæftʌb] = [maʊf]	African American English
Aspirated vowels initiating a word, sounds like an [h] sound	*it*	= [hɪt]	Appalachian English, Ozark English
Intrusive [t]	*cliff*	= [klɪft]	Appalachian English
Devoicing of final [b], [d], and [g]	*lid*	= [lɪt]	African American English
Changes in Consonant Clusters			
Epenthesis	*ghosts*	= [gostəs]	Appalachian English, Ozark English
Metathesis	*ask*	= [æks]	African American English
Word-final reduction of consonant cluster (especially prominent if one of the consonants is an alveolar)	*test*	= [tɛs]	African American English
Deletion of [l] in word-final consonant clusters	*help*	= [hɛp]	African American English, also noted in Appalachian English and Ozark English before labial consonants
Deletion of word-final consonants with nasalization of preceding vowels	*man*	= [m̃æ]	African American English

Sources: Summarized from Christian, Wolfram, and Nube (1988); Fasold and Wolfram (1975); Seymour and Miller-Jones (1981); Wolfram (1994).

potential of language transfer. **Transfer** indicates the incorporation of language features into a nonnative language, based on the occurrence of similar features in the native language. In some Hispanic communities in the Southwest the use of "no" as a generalized tag question (You go to the movies a lot, no?) may be attributable to the transfer from Spanish, as can phonological features such as the merger of /ʃ/ and /tʃ/ (*shoe* sounds like *chew*), the devoicing of /z/ to /s/ (*lazy* becomes [leˡsi]) and the merger of /i/ and /ɪ/ (*pit* and *peat* sound similar or *rip* and *reap* are pronounced with the same vowel quality).

One of the most publicized ethnic dialects is African American Vernacular English. A survey of published research in American English shows that more than five times as many publications are devoted to this dialect when compared to any other group of dialects. The next section will examine some of the general and phonological characteristics of this dialect.

African American Vernacular English.   Sometimes called Black English or African American English, African American Vernacular English is a systematic, rule-governed dialect that is spoken by many but not all African American people within the United States. Although it shares many commonalities with Standard American English and Southern English, there are certain differences that distinguish this dialect. These differences affect the phonological, morphological, syntactical, and semantic systems. In this section only the phonological variations will be addressed.

Not all African Americans use African American Vernacular English and among those who do, the degree of use differs significantly. There are several variables that influence the use of this dialect: age, gender, and socioeconomic status being the most noted. Relative to age, there is evidence that the use of this dialect decreases as the individual becomes older. Elementary school children use a type of dialect that varies the most from mainstream language, whereas dialect features that appear prominently in adolescence level off in adulthood (Washington, 1998).

Gender differences in the use of African American Vernacular English have also been reported. Males often exhibit increased use of vernacular, nonstandard forms relative to females. This increase in use within the male population possibly represents differential socialization along gender lines. More positive values of masculinity are associated with more frequent use of vernacular forms, whereas women, particularly middle-class women, use standard forms more frequently (Labov, Yaeger, and Steiner, 1972).

Differences in the use of this dialect dependent on socioeconomic status are also apparent. Lower- and working-class African Americans reportedly use this dialect more frequently than do middle- or upper-middle-class African Americans. This distinction may also reflect differences in educational background. Terrell and Terrell (1993) suggest that there is a continuum of dialect use from those who do not use the dialect at all to those who use this dialect in almost all communicative contexts. This continuum is significantly influenced by social status variables. In addition, African Americans from middle- and upper-middle-class backgrounds appear to be more adept at **code switching,** changing back and forth between African American Vernacular English and Standard American English, than their lower- and working-class counterparts.

If a comparison is made between the documented phonological features of African American Vernacular English and other dialects within the United States, four types of phonological distinctions can be noted. First, those features may occur in all dialects of American English but are either more frequent in African American Vernacular English or occur in a wider range of communicative contexts. In Table 6.5, the first four items belong to this category. Second, some phonological variations occur not only in African American Vernacular English but also in other nonstandard vernacular dialects. They do not, however, occur in formal or informal standard dialects. Items 5 through 8 in Table 6.5 represent these features. Third, some of the phonological features represent those noted in the phonology of the South. Often these distinctions (items 9 through 12) are old-fashioned features of southern phonology and are rapidly disappearing in present-day speech. Others (items 13 through 17) do not appear or only rarely appear in earlier records of African American Vernacular English or southern dialect but emerged during the last quarter of the nineteenth century and are expanding rapidly in the speech of both dialects. The last set of features (items 18 through 24) seem to be unique to African American Vernacular English.

CLINICAL APPLICATION

African American Dialect: More than Phonological Changes

Although several phonological features of African American dialect have been introduced in this section, semantic, morphosyntactic, and pragmatic variations are also a part of this dialect (see for example van Keulen, Weddington, and DeBose, 1998, or Terrell and Terrell, 1993). Children may use these dialect features during language assessment; it is therefore important that the clinician be aware of these variations. The following is a summary of African American dialect features noted in the grammatical structure of preschoolers (Washington and Craig, 1994).*

Morphological and Syntactic Form	Examples
Zero copula or auxiliary	
Is, are, and modal auxiliaries *will, can,* and *do* are not consistently used.	"the bridge out" "how you do this"
Subject-verb agreement	
A subject and verb that differ in either number or person is used.	"what do this mean"
Fitna/sposeta/bouta	
Abbreviated forms for "fixing to," "supposed to," and "about to."	*fitna:* "she fitna a backward flip"
Ain't	
Ain't is used as a negative auxiliary.	"why she ain't comin?"
Undifferentiated pronoun case	
Nominative, objective, and demonstrative cases of pronouns occur interchangeably.	"him did and him"
Multiple negation	
Two or more negative markers in one utterance.	"I don't got no brothers"
Zero possessive	
Possession coded by word order so that the possessive -s marker is deleted or the nominative or objective case of pronouns is used rather than the possessive.	"he hit the man car" "kids just goin' to walk to they school"

*Other morphological and syntactic variations were noted, but these forms were used by at least one third of the children in the study.

Table 6.5   Frequently Cited Features of African American Vernacular English

Feature	Example
Features that appear in most dialects of American English and appear to be more prevalent in African American Vernacular English	
1. Final consonant cluster reduction	*first girl* → firs' girl
Loss of second consonant	*cold* → col; *hand* → han
2. Unstressed syllable deletion	*about* → bout
Initial and medial syllables	*government* → gov'ment
3. Deletion of reduplicated syllable	*Mississippi* → miss'ippi
4. Vowelization of postvocalic [l]	*bell* → [bɛə]; *pool* → [puə]
Features that appear in vernacular dialects of American English but not in standard dialects	
5. Loss of "r" after consonants	*throw* → [θoʊ]
After [θ] and in unstressed syllables	*professor* → [pəfɛsɚ]
6. Labialization of interdental fricatives	*bath* → [bæf]; *teeth* → [tif]
7. Syllable-initial fricatives replaced by stops	*those* → [doʊz]; *think* → [tɪŋk]
Especially with voiced fricatives	*these* → [diz]
8. Voiceless interdental fricatives replaced by stops	*with* → [wɪt]
Especially when close to nasals	*tenth* → [tɪnt]
Features that appeared in old-fashioned southern dialects	
9. Metathesis of final [s] + stop	*ask* → [æks]; *grasp* → [græps]
10. Loss of r-coloring of stressed central vowel [ɝ]	*bird* → [bɜd]; *word* → [wɜd]
11. Loss of r-coloring of centering diphthongs with [ɚ]	*four* → [foə]; *farm* → [faəm]
12. Loss of r-coloring of unstressed central vowel [ɚ]	*father* → [faðə]; *never* → [nɛvə]
Features that are recently evolving in southern and African American Vernacular English dialects	
13. Reduction of diphthong [aɪ] to [a] before voiced obstruents and in the final syllable position	*tied* → [tad]; *lie* → [la]
14. Centering of offglide in [ɔɪ] to [ɔə]	*oil* → [ɔəl]; *boil* → [bɔəl]
15. Merger of [ɛ] and [ɪ] before nasals	*pen* → [pɪn]; *Wednesday* [wɪnzdi]
16. Merger of tense and lax vowels before [l] ([i] → [ɪ]; [e] → [ɛ])	*bale and bell* → [bɛl]; *feel and fill* → [fɪl]
17. Fricatives become stops before nasals	*isn't* → [ɪdn̩]; *wasn't* → [wʌdn̩]

Features that are apparently unique to African American Vernacular English	
18. Stressing of initial syllables, shifting the stress from the second syllable	*police* → [ˈpoʊ.lis]; *Detroit* → [ˈdi.trɔət]
19. Deletion of final nasal consonant but nasalization of preceding vowel	*man* → [mæ̃]; *thumb* → [θʌ̃]
20. Final consonant deletion (especially affects nasals)	*five* → [fɑ:]; *fine* → [fɑ:]
21. Final stop devoicing (without shortening of preceding consonant)	*bad* → [bæ:t]; *dog* → [dɔ:k]
22. Coarticulated glottal stop with devoiced final stop	*bad* → [bæ:tʔ]; *dog* → [dɔ:kʔ]
23. Loss of [j] after specific consonants (loss of palatalization in specific contexts)	*computer* → [kɑmputə]; *Houston* [hustn̩]
24. Substitution of [k] for [t] in [str] clusters	*street* → [skrit]; *stream* → [skrim]

Sources: Wolfram (1994); Stockman (1996).

Implications for Appraisal. For the dialect speaker, several issues need to be considered during the assessment process. The first and foremost is determining which phonological characteristics constitute dialectal differences. When contrasted to General American English, the noted variations in pronunciation of the dialect speaker may be dialectal differences and not signs of a disordered phonological system.

What to Do?

1. Be sensitive to local dialect patterns and to any regional or cultural dialects that may impact the client's speech. Unbiased assessment of an individual's phonology must account for the norms of the particular dialect. In other words, are these phonological variations also represented in individuals with whom this client interacts? In addition, in a society in which the mobility level is high, clinicians should expect that certain regional dialects will appear outside of their associated geographical areas.

2. Choose assessment instruments that account for dialectal variations or consider dialect features when scoring any standardized measure. Some articulation tests—the Goldman-Fristoe (Goldman and Fristoe, 2000) and Fisher-Logemann (Fisher and Logemann, 1971), for example—have guidelines for scoring certain dialect features. However, many instruments do not. The clinician's knowledge of dialect features (see Table 6.4) will be helpful in scoring these measures.

3. Evaluate not only the presence of specific dialect features but also their frequency of occurrence. The results of research indicate that a judgment of disordered versus different phonological systems is often influenced by the relative frequency rather than just the categorical presence or absence of certain patterns (Bauman-Waengler, 1993a, 1993b, 1994b, 1995, 1996; Kercher and Bauman-Waengler,

1992; Seymour, Green, and Hundley, 1991; Stockman, 1996; Wolfram, 1994).

4. Assess the client's communicative effectiveness in the regional or cultural dialect. If unfamiliar with the dialect, ask other professionals or members of the community about the client's communication skills. The client's teachers are often a good source of information.

The Speaker of English as a Second Language

The number of immigrants to the United States has increased, averaging close to one million a year since 1990 (2003 Yearbook of Immigration Statistics). These individuals come from a wide array of countries and backgrounds. They bring to the United States a wealth of different languages. One way to examine the types and numbers of non-English language backgrounds is through the statistics provided by the Office of English Language Acquisition (OELA) in the data they have collected for **limited English proficient** students within the United States.

According to the OELA's (2002) latest statistics, more than 460 languages are spoken by limited English proficient students nation-

Table **6.6** Top Three Languages Spoken by Limited English Proficient Students (LEPS) by State

States	# LEPS	1st Lang.	%	2nd Lang.	%	3rd Lang.	%
USA	4,552,403	Spanish	79.00	Vietnamese	2.00	Hmong	1.60
Alabama	7,434	Spanish	74.70	Vietnamese	5.80	Korean	1.90
Alaska	19,896	Yup'ik	38.60	Inupiak	11.20	Spanish	10.00
Arizona	198,477	Spanish	85.00	Navajo	7.80	Apache	1.30
Arkansas	10,600	Spanish	87.00	Lao	2.40	Vietnamese	2.20
California	1,511,299	Spanish	83.40	Vietnamese	2.50	Hmong	1.80
Colorado	71,199	Spanish	81.80	Vietnamese	2.60	Asian	unspecified
Connecticut	21,492	Spanish	67.60	Portuguese	5.30	Polish	2.80
Delaware	2,371	Spanish	72.30	Haitian Creole	7.60	Korean	3.30
DC	5,435	Spanish	76.40	Vietnamese	3.90	Amharic	2.50
Florida	249,821	Spanish	75.80	Haitian Creole	12.40	Portuguese	
Georgia	64,849	Spanish	70.10	Vietnamese	4.40	African	unspecified
Hawaii	11,687	Ilocano	31.80	Samoan	12.40	Marshalles	9.10
Idaho	19,298	Spanish	78.80	Native American		unspecified	5.60
Illinois	140,540	Spanish	77.60	Polish	4.40	Arabic	1.70
Indiana	20,467	Spanish	64.40	Penn. Dutch	3.70	Japanese	1.50
Iowa	11,402	Spanish	62.30	Serbo-Croatian	11.60	Vietnamese	6.70
Kansas	19,075	Spanish	81.30	Vietnamese	4.40	Lao	1.60
Kentucky	5,119	Spanish	47.30	Serbo-Croatian	13.00	Vietnamese	6.40
Louisiana	6,346	Spanish	48.50	Vietnamese	25.10	Arabic	4.40
Maine	2,737	French	16.80	Spanish	12.90	Passamaquoddy	10.70
Maryland	12,183	Spanish	53.00	Korean	6.00	Haitian Creole	3.40
Massachusetts	24,165	Spanish	69.40	Portuguese	10.00	Khmer	5.10
Michigan	36,463	Spanish	44.80	Arabic	22.50	Chaldean	5.00
Minnesota	46,601	Hmong	34.10	Spanish	28.30	Somali	6.60

wide. The data submitted indicate that Spanish is the native language of the great majority of limited English proficient students (79.2 percent), followed by Vietnamese (2 percent), Hmong (1.6 percent), Cantonese (1 percent), and Korean (1 percent). All other language groups represented less than 1 percent of the limited English proficient student population. Languages with more than 10,000 speakers include Arabic, Armenian, Chuukese, French, Haitian Creole, Hindi, Japanese, Khmer, Lao, Mandarin, Marshallese, Navajo, Polish, Portuguese, Punjabi, Russian, Serbo-Croatian, Tagalog, and Urdu.

These national figures, however, mask substantial regional variations in linguistic diversity. For example, in nine states Spanish is not the dominant language among limited English proficient students: Blackfoot is the top language in Montana, French in Maine, Hmong in Minnesota, Ilocano in Hawaii, Lakota in South Dakota, "Native American" in North Dakota, Serbo-Croatian in Vermont, and Yup'ik in Alaska. Table 6.6 contains the three top languages spoken by limited English proficient students by state (2001–2002 statistics).

With such a large variety of languages, this section will examine only the phonological systems of the top five languages represented in this survey. Therefore, the following section will contrast the vowel, consonant,

States	# LEPS	1st Lang.	%	2nd Lang.	%	3rd Lang.	%
Mississippi	63,116	Spanish	60.40	Vietnamese	18.80	Choctaw	7.10
Missouri	2,954	Spanish	44.20	Serbo-Croatian	19.20	Vietnamese	6.60
Montana	11,525	Blackfoot	25.20	Crow	15.60	Dakota	10.60
Nebraska	7,575	Spanish	76.80	Vietnamese	6.10	Nuer	3.30
Nevada	10,301	Spanish	91.50	Tagalog	1.90	Chinese	unspecified
New Hampshire	38,902	Spanish	38.70	Serbo-Croatian	10.50	Portuguese	3.80
Ohio	7,190	Spanish	39.20	Arabic	8.20	Somali	8.00
Oklahoma	19,814	Spanish	51.70	Cherokee	20.20	Choctaw	4.20
Oregon	43,410	Spanish	72.50	Russian	8.40	Vietnamese	3.60
Pennsylvania	44,126	Spanish	52.90	Vietnamese	5.00	Khmer	3.60
Rhode Island	31,277	Spanish	69.80	Portuguese	6.70	Kabuverdianu	4.90
South Carolina	10,164	Spanish	77.30	Russian	2.80	Vietnamese	2.40
South Dakota	6,900	Lakota	57.40	Spanish	8.80	German	8.60
Tennessee	5,848	Spanish	61.20	Vietnamese	4.80	Arabic	4.20
Texas	12,350	Spanish	93.40	Vietnamese	1.90	Cantonese	0.70
Utah	558,773	Spanish	65.30	Navajo	6.70	Vietnamese	2.50
Vermont	41,057	Croatian	26.70	Vietnamese	16.70	Spanish	12.30
Virginia	998	Spanish	60.40	Korean	5.20	Vietnamese	4.80
Washington	35,298	Spanish	60.90	Russian	7.50	Vietnamese	6.40
West Virginia	57,409	Spanish	26.30	Arabic	8.60	Khmer	8.50
Wisconsin	1,139	Spanish	47.80	Hmong	40.10	Lao	1.10
Wyoming	29,037	Spanish	90.40	Vietnamese	6.00	Russian	3.60

Source: Adapted from statistics from the Office of English Language Acquisition (2002).

The term *limited English proficient* is used for any individual between the ages of 3 and 21 who is enrolled or preparing to enroll in an elementary or secondary school, who was not born in the United States, or whose native language is a language other than English. Individuals who are Native Americans or Alaska Natives and come from an environment where a language other than English has had a significant impact on the individuals are also included in this definition. The difficulties in speaking, writing, or understanding the English language compromise the individual's ability to successfully achieve in classrooms, where the language of instruction is English, or to participate fully in society (PL 107-110, The No Child Left Behind Act of 2001). Title III funds are provided to ensure that limited English proficient students, including immigrant children and youth, develop English proficiency and meet the same academic content and academic achievement standards that other children are expected to meet.

and suprasegmental systems of Spanish, Vietnamese, Hmong, Cantonese, and Korean to the phonological system of American English. This contrast is provided as a way to possibly predict which sounds or features might be difficult for individuals learning English as a second language when their native language is one of these five languages. Although other factors play a role in second language acquisition, such as the length of time in the United States and the age when the individual came to the United States, it still appears that a primary cause of difficulty is the interaction between the native language and American English (Yeni-Komshian, Flege, and Liu, 2000).

Spanish American English. Many dialects and language variations of Spanish fall under this one large categorization. Immigrants within the United States who speak Spanish seem to fall basically into five categories: those from (1) Mexico, (2) Central and South America, (3) Puerto Rico, (4) Cuba, and (5) other coun-

tries not specifically identified in the 2000 U.S. census. Figure 6.3 gives an estimate of the distribution of Spanish-speaking individuals within the United States according to this census.

This discussion will first examine some basic qualities of the vowel and consonant system of Chicano Spanish and then attempt to note those differences that might occur in the various dialects of Spanish, such as Puerto Rican Spanish and Nicaraguan Spanish.

There are five vowels in Spanish: [i], [e], [u], [o], and [a]. There are no central vowels in Spanish, neither those without r-coloring nor those with r-coloring. In addition, all Spanish vowels are long and tense. Thus, for the Spanish student of English, the contrasts between *beat* and *bit, pool* and *pull, boat* and *bought,* and *cat, cot,* and *cut* are difficult. In addition, the [e] and [o] vowels are monophthongs in Spanish. So, although easily recognizable, they will sound somewhat different. There is some comparability between the diphthongs of Spanish and English: [aɪ], [aʊ], and [ɔɪ]. However, the gliding action between onglide and offglide is quicker and reaches a higher, more distinct articulatory position (González, 1988).

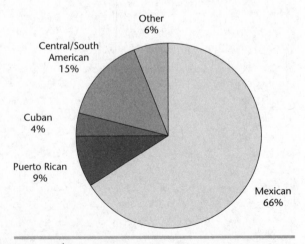

Figure 6.3 Distribution of Spanish-Speaking Individuals within the United States
Source: Adapted from the U.S. Bureau of the Census (2000).

The consonants of Spanish show many similarities. The voiced and voiceless stop-plosives are present in Spanish; however, the [t] and [d] are articulated as dentals as opposed to the alveolar production of the American English [t] and [d]. For the Spanish productions, the tip of the tongue is against the edges of the inner surfaces of the upper front teeth. The production is symbolized as [t̪] and [d̪]. Other shared consonants include [j, w, f, m, l, s, tʃ, and n]; [θ] may occur in some dialects but not in others. The consonants [v, z, h, ð, ʃ, dʒ, ʒ, ŋ] are present in English but not in Spanish. Although [ŋ] and [ð] are allophones of other phonemes, they do not form minimal pairs in Spanish. In addition, the letter *r* is pronounced differently in Spanish. Spanish distinguishes two *r* phonemes: [ɾ] and an alveolar trill. The [ɾ], which was introduced in Chapter 4, is a flap, tap, or one-tap trill that in American English can be an allophonic variation of [t] or [d] when these sounds are produced between two vowels. For example, in casual conversation the word *ladder* or *better* can be pronounced [læɾɚ] or [bɛɾɚ]. The second r of Spanish is an alveolar trill (which according to the IPA is transcribed [r] but to eliminate confusion will be symbolized here as r̄) in which the apex of the tongue flutters rapidly against the alveolar ridge with either two or three vibrations. Therefore, the transference of the Spanish *r* to English will end up with a qualitatively somewhat different sounding *r*. Table 6.7 demonstrates the vowel and consonant sounds of Hispanic Spanish.

Table 6.7 Phonological Inventory: A Comparison of Spanish to General American English (GAE)

Spanish Vowels	Vowel Differences: Spanish and GAE
[i, e, u, o, a]	■ [ɪ, ɛ, æ, ʊ, ʌ, ə, ɝ, ɚ] and diphthongs are not present in Spanish. ■ Spanish speaker may substitute similar vowels in GAE, e.g., *could* → [kud] ■ Spanish speaker may substitute [er] for [ɝ], *bird* → [berd]
Spanish Consonants	**Consonant Differences: Spanish and GAE**
[p, t, k, b, d, g]	■ Because voiceless stops are unaspirated in Spanish, speaker may produce GAE voiceless stops as unaspirated. ■ In Spanish, [t] and [d] are dentalized productions.
[f, x, s, β] ([χ] is a voiceless velar fricative, [β] is a voiced bilabial fricative)	■ [v, z, ð, θ, ʃ, ʒ] not present in Spanish.
[tʃ]	■ [dʒ] not present in Spanish, variable production of [tʃ].
[w, j, l, ɾ, r]	■ [r] is produced as a trilled vibrant production in Spanish.
[m, n, ŋ]	■ [n] is a dentalized production in Spanish. ■ [ŋ] is palatalized in Spanish.

Sources: Goldstein (1995); Perez (1994); Ruhlen (1976).

CLINICAL APPLICATION
Phonological Changes—
Hispanic Spanish

Differences between American English and Hispanic Spanish lead to the following problems, which are noted in Penfield and Ornstein-Galacia (1985) and Perez (1994).

1. Variable production of [tʃ] and [ʃ], thus [tʃoᵘ] for *show* and [ʃɛk] for *check*.
2. Devoicing of [z] in all environments, especially in word-final position.
3. Devoicing of [v] in word-final position, thus [hæf] for *have*.
4. Realization of [v] as [β] (a voiced bilabial fricative) or [b] especially between two vowels, thus, [aβan] for *oven*. Note that the central vowels might be replaced by the Spanish [a] vowel.
5. Realization of [θ] and [ð] as [t] and [d], thus [tɪŋk] for *think* and [deɪ] for *they*.
6. Realization of [j] for [dʒ] in word-initial position, thus [jas] for *just*.
7. Devoicing of [dʒ] between two vowels and in word-final positions, thus, [tineɪtʃɚ] for *teenager* and [læŋwɪtʃ] for *language*.
8. Realization of [a] for [ʌ] in stressed syllables, thus [drag] for *drug*.
9. Tensing of [ɛ] to [e], especially preceding nasals, thus [frend] for *friend*.
10. Inconsistent realizations of [i] – [ɪ], [e] – [ɛ], [ɛ], and [æ], and [u] – [ʊ]. Thus, *speak* may be pronounced [spɪk].
11. Velarization of [h] as [x] (a voiceless velar fricative), thus [xi] for *he*.
12. Reduction of consonant clusters in word-final position, thus *war* for *ward* or *star* for *start*.
13. Deletion of intervocalic flaps and occasionally other consonants, thus [lɪl] for *little* and [læɚ] for *ladder*. Syllables may be reduced as well.
14. Trilling of the *r*, which may result in [ɾ] or [r̄] for *r*, thus, [əɾaᵘnd] or [ər̄aᵘnd] for *around*.
15. Intrusive [h], thus for *and it* the Spanish speaker could say [hændhɪt].
16. Unstressed syllable deletion such as [spleɪn] for *explain*.
17. Shift of major stress on noun compounds from the first word to the second word, thus, instead of 'mini-skirt, mini'skirt.
18. Shift of major stress on verb particles from the second word to the first word, for example, 'show up instead of *show 'up*.
19. Shift of stress on specific words such as 'ac cept for *ac 'cept*.

Cuban American English. The Cuban Americans are considered the oldest population of Hispanic immigrants in the United States. Most of the Cuban Americans today live in New York, New Jersey, California, and Florida. Cuban American Spanish is categorized as a variety of Caribbean Spanish, which includes the three Antillean islands as well as the coastal areas of Mexico, Panama, Colombia, and Venezuela (Otheguy, Garcia, and Roca, 2000).

CLINICAL APPLICATION
Phonological Changes—Cuban American

According to Hidalgo (1987), the following phonological features are problematic for speakers of Cuban American Spanish.

1. Before consonants, [s] is typically aspirated, and in word-final position, [s] is deleted. This could lead to deletion of the final [s] if a transfer is made between Cuban American Spanish and English.
2. The consonants [l] and [r̄] are frequently interchanged before consonants and in word-final position. Inconsistent realizations of [l] and [r] could result in American English.
3. Deletion of intervocalic and word-final [d]-production could lead to a similar deletion pattern for [d] in American English.
4. The Spanish [r̄] may be pronounced like [h] or as a uvular approximate. This could impact the quality of the r-productions in American English.
5. The labio-dental [v] is used as a variant of [b], particularly in words spelled with *v*. This could positively impact the production of American English (see number 4) as the substitution of [b] for [v] is noted in Hispanic Spanish.

Puerto Rican American English. Before the invasion of Puerto Rico by the United States in 1898, this island had belonged to Spain for approximately 400 years (Zentella, 2000). Since that time Puerto Rico has experienced intense Americanization. New York presently has the largest population of Puerto Ricans, although a considerable number of Puerto Ricans also live in Massachusetts, Florida, and Pennsylvania (Zentella, 2000). The use of Spanish and English varies according to the situation; however, the issue of generation will also play an important role. For example, parents who grew up in Puerto Rico speaking Spanish and move to the United States will have a tendency to use Spanish at home with their children, whereas their children will speak both English and Spanish.

CLINICAL APPLICATION
Phonological Changes— Puerto Rican Spanish

The following phonological distinctions were noted by Zentella (2000).

1. The use of [s] for [z] and [tʃ], especially before [i] and [e], pronunciation differences such as [sip] for *cheap* or [sen] for *chain* could result.
2. Similarities noted in numbers 2, 4, and 5 from the Penfield and Ornstein-Galacia (1985) and Perez (1994) list: devoicing of [z] in all environments, especially in word-final position; realization of [v] as [β] (a voiced bilabial fricative) or [b] especially between two vowels, thus [aβan] for *oven*, and realization of [θ] and [ð] as [t] and [d], thus [tɪŋk] for *think* and [deɪ] for *they.*
3. The consonants [l] and [r̄] are frequently interchanged before consonants and in word-final position. Inconsistent realizations of [l] and [r] could result in American English.
4. The Spanish [r̄] may be pronounced as a uvular approximant in the middle of words and in the word-initial position. This could impact the quality of the r-productions in American English.

Nicaraguan American English. Most of the immigration of Nicaraguans to the United States took place during the Somoza regime in the middle of the 1970s with the uprising of the Sandinista group (Lipski, 2000). Nicaraguans are primarily concentrated in New York City, Los Angeles, New Orleans, and Miami. Within the Nicaraguan population there is a group of individuals who speak one of two indigenous languages from this area—Miskito or Caribbean Creole English. This last group of Nicaraguans, due to their English language skills, were able to integrate almost immediately into the job market of the United States (Lipski, 2000). The Spanish of the Nicaraguans shares many similarities with the other noted groups of Spanish speakers within the United States.

CLINICAL APPLICATION
Phonological Changes— Nicaraguan Spanish

According to Lipski (2000), the following phonological features of Nicaraguan Spanish may influence pronunciation of General American English.

1. Weak production of the intervocalic [j]. In words such as *yoyo* and *oh yes* the [j] sound could be impacted and may be perceived as possibly a sound deletion.
2. Velarization of word-final [n] could result in an inconsistent distinction between [n] and [ŋ] at the end of words, thus, *sun* could be produced as *sung.*
3. The Spanish [r̄] may be pronounced as a velar approximate in the middle of words and in the word-initial position. This could impact the quality of the r-productions in American English.

Vietnamese American English. With the end of the Vietnam War in 1975 and the subsequent rule of Vietnam by a Communist government, an influx of immigrants came from

Indochina to the United States in search of political asylum. Vietnamese is part of the Viet-Muong grouping of the Mon-Khmer branch of the Austroasiatic language family. This family also includes Khmer, which is spoken in Cambodia, as well as Munda languages spoken in northeastern India and others in southern China. Vietnamese is a tone language; the variations in tones signify different meanings. Three dialects of Vietnamese are mutually intelligible: North Vietnamese (Hanoi dialect), Central Vietnamese (Hué dialect), and Southern Vietnamese (Saigon dialect). The tones in each of these dialects vary slightly, although the Hué dialect is more markedly different from the others. Table 6.8 demonstrates the vowels and consonants of Vietnamese according to Cheng (1994) and Ruhlen (1976).

CLINICAL APPLICATION

Phonological Changes—Vietnamese

Based on the absence of certain consonants and the discussion by Cheng (1994), the following possible pronunciation difficulties may arise in the Vietnamese speaker of American English.

1. The affricates [tʃ] and [dʒ] do not exist in Vietnamese and may produce difficulties.
2. There is a limited number of final consonants in Vietnamese. The consonants [p, k, m, ŋ] and a [ŋm] consonant combination are the only final consonants used by all three dialects of Vietnamese. Depending on the dialect, there is variable use of [t], [c] (a voiceless palatal stop), [n], and [ɲ] as final consonants. Therefore, the Vietnamese speaker may have problems realizing the other consonants in the word-final position.
3. There are no consonant combinations in Vietnamese. The Vietnamese speaker may either re-

Table 6.8 Phonological Inventory: A Comparison of Vietnamese to General American English (GAE)

Vietnamese Vowels	Vowel Differences: Vietnamese and GAE
[i, u, e, ɛ, o, ɔ, ʌ, æ, ɐ, ɯ, ɤ] ([ɯ] is a high-back vowel without lip rounding; [ɤ] is a mid-back vowel without lip rounding; [ɐ] is a low-central vowel.)	▪ [ɪ, ʊ, ɝ, ɚ] and diphthongs do not exist in Vietnamese. ▪ Vietnamese speaker may substitute similar vowels in GAE, e.g., *hit* → [hit]
Vietnamese Consonants	**Consonant Differences: Vietnamese and GAE**
[p, ɓ, t, ɗ, k, g/ʔ] ([ɓ] is a bilabial implosive; [ɗ] is an alveolar implosive.)	▪ Cheng (1994) notes the presence of [g] in Vietnamese; Thompson (1965) describes it as a glottal stop.
[f, s, z, x, ɣ] ([x] is a velar fricative.)	▪ [v, ʃ, ʒ, ð, θ] do not exist in Vietnamese. ▪ [tʃ, dʒ] do not exist in Vietnamese.
[j, w, l]	▪ r-sounds exist only in some dialects of Vietnamese.
[m, n, ŋ, ɲ] ([ɲ] is a palatal nasal.)	▪ Final consonants are limited to [p, t, k, m, n, ŋ].
Vietnamese is a tone language.	▪ No consonant blends in Vietnamese.

Sources: Cheng (1994); Ruhlen (1976).

duce the combination to a singleton production or insert a schwa sound between the blend. Thus, the word *stew* might become [sətu].

4. Depending on the dialect, an *r* sound might not be present. In addition, there are no central vowels with r-coloring. This sound, especially its prevalence in American English, might be problematic for Vietnamese speakers of American English.

5. Depending on the dialect, other sounds may not be present in the inventory of Vietnamese and may therefore need to be learned. These include [v], [z], [ʃ], [θ], [ð], [ʒ], and [j]. There will be a tendency to substitute the voiceless counterparts [f] and [s], which do exist in Vietnamese, for the voiced consonants. In addition, the voiceless and voiced velar fricatives may be substituted for other fricative sounds.

Cantonese American English.   The majority of Chinese Americans are from the Canton Province in southern China. They originally settled in California but dispersed to cities such as New York City, Chicago, and other large cities. Today, approximately 40 percent of the Chinese Americans reside in California, primarily in the two metropolitan areas of San Francisco and Los Angeles. In the San Francisco Bay area alone, there are approximately 400,000 Chinese Americans.

As one of the Chinese languages, Cantonese belongs to the Sino Tibetan language family, which also includes Tibetan as well as Lolo Burmese and Karen (both spoken in Burma). The major languages within Chinese are Mandarin, Wu, Min, Yue (Cantonese), and Hakka (Li and Thompson, 1987). Given all the dialects that exist within Cantonese, the language is sometimes referred to as a group of Cantonese dialects, and not just Cantonese. Oral communication is virtually impossible among speakers of some Cantonese dialects. For instance, there is as much difference between the dialects of Taishan and Nanning as there is between Italian and French. According to its linguistic characteristics and geographical

distribution, Cantonese can be divided into four dialects: Yuehai (including Zhongshan, Chungshan, Tungkuan), as represented by the dialect of Guangzhou City; Siyi (Seiyap), as represented by the Taishan city (Toishan, Hoishan) dialect; Gaoyang, as represented by the Yangjiang city dialect; and Guinan, as represented by the Nanning city dialect, which is widely used in Guangxi Province. If not otherwise specified, the term *Cantonese* often refers to the Guangzhou Dialect, which is also spoken in Hong Kong and Macao. See Table 6.9 for the vowels and consonants of this dialect.

CLINICAL APPLICATION

Phonological Changes—Cantonese

The following learner difficulties for Cantonese speakers of American English are outlined by Chan and Li (2000).

1. There are no voiced syllable-final plosives in Cantonese; therefore, learners of English tend to substitute [p, t, k] for [b, d, g] in the word-final position. In addition, there is a tendency to not release the voiceless plosives in Cantonese, which is transferred to American English. Thus, *rope* and *robe* or *mate* and *maid* are practically indistinguishable. Cantonese learners of English also have a tendency to devoice plosives in syllable-initiating position.

2. Due to the absence of voiced [v] and [z], Cantonese speakers of English tend to substitute their voiceless counterparts, [f] and [s].

3. As [ʃ] and [ʒ] do not exist in Cantonese, [s] will often be used as a substitute for these sounds.

4. Cantonese does not have "th" sounds and the Cantonese speaker of English will often substitute [t] or [f] for [θ] ([tɪn] for *thin*) and [d] or [f] for [ð] ([deɪ] for *they*).

5. The affricates [tʃ] and [dʒ] do not exist; Cantonese speakers of English will tend to substitute [ts] and [dz] for [tʃ] and [dʒ].

6. Cantonese speakers of English often have trouble distinguishing [l], [n], and [r]. Where the [r] is in a word-initial position, they tend to substitute an l-like sound for [r]. Other speakers may substitute

Table 6.9   Phonological Inventory: A Comparison of Cantonese (Hong Kong) to General American English (GAE)

Cantonese Vowels	Vowel Differences: Cantonese and GAE
[i, y, ɪ, ɛ, œ, ɵ, ɔ, ʊ, u, ɐ, a] ([y] is a high-front vowel with lip rounding, [ɵ] is a central vowel with lip rounding, [œ] is a vowel similar to [ɛ] but with lip rounding.)[1]	■ [e, æ, ɑ, o, ɝ, ɚ, ʌ, ə] are not present in Cantonese. ■ Although Cantonese has long and short vowels, they do not differ qualitatively. Therefore, long and short vowels such as [e] and [ɛ], which are different qualitatively, may be difficult.
Cantonese Consonants	**Consonant Differences: Cantonese and GAE**
[p, p^{h2}, t, t^h, k, k^h, k^{w3}]	■ [b, d, g] do not exist in Cantonese. ■ In Cantonese, phonemic oppositions are signaled by the presence and absence of aspiration. Speakers may have distributional difficulties with aspirated and unaspirated productions in GAE.
[f, s , h]	■ Voiced fricatives [v, z] as well as [ʃ, ʒ, θ, ð] are not present in Cantonese.
[ts, t^hs, dz, d^hz]	■ Affricates are somewhat different. There is phonemic opposition between aspirated and unaspirated [t, d] in affricate productions.
[w, j, l] [m, n, ŋ]	■ [r] is not present in Cantonese.

1. There are long and short variants of many of the vowels and many diphthongs in Cantonese; officially, Cantonese counts fifty-two vowels (Cheng, 1994).

2. The raised [^h] indicates that these sounds have an aspirated and a nonaspirated variation, which is phonemic and therefore distinguishes meaning between words.

3. The [k^w] is a coarticulated consonant, as the [k] and [w] are articulated together.

Source: Lee (1999).

[w] for [r]. In syllable-initial position, [n] may be substituted by [l], whereas in final position, the [l] may be deleted or a [u] sound is used, rendering *wheel* as [wiu].

7. Long and short vowels are problematic for Cantonese speakers of American English. Thus, word pairs with [i] – [ɪ] and [u] – [ʊ] may be difficult.

8. When [i] or [ɪ] occur at the beginning of a word, there is a tendency to add a [j] sound, thus, *east* and *yeast* sound the same. This is a transfer from Cantonese as the vowel [i] in syllable-initial position is preceded by [j].

9. Because Cantonese contains no consonant clusters, speakers will have a tendency to delete these clusters in words or insert a schwa vowel between the consonant sounds of the cluster.

Hmong American English.   Many people think that the Hmong came to the United States to enjoy the economic benefits, but, in fact, most are here to escape the death and horror of a genocidal war against them. The long campaign of the Laotian and Vietnamese governments to destroy the Hmong is vengeance for Hmong support of the United States in the Vietnam War. The Hmong people in the United States are largely concentrated in Wisconsin, Minnesota, and California. Several million Hmong people remain in China, Thailand, and Laos, speaking a variety of Hmong dialects. The Hmong language group is a monosyllabic, tonal language (seven to twelve tones, depending on the dialect). There appear to be two basic dialects of Hmong: Mong Leng and Hmong Der. These two dialects are mutually intelligible. The following consonant and vowel inventories are based on the Mong Leng dialect, which is offered by Mortensen (2004). The phonology of Hmong Der can be found in Ratliff (1992). Table 6.10 depicts the vowels and consonants of Hmong Mong Leng dialect.

Table 6.10 Phonological Inventory: A Comparison of Mong Leng Hmong to General American English (GAE)

Hmong Vowels	Vowel Differences: Hmong and GAE
[i, ɨ, e, æ, a, u, ɔ] ([ɨ] vowel is a rounded centralized vowel with a high tongue position. The tongue position is moved horizontally so that the maximum elevation of the tongue is mediopalatal rather than prepalatal as it is with [i].)	■ [æ] and [a] are variants of one /a/-type vowel; they can be used interchangeably. The Hmong speaker might have trouble realizing the distinctions between these two vowels in GAE.
Three nasalized vowels exist: [ĩ], [ũ], and [ã]	■ The short vowels [ɪ, ɛ, ʊ, o] and the central vowels are not part of the Hmong inventory.
Hmong Consonants	**Consonant Differences: Hmong and GAE**
[p pʰ¹, pˡ pˡᵗ², t tʰ, ʈ ʈʰ, c cʰ¹, k kʰ, q qʰ, ʔ] d dʰ	■ The voiced stops [b, g] do not exist in Hmong.
[ᵐb ᵐbʰ, ᵐbˡ ᵐbˡᵗ, ⁿd ⁿdʰ, ⁿɖ ⁿɖʰ, ᶮɟ ᶮɟʰ, ᵑg ᵑgʰ, ᴺɢ ᴺɢʰ]	■ The voiced stops [b, d, g] are prenasalized stops. Therefore, the nasal is produced prior to the stop. This could create qualitative difficulties in GAE.
[f, v, s³, ʂ, ʐ, ç, ʝ⁴, h]	■ [ʂ, ʐ, ç, ʝ] are retroflexed and palatalized fricatives that may be used as substitutions for [ʃ, ʒ]. [θ, ð] do not exist in Hmong.
[ⁿdz, ⁿdz, ⁿɖ, ⁿɖzʰ]	■ All affricates are prenasalized.
[l, j] [m, mˡ mˡᵗ, n, ɲ, ŋ]	■ [r] and [w] are not part of the Hmong inventory.

1. The elevated [ʰ] indicates that these sounds have aspiration, which has phonemic value.

2. The elevated [ˡᵗ] indicates that these sounds have a lateral release.

3. There is an aspirated [s] that may be produced by some speakers.

4. This sound is a voiceless palatal fricative that is similar (but with a narrower opening between the active and passive articulators) to a voiceless [j].

Sources: Matisoff (1991); Mortensen (2004).

CLINICAL APPLICATION

Phonological Changes—Hmong

Based on the absence of certain consonants, the following possible pronunciation difficulties may arise in the Hmong speaker of American English.

1. Voiced stop-plosives that do not demonstrate prenasalization do not exist. There is the possibility of substituting the prenasalized voiced stops for these sounds.
2. The voiced fricative [z] does not exist in Hmong. Again, the Hmong speaker of American English may substitute the voiceless fricative [s] in words containing [z].
3. The consonant [w] is not within the inventory of Hmong. This may need to be learned.
4. An *r* sound is not present in Hmong. In addition, there are no central vowels with r-coloring. This sound, especially its prevalence in American English, might be problematic for Hmong speakers of American English.
5. The affricates in Hmong are prenasalized. There could be a tendency to substitute the prenasalized affricates for [tʃ] and [dʒ]. In addition, [ʃ] and [ʒ] do not exist.
6. The Hmong language has many stop-plosives with a lateral release such as [pˡ] and [pᵗ]. These might be substituted for [pl], for example.
7. There are no word-final consonants in Hmong. This could be difficult for the Hmong speaker to realize.
8. Most words are monosyllabic in Hmong. This could pose difficulties when trying to pronounce multisyllabic words and manipulating word stress.

Korean American English. In 1903, the first Korean immigrants to the United States arrived in Honolulu, Hawaii. Today, a little over one million Korean Americans live throughout the United States, representing one of the largest Asian American populations in the country. The largest concentration of Korean Americans is found in the five-county area of Los Angeles, which includes Los Angeles, Orange, San Bernardino, Riverside, and Ventura counties.

About one-quarter of all the Korean Americans living in the United States reside in this region. The next largest area of concentration is the New York region, including New York City, northern New Jersey, and the Connecticut–Long Island area. This area constitutes about 16 percent of the entire Korean American population in the United States.

The Korean language belongs to the Altaic language group but contains many words of Chinese origin (Ball and Rahilly, 1999). There are nineteen consonants and eight vowels, which occur distinctively long or short. These vowels and consonants are shown in Table 6.11 from Ladefoged and Maddieson (1996) and Lee (1999).

CLINICAL APPLICATION

Phonological Changes—Korean

The following areas are considered problematic for Korean speakers of American English.

1. Korean differs considerably from English in the phonetic realization of word-final stops. Word-final Korean stops are always unreleased—that is, produced without audible aspiration—whereas English stops are either released or unreleased. This, together with the differences in voicing and aspiration initiating a syllable and intervocalically, can lead to confusion of [p]–[b], [t]–[d], and [k]–[g] pairs of words such as *cap* and *cab*.
2. Several English consonant sounds do not exist in the Korean speech sound system. These include the fricatives /f/, /v/, /θ/, and /ð/. These sounds are produced as /p/, /b/, /t/, and /d/, respectively, and the /p/ and /f/ and the /b/ and /v/ sounds in particular are very often confused.
3. Korean speakers make no distinction between /r/ and /l/. The equivalent Korean consonant is alveolar and is somewhere between the two. This, combined with the fact that there are no central vowels with r-coloring, leads to problems with r-sounds and the stereotyped [r] and [l] mix-up.
4. There are differences in the structure of syllables between Korean and English. In Korean, consonants are not released unless they are followed by

Table 6.11 Phonological Inventory: A Comparison of Korean to General American English (GAE)

Korean Vowels	Vowel Differences: Korean and GAE
[i, e, ø, ɛ, a, ɯ, u, o, ʌ] ([ɯ] is a high-back vowel without lip rounding, [ø] is a close-mid-vowel similar to [e] but with lip rounding.)	■ Korean has a set of short vowels and long vowels that, according to Lee (1999), demonstrate slightly different tongue positions. ■ The vowels [ɪ, æ, ʊ] as well as the central vowels with r-coloring are not present in Korean.
Korean Consonants	**Consonant Differences: Korean and GAE**
[p, pʰ[1], t, tʰ, k, kʰ, d[1]]	■ Voicing is context dependent—initiating a syllable, they are voiceless; intervocalically, they are voiced. This could cause difficulties with voiced and voiceless stop-plosives.
[s, z, h]	■ [f, v, ʃ, ʒ, θ, ð] are not present in Korean.
[tʃ tʃʰ, dʒ dʰʒ[2]] [m, n, ŋ]	■ Affricates appear close to those produced in GAE; however, aspiration has phonemic value.
[l]	■ The consonants [w, r, j] are not present in Korean. The [l] in Korean is productionally in between the GAE [r] and [l], which leads to the typical mix-up of these consonants.

1. Syllable initially, these sounds are voiceless unaspirated or slightly aspirated, whereas intervocalically, they are voiced.

2. Lee (1999) describes this affricate as containing postalveolar stops ([c] and [ɟ]), whereas Ladefoged and Maddieson (1996) use the symbols that are noted above.

Sources: Ladefoged and Maddieson (1996), Lee (1999).

a vowel in the same syllable, and word-final consonants are never released. This causes the insertion of a vowel at the end of every English word that ends with a consonant. For example, *Mark* becomes [maku] and *college* becomes [kalədʒi]. This is a strong characteristic of the speech of beginning learners of English in Korea.

5. Korean is a syllable-timed language, and Korean learners of English are unused to the patterns of stressed and unstressed syllables in English words.

6. Korean is not a stress-timed language. Korean learners of English have little or no experience in using English in communicative situations, where emphasizing and deemphasizing words takes on a meaning in context. Also, Korean has a very different syntactic structure when compared to English. Because of these factors, Korean learners of English tend to pronounce each word in a sentence with equal emphasis. They have difficulty producing and perceiving weak forms in English, and they have little intuitive grasp of where to speed up, slow down, add stress, or deemphasize words in their sentences for communicative effect.

Implications for Appraisal. The native language may impact the client's acquisition of English to varying degrees. Therefore, it is quite possible that the client's irregular pronunciations may be a consequence of native language interference. If so, the differences between the sound inventory, phonemic values, and phonotactic constraints of the native language, on the one hand, and of General

American English, on the other, will provide guidelines for accent reduction. A second possibility is that the client may evidence a phonological disorder in both the native language and General American English. To decide this, tests that assess the phonological systems of both languages should be used. For many of the languages, however, such standardized assessment tools will not be available or the clinician's knowledge of the foreign language will not be adequate enough to administer the test. In these cases, other professionals with knowledge of the language and/or family members can be a valuable portion of the appraisal process.

SUMMARY OF THE DATA

Tables 6.12 and 6.13 can be useful in organizing your data for later analysis.

Table 6.12   Considerations When Collecting Data

Hearing Screening	
Does not pass screening	⟶ Referral
Examination of Speech Mechanism	
Not passing, deviancies	⟶ Additional testing, referral
Initial Impression	
Poor intelligibility	⟶ Need careful planning of further evaluation, especially spontaneous speech sample; see section on the unintelligible child
Articulation Test	
Few errors	⟶ Stimulability, contextual testing
Many errors	⟶ Attempt stimulability
Speech Sample	
Poor intelligibility	⟶ Choose topic, structure situation, gloss utterances
Language Screening	
Not within normal limits	⟶ Do more extensive language testing
Auditory Discrimination Testing	
Noted collapse of phoneme oppositions	⟶ Do auditory discrimination testing
Cognitive Appraisal	
Necessary	⟶ Referral, obtain records

Table 6.13 Checksheet for Data Collection

Hearing Screening	Pass _____ Not Passing _____
Examination of Speech Mechanism	Pass _____ Not Passing _____
	Noted deviancies _____
	_____
Initial Impression	Intelligibility
	Good _____ Fair _____ Poor _____
	Error productions noted
	_____
Articulation Test	Error productions noted
	_____
	Stimulability testing
	Sound _____
	Sound level: Yes _____ No _____
	Syllable level: Yes _____ No _____
	Word level: Yes _____ No _____
	Sound _____
	Sound level: Yes _____ No _____
	Syllable level: Yes _____ No _____
	Word level: Yes _____ No _____
	Sound _____
	Sound level: Yes _____ No _____
	Syllable level: Yes _____ No _____
	Word level: Yes _____ No _____
Contextual Testing	Sound _____
	Word contexts that elicit norm production
	_____
	Sound _____
	Word contexts that elicit norm production
	_____
	Sound _____
	Word contexts that elicit norm production
	_____
Speech Sample	Intelligibility
	Good _____ Fair _____ Poor _____
	Error productions noted
	_____
Language Screening	Pass _____ Not passing _____
Auditory Discrimination Testing	Sound _____
	Does _____ Does not _____ discriminate
	Sound _____
	Does _____ Does not _____ discriminate
Information on Cognitive Appraisal	Necessary _____ Not necessary _____

SUMMARY

First, this chapter summarized the various areas of data collection in the appraisal portion of the assessment process. These include (1) an articulation test, (2) spontaneous speech sampling, (3) evaluation of the oral mechanism, and (4) additional measures exemplified by a hearing screening, language screening, auditory perceptual testing, and cognitive appraisal. Methods and goals for each of these areas were discussed together with limitations that might be inherent in the procedures. For example, an articulation test provides a relatively time-efficient way to evaluate articulation skills; however, it does not provide the clinician with any information about the client's abilities to use these skills in naturalistic contexts. In the second portion of this chapter, special assessment considerations were examined for the child with an emerging phonological system, the unintelligible speaker, the dialect speaker, and the speaker with English as a second language. Each of these groups of clients presents the clinician with challenges that will necessitate changes in the appraisal process and the evaluation of the results. This chapter is seen as a guide to assist the clinician in the selection of appraisal procedures that will maximize clinical decision making within the diagnostic process.

CASE STUDY

According to Table 6.5, which one of the following productions would be indicative of African American English?

house	[haᵘş]	matches	[mætʃəş]	thumb	[tʌm]
telephone	[tɛfoᵘn]	lamp	[wæmp]	finger	[fɪŋgə]
cup	[tʌp]	shovel	[ʃʌvə]	ring	[rĩ]
gun	[gã]	car	[kɑə]	jumping	[djʌmpən]
knife	[nɑˈt]	rabbit	[wæbət]	pajamas	[djæməş]
window	[wɪnoᵘ]	fishing	[fɪʃĩ]	plane	[pweˈn]
wagon	[wædən]	church	[tʃɜtʃ]	blue	[bwu]
wheel	[wiə]	brush	[bwʌʃ]	bath	[bæf]
chicken	[tʃɪkə̃]	pencils	[pɪnsəz]	drum	[dwʌm]
zipper	[zɪpə]	scissors	[sɪzəz]	Santa	[sænə]
duck	[dʌ]	bathtub	[bæftʌb]	street	[skrit]
vacuum	[vækum]				

Answers: thumb (see #7), telephone (see #2), finger (see #12), shovel (see #4), ring (see #19), gun (see #19), car (see #11), fishing (see #19), church (see #10), wheel (see #4), bath (see #6), chicken (see #19), pencils (see #4), zipper (see #12), bathtub (see #6), street (see #24), vacuum (see #23)

THINK CRITICALLY

The following selected words are from the HAPP-3 (Hodson, 2004).

1.	basket	13.	three
2.	glasses	14.	mouth
3.	spoon	15.	screwdriver
4.	zip	16.	truck
5.	boats	17.	thumb
6.	cowboy hat	18.	music box
7.	green	19.	watch
8.	feather	20.	rock
9.	fork	21.	shoe
10.	mask	22.	string
11.	star	23.	crayons
12.	toothbrush	24.	hanger

1. Based on Table 6.5, which of the preceding listed words might be produced differently according to African American English? What might be the characteristic production?
2. Select one of the phonological inventories of either Spanish (Table 6.7), Vietnamese (Table 6.8), Cantonese (Table 6.9), Mong Leng Hmong (Table 6.10), or Korean (Table 6.11). Based on these inventories, hypothesize which difficulties might be encountered with the preceding listed words by children speaking one of these languages.

TEST YOURSELF

1. All of the following pertain to the collection of data in assessment except
   a. interview with parents and other professionals
   b. selection of therapy targets
   c. school and medical records
   d. evaluation by the clinician
2. In an assessment, you begin collecting data about your client
   a. as you greet and observe the client interacting with family
   b. when you begin administering an articulation test
   c. during the spontaneous speech sample
   d. after the speech mechanism evaluation
3. When selecting a measure of articulation for assessment, you should consider
   a. the age and development level of the child
   b. if the test is able to provide standardized scores
   c. how the test analyzes speech sound errors
   d. if the test includes an adequate sample of sounds relevant to the client
   e. all of the above
4. Of the three different scoring systems for sound errors, which is considered to be the most precise and most universally accepted among professionals?
   a. two-way scoring
   b. five-way scoring
   c. phonetic transcription
5. Approximately 80 percent of the clinical population with "delayed speech" also have associated problems with their
   a. hearing
   b. language
   c. vision
   d. oral structure
6. A language variation spoken by the members of a particular region, cultural, or social community is a
   a. second language
   b. dialect
   c. language disorder
   d. speech disorder
7. You observed a clinician who administered an articulation test, completed a speech mechanism evaluation, and a gave a language test to a child. You most likely were observing a
   a. comprehensive evaluation
   b. screening
   c. cognitive evaluation
8. Which of the following is a disadvantage to articulation tests?
   a. the necessary time to administer a test is usually minimal

b. results from these tests usually yield a list of "incorrect" sound productions in different word positions

c. articulation tests examine errors in isolated words

d. these tests provide standardized scores

9. Taking a history, visual inspection, screening audiometry, and acoustic immittance are all portions of a
   a. speech screening   c. language screening
   b. cognitive screening d. hearing screening

10. Since it is often difficult to administer an articulation test to a young child with emerging phonology, you
   a. ask the family for additional information (recorded speech from home, a log of words from home, etc.)
   b. do not evaluate the child for services
   c. examine only the oral structure
   d. evaluate language instead

WEBSITES

www.phonologicaldisorders.com

This website, created by the author of this textbook, contains several articulation test results and conversational samples from children which can be viewed and analyzed. Links are given to other websites and resources.

www.suite101.com/article.cfm/speech_language_disorders/43601/1

This link provides a brief explanation of why oral mechanism exams are important. It is not written by a speech-language pathologist, but it mentions the role of the speech-language pathologist in completing such exams during evaluations.

www.aability.com/qschoolscreen.htm

This website is a question-and-answer site where speech-language pathologist Ruth Alice Jurey provides a forum for parents or the public to ask questions about speech, language, and reading. This particular link provides the answer to a parent's concern regarding speech screenings in schools.

www.superduperinc.com/CEU/ArticPhonology_Demo/handout.pdf

This website provides a link to a pdf file from Super Duper publications. The document is a thorough explanation of choosing articulation assessments and general administration guidelines. The article also touches on stimulability.

www.eurocran.org/content.asp?contentID=1270

This website provides a quick review and tips on how to collect a spontaneous speech sample, including topics such as setting, timing, length of sample, and more.

www.ncbi.nlm.nih.gov/entrez/query.fcgi?cmd=Retrieve&db=PubMed&list_uids=15053086&dopt=Abstract

This site contains the abstract to a recent study from 2004 entitled *Sampling children's spontaneous speech: How much is enough?*

FURTHER READINGS

Bernthal, J., & Bankson, N. (1994). *Child phonology: Characteristics, assessment, and intervention with special populations.* New York: Thieme.

Hegde, M. N. (2001). *Pocketguide to assessment in speech-language pathology* (2nd ed.). San Diego, CA: Singular Publishing.

Shipley, K. G., & McAfee, J. G. (1998). *Assessment in speech-language pathology: A resource manual* (2nd ed.). San Diego, CA: Singular Thompson Learning.

Smit, A. B. (2004). *Articulation and phonology: Resource guide for school-age children and adults.* Clifton Park, NY: Thomson Delmar Learning.

Wolfram, W., & Schilling-Estes, N. (2006). *American English: Dialects and variation* (2nd ed.). Malden/Oxford: Blackwell.

Speech-Motor Assessment Screening Form

Each of the following parameters is assessed using the following system:

Pass	Within normal limits
Deviant	Deviant from norm, divided into "slight" or "marked" deviancy
Not passing	Clearly outside of normal limits

STRUCTURE

Head/Face

Sitting opposite the client, evaluate head and facial structures according to the categories provided.	Pass	Deviant Slight	Deviant Marked	Not Passing
Size, shape of head				
Symmetry of facial features:				
Left half vs. right half				
Absence of drooping or spasticity				
Mandible/maxilla relationship				
Appearance of lips (contact at rest; vermilion)				
Appearance of nose (septum; nares)				
Appearance of philtrum/columella				
Absence of any striking features (e.g., adenoid facies, facial dimensions)				

Comments:

Breathing

Observe and evaluate the client's breathing behavior (as "structural" prerequisite for speaking and voice production) during normal (silent) breathing and during speaking. During silent breathing the client's mouth should be closed and no clavicular movement should be noticeable.	Pass	Deviant Slight	Deviant Marked	Not Passing
Silent breathing				
Mouth closed (mouth open would indicate a deviancy)				
Relationship for the time of inspiration versus expiration is about 1:1				
Lack of clavicular breathing				

Breathing	Pass	Deviant Slight	Deviant Marked	Not Passing
Breathing during speaking				
Breathing through nose (exclusive mouth breathing is a deviancy)				
Relationship for the time of inspiration versus expiration is 1:2+				
Lack of clavicular breathing				
Comments:				

Oral/Pharyngeal Cavity

The head should be bent back slightly for inspection of the palatal areas. A few reminders:

Missing frontal teeth might have a direct effect on sibilant production.
Dentition:
  Class I (normal) occlusion: lower molars (or canine for children without molars) half a tooth ahead of upper molars.
  Class II malocclusion (overbite): Maxilla protruded in relation to mandible, measured by the positions of the first (maxillary and mandibular) molars.
  Class III malocclusion (underbite): Mandibular molar more than half a tooth ahead of maxillary molar.
  Open bite: Gap between biting surfaces. Especially frontally open bites might influence articulation negatively.
  Cross bite: Misalignment of the teeth characterized by a crossing of the rows of teeth.
Macroglossia = tongue appears too large
Microglossia = tongue appears too small
Shrinkage, i.e., a "shriveled" tongue area, might indicate a paralytic condition.
The midline of the hard and soft palates appears normally pink and white; a blue tint suggests a submucous cleft.
Redness of fauces and pharynx might indicate inflammation.

	Pass	Deviant Slight	Deviant Marked	Not Passing
Dentition				
Front teeth present				
Spacing of teeth adequate				
Axial orientation of teeth is adequate				

Oral/Pharyngeal Cavity	Pass	Deviant Slight	Deviant Marked	Not Passing
Dentition				
Class I normal occlusion				
If a malocclusion is noted, indicate the type:				
Tongue				
Normal size in relationship to oral cavity				
Normal color				
No shrinkage				
Absence of fissures, lesions, fasciculations				
Normal resting position				
Palate (hard and soft)				
Normal color				
Normal width of vault				
Absence of fistulas, fissures				
Absence of clefts				
If cleft, circle one: Repaired Unrepaired				
Normal uvula				
If abnormal, circle one: Bifid Other deviations				
Normal length of uvula				
Appearances of fauces, pharynx				
Comments:				

FUNCTION

For older children and adults, these tasks can be elicited by asking the client to complete the task. For younger children (preschool age and below), imitation may be required.

Head/Face	Pass	Deviant Slight	Deviant Marked	Not Passing
Eyes/facial appearance				
Raising of eyebrows is symmetrical				

		Pass	Slight	Marked	Not Passing
Can smile, frown on command					
Smiling, frowning symmetrical					

		Deviant			
Head/Face		**Pass**	**Slight**	**Marked**	**Not Passing**
Lips					
Can protrude lips with mouth closed					
Can protrude lips with mouth slightly open					
Can protrude lips to left/right side					
Can protrude and spread lips ([u]–[i])					
Demonstrates rapid lip movements ("pa-pa-pa")					
Mandible					
Can lower mandible on command					
Can move mandible to left/right side					
Comments:					

		Deviant			
Oral/Pharyngeal Cavity		**Pass**	**Slight**	**Marked**	**Not Passing**
Tongue					
Can stick out tongue					
Can move tongue upward (try to touch nose with tip of tongue)					
Can move tongue downward (try to touch chin with tip of tongue)					
Can move the tip of the tongue from the left to the right corner of the mouth					
Can move the tongue quickly and smoothly from the right to the left corner of mouth					

	Pass	Deviant Slight	Deviant Marked	Not Passing
Can move tongue smoothly around the vermilion of lips (lick around lips) clockwise and counterclockwise				
Can move the tongue from left to right on the outside/inside of the upper teeth				
Can move the tongue from left to right on the outside/inside of the lower teeth				
Can say "pa-pa-pa" quickly, smoothly				
Can say "ta-ta-ta" quickly, smoothly				

Oral/Pharyngeal Cavity	Pass	Deviant Slight	Deviant Marked	Not Passing
Tongue				
Can say "ka-ka-ka" quickly, smoothly				
Can alternate between quick repetitions of "pa-ta" and "ta-pa"				
Can alternate between quick repetitions of "pa-ta-ka," "ka-ta-pa," and "ta-pa-ka"				
Velopharyngeal function				
During short, repeated "ah" phonation adequate velar movement is noted				
Can puff up cheeks				
Can maintain intraoral air (puffed cheeks) when slight pressure is applied to cheeks				
Absence of nasal emission				

Breathing	Pass	Deviant Slight	Deviant Marked	Not Passing
Silent breathing				
During quick inspiration breath intake is through nose				
During quick inspiration breath intake is thoracic/abdominal				
Breathing during speaking				
Can sustain "ah" for 5 seconds				
Comments:				

7

Diagnosis

PHONETIC VERSUS PHONEMIC EMPHASIS

LEARNING OBJECTIVES

When you have finished this chapter, you should be able to:

- Describe how to evaluate the inventory and distribution of speech sounds.
- Explain the advantages of analyzing words into prevocalic, postvocalic, and intervocalic consonants.
- Understand the connection between phonemic contrasts and distinguishing phonetic from phonemic disorders.
- Describe what is meant by a sound preference.
- Differentiate between "consistent loss" versus "inconsistent loss" of phonemic contrasts.
- Explain what signals a primarily phonetic disorder.
- Specify the guidelines for beginning therapy.
- Identify the five areas that are analyzed for a comprehensive phonemic analysis.
- Define early syllable shapes, and what is meant by a syllable constraint.
- Explain how you would analyze error patterns according to place-manner-voicing features.
- Name the idiosyncratic processes found in the speech of children with phonological disorders.
- Distinguish between least and more phonological knowledge.
- Define intelligibility, and list factors that affect intelligibility of an utterance.
- Determine the percentage of consonants correct.

$\mathcal{I}$n Chapter 6, different means of appraisal were outlined that would inform the clinician about the client's articulatory-phonological abilities in several areas. These means included both citation form and spontaneous speech sound performance as exemplified by the gathering of data from an articulation test and a spontaneous speech sample. Supplemental tests that would screen the adequacy of the oral mechanism, hearing, language, auditory perception, and cognitive abilities were also suggested. The next step in the assessment process is to *organize, analyze, and interpret the collected data*. The end product of this assessment portion not only provides the clinician with a solid foundation for diagnostic decisions but also leads directly to treatment goals.

One of the first diagnostic decisions facing a clinician is *how* to organize and analyze the available data. There are many possibilities, which all lead to somewhat different interpretations. It is important to choose the organization and analysis that best suit the individual client. Above all, the client's type and degree of speech sound difficulties will play a major role in this selection process.

The first goal of this chapter is to present some general organizational methods that can be used to give the clinician an overview of the speech sound problems noted on the articulation test and spontaneous speech sample. This organization is suitable for any dependent analysis, regardless of age or the type and degree of impairment. The chapter's second goal is to provide an analysis procedure that will aid the clinician in determining whether the client has primarily a phonetic disorder, an impairment of speech sound form, or a phonemic disorder—that is, deficiencies in phonemic function. This analysis will first take into account the preservation or collapse of phonemic contrasts in the client's speech. Although a clear division into phonetic versus phonemic disorder is not always possible (a client may demonstrate characteristics of both), the clinician needs to be aware of the important differences between the two. A tentative decision as to primarily phonetic versus phonemic difficulties will guide the clinician in further analyses and intervention decisions. The third goal of this chapter is to present additional analysis procedures. For the client with a primarily phonetic disorder, suggestions will be offered for further testing and guidelines will be given on integrating diagnostic results into beginning therapy goals. For the client with a primarily phonemic disorder, a phonological assessment battery will be introduced. Organizational categories for this battery include (1) the inventory and distribution of sounds, (2) syllable shapes and constraints, (3) phonological contrasts, and (4) phonological rules or patterns. Analyzing the patterns or phonological rules of a particular client's speech can be achieved in a number of ways. Several contemporary methods for this analysis will be described.

It should be emphasized that the overall aim of this chapter is to provide information that will aid in clinical decision making. There are no prescribed answers. Based on all assessment data collected, each clinician will need to determine for each and every individual client which analysis procedures need to be completed for a valid diagnosis. This chapter is seen as an aid to making those decisions.

PRELIMINARY ANALYSIS: INVENTORY AND DISTRIBUTION OF SPEECH SOUNDS

One way to organize the results of the articulation test and spontaneous speech sample is to look at the inventory and distribution of speech sounds. The **inventory of speech sounds** is a list of speech sounds that the client can articulate within normal limits. However, for many clients, this is not a simple dichotomy between norm and aberrant productions. Some will show a regular production of a speech sound in one context but not in another. This is exemplified by a child who substitutes [t/s] within a word and at the end of a word but realizes the target sound correctly when the word begins with [s]. Such inconsistencies should be duly noted because they provide important clinical information. In addition, some clients realize a sound normally in contexts in which it does not belong but consistently mispronounce it in contexts in which it should be used. For example, an analysis revealed that a child had no accurate productions of [s] in all words that contained s-sounds. However, in the word *brush,* [ʃ] was replaced by an accurate [s]. This phenomenon has often been reported (Fey, 1992; Pollack and Rees, 1972; Smith, 1973) and frequently occurs in children with phonemic disorders (Fey, 1992). Examples such as these demonstrate that norm articulation of the sound in question is within the client's capabilities; however, the client does not seem to understand the language-specific function and/or organization of speech sounds as phonemes. Such information aids considerably in determining which clients show evidence of a phonemic disorder.

The **distribution of speech sounds** refers to where the norm and aberrant articulations occurred within a word. Articulation tests often categorize according to three word positions: initial, medial, and final. As previously noted, *word-medial position* is an imprecise term. This lack of precision has bothered many practitioners who were interested in a closer look at the client's error patterns.

> Some of the problems inherent in using the term *medial* to refer to all sounds in between the first and last sounds of a word were discussed in the Syllable Structure section of Chapter 2.

In an attempt to introduce more structure and to reflect the hierarchical relationship of the syllable to the word, Grunwell (1987), for example, adopted a categorization that divides each multisyllabic word into its syllables. The sounds within the syllable are then further classified according to whether they initiate or terminate syllables. Although this system is clearly superior to the three-position one used by most articulation tests, dividing words into syllables poses its own problem: where to place the syllable boundaries. There is no clear-cut way to pre-

dict where a particular speaker will divide the syllables of a word. For example, does one say "roo-ster" or "roos-ter"? Ask several people how *telephone* is divided: *te-le-phone* or *tel-e-phone*? The problem of where and how to syllabify words is not a new one. For decades, many scholars have wrestled with the problem (e.g., Jespersen, 1913; Ladefoged, 2006; Rosetti, 1959; Scripture, 1927; Sievers, 1901; Stetson, 1936, 1951). To date, it still cannot be said with any certainty exactly where syllables begin and end.

More recently, syllabication guidelines for General American English have been offered (e.g., French, 1988; Grunwell, 1987; Lowe, 1994). These guidelines are based on where the majority of a given set of normal speakers syllabified specific words. However, they are often based on subjective feelings of where syllables can and cannot be divided. Although most syllabication guidelines contain the warning that syllable divisions may vary from speaker to speaker, they do not solve the problematic aspects of the syllable and its division.

Therefore, the following analysis procedure is based not on where the syllable supposedly begins and ends but rather on where the consonants occur relative to the vowel nuclei. This procedure eliminates the necessity of establishing syllable divisions and can be used on words from an articulation test or from a spontaneous speech sample. The consonants can be divided into three categories:

1. *Prevocalic consonants.* Consonants that occur before a vowel. These may be sin-

> It seems plausible that children with phonological difficulties may syllabify words quite differently from what is normally the case. By imposing predetermined syllabication guidelines on words, which may or may not be accurate in a specific case, any subsequent analysis could be faulty and could lead to wrong conclusions.

gletons (i.e., single consonants) or consonant clusters at the beginning of the word or utterance.

2. *Postvocalic consonants.* Consonants that occur after a vowel. These may be singletons or consonant clusters at the end of a word or utterance.

3. *Intervocalic consonants.* Consonants that occur between two vowels. These may be singletons or consonant clusters at the juncture of two syllables.

Using a Matrix to Examine the Inventory and Distribution of Speech Sounds

Figure 7.1 is a matrix that can be used to record the utterances from both articulation tests and spontaneous speech samples. The entire word is written in the left-hand column. Next, the word is divided into individual sound realizations. Using phonetic transcription, the target production (Targ.) and the client's realization (Prod.) should be recorded for each sound within the word: When applicable, prevocalic, syllable nucleus, and postvocalic sounds are recorded for one-syllable words, while multisyllable words would contain intervocalic sounds. Let's use the word *chicken* [tʃɪkən], for which the client says [tɪtə], to demonstrate the process.

Word: Chicken

Prevocalic		Nucleus		Inter-/Post-vocalic		Nucleus		Inter-/Post-vocalic	
Targ.	Prod.	Targ.	Prod.	Targ.	Prod.	Targ.	Prod.	Targ.	Prod.
tʃ	t	ɪ	ɪ	k	t	ə	ə	n	ø

In this example, the symbol ø is used to indicate deletions. In addition, any type of aberrant productions could be circled by the clinician.

This information is then transferred to the matrix for summarizing phones accord-

ing to pre-, inter-, and postvocalic word positions, found in Figure 7.2. For the purpose at hand, a check mark (✓) will be used to indicate a norm realization, a ø to record deletions, and the appropriate phonetic symbols with diacritics to document substitutions and distortions. Therefore, this matrix is used to record both the norm and the aberrant productions of the client. As can be noted in Figure 7.2, singleton consonant productions are recorded separately from clusters. Using the *chicken* example, [t] would be recorded in the prevocalic matrix under tʃ ([tʃ] → [t]), [t] would be recorded under intervocalic k ([k] → [t]), and a ø would be placed in the postvocalic box under [n]. If the clinician would like to consolidate the results even further, Figure 7.3 depicts a matrix that could be used to record pre-, inter-, and postvocalic realizations on a single form. Results from Figures 7.2 and 7.3 will give the clinician (1) the inventory of consonants, (2) the distribution of phones, and (3) the number of times each consonant occurred.

In order to demonstrate how each of these matrices could be clinically utilized, Table 7.1 presents the results of the Goldman-Fristoe Test of Articulation (Goldman and Fristoe, 2000) for H. H., a 7;4-year-old child who was introduced in Chapter 4. The entire word has been transcribed for each of the utterances. Although spontaneous speech results should also be included in the assessment, for simplification, this introduction will analyze only the results of the articulation test (see Table 7.1). A spontaneous speech sample that could be analyzed according to these procedures is contained at the end of Chapter 4 in Appendix 4.1. Figures 7.4, 7.5, and 7.6 (pages 000 and 000) are examples of how these matrices could be used to record the responses for H. H. A more detailed analysis for H. H. is contained in Appendix 4.1 in Chapter 4.

Figure 7.1 Preliminary Matrix for Recording Utterances

Transcribed Word	Prevocalic	Nucleus	Inter-Postvoc.	Nucleus	Inter-Postvoc.	Nucleus	Inter-Postvoc.	Nucleus	Inter-Postvoc.
	Targ. → Prod.	Targ. → Prod.	Targ. → Prod.	Targ. → Prod.	Targ. → Prod.	Targ. → Prod.	Targ. → Prod.	Targ. → Prod.	Targ. → Prod.

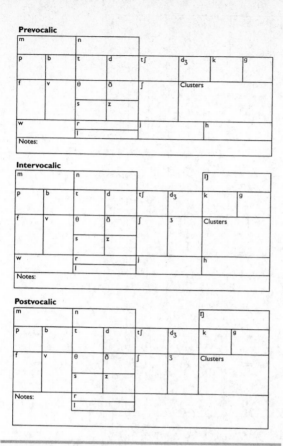

Prevocalic

Intervocalic

Postvocalic

Figure 7.2 Matrix for Recording Phones According to Pre-, Inter-, and Postvocalic Word Positions

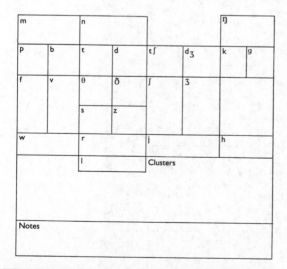

Figure 7.3 Matrix for Recording the Overall Inventory of Phones

Table 7.1 Single-Word Responses to Goldman-Fristoe Test of Articulation for Child H. H.

Target Word	Child's Production
1. house	[haᵁ]
2. telephone	[tɛfoᵁ]
3. cup	[tʌp]
4. gun	[dʌn]
5. knife	[naɪ]
6. window	[wɪnoᵁ]
7. wagon	[wædən]
wheel	[wi]
8. chicken	[tɪtə]
9. zipper	[tɪpə]
10. scissors	[tɪtə]
11. duck	[dʌt]
yellow	[jɛwoᵁ]
12. vacuum	[ætu]
13. matches	[mætət]
14. lamp	[wæmp]
15. shovel	[dʌvə]
16. car	[tɑə]
17. rabbit	[wæbɪ]
18. fishing	[bɪdɪn]
19. church	[tɜ]
20. feather	[bɛdə]
21. pencils	[pɛntə]
this	child would not say
22. carrot	[tɛwə]
orange	[oᵁwɪn]
23. bathtub	[bætʌ]
bath	[bæ]
24. thumb	[bʌm]
finger	[bɪnə]
ring	[wɪŋ]
25. jump	[dʌmp]
26. pajamas	[dæmi]
27. plane	[beɪn]
blue	[bu]
28. brush	[bʌs]
29. drum	[dʌm]
30. flag	[bæ]
31. Santa Claus	[tænə dɑ]
32. Christmas	[tɪtmə]
tree	[ti]
33. squirrel	[twɜə]
34. sleeping	[twipɪn]
bed	[bɛd]
35. stove	[doᵁ]

Figure 7.4 Example of Preliminary Matrix for Recording Utterances for Child H. H.

Transcribed Word	Prevocalic Targ. → Prod.	Nucleus Targ. → Prod.	Inter-Postvoc. Targ. → Prod.	Nucleus Targ. → Prod.	Inter-Postvoc. Targ. → Prod.	Nucleus Targ. → Prod.	Inter-Postvoc. Targ. → Prod.	Nucleus Targ. → Prod.	Inter-Postvoc. Targ. → Prod.
house	h → h	aʊ → aʊ	s → ∅						
telephone	t → t	ɛ → ɛ	l → l	ə → ∅	n → ∅	oʊ → oʊ		unstressed syllable deletion – 2nd syllable	
cup	k → t	ʌ → ʌ	p → p						
gun	g → d	ʌ → ʌ	n → n						
knife	n → n	aɪ → aɪ	f → ∅						
window	w → w	ɪ → ɪ	nd → n	ɪ → ɪ	n → n				
wagon	w → w	æ → æ	g → g	ə → ə	n → n				
wheel	w → w	i → i	l → ∅						
chicken	tʃ → t	ɪ → ɪ	k → t	ɪ → ɪ	n → ∅				
zipper	z → t	ɪ → ɪ	p → p	ɛ → ɛ	z → ∅				
scissors	s → t	ɪ → ɪ	z → t	ɛ → ɛ	z → ∅				
duck	d → d	ʌ → ʌ	k → t						
yellow	j → j	ɛ → ɛ	l → l	oʊ → oʊ					
vacuum	v → ∅	æ → æ	kj → kj	u → u	m → ∅				

Prevocalic

m ✓		n ✓					
p ✓	b ✓ ✓ ✓	t ✓	d ✓	tʃ [t][t]	dʒ [d] [d]	k [t][t] [t]	g [d]
f [b] [b] [b]	v Ø	θ [b]	ð	ʃ [d]	Clusters [pl]→[b] [bl]→[b] [br]→[b] [dr]→[d]	[fl]→[b] [kr]→[t] [skw]→[tw] [sl]→[tw] [st]→[d]	
		s [t][t]	z [t]				
w ✓ ✓ ✓		r [w][w] l [w]		j ✓			h ✓
Notes:							

Intervocalic

m ✓		n ✓					
p ✓ ✓	b ✓	t	d	tʃ [t]	dʒ	k [t]	g [d]
f ✓	v ✓	θ	ð [d]	ʃ [d]	ʒ	Clusters [nd]→[n] [ng]→[n] [kj]→[t] [kl]→[d] [ns]→[nt] [sm]→[tm] [θt]→[t] [st]→[t]	
		s	z [t]				
w		r [w][w] l [w]		j			h
Notes:							

Postvocalic

m Ø ✓ ✓		n Ø ✓ ✓ Ø ✓					ŋ ✓
p ✓	b Ø	t Ø Ø	d ✓	tʃ Ø	dʒ	k [t]	g Ø
f Ø	v Ø	θ Ø	ð	ʃ [s]	ʒ	Clusters [mp] ✓ ✓ [lz]→Ø [ndʒ]→[n]	
		s Ø	z Ø [t] Ø				
Notes:		r l Ø Ø Ø		[ɚz]→[ə] scissors			

Figure 7.5 Matrix for Recording Phones According to Pre-, Inter-, and Postvocalic Word Positions for Child H. H.

Phonemic Contrasts: Differentiating Phonetic from Phonemic Disorders

Clients with phonemic disorders are characterized by impaired phonemic systems; they show difficulties using phonemes contrastively to differentiate meaning. Therefore, if two or more phonemes are represented by the same sound production, this indicates that the contrastive phonemic function has not been realized. The emphasis in this phase of the analysis is on the contrastive use of sounds, not on their accurate production. Loss of

Overall Inventory of Phones

m 4✓ 1Ø		n 5✓ 2Ø					ŋ 1✓
p 4✓ 1Ø	b 4✓ 1Ø	t 1✓ 2Ø	d 2✓	tʃ 3[t] 1Ø	dʒ 2[d]	k 5[t]	g 2[d] 1Ø
f 1✓ 1Ø 3[b]	v 1✓ 2Ø	θ 1Ø 1[b]	ð 1[d]	ʃ 2[d] 1[s]	ʒ 3 not tested		
		s 2[t] 1Ø	z 3[t] 2Ø				
w 3✓		r 4[w]		j 1✓			h 1✓

•Prevocalic 1[pl]→[b] 1[bl]→[b] 1[br]→[b] 1[dr]→[b] 1[fl]→[b] 1[kr]→[t]	l 2[w] 3Ø 1[skw]→[tw] 1[sl]→[tw] 1st→[d]	Clusters •Intervocalic 1nd→[n] 1[kj]→[t] 1[θt]→[t] 1[ng]→[n] 1[kl]→[d]	1[sm]→[tm] 1st→[t] •Postvocalic 2[mp]✓ 1[lz]→Ø 1[ndʒ]→[n]
Notes *Vowel nucleus* 5 [æ]→[ə] 2 [ɝ]→[ɜ]			

Figure 7.6 Overall Inventory of Phones for Child H. H.

phonemic contrast is the central problem of clients with phonemic—that is, phonological impairments.

Depending on the client, the neutralization of specific phonemic contrasts can be consistent or inconsistent. A *consistent loss* is indicated by the exact same realization (the same distortion, substitution, and/or deletion) occurring every time in the client's realizations. Consistent loss of a phonemic contrast can be exemplified by the child who, regardless of the position of the sound in the word, realizes all [s] sounds as [t] ([s] → [t]). The child has neutralized the contrast between /s/ and /t/. Also, the child who always deletes the intended phoneme ([s] → ø) would demonstrate a consistent loss of phonemic contrast as well. *Inconsistent* realizations refer to substitutions or deletions that occur only in certain contexts. The sounds produced by a child who prevocalically realizes [t] for [s] but produces [s] accurately in specific words in postvocalic positions would be indicative of an inconsistent loss of the phonemic contrast. If we examine H. H.'s productions, we see several different inconsistent losses of phonemic contrast. One example is [f]. At the beginning of a word, H. H. realizes [f] as [b] ([f] → [b]) in such words as *fishing, feather,* and *finger*. However, intervocalically in *telephone,* H. H. produces [f] correctly. At the end of the word, such as in *knife,* H. H. deletes [f]. This is an example of an inconsistent loss of a phonemic contrast. The final decision on which speech sounds are indeed employed as contrastive phonemes will often necessitate that the clinician check sound oppositions through minimal pairs, for example.

What to Do? The analysis of phonemic contrasts can begin with the matrices presented in Figures 7.2 and 7.3. These provide an overview, which can be used to fill out Figure 7.7, the Neutralization of Phonemic Contrasts Summary Form (page 000).

1. Look for those sounds that are *consistently* used for another phoneme. For example, [k] was consistently realized as [t] in H. H.'s productions (see Figures 7.5 and 7.6). There were no instances (including consonant clusters) in which [t] was not substituted for /k/.
2. Look for those sounds that are *inconsistently* used—that is, occurring only in certain contexts. Inconsistencies are exemplified by (a) norm productions in some instances and the collapse of the phoneme contrast in others, (b) the production of two or more different sound realizations for one phoneme, or (c) the use of substitutions in certain contexts together with sound deletions in other contexts. For H. H., [f] shows an inconsistent loss of a phonemic contrast. In the

prevocalic position, [f] → [b]; postvocalically, [f] is deleted; the intervocalic production was accurately articulated. Also, check to see whether any pattern can be noted pre-, inter- and/or postvocalically. From Figure 7.5, we see that H. H. does seem to demonstrate a pattern with [tʃ]: in pre- and intervocalic positions, [t] is realized; postvocalically, [tʃ] is deleted.

3. Summarize the collapse of contrasts. The purpose of this overview is to discover any substitutions that represent more than one target phoneme. Therefore, all target phonemes with the same substitution are grouped together. For H. H., [k], [s], [z], and [tʃ] are replaced by [t], for example. In addition, [d] replaced [g], [dʒ], [ð], and [ʃ]. These are summarized for H. H. on Figure 7.8.
4. Look for any *sound preferences*. This is exemplified by a sound or sound combination representing several different phonemes. Sound preferences should be checked to see whether any patterns exist, for example, one phone utilized for a whole class of consonants. For H. H., [t] and [d] seem to represent sound preferences; both were employed as substitutions for four different phonemes. The summary of H. H.'s phonemic contrasts is provided in Figure 7.8. Only consonant singletons were entered in this form, but it could also be used to look at consonant cluster productions.

Further testing may be warranted for sounds that show inconsistent contrasts. This could be easily achieved by having the client name pictures or read minimal pair words.

DECISION MAKING: PRIMARILY PHONETIC EMPHASIS

It is important to analyze all existing data, possibly supplementing them with additional

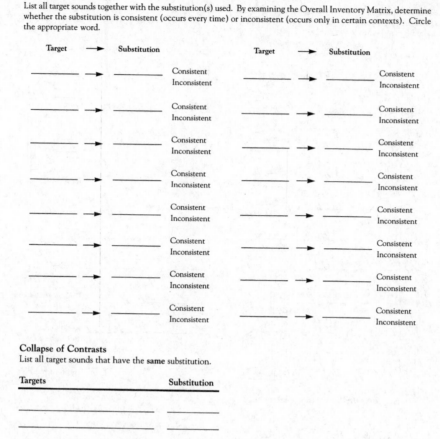

List all target sounds together with the substitution(s) used. By examining the Overall Inventory Matrix, determine whether the substitution is consistent (occurs every time) or inconsistent (occurs only in certain contexts). Circle the appropriate word.

Collapse of Contrasts
List all target sounds that have the **same** substitution.

Sound Preferences
List any speech sounds which are used for a wide range of target phonemes.

Figure 7.7   Neutralization of Phonemic Contrasts Summary Form

information, before arriving at the tentative decision that the client does show evidence of a phonetic disorder. In doing so, it must always be kept in mind that phonetic and phonemic disorders can co-occur. "It would be a mistake to adopt an either/or dichotomy" (Elbert, 1992, p. 242). The following section outlines the factors that will help

the clinician in the process of decision making when considering a primarily phonetic emphasis.

Phonetic disorders are signaled by:

1. *Preservation of phonemic contrasts.* Substitution of one phoneme for another suggests the collapse of phonemic contrasts and

List all target sounds together with the substitution(s) used. By examining the Overall Inventory Matrix, determine whether the substitution is consistent (occurs every time) or inconsistent (occurs only in certain contexts). Circle the appropriate word.

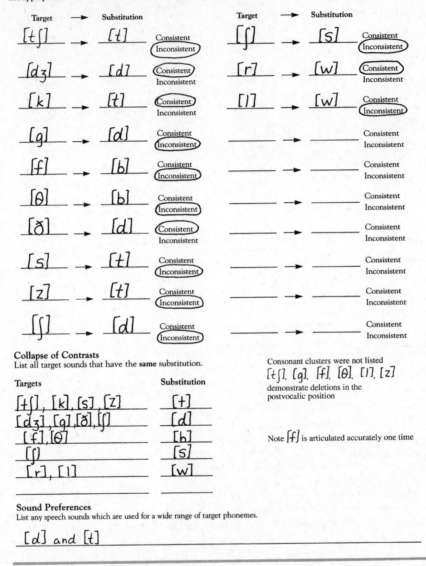

Target	→	Substitution	
[tʃ]	→	[t]	Consistent / **(Inconsistent)**
[dʒ]	→	[d]	**(Consistent)** / Inconsistent
[k]	→	[t]	**(Consistent)** / Inconsistent
[g]	→	[d]	Consistent / **(Inconsistent)**
[f]	→	[b]	Consistent / **(Inconsistent)**
[θ]	→	[b]	Consistent / **(Inconsistent)**
[ð]	→	[d]	**(Consistent)** / Inconsistent
[s]	→	[t]	Consistent / **(Inconsistent)**
[z]	→	[t]	Consistent / **(Inconsistent)**
[ʃ]	→	[d]	Consistent / **(Inconsistent)**

Target	→	Substitution	
[ʃ]	→	[s]	Consistent / **(Inconsistent)**
[r]	→	[w]	**(Consistent)** / Inconsistent
[l]	→	[w]	Consistent / **(Inconsistent)**

Collapse of Contrasts
List all target sounds that have the **same** substitution.

Targets	Substitution
[tʃ], [k], [s], [z]	[t]
[dʒ], [g], [ð], [ʃ]	[d]
[f], [θ]	[b]
[ʃ]	[s]
[r], [l]	[w]

Consonant clusters were not listed
[tʃ], [g], [f], [θ], [l], [z]
demonstrate deletions in the postvocalic position

Note [f] is articulated accurately one time

Sound Preferences
List any speech sounds which are used for a wide range of target phonemes.

[d] and [t]

Figure 7.8 Neutralization of Phonemic Contrasts Summary Form: Application for Child H. H.

therefore a phonological disorder. However, if one sound is being used as a substitution for several phonemes, the client's realizations should be carefully examined to deter-mine if even minimal production differences are being used to signal phonemic contrasts. For example, a child might be using a pala-talized [s], [sʲ], as a substitution for [ʃ]. The

CLINICAL APPLICATION

For H. H., the following neutralization of phonemic contrasts for singleton consonants was established:

1. Consistent neutralization of contrasts: [k] → [t]

[ʤ], [ð] → [d]

2. Inconsistent contrast neutralization: [r] → [w], [tʃ], [z], [s] → [t] (note: [tʃ], [z], and [s] are deleted in the postvocalic position)

[ʃ] → [s] (note: occurs only in postvocalic position)

[ʃ] → [d] (note: occurs in pre- and intervocalic positions)

[g] → [d] (note: [g] is deleted in the postvocalic position)

[f], [θ] → [b] (note: [f] is realized correctly one time in intervocalic position)

[l] → [w] (note: [l] is deleted in the postvocalic position)

3. Sound preferences: [d] is used to represent four other phonemes

[t] is used to represent four other phonemes

palatalized [s] is articulated with the tongue in a more posterior position than is normally the case. In addition, this same child could be using a dentalized [s̪] for [θ]. The dentalized [s̪] demonstrates a more anterior tongue position than is normally the case. Both substitutions would be labeled as [s] distortions; however, in this case the child is demonstrating production variations to signal the phonemic contrasts: [sʲ] for [ʃ] and [s̪] for [θ]. Even minimal form differences, if used consistently, could indicate the preservation of phonemic contrasts. Omissions of sounds should also be carefully evaluated to determine if articulatory changes can be discovered between minimal pairs with and without the deleted sound. Several investigators have demonstrated that omitted sounds may be represented by some other articulatory gesture to preserve the phonemic contrasts (Bauman-Waengler, 2002a, 2002b; Smit and Bernthal, 1983; Weismer, 1984; Weismer, Dinnsen, and Elbert, 1981). Noted changes included variations in vowel duration and a final gliding articulation of the vowel preceding the deleted sound.

What to Do? Use pictures or words representing minimal pairs of the target sound and the substitution or omission. Have the client spontaneously produce each word. If a distinguishable articulatory contrast is realized between the two sounds, utilize narrow transcription to document the variation. Different articulatory gestures might indicate that the client is differentiating

Minimal pair words for the most frequently misarticulated sounds are contained in Chapter 8.

between the two phonemes but not in a conventional manner.

2. *Peripheral, motor-based problems.* By definition, phonetic disorders are characterized by misarticulations—that is, aberrant speech sound form representing disruptions of the relatively peripheral articulatory process and involving inadequate motor learning (Fey, 1992). Speech sound errors within the framework of phonetic disorders are also relatively consistent; that is, inadequate motor learning of the particular sound is generalized throughout the system. Therefore, consistent inventory constraints are noted regardless of the position of the sound within the word (Elbert, 1992). In addition, phonetic disorders are not cognitive-linguistic (organizational) or perceptually based problems (Kamhi, 1992). Organizational difficulties would be reflected in disturbed phonotactics, whereas clients with perceptually based problems may not be able to discriminate between the target sound and its inaccurate production.

What to Do? Examine the client's irregular productions relative to their occurrence pre-, inter-, or postvocalically. If the production remains consistent, occurring in every tested word and position, this would suggest a phonetic disorder. However, if positional constraints are discovered, the organization or phonotactics may not be intact, pointing to a phonemic disorder (Elbert, 1992).

Often, no pattern can be discovered; that is, the client produces the sound correctly in some words and incorrectly in others. In this case, two additional factors should be considered: (1) the phonetic context and (2) the possibility of an emerging sound. Due to the possible influence of coarticulation, specific phonetic contexts may enhance or hinder the production of the target sound. Words that contain accurate sound realizations should be

examined to determine if a common phonetic context exists. Emerging sound patterns in the speech of children can also result in inconsistent realizations. Support for this possibility includes the appearance of the sound in productionally "easy" contexts (e.g., single syllables or familiar words) and its stimulability at the sound or word level. If the production is influenced by the phonetic context or the sound seems just to be emerging, this would suggest a phonetic disorder.

CLINICAL APPLICATION

Phonetic or Phonemic Difficulties

Tommy's parents requested an evaluation of his speech sound skills. They were concerned that he had some misarticulations that were not age appropriate. The initial impression of Tommy, age 7;1, was that of an alert child who was fairly intelligible but seemed to have problems with [s], [z], [r], [θ], and [ð]. Tommy passed a hearing screening, an examination of the speech mechanism, and a language screening test. A spontaneous speech sample and an articulation test revealed the following:

1. Substitution of w/r ([r] → [w]) in all word positions. The r-coloring of central vowels was also not realized. Results were consistent in single-word tasks and spontaneous speech.
2. Substitution of θ/s and ð/z ([s, z] → [θ, ð]) in all word positions with the exception of [st] blends at the beginnings or end of words. In these blends, [s] was accurate. Such an accurate production of [s] in blends was noted only in one-word samples, not in conversational speech.
3. Substitution of t/θ and d/ð ([θ, ð] → [t, d]) in all word positions; consistent in one-word samples and spontaneous speech.

Initial Analysis

Tommy did not seem to fit the typical picture of a child with a phonemic disorder. Due to the age of the child, the clinician was not too concerned about the th-problems. However, she was concerned that Tommy's errors constituted a collapse of phonemic contrasts. Further testing was warranted.

Preservation of Phonemic Contrasts

Minimal pairs were used to test Tommy's productions of [w] versus [r]. The clinician noticed subtle differences in attempted [r]-productions when contrasted to his realization of [w]. For example, there was not as much lip rounding when he tried to say a word beginning with [r] when compared to his [w] realization. Tommy was not stimulable for [r] at the sound level. When Tommy was asked to produce minimal pairs with [s] and [θ], his [s] sounded like a [θ] in certain contexts and like a dentalized [s] ([s̪]) in others. He was stimulable for [s], [z], [θ], and [ð] at the sound and word levels.

Peripheral Motor-Based difficulties

Errors were consistent across word positions. The accurate production of [s] in [st] blends was thought to be the effect of coarticulation. Discrimination of minimal pairs with [s] versus [θ] and [z] versus [ð] demonstrated an accuracy of over 90 percent. Discrimination of [w] versus [r] was 70 percent accurate.

Clinical Decision Making

The clinician decided that Tommy showed more evidence of a motor-based phonetic disorder than of a phonemic disorder. Further testing did not indicate perceptual or cognitive-linguistic-based difficulties. In certain contexts, Tommy distinguished productionally and perceptually between the target sounds and his substitutions.

Guidelines for Beginning Therapy: Phonetic Disorder

The gathering of data is completed and diagnostic decisions have been made. Any diagnosis should also lead directly into the selection of intervention goals and strategies. Although goals and strategies will constantly change, depending on the client and the noted difficulties, specific diagnostic information should aid in deciding where to begin with therapy.

Stimulability. Although stimulability is not an absolute predictor of which error sounds will improve in therapy and at which level therapy should begin (sound, syllable, word level), stimulability can be used as a probe to find out which sounds might be somewhat easier for the client to realize. If a client is stimulable for a particular sound, the clinician could attempt this sound in therapy for a trial period.

Correct Production of the Sound in a Specific Context. The collected data often give evidence of a typically misarticulated sound produced *accurately* within a specific word context. Such a word might appear on an articulation test or in the spontaneous speech sample. It was also suggested that articulation test results be supplemented with additional word lists. These probes could yield such a context as well. Norm productions of a word or words containing a usually misarticulated sound verify that, under certain contextual conditions, the client is able to realize its regular articulation. These words, therefore, offer themselves as a therapeutic point of departure.

Sounds Affecting Intelligibility. Certain sounds affect intelligibility more than others. One main reason is their relatively high frequency of occurrence in conversational contexts. A chart displaying the frequency of occurrence of General American English consonants is provided in Appendix 7.1. Other sounds may affect intelligibility due to their conspicuous aberrant articulation. Therapeutically, high priority should be given to sounds that affect the intelligibility of the client the most.

Developmentally Earlier Sounds. Under comparable clinical circumstances, sounds that are acquired developmentally earlier should be considered first targets. The term *comparable clinical circumstances* means that both sounds were stimulable to the same degree and that the sounds in question seemed to have a comparable impact on the client's intelligibility.

Decision Making: Where to Begin Therapy

The previous Clinical Application with Tommy can be used as an example to illustrate these guidelines for making decisions concerning where to begin therapy.

Sound	Stimulable	Correct Word Context	Intelligibility	Development
[r]	no	no	high frequency	earlier than [s], [z], [θ], [ð]
[s], [z]	yes, sound/word	yes, st-blends	high frequency	relatively late
[θ], [ð]	yes, sound/word	no	[ð] high, [θ] low	later sound

Given these variables, it would appear that in this case, [s] and [z] are good choices for initiating a trial probe in therapy. They were stimulable, appeared correctly in certain word contexts, and have a high frequency of occurrence in General American English. Therefore, they will have a definite impact on Tommy's speech intelligibility. In addition, [s] and [z] are typically developmentally earlier than [θ] and [ð]. However, due to the high frequency of occurrence of [r] in General American English and relative early mastery in the acquisition process, [r] should probably be targeted before [θ] and [ð].

DECISION MAKING: PRIMARILY PHONEMIC EMPHASIS

If a phonemic impairment is suspected, a thorough *phonological assessment* becomes necessary. Data for a phonological assessment can be organized in a number of ways. The following organizational scheme is one that has been described either partially or totally by several authors (e.g., Elbert and Gierut, 1986; Fey, 1992; Grunwell, 1987; Howell and Dean, 1994; Ingram, 1989b; Lowe, 1994). This organization will help the clinician in answering important assessment questions and in the planning of therapy goals. The categories found in this organizational scheme are:

1. inventory of speech sounds
2. distribution of speech sounds
3. syllable shapes and constraints
4. phonological contrasts
5. phonological error patterns

Inventory and Distribution of Speech Sounds

The inventory and distribution of speech sounds were discussed earlier in this chapter. Figures 7.1, 7.2, and 7.3 on pages 212–214 are provided to aid in organizing and analyzing these parameters.

Syllable Shapes and Constraints

The term **syllable shape** refers to the structure of the syllables within a word. Therefore, the unit of analysis is the word; that is, each word is described according to occurring vowels, designated as *V*, and consonants, *C*, within that word.

> More information can be found in the Syllable Structure section of Chapter 2.

Syllable shapes vary, with the productionally easiest ones being open syllables such as *eye* or *go*. Syllable shapes in General American English can be very complex, containing up to three consonants prevocalically and four postvocalically. Syllable shapes are important because clients with phonological disorders may delete syllables, use predominantly open syllables, or demonstrate specific consonant preferences in the production of syllables (Crystal, 1981; Hodson and Paden, 1991; Pollock and Schwartz, 1988).

A **syllable constraint** refers to any restriction or limitation established in the production of syllable shapes. Children acquiring speech in a normal manner use many different syllable shapes at an early age. When Stoel-Gammon (1987) analyzed the speech of thirty-two 2-year-olds, she found that thirty-one of the thirty-two children produced two different types of closed syllables while over half of them demonstrated CVCVC structures and word-initial clusters. Approximately half of the 2-year-olds in this investigation were also realizing word-final clusters. Therefore, even children with an emerging phonological system should demonstrate both open and closed syllable structures.

The information about syllable shapes and any possible constraints can be obtained from the articulation test and the spontaneous speech sample. Both the type and frequency of occurrence of the syllable shapes of each word should be noted. Worthwhile information is also gained by determining whether discrepancies exist between the responses on the articulation test and the conversational speech sample. Specific syllable constraints in the speech sample could in part explain a decrease in the client's intelligibility.

Table 7.2 provides the most frequent one-syllable word shapes reported by French, Carter, and Koenig (1930) in one-syllable words. Several two-syllable shapes are included; more could be added. According to Shriberg and Kent (2003), approximately 77 percent of the words spoken by adult speakers of General American English are one-syllable words, and both one- and two-syllable words comprise almost 94 percent of those spoken.

Table 7.2 Common One- and Two-Syllable Shapes

Shape	Examples
V	a, I
CV	go, he
CCV	grow, tree
VC	up, on
VCC	ask, oops
CVC	hop, doll
CCVC	trees, brush
CVCC	hopped, lamp
CCVCC	stopped, drink
Two-Syllable	
CVCVC	wagon, shovel
CVCCV	window, candy
CVCCVC	bathtub, jumping

The main goal of our analysis is to determine whether the client has basic syllable structures and, if so, which ones. Simple open and closed syllable shapes of one- and two-syllable words should be a portion of the client's repertoire.

What to Do?

1. Analyze the client's sample to determine if one-, two-, and, when appropriate, three- or more syllable words exist. Note if there is a large proportion of any single syllable type. For example, it is remarkable if the client uses primarily only one-syllable words.

2. Analyze any reductions in the syllable number or syllable shapes. Reductions in the number of syllables include multisyllable words in which syllable deletions occur. For example, *telephone*, a three-syllable word, might be reduced to [tɛfoʊn]. Changes in the syllable shape are exemplified by words in which deletion of consonants has altered the original syllable shape. For example, *house*, a

CVC shape, might become [haʊ], a CV shape.

Syllable Shapes with H. H.

Analyzing the data from the Goldman-Fristoe test for H. H. demonstrated:

1. the presence of one- and two-syllable words
2. three-syllable words (*telephone, pajamas*) were reduced to two syllables—however, H. H. could produce three syllables (see *Santa Claus* and *Christmas tree*)
3. syllable shapes of one-syllable CVC words were frequently reduced to a CV structure, although in the majority of cases, the CVC structure was maintained
4. the majority of two-syllable words were reduced in shape by final consonant deletion

Based on this sample, H. H. can produce one- and two-syllable words; however, the syllable shapes were often reduced, that is, produced as open syllables in two-syllable words.

Phonological Contrasts

The organization and analysis of data for determining phonological contrasts were dealt with earlier in this chapter. See the Phonemic Contrasts: Differentiating Phonetic from Phonemic Disorders section on page 215 and Figure 7.7 on page 217.

Phonological Error Patterns

Phonological assessment attempts to evaluate the phonological system of each client as accurately as possible. An accurate assessment leads to both an effective diagnosis and successful subsequent therapy. Although the client's productions must be compared to the adult model, it should also be kept in mind that the client's realizations represent a system in themselves. A **system** refers to an or-

derly combination of parts forming a complex unity. A central goal of any phonological assessment is to understand the client's phonological system. Identifying and categorizing the error patterns are an important aspect of this understanding. Knowledge of existing patterns within the system will lead directly to important therapeutic decisions. On the other hand, a lack of this knowledge can easily result in misinterpreting patterns as inconsistencies in the client's phonological system.

There are a number of methods available for analyzing error patterns. While some techniques are more productionally based—analyzing the speech sound form—others attempt to analyze the client's phonemic system. Recalling that phonetic and phonemic disorders can, and often do, occur together, the following form- and function-based frameworks are offered: (1) place-manner-voice, (2) phonological process, and (3) assessing phonological knowledge as an application of generative phonology.

Place-Manner-Voice Analysis. The place-manner-voice analysis is a productionally based system; it depicts speech sound form. As its name implies, this analysis describes error patterns according to a rather broad phonetic feature classification system. Place, manner, and voicing characteristics of each error sound are compared to those representing the norm production features. This comparison can then be examined to determine whether any patterns emerge within the sound system of the client. In this context, patterns are defined as the frequent use of a specific place-manner-voicing feature. The place-manner-voice analysis is designed only to classify substitutions of one sound for another. Distortions and deletions are not accounted for by this system.

The following place-manner-voice categorization system is taken from Howell and Dean (1994):

Place of Articulation

Labial	[p], [b], [f], [v], [m], and [w]
Dental	[θ] and [ð]
Alveolar	[t], [d], [s], [z], [n], and [l]
Postalveolar	[ʃ], [ʒ], [tʃ], and [dʒ]
Palatal	[j], [r]
Velar	[k], [g], and [ŋ]
Glottal	[h]

Manner of Articulation

Stop-plosives	[p], [b], [t], [d], [k], and [g]
Fricatives	[f], [v], [θ], [ð], [s], [z], [ʃ], [ʒ], and [h]
Affricates	[tʃ] and [dʒ]
Nasals	[m], [n], and [ŋ]
Liquids	[l] and [r]
Glides	[w] and [j]

Voicing

Voiced	[b], [d], [g], [v], [ð], [z], [ʒ], [dʒ], [m], [n], [ŋ], [l], [r], [w], and [j]
Voiceless	[p], [t], [k], [f], [θ], [s], [ʃ], [tʃ], and [h]

Figure 7.9 provides a graph of the consonants of General American English according to this system, and Figure 7.10 presents a Place-Manner-Voicing Summary Sheet.

What to Do? Transfer the information from the Overall Inventory of Phones Matrix (Figure 7.3) to the Place-Manner-Voicing Summary Sheet (Figure 7.10) in the following way:

1. Target sound and its substitution are written in the left-hand column.

2. Compare the substitution to the target sound, noting any place, manner, and/or voicing features that were affected. The appropriate change in feature(s) should be circled. Some substitutions will be only one-feature changes; others could be changes in place, manner, *and* voicing characteristics.

3. List the specific place, manner, and/or voicing change that occurred in the column marked Specific Changes. For example, if a child substituted a [t] for [k] ([k] → [t]) "place" would be circled, and "velar → alveolar" recorded in the blank after the place feature.

4. List the number of times this particular feature change occurred. This should be marked down in the Number of Errors column.

5. List each single-sound substitution according to the prescribed directions. After all

	Labial		Dental		Alveolar		Post-Alveolar		Palatal		Velar		Glottal	
Stops	p	b			t	d					k	g		
Nasals		m				n						ŋ		
Fricative	f	v	θ	ð	s	z	ʃ	ʒ					h	
Affricative							tʃ	dʒ						
Liquids					l					r				
Glides		w								j				

Figure 7.9 Place-Manner-Voice Features of General American English Consonants

Target	→	Substitution	Circle Differences	Specific Changes	No. of Errors
_____	→	_____	Place Manner Voicing	_____ _____ _____	_____ _____ _____
_____	→	_____	Place Manner Voicing	_____ _____ _____	_____ _____ _____
_____	→	_____	Place Manner Voicing	_____ _____ _____	_____ _____ _____
_____	→	_____	Place Manner Voicing	_____ _____ _____	_____ _____ _____
_____	→	_____	Place Manner Voicing	_____ _____ _____	_____ _____ _____

Summary

PLACE		MANNER		VOICING	
Change	No. of Occ.	Change	No. of Occ.	Change	No. of Occ.
_____	_____	_____	_____	_____	_____
_____	_____	_____	_____	_____	_____
_____	_____	_____	_____	_____	_____
_____	_____	_____	_____	_____	_____
_____	_____	_____	_____	_____	_____

Distortions _____

Deletions _____

Figure 7.10   Place-Manner-Voicing Summary Sheet
Additional lines for target → substitution could be added. See Figure 7.11, page 227.

substitutions and feature changes have been listed, look for patterns of errors by using the summary at the bottom of the sheet.

Figure 7.11 is the Place-Manner-Voicing Summary Sheet filled out for H. H.

CLINICAL APPLICATION

Place-Manner-Voicing Analysis for H. H.

Using the summary sheet, H. H.'s place, manner, and voicing substitutions could be summarized as follows:

Target	→	Substitution	Circle Differences	Specific Changes	No. of Errors
[tʃ]	→	[t]	(Place) (Manner) Voicing	postalveolar → alveolar affricate → stop	3 3
[dʒ]	→	[d]	(Place) (Manner) Voicing	postalveolar → alveolar affricate → stop	2 2
[k]	→	[t]	(Place) Manner Voicing	velar → alveolar	5
[g]	→	[d]	(Place) Manner Voicing	velar → alveolar	2
[f]	→	[b]	Place (Manner) (Voicing)	fricative → stop voiceless → voiced	3 3

Summary

PLACE		MANNER		VOICING	
Change	No. of Occ.	Change	No. of Occ.	Change	No. of Occ.
postalveolar → alveolar	8	affricate → stop	5	voiceless → voiced	6
velar → alveolar	7	fricative → stop	12	voiced → voiceless	3
dental → labial	1	liquid → glide	5		
dental → alveolar	1				
palatal → labial	3				
alveolar → labial	2				

Distortions ___ [ʊ] ___

Deletions ___ [m], [n], [b], [t], [tʃ], [g], [f], [v], [θ], [s], [z], [l] ___

Figure 7.11 Place-Manner-Voicing Summary Sheet for Child H. H.
(Continued on page 228.)

Place: High occurrence of alveolars being substituted for postalveolar and velar phones (postalveolar and velar → alveolar).

Manner: High occurrence of stops being substituted for fricatives (fricatives → stops).

Voicing: Errors of both voiced → voiceless and voiceless → voiced consonants.

In summary, place-manner-voice analyses are productionally based. They provide the clinician with information about specific changes in place, manner, and voicing that occur in the speech of the client when compared to norm realizations. Although the system evaluates actual phonetic features of speech sounds, it is rather broad-based. Some important features, such as organ of articulation, and secondary features, such

Target → Substitution	Circle Differences	Specific Changes	No. of Errors
[θ] → [b]	(Place) (Manner) (Voicing)	dental → labial / fricative → stop / voiceless → voiced	1 / 1 / 1
[ð] → [d]	(Place) (Manner) Voicing	dental → alveolar / fricative → stop	1 / 1
[ʃ] → [d]	(Place) (Manner) (Voicing)	postalveolar → alveolar / fricative → stop / voiceless → voiced	2 / 2 / 2
[ʃ] → [s]	(Place) Manner Voicing	postalveolar → alveolar	1
[s] → [t]	Place (Manner) Voicing	fricative → stop	2
[z] → [t]	Place (Manner) (Voicing)	fricative → stop / voiced → voiceless	3 / 3
[r] → [w]	(Place) (Manner) Voicing	palatal → labial / liquid → glide	3 / 3
[l] → [w]	(Place) (Manner) Voicing	alveolar → labial / liquid → glide	2 / 2
→	Place Manner Voicing		

Figure 7.11 Continued

as lip rounding of [ʃ], are not accounted for. Only substitutions of one sound for another can be classified according to place-manner-voicing parameters. Sound deletions, distortions, assimilations, and syllable structure changes are not assessed.

Phonological Process Analysis. This type of analysis procedure was introduced in Chapter

4. A phonological process analysis is a means of identifying substitutions, syllable structure, and assimilatory changes that occur in the speech of clients. Each error is identified and classified as one or more of the phonological processes. Patterns of error are described according to the most frequent phonological processes present and/or to those that affect a class of sounds or sound sequences. The

processes utilized to identify substitutions are again primarily productionally based; however, they do account for sound and syllable deletions as well as several assimilation processes.

Certain processes seem to occur more frequently in the speech of children developing their phonological systems in a normal manner. Others, labeled idiosyncratic processes, occur infrequently in the normal population (Stoel-Gammon and Dunn, 1985). On most protocols, substitution processes are limited to consonants, but vowel processes have been identified as well (Ball and Gibbon, 2002; Pollock and Keiser, 1990; Reynolds, 1990; Stoel-Gammon and Herrington, 1990). Examples

of idiosyncratic processes found in the speech of children with phonological disorders are shown in Figure 7.12. Phonological processes used to identify vowel errors are summarized in Figure 7.13.

Children with phonological disorders use these processes in their speech somewhat differently than do normally developing children. Grunwell (1987) provides five different classifications to account for these differences: (1) persisting normal processes, (2) chronological mismatch, (3) systematic sound preference, (4) unusual or idiosyncratic processes, and (5) variable use of processes.

Persisting normal processes are exemplified by the child who makes active use of

Figure 7.12 Idiosyncratic Processes Found in the Speech of Children with Phonological Disorders

The following are a few examples of the relatively uncommon processes that have been found in the speech of children with phonological disorders:

Process	Example		
Initial consonant deletion	"duck" [dʌk]	→	[ʌk]
Backing of stops	"tub" [tʌb]	→	[kʌb]
Backing of fricatives	"sun" [sʌn]	→	[ʃʌn]
Glottal replacement	"gun" [gʌn]	→	[ʔʌn]
Denasalization	"knee" [ni]	→	[di]
Fricatives replacing stops	"toe" [toʊ]	→	[soʊ]
Stops replacing glides	"yarn" [jɑrn]	→	[dɑrn]
Metathesis (reversal of two sounds)	"nest" [nɛst]	→	[nɛts]
Affrication (a nonaffricate becomes an affricate)	"top" [tɑp]	→	[tʃɑp]
Migration (movement of a sound from one position in the word to another position)	"soap" [soʊp]	→	[oʊps]
Unusual cluster reduction	"plane" [pleɪn]	→	[leɪn]
Unusual substitution processes	"plane" [pleɪn]	→	[reɪn]
Vowel processes, for example, centralization of vowels	"bed" [bɛd]	→	[bʌd]

Sources: Bauman-Waengler and Waengler (1988, 1990); Dodd and Iacano (1989); Leonard and McGregor (1991); Roberts, Burchinal, and Footo (1990); Stoel-Gammon and Dunn (1985); Waengler and Bauman-Waengler (1989).

Figure 7.13 Phonological Processes Used to Identify Vowel Errors

Several common and idiosyncratic substitution processes that describe changes in consonant productions have been identified. However, children with phonological disorders may also evidence impaired vowel systems. The following processes have been used to describe vowel substitutions in children (Ball and Gibbon, 2002; Bauman-Waengler, 1991; Pollock and Keiser, 1990):

1. *Vowel backing.* A front vowel is replaced by a back vowel of a similar tongue height. Example: [ɪ] → [ʊ].

2. *Vowel fronting.* A back vowel is replaced by a front vowel of a similar tongue height. Example: [u] → [i].

3. *Centralization.* A front or back vowel is replaced by a central vowel. Example: [ɛ] → [ʌ].

4. *Decentralization.* A central vowel is replaced by a front or back vowel. Example: [ʌ] → [ɛ].

5. *Vowel raising.* A front vowel is replaced by a front vowel with a higher tongue position, or a back vowel is replaced by a back vowel with a higher tongue position. Example: [æ] → [ɛ].

6. *Vowel lowering.* A front vowel is replaced by a front vowel with a lower tongue position, or a back vowel is replaced by a back vowel with a lower tongue position. Example: [u] → [ʊ].

7. *Diphthongization.* A monophthong is realized as a diphthong. Example: [ɛ] → [ɛɪ]

8. *Monophthongization (or diphthong reduction).* A diphthong is realized as a monophthong. Example: [aɪ] → [a].

9. *Complete vowel harmony.* A vowel change within a word that results in both vowels being produced the same. Example: [tɛdi] → [tɛdɛ]

10. *Tenseness harmony.* A lax vowel becomes tense when there is another tense vowel in the same word. Example: [mɛni] → [meni]

11. *Height vowel harmony.* A vowel is replaced with a vowel that is closer in tongue height to another vowel in the same word. Example: [bæskɪt] → [bɛskɪt]

commonly noted phonological processes but beyond the age at which they are typically seen. Thus, a 4-year-old child demonstrating very early processes, such as reduplication or final consonant deletion, might be considered within this category.

Chronological mismatch is evidenced by a child who demonstrates the persistence of early simplifying processes together with patterns that are characteristic of later stages of phonological development. For example, a child produces all fricative sounds adequately, implying that a relatively late process, stopping of fricatives, has been effectively suppressed. However, at the same time, the child still demonstrates velar fronting ([k] → [t]; [g] → [d]), which is normally suppressed at an earlier age than stopping of [s] and [z]. This early process, which has not yet been suppressed, co-occurs with later developmental speech patterns.

Systematic sound preference pertains to the use of a single phonetic realization for several different phonemes. This sound preference results when both normal developmental processes and idiosyncratic or unusual processes co-occur. Weiner (1981) notes that sound preferences are often limited to replacements for fricatives and operate primarily in initial word positions. An example of systematic sound preference would be the productions of a child who substitutes [d] for [s], [z], [ʃ], [ʒ], [tʃ], [dʒ], and all initial consonant blends.

Unusual or idiosyncratic processes are characterized by patterns that are uncommon in the speech of normally developing children (unusual processes) or those that seem to be characteristics of the speech of individual children with phonological disorders (idiosyncratic processes). Grunwell (1987) suggests that the term *idiosyncratic processes* be used very tentatively because these processes can often be found in the speech of normally developing children as well.

The last category, *variable use of processes,* denotes two possibilities: (1) a process operating on one target sound may in one context still be active and in another already suppressed or (2) depending on the context, different processes may be operating on the same target phoneme. An example of (1) is a child who uses stopping, realizing [tup] for *soup* and [tʌn] for *sun,* but demonstrates a norm production of [s] in *soap* and *saw.* The second possibility, the use of different processes for the same target, would be exemplified by a child who employs velar fronting, pronouncing *cake* as [teɪt] and *wagon* as [wædən]. However, when the same target phonemes /k/ and /g/ occur in other contexts, different processes are noted. For instance, final consonant deletion is evidenced when *bake* is pronounced [beɪ], while glottal realization is used when *Maggie* is articulated as [mæʔi]. The speech of children with phonological disorders is characterized by extreme variability of pronunciation patterns. Often, several different realizations are used to represent one phoneme. The variable use of processes may, therefore, be expected frequently in the speech of children with phonological disorders.

Treatment implications of Stampe's theory of natural phonology include suppression of the phonological processes in order to increase the complexity of the child's phonological patterns. The suppression of these phonological processes occurs naturally in the speech of normally developing children, but for children with phonological disorders, treatment must focus on helping to suppress the age-inappropriate processes as well as processes that are not acceptable for the adult language being learned. Typically, several sounds that demonstrate active use of a specific phonological process are selected. These sounds are trained in close succession to aid the child in suppressing the phonological process. Therapy emphasizes the meaningful use of speech, and words are seen as the smallest units to be contrasted and practiced.

The following are the results of an articulation test from Ryan, age 6;6, who was introduced in Chapter 4. Using a phonological process analysis, we find that Ryan demonstrates a high frequency of occurrence of the processes fronting, gliding, cluster substitution, and cluster reduction. The number of times each process occurred is listed in Table 7.3.

horse	[hoʊɚθ]	cold	[koʊd]
wagon	[wægən]	jumping	[dʌmpən]
monkey	[mʌŋki]	TV	[tivi]
comb	[koʊm]	stove	[θtoʊv]
fork	[foɚk]	ring	[wɪŋ]
knife	[naɪf]	tree	[twi]
cow	[kaʊ]	green	[gwin]
cake	[keɪk]	this	[dɪθ]
baby	[beɪbi]	chair	[ʃɛɚ]
bathtub	[bæftəb]	watch	[waʃ]
nine	[naɪn]	thumb	[fʌm]
train	[tweɪn]	mouth	[maʊf]
gun	[gʌn]	shoe	[su]
dog	[dɑg]	fish	[fɪs]
yellow	[wɛloʊ]	zipper	[ðɪpɚ]
doll	[dɑl]	nose	[noʊθ]
pig	[pɪk]	sun	[θʌn]
cup	[kʌp]	house	[haʊθ]
swinging	[s̠wɪŋɪŋ]	steps	[stɛp]
table	[teɪbəl]	nest	[nɛt]
cat	[kæt]	books	[bʊkθ]
ladder	[læɾɚ]	bird	[bɝd]
ball	[bɑl]	whistle	[wɪθəl]
plane	[pweɪn]	carrots	[kɛɚət]

Table 7.3 Phonological Process Analysis Summary Sheet for Ryan

Processes	Number of Occurrences
Syllable Structure Changes	
Cluster reduction	4
Cluster deletion	
Reduplication	
Weak syllable deletion	
Final consonant deletion	
Initial consonant deletion	
Other _____	
Substitution Processes	
Consonant cluster substitution	8
Fronting	12
Labialization	3
Alveolarization	
Stopping	2
Affrication	
Deaffrication	2
Denasalization	
Gliding of liquids	6
Gliding of fricatives	
Vowelization	
Derhotacization	
Voicing	
Devoicing	2
Other _____	
_____	
_____	
Assimilation Processes	
Labial assimilation	
Velar assimilation	
Nasal assimilation	
Liquid assimilation	
Other _____	
_____	
_____	

Phonological processes provide a means of classifying error patterns noted in disordered speech and suggest a direct and simple way to handle intervention. Although these processes have been labeled phonological, they are based to a large extent on phonetic production features. For example, substitution processes are named after the differences between the production of the target and the error sound. Phonological processes do not give concrete information about the neutralization of specific phonemic contrasts, nor do they account for phonological rules that might be operating. Even more important, the presence of phonological processes in the speech of an individual does not necessarily indicate the presence of a phonological disorder. In their contemporary usage, phonological processes are descriptive terms; the existence of a particular process neither explains the problem nor denotes its etiology (Butcher, 1990; Fey, 1992; Shriberg and Kwiatkowski, 1983; Weismer, 1984). The practice of using phonological processes to *imply* a phonological disorder has been identified by Kamhi (1992) as being the most serious problem associated with this type of analysis.

To summarize, phonological processes, a central aspect of natural phonology, have been extensively used to describe disordered speech patterns and to select treatment goals. The speech of children with disordered phonological systems may show differences in kind and use of phonological processes when compared to the speech of children with normally developing systems. However, caution should be exercised when descriptions of phonological processes are used to imply the presence of a phonological disorder.

Assessing Productive Phonological Knowledge.
Elbert and Gierut (1986) present an approach to analyzing a child's *productive phonological*

Using Phonological Processes

Lillian, age 5;6, was screened by the speech-language pathologist in her kindergarten class. The classroom teacher said that Lillian was at times hard to understand. The speech-language pathologist summarized her screening results according to phonological processes:

Process	Examples	Total Number of Times Used
Velar fronting	[k] → [t] [kʌp] → [tʌp] [g] → [d] [gʌn] → [dʌn]	14 times, all words tested
Final consonant deletion	[beɪk] → [beɪ] [lɑg] → [lɑ]	5 times, only on words ending with [k] and [g]
Cluster reduction and cluster substitution	[klaʊn] → [taʊn] [græs] → [dæs]	5 times, only on words with [k] and [g] clusters

First, the therapist realized that this was a case of chronological mismatch. Lillian had suppressed later processes such as stopping of fricatives; however, she was still using the early process velar fronting. In addition, variable use of processes was noted. When [k] or [g] was produced in the word-initial position or in consonant clusters, fronting was demonstrated. In the word-final position, the sounds were deleted.

knowledge. The authors postulate that "the way in which the child *uses* the sound system allows us to determine what the child *knows* about the sound system" (p. 50). This approach emphasizes first that the child's performance must be described independently of the adult norm system. It is only *after* the child's phonological knowledge is assessed that comparisons are made between the child's phonological system and the adult model. The analysis procedures seem to be particularly useful with children who have severe phonological disorders or complex patterns of errors. This analysis may not be appropriate for children who exhibit only one or two sound errors or for those who produce sound distortions.

The child's productive phonological knowledge is determined by (1) the breadth of the distribution of sounds and (2) the use of phonological rules. The breadth of the distribution of sounds consists of

1. the phonetic inventory,
2. the phonemic inventory, and
3. the distribution of sounds in the phonemic inventory.

The following definitions and examples are given for each:

1. Breadth of the Distribution of Sounds
   A. *Phonetic inventory.* Includes all the sounds that the child produced. Whether these sounds concur with the target sound is unimportant. The phonetic inventory would include sounds and sound substitutions listed on the matrix for recording the overall inventory of phones (Figure 7.3). Thus, all sounds accurately articulated and those used as substitutions would be listed.
   B. *Phonemic inventory.* Lists only those sounds that are used contrastively—

that is, those that signal meaning differences. The Neutralization of Phonemic Contrasts Summary Form (Figure 7.7) could be used as a portion of this analysis. Those sounds that do appear on the summary form should be further tested using minimal pairs. For example, for H. H. [k], [s], [z], and [tʃ] were all realized as [t]. Minimal pairs such as *keys, Cs, Zs, cheese,* and *Ts* could be presented to see whether H. H. produces differences between the pairs.

C. *Distribution of sounds in the phonemic inventory.* Includes an analysis of the distribution of sounds by (1) word position and (2) morphemes. Word position distribution examines whether sounds that contrast meaning are used by the child in *all* versus *some* word positions. This could include a comparison of the articulation test, the spontaneous speech sample, and other selected words to see whether the child does produce some errors inconsistently, that is, correct only in some contexts and incorrect in others. For example, a child who says [wæmp] for *lamp* and [wʊk] for *look* but can realize [l] correctly in *yellow* and *telling* demonstrates a distribution by word position; intervocalically the child can realize a norm [l] production. *Distribution by morpheme* examines whether sounds are used contrastively for *all* versus *some* target morphemes. For example, H. H. substitutes [b] for [f] in *fishing, feather,* and *finger* but articulates [f] correctly in *telephone.*

In addition, the phonological rules operating in the child's system are categorized according to static and dynamic rules.

2. The Use of Phonological Rules
   A. *Static rules.* Describe the phonotactic constraints operating within the child's system. There are three types of static rules:
      (1) *Inventory constraints.* Certain sounds do not occur in the phonetic or phonemic inventories.
      (2) *Positional constraints.* Certain sounds occur only in certain word positions but not in others.
      (3) *Sequence constraints.* Certain sound combinations do not occur.
   B. *Dynamic rules.* Alter the production of sounds by changing segments in specific contexts or environments. There are two types of dynamic rules:
      (1) *Allophonic rules.* Describe phonetic variations in the production of a sound. Free variation and complementary distribution can be employed to provide evidence of whether specific phonetic variations are employed to signal phonemic differences.
         a. *Free variation.* Refers to sounds that co-occur in the same position for the same word. Although these sounds have the potential to signal a difference in meaning, in this phonological system they do not. Therefore, for this particular system, they are not meaning-differentiating phonemes. For example, a child sometimes produces [ta] and sometimes [ka] for *car.* Although the production differences between [t] and [k] are linguistically relevant, they do not signal phonemic differences in the child's system. [t] and [k] are in free variation. Free variations are random, that is,

unpredictable in terms of specific contextual factors.

b. *Complementary distribution.* Refers to those sounds that occur in mutually exclusive contexts. These variations are context-conditioned and their occurrence is predictable. Here again, phonetic differences are not signaling a difference in meaning; the phonetic difference is not phonemically relevant. For example, a child realizes all word-initial stops as voiced and all word-final stops as voiceless. Thus, *pin* and *bin* are produced as [bɪn], while *rip* and *rib* are realized as [rɪp]. Variations such as these are context-conditioned and predictable. Although [p] and [b] can both be produced, they never occur in the same context; they are mutually exclusive. In this example, [p] and [b] would stand in complementary distribution. The child does not use [p] and [b] to signal phonemic differences.

(2) *Neutralization rules.* Refers to the collapse of a phonemic contrast between sounds in certain contexts or environments. According to Elbert and Gierut (1986), three conditions must be met before the neutralization rule is operating:

a. The presence of the phonemic contrast must be evidenced somewhere in the child's system. The underlying assumption is that the phonemic contrast must somehow be there before it can be neutralized.

b. This phonemic contrast must be missing in other environments.

c. There must be evidence of morphophonemic alternations. Such alternations are produced when a specific sound in a specific morpheme is changed in a new morphemic environment. For example, the child says [aɪs] for *ice;* however, when saying *icy,* [s] changes to [t] and the word becomes [aɪti].

Dynamic rules may be optional or obligatory. *Optional rules* are those that are applied only in some cases or to some morphemes. Obligatory rules, on the other hand, are those that always apply to all morphemes when the particular rule conditions are met. Box 7.1 provides additional references that expand on the concepts of free variation and complementary

BOX 7.1   Determining Phonological Rules: Selected References

Dinnsen, D. A. (1984). Methods and empirical issues in analyzing functional misarticulations. In M. Elbert, D. A. Dinnsen, & G. Weismer (Eds.), *Phonological theory and the misarticulating child.* ASHA Monograph No. 22. Rockville, MD: ASHA.

Elbert, M., & Gierut, J. (1986). *Handbook of clinical phonology: Approaches to assessment and treatment.* San Diego, CA: College-Hill Press.

Grunwell, P. (1987). *Clinical phonology* (2nd ed.). Baltimore: Williams & Wilkins.

Hyman, L. (1975). *Phonology: Theory and analysis.* New York: Holt, Rinehart & Winston.

Rvachew, S., & Nowak, M. (2001). The effect of target-selection strategy on phonological learning. *Journal of Speech, Language, and Hearing Research, 44,* 610–623.

Williams, A. L. (1991). Generalization patterns associated with training least phonological knowledge. *Journal of Speech and Hearing Research, 34,* 1318–1328.

distribution. The reader is referred to these sources for additional examples.

Based on information gained from the breadth of distribution of sounds, the use of phonological rules, and the nature of the child's lexical representations, Elbert and Geirut postulate six different levels of productive phonological knowledge. Type 1 knowledge represents the most productive knowledge and Type 6 the least.

Type 1. Adultlike lexical representation for target morphemes in all word positions. No phonological rules are noted. Type 1 knowledge is signaled by norm production of sounds. Elbert and Gierut (1986) note that children generally have Type 1 knowledge of nasals and glides.

Type 2. Adultlike lexical representation for target morphemes in all word positions; however, obligatory or optional dynamic phonological rules may be functioning as well. For the most part, the child's production of these sounds is comparable to the target, but some rule-governed irregular productions do occur.

Type 3. Adultlike lexical representation for target in all word positions but only for some morphemes. This type of knowledge can be described by "fossilized forms"—that is, forms that were produced incorrectly at an early age and are now resistive to change. Fossilized productions of names and pets' names are commonly observed.

Type 4. Adultlike lexical representation in some word positions for all target morphemes. Type 4 knowledge is signaled by positional constraints. Irregular sound realizations are noted but only in certain word positions.

Type 5. Adultlike lexical representation in some word positions for some target morphemes. Type 5 knowledge is signaled by those representations that were noted in both Type 3 and Type 4 levels. Thus, positional constraints and fossilized forms are both operating on a sound.

Type 6. Nonadultlike lexical representation in all word positions of all target morphemes. These sounds reflect inventory constraints; they are always produced in an aberrant manner relative to the target sound.

Figure 7.14 is a schematic drawing of the decision-making process that occurs for each of these six types of productive phonological knowledge.

MEASURES OF INTELLIGIBILITY AND SEVERITY

Measures of severity and intelligibility can be especially helpful in documenting the necessity for or progress in therapy. Measures of severity and intelligibility can be selected that meet the specific needs of the assessment and the age and the speech status of the particular client.

Measures of Intelligibility

Intelligibility refers to a judgment made by a clinician based on how much of an utterance can be understood. Measurements of the degree of speech intelligibility are based on a subjective, perceptual judgment that is generally related to the percentage of words that are understood by the listener. Factors influencing speech sound intelligibility include the number, type, and consistency of speech sound errors (Bernthal and Bankson, 2004). Clearly, the number of errors is related to the overall intelligibility. However, just adding up the errors does not yield an adequate index of intelligi-

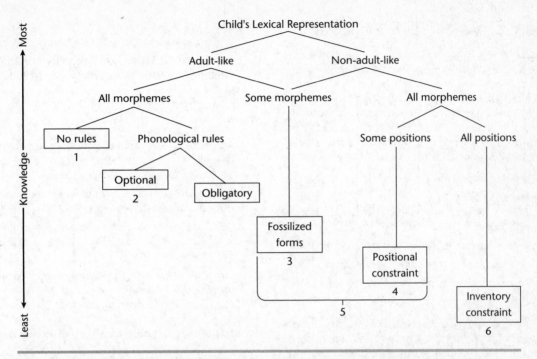

Figure 7.14 Decision Tree for Ranking Child's Phonological Knowledge on a Continuum

Source: From *Handbook of Clinical Phonology: Approaches to Assessment and Treatment* (p. 62), by M. Elbert and J. Gierut, 1986, San Diego, CA: PRO-ED, Inc. Copyright 1986 College-Hill Press. Reprinted with permission.

bility. For example, Shriberg and Kwiatkowski (1982a, 1982b) reported a low correlation between the percentage of consonants correct and the intelligibility of a speech sample.

The intelligibility of an utterance is influenced by several factors. Connolly (1986) lists the following:

1. loss of phonemic contrasts
2. loss of contrasts in specific linguistic contexts
3. the number of meaning distinctions that are lost due to the lack of phonemic contrasts
4. the difference between the target and its realization
5. the consistency of the target-realization relationship
6. the frequency of abnormality in the client's speech
7. the extent to which the listener is familiar with the client's speech
8. the communicative context in which the message occurs

Although intelligibility remains essentially a subjective evaluation, many authors have attempted to quantify it and to apply their results to a wide array of children and adults with communication disorders (e.g., Boothroyd, 1988; Bross, 1992; Gordon-Brannan and Hodson, 2000; Hodson and Paden, 1981; Kent, Miolo, and Bloedel, 1994; Leinonen-Davis, 1988; Ling, 1976; Monsen, 1981; Shriberg and Kwiatkowski, 1982a; Webb and Duckett, 1990; Weiss, 1982; Wilcox, Schooling, and Morris, 1991; Yorkston

BOX 7.2   Measures of Intelligibility

In spite of the fact that there is not a general procedure for measuring intelligibility, the percentage of words understood in a speech sample is a common way to calculate intelligibility (Gordon-Brannan, 1994). Intelligibility can be categorized according to several indices. The following is based on the frequency of occurrence of misarticulated sounds (Fudala and Reynolds, 2000):

Level 6. Sound errors are occasionally noticed in continuous speech.

Level 5. Speech is intelligible, although noticeably in error.

Level 4. Speech is intelligible with careful listening.

Level 3. Speech intelligibility is difficult.

Level 2. Speech is usually unintelligible.

Level 1. Speech is unintelligible.

Kent, Miolo, and Bloedel (1994) summarized a number of procedures that have been used, or could be used, to assess intelligibility. The following are selected for the purpose at hand.

Procedures that emphasize phonetic contrast analysis:

CID Word Speech Intelligibility Evaluation (Word SPINE), for children and adolescents with severe and profound hearing impairments, Monsen, 1981.

CID Picture Speech Intelligibility Evaluation (Picture SPINE), for children and adolescents with severe and profound hearing impairments, Monsen, Moog, and Geers, 1988.

Ling's Phonologic and Phonetic Level Speech Evaluation (PPLSE), for hearing-impaired individuals, Ling, 1976.

Children's Speech Intelligibility Test (CSIT), for children of any age, especially for very young children or children with cognitive or motor limitations, Kent, Miolo, and Bloedel, 1994.

Procedures that emphasize phonological process analysis:

Assessment of Phonological Processes–Revised (APP–R), for children with object-naming competence, Hodson and Paden, 1983.

Functional Loss (FLOSS), for children with limited phonological systems, Leinonen-Davis, 1988.

The RULES Phonological Evaluation, for children with phonological disorders, Webb and Duckett, 1990.

Vihman-Greenlee Phonological Advance Measure, for children, especially those with phonological disorders, Vihman and Greenlee, 1987.

Procedures that emphasize word-level intelligibility:

Assessment of Intelligibility of Dysarthric Speech, for adults and older children, Yorkston and Beukelman, 1981.

Preschool–Speech Intelligibility Measure (P–SIM), for preschool children, but could be used with older children, Wilcox, Schooling, and Morris, 1991.

Weiss Intelligibility Test (WIT), for children and adolescents, Weiss, 1982.

Phonological Mean Length of Utterance (PMLU) and the *Proportion of Whole-Word Proximity* (PWP), for children primarily, Ingram and Ingram, 2001.

and Beukelman, 1981). A summary of intelligibility measures is outlined in Box 7.2.

Measures of Severity

Articulatory competency can also be measured by different severity classifications. Severity measures are attempts to quantify the degree of involvement. Shriberg and Kwiatkowski (1982a, 1982b) developed a metric for measuring the severity of involvement in children with phonological disorders. They suggest calculating the *percentage of consonants correct* (PCC). Based on research, this type of calculation was found to correlate most closely to listeners' perceptions of severity. Quantitative estimates of severity using the PCC give the clinician an objective measure to establish the relative priority of those who might need therapy, for example. The PCC calculations can be translated into the following severity divisions:

>90%   mild
65–85%   mild–moderate
50–65%   moderate–severe
<50%   severe

Box 7.3 provides the procedure for determining the percentage of consonants correct.

Shriberg, Austin, Lewis, McSweeny, and Wilson (1997) have expanded the original concept of Percentage of Consonants Correct (PCC) to other measures that examine the percentage of vowels correct (PVC) and a matrix that weights distortion errors, the Articulation Competence Index (ACI), to mention just two of the ten total indexes. A conversational speech sample is the basis for all calculations. For information on the various metric values, see Shriberg and colleagues (1997).

BOX 7.3   Determining the Percentage of Consonants Correct (PCC)

What is measured?   A five- to ten-minute conversational sample is tape-recorded and analyzed.

What to score?   Only consonants are scored using this metric. The examiner is required to make correct versus incorrect judgments on individual consonant productions. The following sound changes are considered incorrect:

1. deletion of a target consonant
2. substitution of a target consonant, including the substitution of a glottal stop or a cognate
3. partial voicing of a prevocalic consonant
4. any distortions
5. addition of a sound to a correct or incorrect target sound
6. initial [h] deletion and final n/ŋ substitutions in stressed syllables only. For example [ɪt] for *hit* and [rɪn] for *ring* would be incorrect. However, in unstressed syllables—for example, saying [fɪʃən] for *fishing*—would be considered correct. Acceptable allophonic variations are considered correct. For example, the intervocalic allophonic variation of [t] in *water* [wɑɾɚ] is considered correct.

What not to score?   Do not score utterances that are unintelligible or consonants in the second or successive repetitions of a syllable. For example, if the child says [bə beɪbi], score only the first [b]. Also, do not score target consonants in the third or successive repetitions of adjacent words unless the articulation changes. For example, if the child says [trit], [trit], [trit], only the consonants in the first two words are counted. However, if the child changes the articulation saying [trit], [twit], [trit], then the consonants in all three utterances are counted.

Calculation: The percentage of consonants correct is calculated in the following manner:

$$\frac{\text{Number of correct consonants}}{\text{Number of correct plus incorrect consonants}} \times 100$$

SUMMARY

The goal of this chapter was to show how the data gathered in the appraisal section of our assessment could be utilized for several different types of analyses. The first portion of this chapter demonstrated how to organize the data collected from the appraisal portion outlined in Chapter 6. A preliminary analysis included forms and procedures to determine the distribution of speech sounds. These procedures were exemplified using a case study of the child H. H. The next step in the diagnostic process examined the data to determine whether a neutralization of phonemic contrasts existed. Based on the definitions of phonetic-articulatory versus phonemic-phonological impairments, the possibility of differentiating characteristics of these two disorders was discussed. The following section of this chapter outlined further testing that might be necessary for children presenting a phonetic disorder.

The remaining portion of this chapter outlined the procedures for a comprehensive phonological assessment. These included the inventory and distribution of speech sounds, analysis of the syllable shapes and constraints, phonological contrasts, and analyzing phonological error patterns. There are several different ways to analyze the patterns of errors in a phonological assessment. The following means were exemplified: place-manner-voicing, phonological process, and the assessment of productive phonological knowledge. Each of these analyses offers differing results. For each one, sample forms and procedures were supplied as well as a continued implementation of each analysis using the case study of H. H. Finally, measures of severity and intelligibility were described. These measures can be used to document the need for, and progress in, therapy as well as serve as a basis for clinical research.

CASE STUDY

The following spontaneous speech sample is from H. H. Using the directions from Box 7.3, determine the PCC.

Spontaneous Speech Sample for H. H.

Looking at pictures:

[dæ ə pɪtə əv ə tɑ]
That a picture of a dog.

[oᵘ dæ ɪt ə tɪti]
Oh, that is a kitty.

[hi ə bɪ dɑ]
He a big dog.

[wi hæf ə tɪti]
We have a kitty.

[hi baᵘ ən hæ ə tɑwə]
He brown and has a collar.

[wi dɑt aᵘ tɪti ə waːŋ taˈm]
We got our kitty a long time.

Conversation with Mom:

[tæn wi do tu mədɑnoᵘ]
Can we go to McDonald?

[hi tʌm tu mədɑnə wɪt ʌt]
He come to McDonald with us?

[aɪ wʌ ə tibɜdə]
I want a cheeseburger.

[aɪ wʌ fɛnfaɪθ]
I want french fries.

[wɛ ɪt bɪwi]
Where is Billy?

Talking about summer vacation:

[wi doᵘf tu dæma]
We drove to Grandma.

[si wɪf ɪn oᵘ +haɪo]
She live in Ohio.

[si hæt ə fɑm]
She has a farm.

[xxxxx mɑɪ haᵘ]
xxxx My house.

[mɑmi lɛ do]
Mommy let go.

[lɛ do naᵘ]
Let go now.

[si hæt watə taᵘt]
She has lot'a cows.

[taᵘt ju noᵘ mu taᵘ]
Cows, you know, moo cow.

[deɪ it ə ho wɑt]
They eat a whole lot.

	Correct Consonants	Incorrect Consonants
That a picture of a dog.	2	6
He a big dog.	3	2
He brown and has a collar.	4	6
Oh, that is a kitty.	1	4
We have a kitty.	3	2
We got our kitty a long time.	6	3
Can we go to McDonald?	6	5
I want a cheeseburger.	2	5
I want french fries.	4	6
Where is Billy?	2	2
He come to McDonald with us?	7	6
My house.	2	1
Mommy let go.	2	2
Let go now.	2	2
We drove to Grandma's.	3	4
She live in Ohio.	2	3
She has a farm.	3	2
She has lot'a cows.	2	5
Cows, you know, moo cow.	3	3
They eat a whole lot.	3	3

Number of correct consonants = 59

$$\frac{\text{Number of correct consonants} = 59}{\text{Number of correct plus incorrect consonants} = 134} \times 100$$

PCC = 46.3%   < 50% = severe

The following results are from Brandon, age 5;6:

house	[haᵘʂ]	matches	[mætəʂ]	thumb	[tʌm]
telephone	[tɛfoᵘn]	lamp	[wæmp]	finger	[fɪnə]
cup	[tʌp]	shovel	[tʌvoᵘ]	ring	[wɪŋ]
gun	[ɣʌn]	car	[tɑə]	jumping	[djʌmpən]
knife	[nɑˈf]	rabbit	[wæbət]	pajamas	[djæməʂ]
window	[wɪnoᵘ]	fishing	[fɪtsʲən]	plane	[pweˈn]
wagon	[ʍæɣən]	church	[tsʲɜtsʲ]	blue	[bwu]
wheel	[ʍiə]	feather	[fɛdə]	brush	[bwʌsʲ]
chicken	[tsʲɪtən]	pencils	[pɪntoʂ]	drum	[dwʌm]
zipper	[ʑpə]	this	[dɪʂ]	flag	[fwæɣ]
scissors	[sʲɪtə]	carrot	[tɛwət]	Santa	[ʂænə]
duck	[dʌ]	orange	[ɔwɪntsʲ]	tree	[twi]
yellow	[jewoᵘ]	bathtub	[bæftʌb]	squirrel	[tw3woᵘ]
vacuum	[væɣum]	bath	[bæf]	sleeping	[ʂwipən]
bed	[bɛd]	stove	[ʂtoᵘf]		

1. Which sounds are in the phonetic inventory and which ones are in the phonemic inventory for Brandon?
2. Use Figure 7.7, Neutralization of Phonemic Contrasts Summary Form, to list the neutralization of phonemic contrasts for Brandon. Do you notice the collapse of contrasts or any sound preferences?
3. Do you think that Brandon has a phonetic or a phonological disorder or do you see characteristics of both a phonetic *and* a phonological disorder? State your reasoning.
4. Do you notice any idiosyncratic processes in the results of Brandon's articulation test?

TEST YOURSELF

1. Clients with phonemic disorders show difficulty using
   a. appropriate stress in words
   b. phonemes to contrastively differentiate meaning
   c. s-sounds in a word
   d. articulatory motor movements to produce speech sounds
2. Which one of the following factors is not important when considering the guidelines for beginning therapy?
   a. stimulability
   b. sounds affecting intelligibility
   c. whether the sound is a fricative
   d. developmentally earlier sounds
3. A comprehensive phonological assessment includes all of the following except
   a. inventory of speech sounds
   b. distribution of speech sounds
   c. syllable shapes and consonants
   d. stimulability
4. Which of the following is an example of an open syllable shape?
   a. VCC   c. CCV
   b. CVC   d. CCC
5. A child substitutes a [t] for a [θ] ([θ] → [t]). According to place-manner-voicing analysis this would be the following
   a. dental → labial, fricative → stop
   b. dental → alveolar, fricative → stop

c. dental → postalveolar, fricative → stop, voiceless → voiced

d. dental → alveolar, fricative → stop, voiceless → voiced

6. Phonological process analysis is a means of identifying all of the following except
   a. substitutions
   b. contrastive use of phonemes
   c. syllable structure changes
   d. assimilatory changes

7. Which one of the following would be considered an idiosyncratic process?
   a. [k] → [t]   c. [ʃ] → [s]
   b. [t] → [s]   d. [tʃ] → [ʃ]

8. A subjective judgment made by a clinician based on how much of an utterance can be understood is referred to as
   a. severity

b. intelligibility
   c. percent consonants correct
   d. articulatory competency

9. Phonetic and phonemic disorders
   a. can co-occur   c. never co-occur
   b. always co-occur   d. are unrelated

10. Least phonological knowledge would be represented by which of the following?
    a. adultlike lexical representation for target morphemes, but some irregular productions occur
    b. nonadultlike lexical representation in all word positions of all target words
    c. adultlike lexical representations with positional constraints and fossilized forms
    d. adultlike lexical representation, but positional constraints are noted

WEBSITES

www.speech-language-therapy.com/2006cas_dpd_2.htm

This website contains a list of articles related to phonological disorders with a thorough summary of each. Specifically, there are several articles focusing on stimulability that are highlighted.

http://en.wikipedia.org/wiki/Intelligibility

This online dictionary gives a brief definition of speech intelligibility. It is interesting to compare this definition from an ordinary dictionary versus that in the text of this chapter. The text provides a much more accurate description for the field of speech-language pathology, but the website describes the same term in a way that people outside the field may view it.

www.ic.arizona.edu/~lsp/Phonology/Syllables/Phonology3.html

This site, created by the University of Arizona, provides a thorough description of syllables, including an in-depth explanation of syllabication.

www.reference.com

This website has a dictionary and an encyclopedia that give rather complete definitions of such terms as *complementary distribution, free variation, phonological rules,* and more. The explanations are easy to read and follow and there is a wide array of topics that can be accessed.

www.computerizedprofiling.org/downloads_cpvershistory.html

This site, developed by Stephen Long of Marquette University, provides word lists of several articulation tests as well as phonological process analysis features that can be downloaded. The site can be used by students and clinicians to accurately assess diagnostic results.

FURTHER READINGS

Bernthal, J., & Bankson, N. (2004). *Articulation and phonological disorders* (5th ed.). Boston: Allyn & Bacon.

Bleile, K. (2004). *Manual of articulation and phonological disorders: Infancy through adulthood* (2nd ed.). Clifton Park, NY: Thomson-Delmar Learning.

Halle, M. (2002). *From memory to speech and back: Papers on phonetics and phonology, 1954–2002.* Berlin: Walter de Gruyter.

Hudson, G. (1999). *Essential introductory linguistics.* Malden, MA: Blackwell.

Williams, A. L. (2003). *Speech disorders: Resource guide for preschool children.* Clifton Park, NY: Thomson-Delmar Learning.

APPENDIX 7.1

Proportional Occurrence of Consonant Phonemes in First-Grade, Third-Grade, and Fifth-Grade Children's Speech[1]

| | *Percent of All Consonants* | | | | | |
| | *1st Grade* | | *3rd Grade* | | *5th Grade* | |
Rank	Consonant	Percent	Consonant	Percent	Consonant	Percent
1	n	13.63	n	13.46	n	12.59
2	r	8.20	r	8.73	r	9.01
3	t	7.91	t	7.77	t	7.69
4	m	7.49	s	7.48	s	7.31
5	s	6.94	d	6.53	d	6.81
6	d	6.31	m	6.30	m	5.43
7	w	5.57	w	5.22	l	5.33
8	l	4.96	l	5.05	w	5.05
9	k	4.96	ʔ[2]	4.92	k	4.82
10	z	4.58	k	4.76	z	4.62
11	ʔ[2]	4.49	ð	4.58	ð	4.52
12	ð	4.42	z	4.28	ʔ	3.65
13	h	3.37	b	3.13	h	3.04
14	b	3.18	h	3.07	b	2.94
15	g	2.90	g	2.52	g	2.56
16	f	2.21	p	2.34	j	2.53
17	p	2.12	f	2.18	p	2.49
18	v	1.64	j	1.88	f	2.30
19	j	1.41	v	1.58	v	2.12
20	ŋ	1.05	ŋ	1.19	ŋ	1.38
21	θ	1.03	θ	.96	ʃ	1.33
22	ʃ	.84	ʃ	.94	θ	1.04
23	ʤ	.53	ʧ	.57	ʧ	.74
24	ʧ	.51	ʤ	.57	ʤ	.69
25	ʒ	0	ʒ	0	ʒ	0

1. These data are adapted from Carterette and Jones (1974).

2. /ʔ/ is included as a "phoneme" of English in the original data.

Therapy for Phonetic Errors

LEARNING OBJECTIVES

When you have finished this chapter, you should be able to:

- Contrast traditional-motor approaches and multiple-sound approaches.
- Define sensory-perceptual training.
- Identify the different phases of sensory-perceptual training.
- Differentiate between phonetic placement and sound modification techniques.
- Explain facilitating context.
- Define the term *tongue thrust*.
- Describe the phonetic placement and sound modification techniques for the sounds mentioned in this chapter.
- Explain the importance of coarticulatory contexts.
- Identify the easy to hard coarticulatory conditions for the sounds mentioned in this chapter.

This chapter describes techniques that can be used to treat phonetic errors in the speech of children and adults. As previously defined, phonetic errors are motor production problems. This chapter emphasizes a *phonetic approach*, which has also been referred to in the literature as a *traditional* or *motor approach* (e.g., Bernthal and Bankson, 2004; Creaghead, Newman, and Secord, 1989; Klein, 1996; Lowe, 1994; Pena-Brooks and Hegde, 2000; Van Riper, 1978; Weiss, Gordon, and Lillywhite, 1987). Using this approach, the client is directed to position the articulators in such a way that a speech sound, considered to be, within normal limits, is produced. Therapy progresses from one error sound to the next. In addition, several of the treatment protocols cited in the literature also include tasks used to improve auditory discrimination skills (e.g., Van Riper and Emerick, 1984; Weiner, 1979; Winitz, 1975, 1989).

The goal of this chapter is to provide an information base for clinicians to use in their efforts to help their clients achieve a norm production of specific speech sounds. This foundation entails an understanding of how the sound is normally produced and knowledge of the client's misarticulation. In a continuing attempt to unite phonetic and phonological treatment principles, the linguistic function (exemplified by sound frequency, phonotactics, and examples of minimal pairs) will be provided for several of the sounds.

The sounds chosen for inclusion in this chapter represent the most frequently misarticulated sounds noted by McDonald (1964). Where applicable, the voiced or voiceless cognates are also treated. For each individual sound, not all possible misarticulations are addressed. Rather, only the most frequent misarticulations referenced in the research or as a result of personal clinical experience are included. Therefore, for some sounds, [s] for example, most of the misarticulations treated are distortions. For other sounds, such as [l], the majority of the errors are sound substitutions.

*D*ECISION MAKING: WHEN TO USE A PHONETIC APPROACH

Historically, phonetic approaches were first described in Europe around the turn of the century (Gutzmann, 1895; Kussmaul, 1885). Their first documentation within the United States is attributed to Scripture (1902), Ward (1923), and Scripture and Jackson (1919). Through the years, many authors have added to and modified these beginnings, including Mosher (1929); Nemoy (1954); Nemoy and Davis (1937); West, Kennedy, and Carr (1937); Van Riper (1939a, 1939b); Young and Hawk (1955); Mysak (1959); West and Ansberry (1968); and Winitz (1969), to mention just a few. Van Riper's *Speech Correction* (1939b) is often cited as

the text that popularized these techniques that have been used by clinicians for decades.

Any contemporary view of treatment needs to stress what is new. Thus, due to their noncontemporary roots, one might hesitate to take traditional-motor approaches seriously. In addition, after so much emphasis has been placed on analyzing the phonemic systems of our clients, the question arises: Should a traditional phonetic approach still be used? The answer to this question is yes. There is definitely a place for these methods within our contemporary understanding of phonetic-phonological disorders and their remediation.

Phonetic Errors

In **phonetic** or **traditional-motor approaches**, each error sound is treated individually, one after the other. This treatment principle stands in contrast to a **multiple-sound approach**, which attempts to influence several error sounds simultaneously. Traditional-motor approaches should not be automatically used with all clients who exhibit a single-sound error. A client with a single-sound error who has problems with the *function* of the sound within the language system, that is, with the underlying system that governs the use of this particular sound, is probably demonstrating a phonemic disorder. Omissions and substitutions of an isolated speech sound can be phonemic disorders. In such cases, other therapy options may be more suitable. The question is never how many sounds are involved but rather whether the errors, single or multiple, are phonetic or phonemic in nature. If they are phonetically based, the best treatment option may be a traditional-motor, phonetic approach.

Decision Making: A Phonetic Approach with Phonemic Disorders?

As previously discussed, a phonetic approach will probably be chosen if the client demon-

A simplistic solution defines phonetic and phonemic problems according to the number of error sounds observed: If only one or possibly a couple of sounds are in error, we have a phonetic problem; multiple sound errors are phonemic (Paul, 2007). However, the assumption that single-sound errors must be motoric, phonetic in nature, while multiple-sound errors reflect conceptual, phonemic problems has been refuted (Locke, Bleile, Fey, and Folkins, 1996).

strates a phonetic disorder. This does not necessarily mean that it is unsuitable for clients with phonemic disorders. Certain portions of these techniques may prove helpful when working with children who demonstrate phonemic disorders.

Phonological approaches emphasize the function of sounds within a specific language system. Consequently, the internalization of phonological rules and contrasts are the main goals of phonological therapies. If, however, the sound is not in the child's repertoire, and remains elusive in spite of phonological treatment attempts, the phonetic approach could be implemented to establish its norm articulation. This does not mean that a clinician needs to go through all steps of the phonetic approach but that certain ideas and procedures of the phonetic approach can prove useful. Thus, one of the treatment goals would be to help the child produce the appropriate phonetic features of the speech sound. This in turn could facilitate the primary goal: increasing the child's ability to understand and utilize the phonological rules and contrasts with that particular sound.

Bernthal and Bankson (2004) report that the traditional-motor or phonetic approach can also be incorporated into treatment programs for clients who demonstrate linguistic or pattern-based errors, especially if the patterns reflect motor constraints (e.g., prevocalic voicing or certain cluster simplifications). Based on these authors' recommendation, if motor constraints can be identified in the patterns of clients with phonemic disorders, the traditional, phonetic approach constitutes a viable option.

THERAPY SEQUENCE

This section outlines possibilities for sequencing therapy when working with phonetic disorders. These sequences have been described by numerous authors (e.g., Secord, 1989; Van Riper, 1978; Van Riper and Emerick, 1984; Van Riper and Irwin, 1958; Waengler and Bauman-Waengler, 1984; Winitz, 1975) and have been utilized by clinicians for decades. Although the following sequencing is presented, clinicians will find that certain training items will be necessary for some clients, whereas they might prove unnecessary for others. The specific client's needs and capabilities will cause changes in the sequencing of every therapy program.

Each of the treatment phases assumes that the client enters that particular stage with minimal competency and moves to the next stage when a certain level of accuracy has been achieved. The necessary level of accuracy before preceding to the next stage of treatment is usually relatively high. Paul (2001) notes that correct usage is typically set at 80 to 90 percent in structured intervention contexts. Therefore, during structured activities within a therapy setting, 80 to 90 percent accuracy would be needed before proceeding to the next stage. However, is this high accuracy necessary in spontaneous speech before a client is dismissed from therapy? As dismissal criteria, Lee, Koenigsknecht, and Mulhern (1975) have suggested a much lower level of accuracy for spontaneous, natural contexts. They argue that termination criteria in spontaneous contexts should be set at 50 percent accuracy.

It appears that once children use targeted behaviors in spontaneous speech the majority of the time, it is probable that progress will continue toward more consistent usage. These percentages appear reasonable but, again, may vary according to the individual clinician's expectations and client's capabilities.

General Overview of Therapy Progression

Sensory-Perceptual Training/Ear Training. In this phase of therapy, the client develops the ability to discriminate between the target sound and other sounds, including the irregular production that he or she uses. During sensory-perceptual training, the client is not asked to attempt a production of the target sound but only to judge its distinctness from other sounds. The stages of this phase are those outlined by Van Riper and Emerick (1984).

Identification. The clinician describes and demonstrates knowledge of the sight, sound, and feel of the target sound. For young children, the target sound is often given a name, such as naming [s] the hissing-snake sound. For older children and adults, models and diagrams along with more complex articulatory descriptions can be employed. The goal is recognition and discrimination of the sound in isolation when contrasted to other similar and dissimilar sounds. Winitz (1975) adds that discrimination contrasts should at first address speech sounds that are productionally and, therefore, acoustically very different; only later should the client be asked to discriminate between the target sound and the error production. For example, if the client substitutes [θ] for [s], phonetically very different sounds should be presented at first—[s] versus [m], for example. Only at the end of the training period should [s] versus [θ] be introduced. Winitz (1975) believes that phonemic contrasts arranged in a hierarchical order from dissimilar to similar are more efficient than just contrasting the error production to the target sound.

Isolation. Next, the target sound is produced by the clinician in a variety of contexts that vary in word position (initially, medially, and finally) and context complexity (words, phrases, and sentences). The client must indicate when the target sound is heard. The goal of this phase is recognition of the target sound in words and identification of the position of the target sound within that word.

Stimulation. In this phase, variations of the target sound are presented in large quantities; that is, the client is bombarded with them. Variations might include louder or softer and slower or faster presentations of words containing the target sound. In addition, longer or shorter durations of the target sound within words could be presented. The client should also be able to identify the target sound when various speakers (with a tape recorder or in a group setting) say words, sentences, and finally paragraphs that contain it. The goal of this phase is continued identification of the target sound as context and speaker change.

Discrimination. Here, norm and error productions of the target sound are presented by the clinician. The error productions should mirror those of the client. These specific misarticulations are presented by the clinician in contexts of varying complexity, from words to sentences to tongue twisters with several of the misarticulations within one utterance. Van Riper and Emerick (1984) label this *error detection*. The second part of this sensory perceptual training phase is *error correction*. Here, the client is asked to explain why the sound is in error and, possibly, what needs to be done to correct it. For example, the clinician says [θoᵘp] for the word *soap*. The client must identify the error and explain that the tongue was peeking between the teeth, which is wrong for *soap*. For children, the error correction phase must be preceded by careful preparation so that they are capable of making these types of observations. The final goal of this stage is to emphasize the client's ongoing self-monitoring skills. Now, clients must recognize an error every time it occurs in their speech. For this self-monitoring phase, Winitz (1975) suggests that when the client misarticulates, the clinician should wait a few seconds and then imitate the client's production. This should be followed by the clinician correctly repeating the word several times.

Whether sensory-perceptual training is necessary for every client remains a controversial issue (see, for example, Briere, 1966; Dickson, 1962; Monnin, 1984; Sonderman, 1971; Williams and McReynolds, 1975). At least two factors should be considered before implementing these procedures: the age of the client and whether specific auditory discrimination difficulties are noted for the individual client. Age becomes a factor because many of the tasks used to achieve the goals of the training are metalinguistic skills. Metalinguistic skills require the child to think and talk about language. Identifying the position of a sound in a word is a metalinguistic skill, for example. The child must first understand the concept that a "word" is made up of individual "sounds" and their relative relationship to one another. The ability to segment words into sounds develops during the early school-age years (Fox and Routh, 1975; Liberman, Shankweiler, Fischer, and Carter, 1974). Therefore, for younger children, certain aspects of sensory-perceptual training may not be appropriate. Sec-

Auditory perceptual testing was discussed in Chapter 6 and guidelines and assessment protocols were provided.

ond, clinicians should carefully evaluate the specific auditory perceptual skills of their clients. The term *specific perceptual skills* refers to clients' abilities to differentiate between their error production and the target sound. If testing reveals no difficulties with specific discrimination tasks, sensory-perceptual training does not seem warranted.

In the previous discussion, sensory-perceptual training is seen as a phase before production training that, depending on the client's capabilities, may or may not be implemented. However, sensory-perceptual training in the form of self-monitoring remains a necessity during the next phases of therapy. Clinicians will constantly need to help their clients develop discrimination of "correct" versus "incorrect" productions. This type of self-monitoring is not an optional portion of therapy.

Production of the Sound in Isolation. The goal of this phase of therapy is to elicit a norm production of the target sound alone, not in combination with other sounds. An isolated production can easily be achieved with fricatives, glides, and liquids, for example, sounds that can be prolonged. For stop-plosives, young children might find it easier to articulate the target sound together with a central vowel, [kʌ], for example, or with a noticeable aspiration: [kʰ].

There are several possibilities for eliciting the target sound. Beginning clinicians often have the idea that this will be a task that can be achieved in a very short time. This is indeed often the case. However, if norm or near-norm articulation is not obtained within a reasonable time frame (five to ten minutes), persisting with the procedure will probably cause frustration to both the client and the clinician. In this case, either the technique should be changed or other preexercises should be initiated to prepare the client for the correct articulation. The following possibilities are offered for eliciting the target sound in isolation.

Auditory Stimulation/Imitation.   In this procedure, the clinician provides examples of the target sound and the client is asked to imitate the sound. A similar procedure is implemented for stimulability testing (see Chapter 6). Many authors (e.g., Irwin, 1965; Milisen, 1954; Powers, 1971; Van Riper, 1978; Weiss et al., 1987) have suggested that this method be used first to elicit a new sound. The client is instructed to "watch me and do exactly what I do." If this works, it is perhaps the easiest and quickest way to achieve the target sound. Unfortunately, though, it does not always succeed.

Phonetic Placement Method.   In the **phonetic placement method,** the clinician instructs the client how to position the articulators in order to produce a typical production. The phonetic production features of the target sound and the error production are analyzed to determine which articulatory changes need to be initiated so that an accurate production results. In the next section of this chapter, these methods will be described in detail for the most common misarticulations.

Sound Modification Method.   The **sound modification method** is based on deriving the target sound from a phonetically similar sound that the client can accurately produce. The phonetically similar correctly articulated sound is used as a starting point. Specific adjustments to the articulators are then suggested, which should result in the target sound.

   Once the target sound has been produced acceptably in isolation, the next task is to stabilize it. This is typically achieved by having the client repeat it immediately. At first, this will probably need to be carried out in front of a mirror with careful monitoring and feedback

by the clinician. When the production is more stable, the client should articulate the sound a number of times successively, with a softer or louder voice, for example, and when possible, with different durations. This does not need to develop into a tedious drill for client and clinician but can easily be achieved in activities that are fun and motivating. For example, the clinician could hide colored cards or favorite objects around the room. Every time the client finds the object, the target sound could be repeated. The clinician constantly provides feedback as to the acceptability of the productions, also asking the client to attempt judgments about the accuracy of his or her own productions.

Is an Isolated Production Necessary? Using Facilitating Contexts.

Some clients can produce the target sound quite accurately in some word contexts but not in others. These coarticulatory context conditions seem to aid the client's production of a target sound. Supporting contexts have been labeled facilitating contexts (McDonald, 1964). Van Riper (1978) introduced the term *key words* for those words in which the target sound was correctly produced.

   Facilitating contexts or *key words* are often found in the analysis of the client's articulation test or a conversational speech sample. Additional materials examining facilitating contexts include McDonald's (1964) deep testing and Secord's (1981a) probes of articulatory consistency. Van Riper (1978) describes how these key words can be used to move directly to the production of the target sound in isolation. In this case, the target sound is isolated by prolonging the sound within the word or by using the natural syllable structure of the word. In one case, results of an evaluation demonstrated a d/g substitution. However, the word *finger* was found with a correct production of [g]. The facilitating context of a postdorsal-velar nasal [ŋ] aided the client in producing a postdorsal-velar stop. To take advantage of this situation for the purpose of producing an isolated [g], the client first says *fin-ger,* separating the word between [ŋ] and [g]. The *ger* is then reduced to [gʌ].

Facilitating contexts can also be used to begin therapy at the word level. For example, if a small core of words is found with an acceptable production of the target sound, these words can be employed to stabilize the production. As Van Riper (1978) pointed out, key words can be used as a model for the client. Acoustic and articulatory differences are then pointed out between the articulation of these key words and aberrant target sound productions in other words. When the client can feel and hear the target sound, a transition is attempted to other words. For this transition, it is important that the clinician understand the facilitating context(s) in which the sound occurs. For example, is the target sound always preceded or followed by certain vowels or consonants? Are the key words one- or two-syllable words? Does the target sound occur in a stressed or unstressed syllable? If the clinician can predict the facilitating context, words can be added with similar coarticulatory conditions.

CLINICAL APPLICATION
Using Facilitating Contexts

Using the example of *finger,* an analysis suggests that the abutting [ŋ] had a facilitating effect on a norm [g] production; both organ and place of articulation are the same for both sounds. Additional words satisfying this coarticulatory context condition include *singer, linger, hunger,* and *longer.* After these words are accurately articulated, a logical sequence might be to proceed to [ŋ] + [k]: *monkey, stinky, thinker.*

Facilitative contexts can be very effective in therapy. If appropriate words can be found, it is relatively easy to isolate the sound in question: an excellent start for the isolation phase of production. If, in a given situation, the use of meaningful words is especially important, facilitative contexts can also be employed for work at the word level. As always, the final clinical choice will depend on the circumstances and capabilities of the individual client.

Nonsense Syllables. The goal of this therapy phase is to maintain accuracy of the production of the target consonant when it is embedded in varying vowel contexts. The therapeutic efficacy of this phase can be greatly increased by ordering the nonsense syllables from those that are easiest for the client to produce to those that are more difficult. The typical sequencing is target sound + vowel (CV), vowel + target sound (VC), and vowel + target sound + vowel (CVC). However, this sequence may change based on the difficulty the individual client demonstrates with each type of nonsense syllable. Vowels can be arranged in a hierarchical order from those that provide favorable coarticulatory conditions to those that do not. Suitable vowel sequences will be suggested for each of the misarticulations noted in the following section. However, articulatory ease and production accuracy of the individual client will ultimately determine the sequencing of vowels.

Many clinicians skip the nonsense syllable phase of treatment and move directly to the target sound produced in words. One reasoning is that words are more meaningful and interesting to the client than drill work with nonsense syllables. Work with nonsense syllables does not need to be a tedious exercise. Coming up with motivating and enjoyable activities that incorporate nonsense syllables requires only clinical imagination. In addition, although words are more meaningful to children than nonsense syllables, the word material should always be carefully evaluated. Some of the small "articulation cards" with black-and-white line drawings depicting words, for example, are not easily recognizable to the clinician nor the client. Such material stretches the concept of meaningfulness. Finally, and probably most importantly, some clients need work with nonsense syllables before they can produce words with any acceptable level of accuracy. If the client produces under 50 percent accuracy in two to three practice sessions, the word level is probably still too difficult. The clinician could then work with nonsense syllables or utilize consonant–vowel words such as *see, sow,* and *saw* until the production has stabilized. In addition, working with nonsense syllables eliminates the interference of the "old" error with the "new" production of the target sound that is inherent in meaningful word material. Years of practice with the old aberrant articulation of the target sound will often override the new articulation, especially in familiar words. For example, a child may be quite able to produce the nonsense syllable [ki] accurately in the context of other nonsense syllables. However, when attempting the word *key,* the child might suddenly revert back to the "old" substitution and produce [ti].

Words. The goal of this therapy phase is to maintain productional accuracy of the target sound within the context of words. A large variation exists within this category from one-syllable CV structures to multisyllabic words in which the target sound appears several times, often in consonant clusters. Organizing words from relatively easy to more difficult to produce will prove helpful. This should be done in a systematic manner using the articulatory complexity of the word as a guideline. Several factors affect the articulatory complexity of words. These include the length of the word, the position of the sound within the word, the syllable structure, the syllable stress, coarticulation factors, and the client's familiarity with the word.

The Length of the Word. Typically, the fewer the number of syllables, the easier the word is to produce. This would indicate that one-syllable words should be attempted before two- and three-syllable words (Secord, 1989).

The Position of the Sound within the Word. A sound in the initial position of a word or syllable appears to be the easiest. Word- and syllable-final sounds are typically more difficult. Thus, target sounds should generally be placed at the beginning of a word before attempts are made to realize the target sound at the end of a word (Secord, 1989).

The Syllable Structure. Open syllables (CV) are generally easier than closed syllables (CVC). Considering ease of production, the syllable structure may on occasion have precedence over the length of the word. Two-syllable words with a reduplicated CVCV structure, such as *Daddy* or *teddy,* may be easier than CVC words such as *bed* or *mad* (Bernthal and Bankson, 2004).

The Syllable Stress. A target sound is easier to produce in a stressed syllable than in an unstressed one. Therefore, when choosing two-syllable words, the target sound should first appear in the stressed syllable (McDonald, 1964).

Coarticulation Factors. Certain words may be easier to articulate than others due to the influence of coarticulation. This relates not only to preceding and following vowels but also to the neighboring consonants within the word. Knowledge of the vowel and consonant articulations will aid in developing a list of words ordered from relatively easy to produce to more difficult (Winitz, 1975). However, the final decision as to ease and difficulty of production will depend on the client when these words are implemented. Clinicians may find that certain words will be "too difficult"; that is, the target sound is consistently misarticulated within that word. These words should then be attempted at a later time when the regular articulation of the target sound is more stabilized.

Coarticulatory factors also include the number of times the target sound appears in a word and whether it appears as a singleton or as a portion of a consonant cluster. Words that contain the target sound only once are normally easier to articulate than those that might have the target sound more than once. Thus, *cape* is easier than *cake*. Also, words that contain the target sound as a singleton will typically be easier than if the target sound is a portion of a consonant cluster. Thus, *tea* is productionally easier than *tree*.

Familiarity.   Familiar words are usually articulated more accurately than unfamiliar words (Secord, 1989). Therefore, clinicians should begin with words that the client knows well or those that are high-frequency words. With some clients, however, familiar words may also prove to be more difficult. The impact of years of practice misarticulating a familiar word in a multitude of settings may prove hard to overcome. These words may then need to be targeted later when the production and self-monitoring skills of the client have improved.

Structured Contexts—Phrases and Sentences. The goal of this therapy phase is to maintain accuracy of production of the target sound as words are placed into short phrases and sentences. However, at this point, phrases and sentences should not yet be spontaneous but rather structured and elicited. If spontaneous sentences are used, it is possible that the client will choose words containing combinations with the target sound that are still too difficult. This presupposes that clinicians will begin work at this phase while still continuing the work at the word level. This is a logical

supposition because clinicians will typically select a core set of words that can be accurately produced and then put these words into short phrases and sentences.

A *carrier phrase* with a target word at the end is one of the easiest ways to elicit a short phrase. At the beginning, the carrier phrase should probably not contain any other words with the target sound. Another relatively simple way to elicit an utterance is to embed one target word within the carrier phrase, which can be modified to create some degree of spontaneity. For example, if a child is working on [s], the carrier phrase could be "I see a _____." The clinician could have objects or pictures prepared (at first without any s-sounds) that the client identifies to complete the phrase.

During this therapy phase, the clinician moves from highly structured to less structured tasks. At the same time, the clinician might begin to implement target words with more syllables and consonant clusters.

Spontaneous Speech.   The goal of this phase is to maintain accuracy of production when the target sound appears spontaneously in conversation. This goal is first addressed within the therapy setting; however, the client needs to transfer this production accuracy to more and more situations outside therapy. This transfer of behavior to conversational speech in various settings is often referred to as *carryover*.

Both within and outside the therapy setting, this therapy phase should proceed in a systematic manner. One way of accomplishing this is to vary the length of conversation time. Clinicians could start with five minutes of conversation, increasing the time interval as the client's accuracy increases. Initially, before the conversation begins, the client should be aware that the clinician is "listening for our sound." Later, the time interval can be extended and specific contexts that trigger the production of the target sound in many different words included. For example, pictures are available containing words with the target sound that could serve as the basis for conversation. Also, certain topics might lend themselves to the production of specific sounds. For example, a topic that includes racing, race cars, and race car drivers would probably trigger [r] in a variety of contexts.

After a relatively high level of accuracy is achieved within the therapy setting, the next decisive step is correct production of the sound outside, in the real world. Parents and teachers can serve as valuable assistants during this phase of therapy. When working outside the therapy setting, the amount of time implemented and the specific tasks should be discussed with the assisting helper. This phase can become overwhelming to both the helper and the client if both suddenly think that the sound needs to be produced accurately all the time in every outside setting.

CLINICAL APPLICATION

Structuring a Home Program

When structuring a home program, the clinician needs to make sure that the speech assistant (caregiver, teacher, relative, etc.) is informed of several variables:

1. When? Which portion of the day should be set aside for the program?
2. How long? How many minutes should be spent on this program?
3. How often? How many times per day should this program be implemented? Should it be a daily occurrence?
4. What should be done? In detail, what should the assistant do? Does the assistant have written instructions as well as words, phrases, and topics that should be used in the home program?
5. How should accuracy be judged? How should the assistant determine which productions are acceptable and which not?
6. What should be done if a production is considered unacceptable? How should the assistant react to an aberrant production?

7. How should the assistant motivate and reward the client? What type of reward system should be implemented so that the client stays motivated and continues to work within the home program?

One question that the clinician needs to ask is: How can I be sure that the assistant understands what is to be done? This is an important question. If the assistant does not really understand in detail what has to be accomplished, this can often lead to frustration for both the client and the assistant. (The author had a caregiver assistant who, rather than implement two five-minute sessions during the day, thought that one thirty-minute session twice a week would be better. After two long sessions, the child refused to work at home.) Bringing the assistant into therapy can partially solve this problem. The assistant can see and hear which productions are considered accurate and which are not acceptable. After a period of observation, have the assistant take an active role in the therapy session. Helpful advice can then be given to the assistant to guide in making decisions about correct and incorrect productions as well as implementation of activities.

Katie, who was in second grade, was working on [s] in structured conversation. Katie's mother expressed her willingness to work at home with her.

1. When? After discussing this with the mother, a quiet one-on-one time after dinner was considered the best way to begin.
2. How long? Ten minutes was a good time frame to begin with.
3. How often? Every weekday.
4. What should be done? Written instructions were put into a small spiral notebook that the mother could transport in her purse between therapy and home. The clinician described in some detail what the topic of the conversation should be. These topics had been practiced in therapy, and Katie was able to reach a fairly high degree of success with them.
5. How should accuracy be judged? After participating in two therapy sessions, the mother knew what to listen for. Reminders were also written into the notebook. Katie originally had a θ/s substitution. The mother was aware that [s] should have a clear, sharp quality and not sound like [θ].
6. What should be done if a production is considered unacceptable? It was decided that a small stop sign that was constructed in therapy would be used to signal any unacceptable [s]-productions.

The mother would simply hold up the sign when she heard [θ]. Katie knew that when the sign went up, she should repeat the whole sentence and try to monitor her [s]-production.

7. How should the assistant motivate and reward the client? It was decided that if Katie participated for the ten minutes of therapy, she could play on the computer, uninterrupted by her two brothers, for fifteen minutes. Also, at the end of each week of therapy, Katie could pick out one of the videos that the family would watch on the weekend.

Even when an assistant is employed, the clinician should also monitor the client's level of accuracy in situations outside the immediate therapy setting. This can be accomplished in a variety of ways. For example, tape recordings can be brought from home, the clinician and child could go to buy an ice cream, or go window shopping at a toy store. The clinician could also drop by the child's classroom or call on the telephone to check on the accuracy of sound production outside the therapy setting.

Dismissal and Reevaluation Criteria. The last phase of therapy examines dismissal and reevaluation criteria. Fifty percent accuracy during natural spontaneous speech was mentioned earlier as criterion for dismissal. This relatively low percentage was suggested under the assumption that the client's competency will continue to increase on its own. Such a supposition needs to be checked by some type of reevaluation process. A reevaluation can be as simple as stopping by the child's classroom and listening to conversation, or it can be more structured, involving administration of an articulation test and obtaining a conversational speech sample. Whichever means is employed, *reevaluation* is a portion of our clinical responsibility. It is the only way to ensure that therapy was indeed successful, that the client has continued to generalize across situations. The ultimate therapeutic goal is norm production

within all natural, conversational settings. A reevaluation is a way of documenting this.

INDIVIDUAL SOUND ERRORS

This section will not revisit the multitude of traditional-motor approaches that have been suggested throughout the years but focus on those based on the phonetic features of the target sound in relationship to the error production. Knowledge of the correct phonetic placement and the existing differences between the norm production and the misarticulation will be instrumental in facilitating these techniques. Other traditional-motor approaches that may not be quite as "phonetically" oriented are referenced in numerous sources. For example, a compilation of phonetic placement, moto-kinesthetic, and sound approximation techniques can be found in Secord's *Eliciting Sounds* (Secord, 1981b).

This section will contain both phonetic placement and sound modification techniques for the following: s-sounds ([s] and [z]), sh-sounds ([ʃ] and [ʒ]), k-g sounds, l-sounds, r-sounds (including [r] and the central vowels with r-coloring, [ɝ] and [ɚ]), th-sounds ([θ] and [ð]), f-v sounds, affricates, voicing problems (e.g., [p] for [b] substitution), and consonant clusters. The discussion is seen as a reference. It contains a considerable amount of detail that will become necessary when a clinician is actually working with a client and encountering difficulties achieving an accurate production. The proposed methods also allow the clinician several possibilities for establishing a norm realization for each of the previously noted sounds.

MISARTICULATIONS OF [s] AND [z]

One of the most common speech sound errors is the aberrant production of [s] (McDonald,

1964; Weiss, 1980). Most children at some point in their development have difficulty with [s] realizations. Because [s] and [z] are counted among the latest developing speech sounds, they may pose difficulties into the first school year for some children. It is also a frequent deviation heard in the speech of adults. Whether at the grocery store or on television, one can often hear adults with irregular [s] articulations.

The phonetic production characteristics of [s] and [z] consist of several related physiological factors that make their articulation somewhat complicated. First, [s] and [z] are both fricatives. All fricatives are physiologically complex because a rather narrow opening between place and organ of articulation must be maintained over a longer period of time. In fact, the fricatives are also the longest sounds in duration (Bauman and Waengler, 1977; Lehiste, 1970). Throughout this time frame, production requirements necessitate not only a narrow opening between the organ and place of articulation but also maintenance of the right amount of expiratory air flow. There is a precise balance between the articulatory effort required to create the narrow opening and the expiratory air pressure. If this balance is off, even to a small degree, it becomes perceptually noticeable. In addition, aberrant productions can easily cross phonemic boundaries. Thus, if the tongue is too far forward, [s] might sound like [θ]. The same relationship exists between [z] and [ð]. In addition, the voiceless [s] occurs very frequently in General American English. In summary: [s] and [z] are physiologically difficult, perceptually sensitive, and produced in practically every utterance.

Phonetic Description

Norm productions of [s] and [z] are articulated in essentially two different ways: as an apico-alveolar or as a predorsal-alveolar fricative (Carrell and Tiffany, 1960). These differences are delineated in Table 8.1. The apico-alveolar variation is produced with the tongue tip up, while the predorsal-alveolar [s] is realized with the tongue tip down behind the lower incisors. Sagittal grooving of the tongue, which

Table 8.1 Production Differences: Apico-Alveolar versus Predorsal-Alveolar [s] and [z]

	Phonetic Description	
	Apico-alveolar fricative	*Predorsal-alveolar fricative*
	[s] voiceless [z] voiced	[s] voiceless [z] voiced
Notable Differences	Tongue tip up	Tongue tip down behind lower incisors
Organ of Articulation	Apex (tip of tongue)	Predorsal (front portion of tongue)
Place of Articulation	Alveolar ridge	Alveolar ridge
Productional Notes	Narrow opening between tongue tip and alveolar ridge	Tongue arches toward alveolar ridge, narrow opening between predorsal section of tongue and alveolar ridge
	Sagittal grooving of tongue Lateral edges of tongue elevated	Sagittal grooving of tongue Lateral edges of tongue elevated

directs the airstream toward the opening between organ and place of articulation, is essential for both types of productions. In order to achieve this, the lateral edges of the tongue are elevated and touch the first molars to avoid lateral air escape. Although the apico-alveolar articulation is probably the most common, many speakers produce predorsal-alveolar [s] and [z]. Each type of s-production has its therapeutic advantages and disadvantages, which will be discussed in a later section.

Linguistic Function

Frequency of Occurrence. [s] ranks among the top five sounds in frequency of occurrence. Although not as frequent as [s], [z] ranks eleventh within the twenty-four consonants of General American English. The most frequent

word-initial clusters include [st], [str], and [sp]; the most frequently encountered word-final clusters are [st], [ns], [nz], [ks], [ts], [rz], and [nts] (Dewey, 1923; French, Carter, and Koenig, 1930; Roberts, 1965).

Phonotactics. Both [s] and [z] can occur initiating and terminating a syllable. However, in spontaneous speech, the frequency of occurrence of [s] and [z] in initial, medial, and final word positions is not comparable. In the speech of first-, second-, and third-grade children, half of the [s]-sounds occurred initiating a word; the other half were divided fairly equally between medial and final positions. On the other hand, over 90 percent of the [z] sounds were found in word-final position (Mader, 1954).

Tables 8.2 and 8.3 provide the more frequent consonant clusters with [s] and [z]. Word

Table 8.2 Consonant Clusters with [s]

Word-Initiating		Word-Terminating			
[sf]	sphere (a very infrequent cluster)	[fs]	coughs, roofs		
[sk]	school, skate	[sk]	mask, desk	[ks]	blocks, books
[sl]	sled, sleep	[ls]	false, pulse		
[sm]	small, smile				
[sn]	snow, snack	[ns]	dance, bounce		
[sp]	speed, spin	[sp]	wasp, crisp	[ps]	mops, tips
[st]	stop, stove	[st]	ghost, fast	[ts]	kites, cats
[sw]	sweet, sweater				
[skr]	scratch	[rs]*	horse, nurse		
[skw]	square	[lts]	melts, belts		
[spl]	splash	[mps]	lamps, jumps		
[spr]	spring, spray	[nts]	ants, presents		
[str]	street, string	[rst]	first, worst	[rts]	hearts, skirts
		[sks]	desks, masks		
		[sts]	nests, tastes		

*Consonant clusters with [r]. These are considered centering diphthongs. Therefore, these examples do not really represent consonant clusters. However, because they are included in most consonant cluster lists, they have been included in this one as well.

Table 8.3 Consonant Clusters with [z]

Word- or syllable-initiating clusters with [z] do not exist in General American English.

Word-Terminating			
[bz]	ribs, tubs	[vz]	knives, waves
[dz]	adds, toads	[zd]	closed, sneezed
[gz]	bags, bugs	[ldz]	builds, folds
[lz]	bells, shells	[lvz]	wolves, elves
[mz]	teams, games	[rdz]	birds, cards
[nz]	cans, rains	[rlz]	girls, curls
[ŋz]	wings, rings	[rvz]	curves, dwarves
[rz]*	bears, ears		
[ðz]	bathes, breathes		

*Consonant clusters with [r]. These are considered centering diphthongs. Therefore, these examples do not really represent consonant clusters. However, because they are included in most consonant cluster lists, they have been included in this one as well.

examples are also given. All consonant clusters are based on the lists provided by Blockcolsky, Frazer, and Frazer (1987).

Morphophonemic Function. Word-final clusters ending in [s] or [z] can be used, for example, to signal (1) plurality, as in boo<u>ks</u>, goa<u>ts</u>, ne<u>sts</u>; (2) third-person singular, as in he ju<u>mps</u>, she bui<u>lds</u>; and (3) possessives, as in Mo<u>m's</u>, Da<u>d's</u>. Within phrases, contractible auxiliaries and copulas with the verb *to be* also demonstrate consonant clusters with [s] and [z]. Examples include "the ma<u>n's</u> happy" and "the ca<u>t's</u> eating."

Minimal Pairs. Minimal pairs are often used to test the perceptual accuracy of the error production versus the norm production of clients. Several authors (e.g., Grunwell, 1987; Locke,

1980c; Winitz, 1984) have devised protocols to test these types of auditory perceptual skills. In addition, minimal pair contrast therapy, which will be discussed in Chapter 9, employs pairs of words that differ by only a single phoneme. Sounds that are frequently contrasted to [s] and [z] include [θ] and [ð], [ʃ] and [ʒ], and [t] and [d]. Tables 8.4 and 8.5 contain a few examples of minimal pair words and sentences incorporating sound oppositions with [s] and [z]. Sound oppositions contrasting [s] and [z] to [ʃ] and [ʒ] are contained in the next section on [ʃ] and [ʒ] misarticulations.

Initial Remarks

Several important variables must first be considered when confronted with a child or adult displaying an [s] problem. First, the disorder may be the result of a hearing loss, specifically a high-frequency hearing loss. Acoustically, both [s] and [z] have high-frequency components (6,000 to 11,000 Hz). Because all sound productions are monitored auditorily, even a moderate loss in these frequency areas might impair intensity relationships between formant regions and, therefore, lead to a distorted production. This makes a hearing evaluation prior to our conventional diagnostic testing indispensable. If a high-frequency hearing loss is present, our diagnostic evaluation and the subsequent therapy planning need to be organized quite differently.

Second, certain minor structural changes may affect [s] as well. This might include missing teeth in a school-age child or new dentures in an adult. Although circumstances such as these may not cause [s] problems per se, an individual's inability to compensate for such structural deviations can result in unusual production characteristics.

Third, such diagnoses as "tongue thrust" or "tongue thrust swallow" also need to be considered. The term **tongue thrust** refers to excessive

Table 8.4 Minimal Pair Words and Sentences Contrasting [s] and [z] to [θ] and [ð]

[s] versus [θ]		[z] versus [ð]		[s] versus [θ]		[z] versus [ð]	
sank	thank	Zen	then	bass	bath	breeze	breathe
sick	thick			Bess	Beth	close	clothe
sink	think			face	faith	seize	seethe
sing	thing			mass	math	she's	sheathe
saw	thaw			miss	myth	Sue's	soothe
sigh	thigh			moss	moth	tease	teethe
sin	thin			mouse	mouth		
song	thong			pass	path		
sought	thought						
sum	thumb						

He was *sicker* after dinner.
He was *thicker* after dinner.

He had to *saw* the pipes.
He had to *thaw* the pipes.

The captain was *sinking*.
The captain was *thinking*.

Something was wrong with his *sum*.
Something was wrong with his *thumb*.

Did he *breeze* close by her?
Did he *breathe* close by her?

They walked by the *closing* store.
They walked by the *clothing* store.

There's a strange-looking *moss* on the tree.
There's a strange-looking *moth* on the tree.

The boy had a big *mouse*.
The boy had a big *mouth*.

Table 8.5 Minimal Pair Words and Sentences Contrasting [s] and [z] to [t] and [d]

[s] versus [t]		[s] versus [t]		[z] versus [d]		[z] versus [d]	
sell	tell	ace	ate	Z	D	as	add
cent	tent	base	bait	zing	ding	bees	bead
sack	tack	brass	brat	zip	dip	buzz	bud
sag	tag	case	Kate	zoo	do	cries	cried
sail	tail	kiss	kit	zoom	doom	dries	dried
sank	tank	hiss	hit	zipper	dipper	knees	need
sea	tea	lice	light			rose	rode
seam	team	mice	might			size	side
sew	toe	nice	night			toes	towed
sip	tip	peace	Pete			ways	wade
sock	talk	rice	write			trays	trade

He wanted to *sell* his story.
He wanted to *tell* his story.

The *seam* was split.
The *team* was split.

He thought it was *nice*.
He thought it was *night*.

She gave him a large *kiss*.
She gave him a large *kit*.

He looked at the big *zipper*.
He looked at the big *dipper*.

The airplane *zipped* through the clouds.
The airplance *dipped* through the clouds.

It wasn't the right *size*.
It wasn't the right *side*.

The *bees* can't be lost.
The *bead* can't be lost.

anterior tongue movement during swallowing and a more anterior tongue position during rest (Christensen and Hanson, 1981). Hanson (1988) suggests that a more appropriate term would be *oral muscle pattern disorders;* this would avoid the misconception that clients forcefully push their tongues forward. Controversy continues to surround these disorders and their impact on articulation, especially the articulation of [s] and [z]. Not everyone with a tongue thrust does develop [s] problems. On the other hand, there is a higher incidence of children with s-distortions who do demonstrate an oral muscle pattern disorder (Fletcher, Casteel, and Bradley, 1961; Hanson, 1988). Although an interdisciplinary approach is strongly urged, it is within the scope of practice of speech-language pathologists to diagnose and treat oral muscle pattern disorders (ASHA, 1991). Prior to ASHA's 1991 position statement, an ad hoc committee report (ASHA, 1989) suggested, as do several clinicians (Hanson, 1988, 1994; Hanson and Barrett, 1988; Hilton, 1984), that treatment, often called oral myofunctional therapy, may facilitate the correction of [s] difficulties. Knowledge of the diagnostic and treatment procedures of oral muscle pattern disorders will at times be necessary to complement work with [s] and [z] misarticulations. Box 8.1 contains literature citations that refer to the topic of tongue thrust.

Finally, the auditory discrimination abilities of the client need to be carefully evaluated. One portion of a clinician's assessment

---

BOX 8.1 Examples of Tongue Thrust Literature

Bigenzahn, W., Fischman, L., & Mayrhofer-Krammel, U. (1992). Myofunctional therapy in patients with orofacial dysfunctions affecting speech. *Folia Phoniatrica, 44* (5), 235–242.

Cayley, A., Tindall, A., Sampson, W., & Butcher, A. (2000). Electropalatographic and cephalometric assessment of myofunctional therapy in open-bite subjects. *Australian Orthodontic Journal, 16,* 23–33.

Christensen, M., & Hanson, M. (1981). An investigation of the efficacy of oral myofunctional therapy as a precursor to articulation therapy for pre-first-grade children. *Journal of Speech and Hearing Disorders, 46,* 160–167.

Forrest, K. (2002). Are oral-motor exercises useful in the treatment of phonological/articulatory disorders? *Seminar in Speech and Language, 23,* 15–26.

Gommerman, S., & Hodge, M. (1995). Effects of oral myofunctional therapy on swallowing and sibilant production. *International Journal of Orofacial Myology, 21,* 9–22.

Hale, S. T., Kellum, G. D., Richardson, J. F., Messer, S. C., Gross, A. M., & Sisakun, S. (1992). Oral motor control, posturing, and myofunctional variables in 8-year-olds. *Journal of Speech and Hearing Research, 35,* 1203–1208.

Hannuksela, A., & Vaananen, A. (1987). Predisposing factors for malocclusion in 7-year-old children with special reference to atopic diseases. *American Journal of Orthodontal-Dentofacial Orthopedics, 92,* 299–303.

Hanson, M. L. (1994). Oral myofunctional disorders and articulatory patterns. In J. E. Bernthal & N. W. Bankson (Eds.), *Child phonology: Characteristics, assessment, and intervention with special populations* (pp. 29–53). New York: Thieme.

Hanson, M. L., & Barrett, R. H. (1988). *Fundamentals of orofacial myology.* Springfield, IL: Charles C. Thomas.

Lindner, A., & Modeer, T. (1989). Relation between sucking habits and dental characteristics in pre-school children with unilateral crossbite. *Scandinavian Journal of Dental Research, 97,* 278–283.

Subtelny, J. D., Mestre, J. C., & Subtelny, J. (1964). Comparative study of normal and defective articulation of /s/ as related to malocclusion and deglutition. *Journal of Speech and Hearing Disorders, 29,* 269–285.

battery should include specific auditory perceptual testing (see Chapter 6). If the client demonstrates auditory discrimination problems between norm productions of [s] and [z] and the client's specific error realization, auditory discrimination training should probably be implemented.

Types of Misarticulation

As with all treatment plans, a solid diagnostic foundation needs to be established before treating misarticulations of [s] and [z]. It is important to find out exactly what the client does articulatorily during the sound realization—that is, how the client produces the error sound. Although the term *distortion* is often used to label abnormal sound changes, this seldom provides enough diagnostic information. The following guidelines are presented to help distinguish between different [s] and [z] "distortions."

  1. *Interdental [s] problems.* This is a frequent form of distortion. As the name interdental implies, the tongue is actually placed between the upper and lower incisors during this /s/ realization. The visibility of the tongue tip between the teeth is a diagnostic indicator for this aberrant production. Interdental [s] and [z] productions sound very much like [θ] and [ð].

  Phonetic transcription of the error: If the misarticulation does cross phonemic boundaries, [θ] or [ð] are transcribed.

  2. *Addental [s] problems.* This is probably the most frequently encountered s-distortion. Although *addental* actually means "at the teeth," the tongue tip may be positioned either touching or too closely approaching the posterior surface of the upper incisors. In both cases, the tongue is too far forward for norm [s] and [z] productions. Auditorily, /s/ and /z/ may again sound close to /θ/ and /ð/ real-

izations. If the tongue tip is not touching but merely too closely approaching the upper incisors, the [s] may simply lose its sharp, clear tone and sound "dull" or "flat." Although the auditory impression is helpful, it can be misleading. More accuracy is afforded if the clinician can peek into the client's mouth, possibly by tilting the head back during the [s] realization. The forward positioning together with the flattened edges of the tongue might then become visible. The flattened edges of the tongue would indicate the absence of the sagittal groove necessary for regular [s] and [z] realizations.

  Phonetic transcription of the error: [s̪] or [z̪].

  3. *Lateral [s] problems.* As the name suggests, this [s] misarticulation is characterized by a lateral airflow during /s/ realizations. The tip of the tongue is in direct contact with the alveolar ridge (or may even be located more anteriorly, that is, in contact with the upper incisors). In addition, there is no sagittal grooving. The lateral edges of the tongue are flattened, not touching the upper molars as they should be. Under these conditions, the air can freely flow laterally into the cheeks. This lateral escape of air can occur on both sides (bilaterally) or on one side only (unilaterally). If unilateral, one of the tongue's lateral edges is in a normal position for [s] articulation. Auditorily, lateral lisps are very noticeable. There is an unusual, openly conspicuous "slurping" noise component associated with lateral [s] and [z] production.

  Phonetic transcription of the error: [ɬ] or [ɮ].

  4. *Palatal [s] problems.* This faulty [s] articulation is characterized by a more palatal placement of organ and place of articulation than is normally the case. Therefore, predorsal or even mediodorsal portions of the tongue become the organ of articulation. The place of

articulation is no longer the alveolar ridge but palatal areas. Palatal [s] lacks a sharp, clear friction noise; it approaches [ʃ]-quality. Their closest qualitative approximation is to a whispered (voiceless) [j] sound. One can achieve this effect by moving the tongue slightly posteriorly during a regular [s] production.

Phonetic transcription of the error: [sʲ] or [zʲ].

5. *Strident [s] problems.* Unlike all the previously noted [s]-sound deviations, the strident is named not for its phonetic production features but for the auditory impression it creates. This [s] sounds "strident," which, by definition, amounts to a shrill, irritating quality. Strident [s] articulations often have a whistle-like component. This whistle is achieved by an imbalance between air pressure and the opening through which the air must flow. In general, there are many ways to whistle: Some do it through their fingers, whereas others pucker their lips to form various degrees of small openings, for example. The same is true for strident [s] formations: There are many ways to produce this effect. The whistling component can be caused by too much air pressure through an adequate opening or adequate air pressure through a very narrow opening. This narrowed opening may be caused by too deep of a groove across the tongue tip. Sometimes, during a phase of therapy, a clinician may well discover with alarm that the client's [s] suddenly sounds strident. This is usually not due to inadequate tongue placement but rather to an increased overall effort. The child is consciously trying to produce a correct [s] and, in effect, overdoes it with either too much air pressure or an overtensed narrow opening. Luckily, as the child continues to practice, the intermittent stridency normally disappears.

Stridency may also be caused by a lack of airstream concentration across the front teeth due to certain dental anomalies, such as the separation of the upper incisors or an irregular dental position (Luchsinger and Arnold, 1965). For some adults, stridency may result when new dentures are acquired. As the alignment of new dentures is always somehow different from the original set of teeth, certain motoric modifications need to be made. Until this compensation becomes routine, articulatory efforts may result in a strident [s] and/or [z].

Phonetic transcription of the error: [s̝] or [z̝].

6. *[t/s] substitution.* This misarticulation is marked by the substitution of [t] for [s], as in [tʌn] for *sun;* it involves a change in the manner of articulation from a fricative to a stop. According to phonological processes, the term *stopping* is the label used for t/s substitutions. This type of substitution is often seen in the speech of very young normally developing children. However, for some children, it persists. Because this misarticulation represents the substitution of one phoneme for another, clients with a t/s substitution should be evaluated for a phonemic disorder.

Phonetic transcription of the error: [t] or [d].

7. *Nasal [s] problems.* These deviations are characterized by nasality during the produc-

The so-called tapping method can be used to determine the exact location of airflow during lateral [s]-productions. For this method, the fingertips are used to apply intermittent pressure lightly at different points along each side of the cheek by moving horizontally from the back to the front of the cheek at the level where upper and lower teeth approximate one another. By placing pressure on the portion of the cheek where the faulty air escape occurs, the lateral airflow will be momentarily interrupted. If the air escape is one-sided, a sudden cessation of the lateral airflow will be heard only when tapping at the specific point on the respective side. If it is bilateral, it should be heard on both sides.

tion of [s] and [z]. Nasal [s] and [z] problems may be organic or functional in nature. Organic ones result from physical anomalies or neuromotor disorders that affect the structure or function of the velum. Examples include the speech characteristics of individuals with cleft palate or specific dysarthrias. Functional problems are marked by the absence of any known physical anomalies or neuromotor problems. Noted etiologies for functional nasal deviations include articulatory dyspraxia and the imitation of faulty sound patterns, for example, the imitation of a parent with a cleft palate. Also considered functional is the maintenance of learned patterns that originally had an organic cause (Luchsinger and Arnold, 1965; Stern, 1927).

Phonetic transcription of the error: [š] and/or [ž].

Distinguishing functional from organic velopharyngeal competency is the work of a team of professionals. Although an in-depth account of these procedures is not within the scope of this chapter, a few guidelines will be given. First, there is a higher degree of probability that a functional problem exists if the nasality is restricted to [s] and [z]. Organic problems will usually have an effect on *all* speech sounds, particularly those consonants that require a high degree of intraoral occlusion and the buildup of air pressure (stops, fricatives, affricates). Second, most of the functional nasal distortions demonstrate air escape through the nose only. Simultaneous oral and nasal airflow during [s] articulation is not as frequent (Arnold, 1943, 1954). Nasal airflow and its influence on [s]-productions can be verified by pinching the nostrils closed. The nasal resonance will immediately disappear during the occlusion of

> For a discussion of nasality due to organic problems and its impact on articulation, see the Clefting: Cleft Palate and Cleft Lip section of Chapter 10.

the nasal passageway and be audible again if the nostrils are released. Third, functional nasal productions are usually accompanied by a normal tongue placement for [s] and [z].

CLINICAL APPLICATION
A Strident Problem

Josh was a bright child who was doing well in first grade. His teacher was satisfied with the skills that he was acquiring in reading and writing. However, several children had recently started to tease Josh about his conspicuous [s]-production. Josh was aware of his irregular pronunciation and was beginning to withdraw from speaking situations and become aggressive when he was teased. The teacher referred Josh to the speech-language pathologist.

Assessment revealed that Josh's only speech-language problem appeared to be this [s], which was articulated with a clear and shrill whistle in all contexts. The clinician began to analyze the phonetic characteristics this child was demonstrating. Organ, place, manner, and voicing were appropriate. However, it appeared that the more Josh tried to say the sound correctly, the louder the whistle-like component became. Using her phonetic skills, the clinician remembered that there must be a precise balance between the air pressure and the narrow opening between organ and place of articulation for [s]-productions. If there is an imbalance between air pressure and the opening through which the air must flow, a whistling component could result. This whistling component, often referred to as a "strident s," can be caused by too much air pressure through a slightly narrowed opening or normal air pressure through a very narrow opening. Thinking about Josh's efforts when attempting to articulate this sound correctly, the clinician was confident that she had found the phonetic reason for Josh's problem. After explanations, some exercises, and some experimenting with openings and air pressure, Josh could say [s]-sounds without a whistle.

Therapeutic Suggestions

Two approaches seem viable when working with a child or adult displaying an isolated [s] misarticulation: the phonetic placement method (Scripture and Jackson, 1919) and the sound modification method (Van Riper, 1978). Simply stated, phonetic placement amounts to describing the organ, place, and manner of production of the sound in question to the client. Systematic work toward realizing that goal is then implemented in an attempt to change the aberrant production characteristics. Naturally, with children, this needs to be accomplished in an age-appropriate manner. A mirror might be used as visual feedback, while the clinician serves as an auditory feedback system. Although this approach is widely used, it is often not easy to describe what exactly needs to be done with the tongue and the airflow in a manner that the child can easily understand and follow. The sound modification method, on the other hand, uses another sound or sounds that the child can produce in a regular manner as a point of departure for achieving the target sound (Secord, 1981b). Therefore, [t], which the child can produce, might be used to achieve [s], which the child misarticulates. The sound modification method is easier to apply if the speech sound chosen as a starting point has certain phonetic similarities to the misarticulated sound. This way, a bridge is built between the similar sound that can be correctly articulated by the child and the target sound that is in error. Both methods will be discussed for problems encountered with [s] and [z].

Phonetic Placement

Decision Making: Apico- or Predorsal Placement. Although most people produce [s] and [z] as apico-alveolar productions, a predorsal articulation is not without merit. For the apico-alveolar [s], the tongue tip is hovering, so to speak, near the alveolar ridge. This precarious position must be precisely maintained over the entire duration of the sound. In contrast, for the predorsal [s], the tongue tip is resting behind the lower incisors. This provides an easily

identifiable spot for the tongue tip, which does not waver or fluctuate; it is something definite to "hold on to." For this reason, the predorsal [s] is noted as being a more stable production (Kramer, 1939; Krech, 1969; Waengler and Bauman-Waengler, 1984). Such relative stability is often especially important for children whose motor capabilities are not yet fully developed. In addition, a large percentage of [s] and [z] misarticulations are interdental or addental in nature; that is, the tongue tip is elevated but too far forward. To now move the tongue tip down for the predorsal-alveolar version provides a solution that is quite different from the child's previous attempts. The natural tendency to return to the previous incorrect [s] is diminished. It is often easier for a child to accomplish a different, new production task than to attempt minor adjustments of a previous one. The final decision of apico-alveolar or predorsal-alveolar [s] will depend on the client's motor abilities or restrictions and on the type and degree of [s] misarticulation.

Phonetic Placement: Apico-Alveolar [s].   For interdental or addental [s] misarticulations, the tongue tip must be moved back. The client, after instruction, glides the tongue posteriorly from the interdental or addental [s] position to the alveolar ridge. This necessitates visual aid, such as an articulation mirror, and reliable auditory feedback in the form of the therapist noting the exact time during this procedure when [s] is perceived as being appropriate. In addition, the lateral edges of the tongue need to be elevated. This might be aided by implementing specific tongue awareness activities (see Box 8.2) prior to the phonetic placement. One could practice slightly "rolling the tongue," for example, prior to this manipulation so that the client becomes aware of the necessary elevation of the lateral edges.

BOX 8.2   Tongue and Lip Awareness Activities

Tongue and lip awareness activities can often be utilized with beneficial results. They are employed not to strengthen the articulators or increase their coordination per se but rather to heighten the child's *awareness* of tongue and lip movements. Van Riper (1963) states that "they can be said to be useful in teaching the student to manipulate his articulatory apparatus in many new and unaccustomed ways" (p. 267). Many clinicians question or flatly deny the therapeutic benefit of these activities. A decision to use these activities will, therefore, be based on the clinician's philosophy and the needs of the individual client. If used, these exercises should be practiced for a limited time only and should always be specifically selected to reflect the problem at hand. The following are examples of tongue and lip awareness activities.

Tongue Awareness Activities

1. Stick the tongue out flat and wide.
2. Stick the tongue out narrow and long.
3. Stick the tongue out slightly with its tip up then down.
4. Tongue out as far as possible, then tongue tip up and down.
5. Tongue out as far as possible, move the tongue in and out.
6. Tongue out, then move to the left, center, right, center.
7. Tongue out, then move to the far right then far left.
8. Tongue out, then move to the right, the left; next up, then down.
9. Push the tongue tip against the cheeks, bulging out the cheeks to look like you have a golf ball in your mouth.

10. Move tongue slowly on the outside of the mouth around the red of the lips, first clockwise, then counterclockwise.
11. Move tongue slowly on the inside of the mouth from right to left passing by the closed lips. (This can be combined with number 9.)
12. Move tongue slowly on the inside of the lips in a clockwise, then counterclockwise direction.
13. Let the tongue "wash" the outside of the teeth from incisors to molars.
14. Let the tongue "wash" the inside of the teeth from incisors to molars.
15. Tap the tongue against the palate.
16. Move the tongue along the palate from behind the upper incisors posteriorly to the soft palate.
17. Move the tongue around the palate in circles, first clockwise then counterclockwise.
18. Let the tongue tip push against the inside of the lower incisors.
19. Roll the tongue.
20. Hold the tongue roll while you stick the tongue out.

Lip Awareness Activities

1. Pucker lips, then relax; repeat.
2. Spread the lips, then relax; repeat.
3. Round the lips in a wide O, relax; repeat.
4. Use combinations of 1, 2, and 3. Round to spread, round to pucker, pucker to spread.
5. Use combinations of 1, 2, and 3 with articulation: *o* to *i, o* to *u, u* to *i.*
6. "Bite" the lips. First the upper and then the lower lips are "sucked into" the slightly open rows of teeth. Relax by bringing the teeth together in a neutral position.
7. "Rub" both lips together. First right and left, then forward and backward.
8. Make a "crooked" mouth, first to the right and then to the left.

For some children, the phonetic placement technique may be too demanding. They seem unable to manipulate the tongue while simultaneously trying to produce a sound. In these cases, it could be less frustrating to have the tongue tip pushed back passively during the production of the "old" [s] articulation. This can be accomplished by using a tongue depressor, which is placed between the upper and lower teeth and gently pushing the tongue tip back until the appropriate position is reached. The client should be instructed to focus attention on how the new tongue position feels and which changes had to be made to achieve this regular production. In addition, the clinician must serve as a reliable feedback system until the child can correctly discriminate, both auditorily and motorically, between the "new" and the "old" sound.

For lateral [s] realizations, the edge(s) of the tongue is not elevated and the tongue tip is in direct contact with the alveolar ridge. Therefore, the client must learn (1) to raise the lateral edges and (2) to direct the airstream over the tip of the tongue, thus releasing the previous contact. To heighten awareness of raising the lateral edges, one could start with tongue rolling activities. To demonstrate contact versus no contact of the tongue tip with the alveolar ridge, one could use a rather forceful [t] sound (contact) with excessive aspiration (no contact). During the release phase, the client should be directed to notice the airflow over the front edges of the tongue. To develop the necessary central airflow, Secord (1981b) suggests that the client blow through a straw that has been placed along the sagittal groove of the tongue. A smaller cylindrical object (such as a small bamboo stick) can also

be used to aid central airflow while simultaneously creating more of a medial grooving of the tongue. The stick is placed sagitally on the tongue. During [s] attempts, the clinician pushes slightly downward on the stick. This should help create more of a grooving effect while also hindering the contact of the tongue with the alveolar ridge.

The palatal [s]-production is characterized by a too posterior tongue position. Therefore, the client must slowly glide the tongue forward, being careful to maintain the grooving of the tongue. Tongue activities such as numbers 15 and 16 in Box 8.2 could prove helpful prior to this manipulation.

A lack of balance between expiratory airflow and the degree of opening necessary for the production causes a strident [s]. Thus, the client needs to experiment with reducing the air pressure during the production and/or slightly increasing the opening between the organ and place of articulation. Air pressure can be reduced by having the client say the sound softly. Increasing the opening can be accomplished by a slight lowering of the tongue, possibly by lowering the mandible slightly. Table 8.6 provides an overview of

Table 8.6 Overview of Error Productions and the Necessary Articulatory Adjustments for an Apico-Alveolar [s]

Error Production	Articulatory Adjustments
Interdental	Tongue tip must be moved posteriorly. Lateral edges of the tongue may require elevation.
Addental	Tongue tip must be moved posteriorly. Lateral edges of the tongue may require elevation.
Lateral	Tongue tip contact with the alveolar ridge must be released. Raise the lateral edges of the tongue. Direct airflow over the tip of the tongue.
Palatal	Tongue tip must be moved anteriorly.
Strident	Reduce air pressure or increase the opening between the organ and place of articulation.

necessary articulatory adjustments for the various error productions of [s].

Phonetic Placement: Predorsal-Alveolar [s].
With the predorsal-alveolar [s], the client must understand that the tip of the tongue must always stay behind the lower teeth. With visual or tactile aids (the specific portion of the tongue and the alveolar ridge can be touched while looking in a mirror), the client should be directed so that the front or blade portion of the tongue approximates the alveolar ridge. The lateral edges are again elevated.

Particularly for lateral misarticulations, the predorsal [s] has advantages over the apico-alveolar type. Moving the tongue tip down behind the lower incisors eliminates the problem of the contact between the tongue tip and the alveolar ridge, which not only characterizes this misarticulation but is often the reason for the relaxed lateral edges. Palatal [s] misarticulations with their characteristic posterior positioning of both organ and place of articulation may also benefit from the placement of the tongue behind the lower incisors. By choosing the predorsal-alveolar production, the whole tongue is more anteriorly situated.

Sound Modification Methods. Sound modification methods are based on the concept of utilizing a similar, appropriately articulated sound to aid in the production of the misarticulated sound. A similar sound refers to one that is comparable in some of its phonetic production features. This method is easiest to implement when several direct phonetic similarities exist between the sound to be modified and the target sound. However, some successful techniques have evolved out of very limited articulatory similarities.

1. *[t]-[s] method.*
   a. Begin with a series of rapid [t] repetitions, which typically produce inter-

mittent [s]-like fricatives. This effect is increased if the child is asked to produce [t] with lots of air pressure. Have the child listen for the sound in between the [t] repetitions; then ask the child to try to prolong this intermittent [s].
   b. Begin with a [t]-production in which the stop phase is prolonged, building up air pressure behind the occlusion. The client is then instructed to release the [t] very slowly. The result should approximate [s].

2. *[ʃ]-[s] method.* Three steps are necessary to change [ʃ] to a normal [s]-production:
   a. Eliminate the lip rounding associated with the production of [ʃ]. Have the client smile while saying [ʃ].
   b. Move the friction that occurs between organ and place of articulation more anteriorly. Have the client move the tongue slightly forward.
   c. Increase the sagittal grooving of the tongue. Have the client raise the lateral edges of the tongue toward the upper molars.

3. *[f]-[s] method.* This method assumes that the tongue tip for [f] is already situated behind the lower incisors; therefore, a predorsal [s] is the goal.
   a. Pull the middle of the lower lip away from contact with the upper incisors during the production of [f].
   b. Raise the front portion of the tongue slightly as the upper and lower incisors come closer together.

For this modification, the client must be aware that a friction sound should be maintained during the entire attempt.

4. *[i]-[s] method.* Phonetic similarities between [i] and [s] consist of the lip spreading and the high, anterior tongue placement for both sounds. For [i], the tongue tip is typically

The [i] could easily be modified to a voiced [z] if a decision has been made to initiate work with that sound. In addition, the [i]-[z] method has the advantage of maintaining voicing throughout the modification, which is not the case with the [i]-[s] method. See the section on Where to Begin: [s] or [z].

in a lowered position while the anterior portion of the body of the tongue is elevated toward the palate (Shriberg and Kent, 2003). Thus, this modification will normally result in a predorsal (tongue tip down) [s].

    a. Instruct the client to bring the teeth slightly closer together during the [i] production.

    b. Elevate the front portion of the tongue until a friction-type sound is heard.

    c. Raise the lateral edges of the tongue toward the upper molars.

Functional Nasal [s] and [z] Problems.   Therapy for functional nasal [s] and [z] problems does not fit readily into the categorizations of phonetic placement or sound modification methods. The reason for the aberrant nasal [s] is not a deviant tongue placement but rather the inadequate velopharyngeal closure leading to nasal emission. Specific consonants can be used as a bridge to promote sufficient velar closure.

1. *[t]-[s].* If [t] can be produced without hypernasality, instruct the client to hold the stop phase of the [t], building up pressure during the occlusion. [t] is then *slowly* released, producing [s]. Complete velopharyngeal closure is normally necessary when producing [t]. By increasing the air pressure, the occlusion is strengthened due to the higher degree of production effort. This heightened effort may promote more velopharyngeal closure for the following [s] approximation as well. Visual

and auditory feedback should also be implemented to increase the client's awareness of nasal emission versus no nasal emission.

2. *[f]-[s].* Requisites for this method are an [f] production without hypernasality and the correct tongue placement for [s]. During [f], the client removes the labiodental contact (similar to the previously noted [f]-[s] method), gliding the tongue to an [s] approximation. Important here is that the client should continue to think about the [f] noise and keep that noise going. This method is based on the assumption that adequate velopharyngeal closure for [f] will now extend to [s]. Again, visual and auditory feedback should be implemented.

Where to Begin: [s] or [z]?   When attempting to achieve an isolated sound production, most clinicians automatically begin with voiceless [s]. The reasoning seems to be that the fricative, while complicated enough for the client, should not be further burdened with the addition of voicing. However, beginning with [z] could be advantageous under certain conditions.

First, voiced consonants normally are produced with less air pressure than the voiceless ones. An increased air pressure can at times be counterproductive to establishing norm articulations. Especially with an apico (tongue tip up) [s], this increased air pressure could lead to the client "losing" the precariously new approximation between organ and place of articulation.

A second factor that supports a choice of [z] is the ability of the voicing component to mask minor productional differences. Listeners seem to be more critical of even slight deviations of the voiceless [s]. The same articulatory features used for the production of [z] are not as noticeable. Naturally, we do not want the client to acquire an [s] that is somehow not acceptable.

The following scenario can serve as an example. We have begun work on [s]; however, even with our best efforts and those of the child, the production is still slightly off target. We have tried several times to correct for the minor mispositionings, but the articulation is still not quite accurate. We are becoming somewhat frustrated; the child, we feel, is already frustrated. This could be a good time to attempt a voiced [z]. If the articulatory variation is minor enough, the voicing should provide us with an acceptable sound. While giving the child success (finally), it also allows practice time for the new sound. This practice with [z] is often all the child needs to achieve an acceptable [s] articulation.

A third consideration in favor of [z] is a coarticulatory consideration. If the voiceless [s] is placed in a consonant–vowel (or vowel–consonant) context, the client must change the voicing halfway through the utterance. This sudden change in voicing could strain an already difficult articulatory-motor task. By utilizing [z], voicing can be maintained throughout the production. To attain [s] once [z] is acceptable is relatively easy. If the child whispers [z], [s] will result. The next task is to put the isolated sound production into specific contexts.

Coarticulatory Conditions

The phonetic context in which a target sound is placed can have a considerable impact on the production of that sound. There are certain contexts that can support the production features of the target sound and others that might undermine them. Phonetic contexts that support the production of a target sound can be used effectively by clinicians in certain phases of therapy. On the other hand, ignoring coarticulatory contexts may lead to endangering a "new" sound production that is still relatively unstable. Facilitative coarticulatory conditions rely on knowledge of, and comparison between, phonetic features.

If the newly acquired [s] is practiced in syllables or words, the vowels that precede or follow it should be considered. Recall that [s] is articulated with the tongue in a relatively anterior position and with some degree of lip spreading; [i] seems phonetically comparable. Both [s] and [i] require unrounding of the lips while the anterior portion of the tongue is elevated toward the palate. This is not the case with [u]. This vowel is produced with the back of the tongue elevated and requires lip rounding. The coarticulatory effects of the lip rounding on [s] can be demonstrated by saying the word *Sue*. The lip rounding for [u] is already present as one begins to say the initial [s]. This lip rounding and the additional posterior tongue placement could actually work against a newly acquired [s] articulation.

Examining phonetic comparability, it would seem that the front vowels are better suited for our initial context work with [s]. The front vowels [i], [ɪ], [eɪ], [ɛ], and [æ] support the relatively forward tongue placement and the lack of lip rounding. The back vowels have specific features that lack support for [s] and [z]. First, a more posterior tongue placement is associated with all back vowels. In addition, the degree of lip rounding increases from [ɔ] to [oʊ] and from [ʊ] to [u]. The [ɑ] is considered to be an unrounded vowel. Thus, if lip rounding presents a problem for [s], the low-back vowel [ɑ] should demonstrate more favorable coarticulatory conditions than the mid- and high-back vowels.

The phonetic context should be kept in mind when moving through every stage of therapy. By contrasting the phonetic features of the target sound and the surrounding consonants and vowels, a hierarchy of contexts can be established that move step-by-step from more to less supportive coarticulatory conditions. Not every client will need such small steps. However, for those who do, this hierarchy will prove invaluable. On the other hand, some clients may demonstrate phonetic contexts that may be more facilitating for them than those previously mentioned. The clinician should then use those specific contexts. The suggested sequence should not be seen as part of a "therapy cookbook" approach to be followed with every client but as one possibility that incorporates phonetic comparability.

Word Examples. The following one-syllable words are ordered from relatively easy to more difficult coarticulatory conditions:

[s] Words	[z] Words
see - seap - seam - seat - seed - seen	zee - zeal - Zeke
sip - sit - sin - sing	zip - zing - zipped - zinc
say - same - save - sail	Zane
set - said - sell	Zeb - Zed - Zen
sap - Sam - sat - sash - sang	zap - zag - zapped - zagged
sum - sun - suck - sung	
sob - sod - sock - song	czar
sow - soap - sewed - soak	zone - zoned
soot	
Sue - soup - suit - soon	zoo - zoom - zoomed

CLINICAL APPLICATION

Analyzing Coarticulatory Conditions

When analyzing words according to coarticulatory conditions, several factors should be kept in mind:

1. *The vowel following or preceding the target sound.* Consider the comparability of production features of certain vowels relative to the target sound. Some vowels will have production features that are phonetically similar to the target sound, whereas others will be clearly different.

For example, the lip rounding of the high-back vowels and the lip spreading of [s] are dissimilar articulatory conditions.

2. *The syllable structure of the word.* Consider the articulatory gesture as a whole. A word that contains a consonant followed by a vowel (CV) is a less complex articulatory unit than one with a CVC structure. CVCC words are relatively more complex than either CV or CVC structures.

3. *The phonetic features of the surrounding consonants.* Consider the movement of the articulators for the production. Organ, place, manner, and voicing of the target sound can be compared to the other consonants within the word. Again, production similarities may be used to create favorable coarticulatory conditions. For example, the organ, place, and voicing of [s] and [t] are phonetically the same. This is not the case for [s] and [k].

Other consonants may provide supportive coarticulatory conditions based on the absence of specific production features. For example, the tongue is not directly involved in the articulation of the bilabials and [h]. Within an articulatory unit, if [s] precedes or follows a sound that does not require tongue movement, then the coarticulatory effects on [s] are minimal. The tongue movement for [s] is not influenced by any preceding or following articulatory necessities. Therefore, [m], [p], [b], and [h] can provide supportive coarticulatory conditions for those consonants in which the tongue is the active organ of articulation.

4. *The misarticulation of the client.* Consider the type of misarticulation the client demonstrates. The client is accustomed to this motor pattern; it has been practiced for a longer period of time. The new motor task, the norm articulation of the target sound, is relatively new. If the new motor task is put into a phonetic environment similar to the misarticulation, the newly established articulation could be jeopardized. For example, a child's misarticulation of [s] involves a tongue position that is too anterior, an addental or interdental [s] problem. If this [s] is in a word together with [θ], this could trigger the original misarticulation. Or, if the child has a lateral [s], it is probably not a good idea to practice words that contain [l] initially, a lateral sound that might trigger the lateral [s] misarticulation.

$\mathcal{M}$ISARTICULATIONS OF [ʃ] AND [ʒ]

In the following section, typical norm and aberrant productions of [ʃ] and [ʒ] are described. Specific phonetic placement and sound modification methods are then addressed. Because [s] and [ʃ] show many similarities in error productions as well as in the diagnostic procedures that would be implemented, the reader is referred back to the section on [s] misarticulations at several points.

Phonetic Description

Phonetically, [s] and [ʃ] are closely related. However, the sagittal groove is considerably wider for [ʃ] than it is for [s] (Fletcher and Newman, 1991). Therefore, the tongue is somewhat flatter for [ʃ] than for [s]. This is one reason why the friction noise for [ʃ] is not as "sharp" as that for [s]. In addition, the place of articulation is not the alveolar ridge, as with the [s]; it is located slightly posterior to it, at the anterior portion of the palate, the postalveolar or prepalatal area. Finally, [ʃ] has lip rounding rather than the lip spreading common for [s]-productions. Putting this all together, the phonetic description of [ʃ] is a voiceless coronal-postalveolar or coronal-prepalatal fricative with lip rounding. The voiced counterpart of [ʃ] is [ʒ].

Linguistic Function

Frequency of Occurrence. The voiceless [ʃ] is an infrequent sound ranking twentieth out of the twenty-four General American English consonants. The voiced [ʒ] is the most infrequent sound in General American English, occurring only in words of foreign origin, such as *beige* or *rouge* (Dewey, 1923; French, Carter, and Koenig, 1930; Roberts, 1965).

Phonotactics. Both [ʃ] and [ʒ] can occur initiating and terminating a syllable. There are very few consonant clusters with [ʃ] and [ʒ]. Table 8.7 provides the more frequent consonant clusters. Word examples are also given.

Morphophonemic Function. Word-final clusters that end in [ʃ] or [ʒ] can be used to signal past tense in regular verbs that end in these sounds, such as *splashed* and *massaged*.

Minimal Pairs. Frequent sounds that are substituted for [ʃ] and [ʒ] include [s] and [z] and [t] and [d]. Examples of minimal word pairs and sentences are contained in Tables 8.8 and 8.9.

Initial Remarks

Preliminary considerations are similar to those presented for [s]. Thus, hearing acuity, minor structural or functional deviations, and the auditory discrimination abilities of the client need to be assessed before beginning work on the isolated articulation of [ʃ] and [ʒ].

Types of Misarticulation

The most common forms of [ʃ] and [ʒ] misarticulations fall into these categories:

Table 8.7 Consonant Clusters with [ʃ] and [ʒ]

Word-Initiating [ʃ]	Word-Terminating [ʃ]	Word-Terminating [ʒ]
[ʃr] shrimp, shrub	[rʃ] marsh, harsh	[ʒd] rouged, massaged
	[ʃt] washed, wished	

Table 8.8 Minimal Pair Words and Sentences Contrasting [ʃ] and [ʒ] to [s] and [z]

[ʃ] versus [s]		[ʒ] versus [z]	[ʃ] versus [s]		[ʒ] versus [z]	
shack	sack	no words found	bash	bass	beige	base
shag	sag		clash	class		
shame	same		gash	gas		
shave	save		leash	lease		
she	see		mesh	mess		
shed	said		plush	plus		
sheep	seep					
sheet	seat					
shell	cell					
shine	sign					
ship	sip					
shock	sock					
shoe	Sue					
shoot	suit					
show	sew					
shy	sigh					
What a *shine*! What a *sign*!			It was a big *bash*. It was a big *bass*.			
The *shell* was very small. The *cell* was very small.			He broke the *leash*. He broke the *lease*.			
It was a large *shock*. It was a large *sock*.			The *clash* was over. The *class* was over.			

1. *Lateral* [ʃ] *problems.* Lateral [ʃ] misarticulations demonstrate lateral airflow. This is triggered by (a) a firm contact of the frontal portions of the tongue with the prepalatal area and (b) a lowering of the lateral edges of the tongue. The resulting [ʃ] is auditorily highly conspicuous; there is a noticeable noise component to the sound. Lateral [ʃ] errors can be bilateral or unilateral. Means of verifying laterality have been discussed in the section on [s] problems.

Phonetic transcription of the error: typically [ɬ] or [ɮ].

2. *Addental* [ʃ] *problems.* For these misarticulations, the tongue placement is too far forward with the tongue approximating the alveolar ridge rather than the prepalatal area. Reduced medial grooving of the tongue may also be present. If a child demonstrates an addental [s]-production, the likelihood exists that [ʃ] may also be addental.

Phonetic transcription of the error: [ʃ̪] or [ʒ̪] or possibly [s], [z].

3. *Palatal* [ʃ] *problems.* These productions are characterized by a more posterior tongue articulation: Organ and place of articulation are too

Table 8.9   Minimal Pair Words and Sentences Contrasting [ʃ] and [ʒ] to [t] and [d]

[ʃ] versus [t]		[ʒ] versus [d]	[ʃ] versus [t]		[ʒ] versus [d]	
shack	tack	no words found	bash	bat	rouge	rude
shag	tag		cash	cat	beige	bade
shake	take		fish	fit		
shape	tape		flash	flat		
sharp	tarp		hash	hat		
she	tea		mash	mat		
shed	Ted		rash	rat		
shell	tell		rush	rut		
ship	tip		wish	wit		
shop	top					
shoe	two					
shoot	toot					

He found a large *shack* in the woods.

He found a large *tack* in the woods.

The *ship* was broken.

The *tip* was broken.

He tried to *shake* it.

He tried to *take* it.

It was a long *shape*.

It was a long *tape*.

She had a funny *wish*.

She had a funny *wit*.

He couldn't find his *cash*.

He couldn't find his *cat*.

What a *fish* he had.

What a *fit* he had.

It was a large *flash*.

It was a large *flat*.

far back. There is a shift from coronal-postal-veolar or prepalatal to predorsal-mediopalatal (or possibly even mediodorsal-mediopalatal) tongue placement. Because of this, these misarticulations are often perceptually similar to a voiceless [j].

Phonetic transcription of the error: [ç], a voiceless palatal fricative or [ʝ], a voiced palatal fricative.

4. *Nasal [ʃ] problems.* These productions are characterized by nasality during the production of [ʃ] and [ʒ]. Comparable to the nasal [s] problems, the nasality can be functional or organic in nature. The previous discussion for functional nasal [s] problems applies to nasalized [ʃ] as well.

Phonetic transcription of the error: [ʃ̃] or [ʒ̃]

5. *Unrounded [ʃ] productions.* Frequently, children produce [ʃ] with acceptable positioning of organ and place of articulation but without the necessary lip rounding. These productions remain auditorily conspicuous; the sound is "off." When noticing the lips of the client during [ʃ], it will become clear that there is no (or not enough) lip rounding.

Phonetic transcription of the error: [ʃ] or [ʒ]

Therapeutic Suggestions

Phonetic Placement.   Although most [ʃ] and [ʒ] realizations are produced with the tongue tip up, approximating the area directly behind the alveolar ridge, [ʃ] can also be produced with the tongue tip down behind the lower incisors. As with the tongue tip down [s], the tongue arches upward with the front portion of the tongue approximating the postalveolar or prepalatal area. The following descriptions are given for both tongue tip up (coronal-postalveolar or prepalatal) and tongue tip down (predorsal-prepalatal) [ʃ] and [ʒ].

Phonetic Placement: Coronal-Postalveolar or Prepalatal Placement.   For lateral [ʃ], the contact between organ and place of articulation needs to be released. In addition, the lateral edges of the tongue should be elevated, creating a medial groove of the tongue. Techniques suggested for lateral [s] problems can also be used here. However, differences between the production of the [s] and [ʃ] should be kept in mind: For [ʃ], the coronal, as opposed to the apical, placement of the tongue is approximating an area slightly behind the highest point of the alveolar ridge. In addition, there is not as much medial sagittal grooving of the tongue and lip rounding is required.

If the client is demonstrating an addental [ʃ]-production, the tongue needs to be slightly retracted. This can be achieved by having the client prolong the addental [ʃ] and then glide the tongue slowly back. The clinician will need to monitor and identify when the change results in an acceptable [ʃ]. Another way to achieve this goal is to push the tongue back with a tongue depressor.

Its flat portion is placed interdentally and a gentle attempt is made to move the tongue posteriorly.

The tongue placement for a palatal [ʃ] misarticulation is too far back. Thus, during the prolongation of [ʃ], the client should be directed to glide the tongue forward. Medial grooving of the tongue as well as lip rounding should be maintained.

[ʃ] problems resulting from not enough lip rounding require only the addition of lip protrusion during this production. By placing both hands on the cheeks, the client can push the lips forward during the [ʃ] attempts. This manipulation paired with visual and auditory feedback should give the client initial success in achieving a [ʃ] with lip rounding.

Phonetic Placement: Predorsal-Prepalatal Placement.   First, the tip of the tongue is placed down, touching the inside of the lower incisors. Second, the front portion of the tongue has to arch upward, creating a narrow opening between the predorsal portion of the tongue and the area directly behind the alveolar ridge. A slight medial groove is also necessary; therefore, the lateral edges of the tongue have to come into contact with the upper molars. If these conditions are met, only lip protrusion must be added in order to realize an acceptable [ʃ].

Sound Modification Methods

1. *[s]-[ʃ] method.*   Because [s] and [ʃ] sounds are phonetically similar, clients who have difficulty with [ʃ] often demonstrate [s] problems as well. If that is the case, this method cannot be used. If [s] is intact, though, the [s]-[ʃ] method would certainly be a good choice. Only lip rounding and a slight retraction of the tongue are initially required. Fortunately, both requirements are often fulfilled simultaneously. If the lips are clearly protruded, the tongue tip has a tendency to retract a bit (Goguillot, 1889; Weinert, 1974). If this natural retraction is still not enough, the client should be instructed to glide the tongue back slightly. If the [ʃ] is still auditorily somewhat off, slight adjustments may need to be made.

2. [t]-[ʃ] method. The main phonetic dissimilarity between [t] and [ʃ] pertains to the manner of articulation: stop versus sibilant fricative. Organ and place of articulation are close enough to be usable.

  a. Begin with a prolonged [t] production (prolonging the implosion phase) with lip protrusion.
  b. Maintaining the lip protrusion, instruct the client to slowly release the [t] while gliding the tongue back slightly.

3. [tʃ]-[ʃ] method. The goal of this method is to isolate the friction portion of the affricate. This can be done in the following manner:

  a. Begin with a very slow production of [tʃ], making sure that lip protrusion is realized.
  b. Instruct the client to lengthen the final fricative portion of the affricate.

Functional Nasal [ʃ] Problems. Each of the following methods must first be evaluated to see whether adequate velopharyngeal closure, that is, no hypernasal resonance is noted for the sounds coupled with [ʃ].

1. [t]-[ʃ]. This is similar to the technique described in functional nasal [s] problems. The addition of lip rounding will be necessary for [ʃ] realizations.

2. [tʃ]-[ʃ]. First, a forceful [tʃ] is produced, one with an increased buildup of air pressure behind the point of closure. The [t] portion is then slowly released. The client should be instructed that this release should

be only minimal. Our goal is a slightly narrower opening between organ and place of articulation than is normally the case with [ʃ]-productions. This narrow opening with its increased air pressure should help support the velopharyngeal closure necessary for [ʃ].

Coarticulatory Conditions

When describing context conditions that support regular [ʃ]-productions, two questions must be considered: First, is the problem based on difficulties with the tongue placement or is it primarily due to not enough lip rounding? The answer will play a role in the selection of coarticulatory conditions.

If the problem is a result of faulty tongue placement—that is, if addental, palatal, or lateral [ʃ] realizations result—the sequence of supportive vowel coarticulations follows those described for [s]. Thus, the front vowels [i], [ɪ], [eⁱ], [ɛ], and [æ], particularly the high-front vowels [i] and [ɪ], support the relatively high anterior position of the tongue during regular [ʃ]-productions.

If the [ʃ] misarticulation is primarily due to a lack of lip rounding, a different coarticulatory sequence is proposed. Now the natural lip rounding of the back vowels would support the articulatory necessities for [ʃ]. The high-back vowels [u] and [ʊ] with the most lip rounding would be especially helpful, followed by [oᵘ] and [ɔ]. Even the central vowels [ɝ] and [ɚ], which are produced with some degree of lip rounding, could support the lip protrusion necessary for [ʃ]. The unrounded features of the low-back vowel [ɑ] and the front vowels would initially not be indicated.

Word Examples. The following one-syllable words are ordered from relatively easy to more difficult coarticulatory conditions:

[ʃ] Words

Primary Problem: *Tongue Placement*	*Primary Problem:* *Lip Rounding*
she - sheep - sheet - she'd - shield	shoe - shoot
	should - shook
ship - shin - shipped - shift	show - showed - shown - shore
	sure - shirt
shape - shame - shade - shave - shake	shot - shawl - shock - shocked - shop
shed - chef - shell - shelf	shack - shag - shaft
	shed - shell - chef - shelf
shack - shag - shaft	
shut - shove	shade - shave - shake - shape - shame
shop - shot - shawl - shock - shocked	shin - shift - ship - shipped
show - showed - shown - shore	she - sheet - she'd - shield - sheep
should - shook	
shoe - shoot	

Misarticulations of [k] and [g]

Many children go through a phase of substituting [t] for [k] and [d] for [g]. For example, Preisser, Hodson, and Paden (1988) reported that this is the most common deviation involving the [k] and [g] sounds in children from 18 to 29 months of age. Some children seem to "get stuck" in this usually short transient period. In spite of a normal progression in other aspects of their speech-language development, they might retain the [t/k] [d/g] substitution into their preschool or even school years. This poses obvious dangers because the child's enormous increase in vocabulary during this time necessitates the understanding and observation of the phoneme oppositions /t/ versus /k/ and /d/ versus /g/. Many minimal pairs exemplify these contrasts in General American English—*tea* versus *key*, for instance.

Phonetic Description

[k] and [g] are voiceless or voiced postdorsal-velar stops: The back of the tongue is raised, creating a complete blockage of the expiratory airflow at the anterior portion of the velum. A buildup of air pressure occurs until the tongue suddenly moves away from the velum, releasing the air into the oral cavity. Typically, [k] is produced with higher pressure and more tension than [g]. That makes [k] in most cases aspirated and [g] unaspirated. However, the [k] is not usually aspirated in certain context conditions—in word-medial position and as a component of a consonant cluster, for example.

Linguistic Function

Frequency of Occurrence. [k] and [g] occur fairly frequently in General American English. Out of twenty-four consonants, [k] is ranked within the top ten most frequent consonants, while [g] ranks approximately fifteenth (Carterette and Jones, 1974; Mader, 1954; Mines, Hanson, and Shoup, 1978). Frequent word-initiating consonant clusters include [gr], [kw], [kl], and [kr]. Frequent word-final clusters with these sounds are [ks] and [kt] (Dewey, 1923; French, Carter, and Koenig, 1930).

Phonotactics. Both [k] and [g] can occur initiating and terminating a syllable. Most [g] sounds occur initiating words, whereas [k] sounds are fairly equally distributed across initial, medial, and final word positions (Mader, 1954). Tables 8.10 and 8.11 list the more frequent [k] and [g] consonant clusters with word examples.

Morphophonemic Function. Word-final clusters that end in [ks] or [gz] can be used to signal plurality, as in boo<u>ks</u>, le<u>gs</u>, or do<u>gs</u>. In number and tense marking, [k] occurs with [t] or [s] to produce words such as pi<u>cked</u> and pi<u>cks</u>. The [g]

Table 8.10 Consonant Clusters with [k]

Word-Initiating		Word-Terminating	
[kl]	clown, clean	[kl]	uncle, tickle
[kr]	cry, crumb	[ks]	box, six
[sk]	school, sky	[kt]	backed, looked
[skr]	scream, scrape	[lk]	milk, silk, elk
[skw]	squeak, squirt	[rk]	dark, work
		[rkt]	worked, parked
		[sk]	ask, desk
		[sks]	asks, disks

Table 8.11 Consonant Clusters with [g]

Word-Initiating		Word-Terminating	
[gl]	glad, glue	[gz]	pigs, bugs
[gr]	grape, grouch	[gd]	wagged, flagged
[gw]	Gwen, very infrequent		

copulas with the verb *to be* also demonstrate clusters with [k] and [g]. Examples include "the duck's waddling" and "the dog's barking."

Minimal Pairs. The most common substitutions for [k] and [g] are [t] and [d]. Table 8.12 provides examples of minimal pairs and sentences contrasting these sounds.

preceding either [d] or [z] can also mark number and tense in verbs such as logged or wags. Within phrases, contractible auxiliaries and

Table 8.12 Minimal Pair Words and Sentences Contrasting [k] and [g] to [t] and [d]

[k] versus [t]		[k] versus [t]		[g] versus [d]		[g] versus [d]	
cake	take	ache	ate	gate	date	bag	bad
cop	top	back	bat	gown	down	beg	bed
cape	tape	bake	bait	go	doe	bug	bud
cub	tub	beak	beat	got	dot	leg	led
key	tea	bike	bite	gull	dull	sag	sad
kite	tight	knock	knot				
cool	tool	lake	late				
car	tar	like	light				
corn	torn	neck	net				

They didn't like the cold *coast.*	The *cub* was small.	They had a *bake* sale.
They didn't like the cold *toast.*	The *tub* was small.	They had a *bait* sale.
The teacher *caught* the boy.	The *gate* was fixed.	He twisted his *neck.*
The teacher *taught* the boy.	The *date* was fixed.	He twisted his *net.*
He was stuck in the *car.*	There is a scratch on her *back.*	He *likes* it.
He was stuck in the *tar.*	There is a scratch on her *bat.*	He *lights* it.
Hand me the *key.*	The *lock* was big.	Her big brother made her *beg.*
Hand me the *tea.*	The *lot* was big.	Her big brother made her *bed.*

Initial Remarks

Due to the fact that [k] and [g] misarticulations are often substitutions of one speech sound for another, it is especially important that the client be evaluated for a phonemic disorder.

Types of Misarticulation

1. *[t] and [d] substitutions.* These are the most common aberrant productions noted for [k] and [g]: [t] replaces the voiceless [k], while [d] is substituted for the voiced [g]. Thus, the manner of articulation is maintained but the point of contact between organ and place of articulation is moved anteriorly: a coronal-alveolar replaces a postdorsal-velar articulation.

Phonetic transcription of the error: [t] or [d].

2. *Substitution of a postdorsal-velar fricative.* Here, the manner of articulation is affected: A narrow opening between organ and place of articulation replaces the complete contact necessary for a stop-plosive production. Thus, the back of the tongue is not raised sufficiently to form the necessary closure. Organ and place of articulation remain the same.

Phonetic transcription of the error: [x], a voiceless postdorsal-velar fricative, and [ɣ], a voiced postdorsal-velar fricative.

3. *Substitution of a postdorsal-uvular stop.* The client produces a stop-plosive but the place of articulation is too far back in the mouth. The result is a [k] or [g] that sounds "guttural."

Phonetic transcription of the error: [q], for voiceless and [ɢ] for voiced postdorsal-uvular stops.

Therapeutic Suggestions

Phonetic Placement. In cases of [t] for [k] substitutions, it is necessary to prevent the tip of the tongue and/or its neighboring frontal portions from reaching the alveolar ridge. Therefore, the tip of the tongue must remain down, behind the lower incisors. Visibility offered by a relatively wide opening of the mouth and subsequent observation in an articulation mirror during all phases of the activity can be helpful. This placement may be preceded by tongue activities that emphasize identifying the front versus the back portions of the tongue, hard palate, and velar areas. Some clinicians have suggested that the child cough or gargle in an attempt to demonstrate the area of the mouth and tongue involved in the articulation.

One way to obtain a [k] is to place the client's little finger sagittally holding down the front half of the tongue while the client produces the "old k-sound." Under this condition, the tip of the tongue is prevented from making contact with the alveolar ridge. If enough of the tongue body is held down (not just the tongue tip but the entire length of the client's little finger should be positioned on the tongue), and the client continues to make a stop-plosive sound, [k] should result.

A similar procedure uses a tongue depressor placed flat and transversely into the child's mouth, the edge of the tongue depressor pushing at the corners of the mouth. The anterior portions of the tongue rest under the tongue depressor. This method is again an attempt to hinder the elevation of the front part of the tongue. With this part of the tongue secure under the tongue depressor, a [t] for [k] substitution is difficult to attain.

If the client produces a *postdorsal-velar fricative* instead of the regular stop production, the manner of articulation must be changed. The client should be instructed about the necessary elevation of the back of the tongue and the explosive release of the obstructed airstream. [t] could be used initially to illustrate the buildup of air pressure and the quick release. During a rather forceful [t]-production, the client should note the feeling of the air pressure followed by the burst of air. The emphasis should be on the close contact between organ and place of articulation. The client then tries to duplicate this feeling when producing [k].

For a postdorsal-uvular substitution, the place of articulation must be more anteriorly placed in the oral cavity. Nemoy and Davis (1937) suggest that the client repeat in a rapid sequence [i]-[k], [i]-[k], [i]-[k], trying to keep the tongue in the [i] position while saying the [k] sound. The pairing of the front vowel [i] with the postdorsal-uvular substitution has a tendency to create a more forward positioning of the tongue.

Sound Modification Methods

1. *[ŋ]-[g] method.* These two speech sounds are phonetically very similar: organ and place of articulation are directly comparable; however, [ŋ] is a nasal while [g] is a stop. The easiest way to use this modification method is to have the client:

a. Prolong [ŋ] sound while holding the nostrils closed.

b. Release the buildup of air pressure into the oral cavity; [g] should result. If [k] is the goal, have the child whisper [ŋ] with the same procedure but with an increase in air pressure.

2. *[u]-[k] method.* This method is based on using the high-back vowel [u] to facilitate the tongue positioning for [k]. Have the client:

a. Prolong [u] and then elevate the back of the tongue.

b. Suggest that the client try to "stop" the sound by blocking it with the back portion of the tongue. The goal is to obtain complete closure between the posterior portion of the tongue and the soft palate.

c. Release the sound. If the tongue positioning for [u] is maintained, an acceptable [k] or [g] should result.

Coarticulatory Conditions

[k] and [g] also demonstrate context-dependent modifications during their productions. In the context of back vowels such as [u] or [ɑ], the articulation is made farther back in the mouth. In the context of front vowels, such as in the word *key,* the point of contact is more frontally located (Shriberg and Kent, 2003). These modifications can be used to structure coarticulatory conditions that support specific production goals.

If the goal is to move the organ and place of articulation posteriorly, for example, when a [t] for [k] substitution is realized, combining [k] with the back vowels [u], [ʊ], [oʊ], [ɔ], and [ɑ] will be advantageous. During the production of back vowels, the posterior portion of the tongue is elevated, supporting the placement necessary for [k]. The front vowels do not provide this coarticulatory support. In fact, the high-front vowels pose an additional danger in this respect. Due to the influence of the high-frontal tongue placement for these vowels, the client might be tempted to revert back to the [t] substitution. With a t/k substitution, the phonetically supportive vowel sequence follows the order high-back, mid-back, low-back, central, low-front, mid-front, high-front.

If the goal is a more anterior tongue position, as in the substitution of a postdorsal-uvular stop for [k] and [g], the opposite vowel sequence would be indicated. In this case, the front vowels would aid a more anterior placement with the sequence high-front, mid-front, low-front, central, low-back, mid-back, followed by high-back vowels.

It seems advisable to let [g] follow [k] in the sequencing of therapy; the lesser degree of overall muscular effort together with the voicing component make [g] usually more difficult to achieve. According to personal clinical experience, a coarticulatory condition that seems to support [g] articulation is not a vowel context but an abutting consonant. Often in the context of [ŋ], as in the word *finger,* clients have produced a standard [g] that was not evidenced in other g-words. Verification of this observation will come from the particular client. It is always worth a trial period to search for individually based starting points.

Word Examples. The following one-syllable words are ordered from relatively easy to more difficult coarticulatory conditions for a child with a t/k substitution.

[k] Words	[g] Words
coo - coop - cool - cooed* - cooled*	goof - goose - goofs
could*	good* - goods*
cope - comb - cove - coal - coach - coat*	go - goal - goes - ghost* - gold*
cop - cob - cough - call - caught* - cart*	gong - gob - gone - gauze - got*
cup - cub - come - cuff - cut*	gum - gull - Gus - gush - gulp
curb - curve - curl - Kurt*	girl
cap - cab - can - car - calf - cash - cat*	gang - gap - gab - gas - gash
Ken - kept* - Kent*	guess - get* - guest*
Kay - cape - came - cane - cave - cage	gay - game - gave - gain - gate*
king - Kim - kiss - kit* - kid*	give - gill - gift* - guilt*
key - keep - keen - keel	geese

Words marked with an asterisk (*) are those containing [t] and [d]. These words will probably need to be evaluated to determine whether the coarticulatory influence of [t] and [d] will have an impact on the newly acquired [k] and [g].

MISARTICULATIONS OF [l]

Problems with [l]-productions are common in the speech of 3- and 4-year-old children (Prather, Hedrick, and Kern, 1975; Sander, 1972; Vihman and Greenlee, 1987). By age 4;6 to 5, normally developing children demonstrate a decrease in [l] misarticulations (Haelsig and Madison, 1986). Aberrant articulations include substitutions of [w] and [j] for [l]. Due to the relatively high frequency of occurrence of [l] in General American English, misarticulations are also fairly conspicuous errors.

Phonetic Description

[l] sounds are phonetically described as voiced apico-alveolar laterals. During most [l] realizations, the tip of the tongue, the most frontal part of the corona, touches the alveolar ridge. The neighboring coronal areas are relaxed, allowing air to escape laterally. Whereas some articulatory modifications do occur—for example, typical changes take place when [l] is in word-initial versus word-final positions—the main feature for [l], which is a laterally free passage for the expiratory airway, remains constant.

Common descriptions of [l] realizations state that the free lateral passage exists on both sides (bilaterally). However, Faircloth and Faircloth (1973) confirm that during spontaneous speech and under certain articulatory conditions, [l] can be realized unilaterally. Heffner (1975) describes the unilateral production as a common [l] realization. Because very little air actually escapes through the lateral openings, a unilaterally free passage will usually result in a perfectly acceptable auditory [l] impression. Quite in contrast to the escape of air during lateral [s] misarticulations, the lateral airflow during [l] realizations is so minimal, its pressure so low, that our tapping method (see the section concerning lateral [s] misarticulations on p. 000) will not suffice to detect it.

There are two [l] varieties in English: the "light" (or "clear") and the "dark" [l]. Different authors have categorized the production features of the two types in various ways. Some distinguished between them using the location of the tongue tip (Wise, 1958), whereas others have discussed the qualitative differences (Heffner, 1975). The "light" [l] has an [ɪ] quality that results from a convex shape of the tongue, especially its frontal portion near the palatal or prepalatal area (Heffner, 1975). The "dark" [l] has an [ʊ] or [o] quality that is caused by the elevation of the tongue's posterior portion (Shriberg and Kent, 2003). This high-back elevation produces a concave upper surface of the tongue behind the alveolar occlusion. Light l-sounds are transcribed [l], whereas dark l-sounds are symbolized [ɫ].

Although both [l] varieties represent one single phoneme in English, /l/, their usage is nevertheless regulated: Light [l] is typically realized in the initial word position when /l/ precedes a vowel or follows an initial consonant—for example, in the words *like, leap, play,* and *sleep.* Dark [ɫ] is found in word-final positions, as syllabics, and when it precedes a consonant (Heffner, 1975). Examples include the words *full, bottle,* and *told.* Occasional lack of tongue tip contact has also been noted in [l] following a vowel in word-final position (Giles, 1971). This becomes important to clinicians when evaluating children. If the tongue tip contact is not established—for example, in the word *wheel*—the final [l] might assume an [o] or [ʊ] quality. Shriberg and Kent (2003) note that "caution should be observed in evaluating the child's proficiency for /l/ articulation. It is prudent to test /l/ production in more than one context or syllabic position before ascribing the /o/-like sound to an articulatory error" (p. 71).

Linguistic Function

Frequency of Occurrence. [l] is a frequent sound in General American English, ranked eighth in children's speech and fifth in adult's speech (Carterette and Jones, 1974; Mines, Hanson, and Shoup, 1978). Frequent word-initial clusters include [pl], [kl], and [bl], and [ld] and [lz] are commonly occurring word-final clusters (Dewey, 1923; French, Carter, and Koenig, 1930; Roberts, 1965).

Phonotactics. [l] is realized in all word positions, although, as previously noted, allophonic variations exist that are in part dependent on the sound's position within the word. According to Mader (1954), [l] occurs more frequently in medial and final word positions than when initiating a word. Table 8.13 lists the most frequent consonant clusters with [l].

Table 8.13 Consonant Clusters with [l]

Word-Initiating		Word-Terminating	
[bl]	black, blue	[lb]	bulb
[fl]	flower, flake	[ld]	mild, gold
[gl]	glue, glad	[lf]	Ralph, golf
[kl]	clean, clown	[lk]	milk, elk
[pl]	play, plane	[lm]	film, elm
[sl]	sled, slide	[lp]	help, gulp
[spl]	splash, splinter	[ls]	false, pulse
		[lt]	belt, salt
		[lθ]	health, filth
		[lv]	shelve, twelve
		[lz]	bells, dolls
		[ldz]	folds, worlds
		[lts]	belts, adults
		[lvd]	solved, shelved
		[lvz]	shelves, wolves

Morphophonemic Function.   Consonant clusters with [l] are used to signal plurality (do<u>ll</u>s, ha<u>ll</u>s), possessive (Ji<u>ll</u>'s, Bi<u>ll</u>'s), third-person singular (he sai<u>l</u>s, she ro<u>ll</u>s), and contractible auxiliaries and copulas (the ba<u>ll</u>'s rolling, the do<u>ll</u>'s little). The consonant clusters [ld] and [lvd] signal past tense, as in sai<u>led</u> or so<u>lved</u>.

Minimal Pairs.   Common substitutions for [l] are [r], [w], and [j]. Table 8.14 contains minimal pair words and sentences exemplifying these substitutions.

Initial Remarks

Distortions and substitutions are common [l] errors. Typical substitutions include w/l, j/l, and r/l. Because these substitutions are pho-

nemically relevant, it is important to establish whether they represent phonemic difficulties. This information should be the basis for any therapeutic decision. Also, knowledge of the articulatory features of the misarticulated [l] needs to be secured. This should include probes into contexts that would promote light and dark [l] realizations. Because their articulation is different, one type may be closer to norm production than the other.

Types of Misarticulation

1. *[w/l] substitution.*   In word-initial position, this production is marked by the substitution of [w] for [l], as in [wæmp] for *lamp*. Because of the elevation of the back of the tongue for dark /l/ in word-final position, the substitution

Table 8.14   Minimal Pair Words and Sentences Contrasting [l] to [r], [w], and [j]

[l] versus [r]		[l] versus [ɚ]		[l] versus [w]		[l] versus [j]	
lace	race	bowl	boar	lag	wag	lung	young
lane	rain	Dale	dare	life	wife	loose	use
led	red	feel	fear	lake	wake	lard	yard
lick	Rick	male	mare	leave	weave	Lou	you
long	wrong	mole	more	leap	weep	less	yes
lie	rye	owl	our	leak	weak	let	yet
light	right	tile	tire	light	white		
lead	read			let	wet		
lock	rock						

She knew it was the *long* way home.	He didn't want to *leave*.
She knew it was the *wrong* way home.	He didn't want to *weave*.
He stumbled on the *lock*.	*Lou* cannot come to the party.
He stumbled on the *rock*.	*You* cannot come to the party.
What a *deal* !	It was a *light* coat.
What a *dear* !	It was a *white* coat.
The *tile* needed to be replaced.	The *lung* fish swam in the aquarium.
The *tire* needed to be replaced.	The *young* fish swam in the aquarium.

often has a back vowel quality, as in [teˈboʊ] for *table*.

Phonetic transcription of the error: initiating a word or syllable: [w]; terminating a word or syllable: typically a mid-back vowel

2. *[j/l] substitution.* In this substitution, a [j]-like sound replaces [l], thus, [jæmp] for *lamp*. [j] substitutions are usually heard only in word- or syllable-initial position, as in [hɛjoʊ] for *hello*. [j] does not exist in word-final position in General American English. Clients with a phonetic disorder will not violate this phonotactic constraint. Therefore, in word-final position, the client will try to modify [l] accordingly. The result may again resemble a back vowel.

Phonetic transcription of the error: initiating a word or syllable: [j]; terminating a word or syllable: typically a mid-back vowel

3. *[r/l] substitution.* In this substitution, a sound resembling [r] replaces [l], as in [ræmp] for *lamp*. [r] substitutions are typically heard in word- or syllable-initial positions only. Although [r] realizations show a considerable amount of variability in their articulatory features, [r] never has coronal contact with the alveolar ridge as [l] does.

Phonetic transcription of the error: initiating a word or syllable: [r]; terminating a word or syllable: typically a back or central vowel

4. *[l]-distortion.* A common [l] distortion is created by too small an opening for lateral air escape. Lateral openings that are too small, when combined with increased air pressure, can often cause an undue friction noise during [l]-productions.

Phonetic transcription of the error: [ɮ], a voiced lateral fricative

Therapeutic Suggestions

Phonetic Placement. For norm productions of [l], the apex and coronal edges of the tongue are in direct contact with the alveolar ridge. The lateral edges of the tongue are not elevated but rather relaxed, allowing free passage of the air to the right and left of the contact at the alveolar ridge. Visibility of the articulatory events is often very helpful when establishing the placement of an isolated sound. Because visibility for most [l]-productions is limited, a wide open-mouth posture can enhance it. Under this condition, the tip of the tongue should touch the alveolar ridge in such a way that a good portion of the tongue's underside becomes visible.

For w/l substitutions, the client must first realize that the lip protrusion of [w] is not present on [l]. Lip activities numbers 1 through 5 (Box 8.2) or observation of the lips during production of [u]-[i] might help the client understand that there is no lip rounding during [l]-productions. Next, tongue contact with the alveolar ridge needs to be established. The edges of the tongue should be relaxed; for example, the client could be instructed to make a "flat tongue" and then to raise the tip of the flattened tongue to the alveolar ridge. If the posterior elevation of the tongue for [w] is carried over to the [l], the client's initial realization might resemble the dark l-sound. Although this [ɫ] may sound somewhat "off" in word- or syllable-initial positions, the quality should become auditorily more acceptable if it is preceded by a vowel.

If a [j/l] substitution is used, the client must be instructed that the tongue tip needs to touch the alveolar ridge. Because the placement of the dorsum of the tongue is fairly similar for [j] and [l], this may be the only articulatory adjustment necessary. If the resulting [l] approximation has a frictionlike component, the lateral edges of the tongue will need to be lowered to allow more airflow.

The primary consideration for r/l substitutions is contact of the tip of the tongue with the alveolar ridge. In addition, the dorsum of the tongue may need to be more forward. This more forward placement could be established by using the following [i]-[l] sound modification method.

For [l]-distortions caused by limited lateral airflow, the main goal is lowering the lateral edges. The edges of the tongue need to be relaxed and somewhat flattened. With a mirror and a wide-open mouth posture, the client should first practice a flattened tongue versus a rolled tongue. When this has been achieved, the tongue tip should be placed on the alveolar ridge, again trying to distinguish between a flattened versus a rolled tongue posture.

A passive method of lowering the lateral edges of the tongue is as follows. First, place a narrow ribbon (approximately ½-inch wide) flat crosswise over the front of the tongue so that the ends hang down on each side to at least the bottom of the client's chin. Next, have the client place the tip of the tongue firmly against the alveolar ridge. During the client's attempts to produce [l], both ends of the ribbon are pulled down gently. If everything is introduced and executed properly, this will bring the edges of the tongue down, allowing lateral airflow (Gutzmann, 1912; Waengler and Bauman-Waengler, 1985).

Sound Modification Methods

1. *[d]-[l] method.* Organ and place of articulation for these two sounds are very similar; the manner of articulation, though, is different.

    a. Use the previously mentioned method of pulling the lateral edge of the tongue down during [d]-production. A second possibility:

    b. During the stop phase of [d], the client should release the air without losing the tongue tip–alveolar contact.

2. *[n]-[l] method.* Again, only the manner of articulation distinguishes these two sounds: nasal versus lateral.

    a. Utilize the same procedure as described for the [d]-[l] method, but the client's nostrils need to be pinched closed during the [n]-production.

By employing the nasal [n], an additional factor is introduced—the change from nasal to oral resonance. This needs to be considered before implementing this modification method.

3. *[i]-[l] method.* This method is based on similarities between the [i] and the light [l] productions.

    a. Prolong [i] ([ɪ] can also be used) while moving the tongue tip to the alveolar ridge. Although production similarities exist between [i] or [ɪ] and the light [l], this method does not offer much visual feedback for the client if an articulation mirror is being used. If visibility is important, the [ɑ]-[l] method might be a better choice.

4. *[ɑ]-[l] method.*

    a. Prolong [ɑ] with a wide open-mouth posture.

    b. Elevate the tongue tip to the alveolar ridge. Not only is visibility good with this open-mouth posture but it also helps to lower the lateral edges.

Coarticulatory Conditions

Favorable coarticulatory conditions, specifically the sequence of vowels that support regular [l] articulations, will depend on the goal to be achieved. If visibility is important, low vowels might be our choice. This allows the client a means of visual control that can be continued until [l] is somewhat stabilized. A desirable sequence of context exercises might begin with the low-back vowel [ɑ], continuing with the low-front vowel [æ]. Mid-front vowels [ɛ] and [eɪ] and mid-back vowels [ɔ] and [oʊ] would still offer some visibility if produced with a relatively open-mouth posture.

Because of the possible coarticulatory influence of the lip rounding, if the client demonstrates a [w/l] substitution, the mid- and high-back vowels will probably be the last in our sequence.

In the case of [l] distortions based on too small an opening for lateral air escape, the back vowels will probably be our choice. The slightly concave shape of the tongue supports the relaxing of the lateral edges. Here, the dark [l] in word-final position may be easier for our client to achieve.

If a later goal is production of both light *and* dark /l/, two coarticulatory conditions need to be considered; first, the position of /l/ within the word, and second, the tendency for certain vowels to promote light versus dark [l] sounds. Back vowels, especially high-back vowels, coarticulatorily support the dark [l], whereas front vowels, especially high-front vowels, aid the production of light [l]. Depending on our momentary goal, light [l] or dark [ɫ], the sequence of vowels will have to vary. For the coarticulatory support of light [l] articulations, the sequence could be [l] + : high-front, mid-front, low-front, central, low-back, mid-back, and high-back vowels. The opposite sequence is suggested preceding dark [ɫ] realizations: high-back, mid-back, low-back, central, low-front, mid-front, and high-front vowels.

Several supportive coarticulatory possibilities have been suggested. Based on our momentary goal, different vowel sequences were considered. However, the order of supporting coarticulatory circumstances for the new sound achievement must be determined by whatever is easiest for our client to attain.

Word Examples. The following one-syllable words are ordered from relatively easy to more difficult coarticulatory conditions for a child with an [l] problem. Word examples are given for both light and dark /l/.

Words with Light l-sounds	Words with Dark l-sounds
Lee - leap - leaf - leave - leak - leash	pool - tool - fool - cool - school - spool
limb - lip - lid - lit - lick - live	wool* - bull - pull - full
lay - lame - late - laid - lake - lace	bowl - pole - foal - goal - coal
led - let - leg - ledge - left - lend	all - hall - ball - mall - doll - fall - call
lamb - lad - laugh - lag - lamp	hull - dull - gull - skull - pal
lug - luck - love - lump - lunch	bell - tell - fell - sale - shell
law - lot - loss - log - long - lock	mail - bale - pail - Dale - nail - sale - jail
low - load - loan - loaf - loaves	ill - hill - will* - Bill - pill - fill - gill
look - looked	eel - heel - meal - deal - kneel - feel
Lou - loom - loop - loon - loot - Luke	

*If the child had a [w/l] substitution, the words indicated with an asterisk (*) would need to be evaluated to see whether the initial [w] might negatively impact [l] articulations.

*M*ISARTICULATIONS OF [r] AND THE CENTRAL VOWELS WITH R-COLORING

The misarticulations in this section include those occurring with the consonantal r-sound, as in *rabbit* or *red* and/or the central vowels with r-coloring, [ɝ] and [ɚ] as in *bird* or *father*. If children have difficulty producing "r-qualities," they typically demonstrate problems with both consonantal [r] and central vowels with r-coloring (Shriberg, 1975, 1980).

Consonantal [r] develops relatively late; it is frequently still in error during the preschool years (Irwin and Wong, 1983; Kenney and Prather, 1986; Olmsted, 1971). Irwin and

Wong (1983) reported that, even at age 6, only 82 percent of all [r] realizations were correct in spontaneous speech.

The central vowels with r-coloring appear to be among the last, if not the last, vowels to be mastered. Data from the Irwin and Wong (1983) study using spontaneous speech demonstrated that the central vowels with r-coloring were the last vowels to reach a fairly high percentage of norm realization. At age 3, children attained accuracy with both of these vowels only 70 percent of the time; at age 4, accuracy levels with [ɚ] were still below 90 percent.

Although it is expected that r-sounds (both consonantal and central vowels with r-coloring) are "mastered" by school age, there are children who continue to have difficulties with them. Typical problems include substitutions of consonantal [r] in word- or syllable-initial positions and derhotacization or vowelization of the central vowels with r-coloring.

Phonetic Description

Consonantal [r]. There are many forms of [r] articulations in General American English. In fact, /r/ might well be the most variable consonant of our language. In different contexts, the same speaker may use various tongue and lip positions when producing this sound. The different types of [r]-productions are usually placed into two broad categories: the bunched and the retroflexed [r] (Shriberg and Kent, 2003).

The bunched [r] is phonetically classified as a voiced mediodorsal-mediopalatal central central approximant. For this production, the corpus of the tongue is elevated toward the palate while the tongue tip points downward. The voiced expiratory air escapes sagittally through this fairly wide passage. The sides of the tongue touch the bicuspids and molars. This tongue position may vary with the vowel context and lip rounding may be present.

The retroflexed [r] is phonetically classified as a voiced apico-prepalatal central approximant. The tip of the tongue points to the alveolar ridge or its neighboring prepalatal areas. Because the lateral edges of the tongue are raised, preventing lateral air escape, the voiced expiratory air is again channeled sagittally out of the oral cavity. During this action, the dorsum of the tongue is somewhat depressed. This makes the elevation of the tip of the tongue appear even more pronounced. Often, the tip of the tongue might even be slightly bent backward or curled up. Such an articulatory position gave these [r] realizations their characteristic name: retroflexed.

Although [r] is extremely variable in its production features, it is therapeutically helpful to recognize some frequent allophonic variations that occur in General American English. After [θ], the [r] can be produced as a trill. The term **trill** depicts a sound produced by the vibratory action of an organ of articulation tapping rapidly against a place of articulation, in this case the tongue tip against the alveolar ridge. After [t], [r] may have a fricative-like quality. This is caused by the preceding [t], which in its release phase creates a closer approximation between organ and place of articulation than is normally the case. Also, following voiceless consonants, such as in the words *try, cry,* and *fry,* [r] may be partially devoiced.

Central Vowels with R-Coloring. [ɝ] and [ɚ] have been called rhotic or rhotacized vowels and retroflexed vowels. The term *r-colored* or *rhotacized vowels* describes their perceptual quality: they appear to contain r fea-

There is some disagreement as to the exact nature of the r-substitutions in children. Very often the misarticulation is simply called a w/r substitution. Shriberg and Kent (2003) argue that most [w/r] substitutions are actually derhotacized r-productions. Based on extensive clinical experience, Gibbon (2002) states (based on intuition and not clinical data) that most typically developing children acquiring [r] pass through a stage in which they produce [w] substitutions, and some seem to go through another stage in which they progress from [w] to [ʋ], a labiodental approximant, before reaching [r]. Children with speech disorders seem to follow the same path, but more slowly, and some may stick with [ʋ] into adulthood. However, Gibbon believes that [r] realized as [w] may be more common in children with articulatory/phonological disorders.

Linguistic Function

Frequency of Occurrence.   Both consonantal [r] and the central vowels with r-coloring are frequent sounds in General American English. According to Carterette and Jones (1974), they are the second most frequently occurring sound category. There are many consonant clusters with [r], which are also prevalent. These include [pr], [tr], [fr], and [gr] in the word-initial position. The central vowels with r-coloring also occur with final consonants exemplified by [rd], [rt], [rn], and [rz] (Dewey, 1923; French, Carter, and Koenig, 1930; Roberts, 1965).

Phonotactics.   Whereas the consonantal [r] occurs in initiating syllables or in specific clusters, the central vowels with r-coloring function as syllable nuclei. The noted word-final [r] "clusters," such as [rn] and [rt], contain [ɝ] (e.g., *turn, hurt*) or centering diphthongs preceding a consonant (e.g., *barn, farm*); they are therefore technically not consonant clusters. They are also included in Table 8.15.

Minimal Pairs.   The most frequent substitutions for [r] include [w], [j], and [l]. Table 8.16 contains examples of minimal pair words and sentences with these phonemic oppositions.

tures. The second term, *retroflexed,* refers to a possible tongue position during their production. Because these vowels are by no means always produced with a retroflexed tongue articulation, this label is somewhat imprecise.

The central vowel [ɝ] is a stressed vowel and is usually produced with some degree of lip rounding. [ɚ] is the unstressed counterpart of [ɝ]. Both vowels show similar articulations, although lip rounding may be lacking when producing [ɚ]. Based on the results of palatography, Fletcher (1992) noted that tongue actions for the rhotic vowels are similar to those for the rhotic approximants. The r-like vowels can be produced in two ways. First, the tongue might be curled upward and backward in a retroflexed position. Second, the tip might be dropped down, the body of the tongue bunched and moved posteriorly in the mouth. These articulations are comparable to the "retroflexed" and "bunched" consonantal [r]-productions previously discussed.

Initial Remarks

Because several misarticulations of the consonantal [r] include substitutions of one phoneme for another, it is important that the phonemic system of the client be evaluated. Dialectal variations should also be examined. Dialects that characteristically lose r-coloring on central vowels include Southern, South Midland, eastern New England, and African American Vernacular English (Flexner, 1987; Iglesias and Anderson, 1995; Williams and Wolfram, 1977).

Table 8.15 Word-Initiating Consonant Clusters
with [r] and Final Consonants Following Rhotic Vowels

Word-Initiating		Word-Terminating	
[br]	bread, broom	[rb]	Herb, curb
[dr]	dream, drink	[rd]	bird, card
[fr]	frog, friend	[rg]	iceberg, Pittsburgh
[gr]	grass, grouch	[rk]	fork, Mark
[kr]	Craig, cry	[rl]	Karl, girl
[pr]	prune, prince	[rm]	arm, worm
[ʃr]	shrimp, shrub	[rn]	barn, learn
[tr]	train, truck	[rp]	burp, chirp
		[rs]	nurse, horse
[skr]	scream, scratch	[rʃ]	harsh, kirsch
[spr]	spring, sprite	[rt]	dirt, short
[str]	straw, strong	[rv]	serve, starve
		[rz]	doors, ears
		[rdʒ]	large, George
		[rkt]	worked, parked
		[rlz]	girls, Charles
		[rst]	first, pierced
		[rts]	shirts, sports
		[rtʃ]	March, birch

CLINICAL APPLICATION
Dialect and R-Problems

The dialect of the family should always be considered when evaluating younger clients. For example, in the Midwest, a diagnostic situation presented itself in which the client demonstrated a lack of r-coloring on all rhotic vowels. The clinician was first convinced that the child had "r problems" until she met the mother and father. Both parents, who had lived most of their lives in Boston, spoke in a similar manner. Derhotaci-zation was a characteristic of their eastern New England dialect.

Types of Misarticulation

1. *[w/r] substitutions.* [w/r] substitutions represent the most common substitution for consonantal [r]. In some cases, perceived substitutions may not be actual substitutions of [w] for [r]. See marginal note on page 287.

Phonetic transcription of the error: If it is a sound substitution, [w]; if the quality is somewhere between [w] and [r], then [ʋ], indicating a labiodental approximant might be a better choice.

2. *[j/r] substitutions.* With this substitution, a [j]-like sound is produced instead of the consonantal [r].

Phonetic transcription of the error: [j].

3. *[l/r] substitutions.* This misarticulation is characterized by [l] replacing the consonantal [r], as in [lɛd] for *red*.

Transcription of the error: [l].

4. *Derhotacization of the central vowels with r-coloring.* Rhotacized central vowels can also lose their r-quality; [ɝ] is perceived as [ɜ], while [ɚ] sounds like [ə]. The articulatory component necessary to produce the particular [r] resonance is lacking. Fletcher (1992) stated that children often substitute lip rounding for front tongue actions during attempts to produce the rhotics. This results in an [o]- or [ʊ]-like quality.

Therapeutic Suggestions

Phonetic Placement: [r]. Two possibilities offer themselves for phonetic placement therapy with [r]: (1) the apical-alveolar "retroflexed" [r] articulation or (2) the mediodorsal-mediopalatal "bunched" [r] articulation. The retroflexed [r] is often easier to implement

Table 8.16   Minimal Pair Words and Sentences Contrasting [r] with [l], [w], and [j]

[r] versus [l]		[r] versus [l]		[r] versus [w]		[r] versus [j]	
race	lace	boar	bowl	rag	wag	rung	young
rain	lane	dare	Dale	rail	whale	ram	yam
red	led	fear	feel	rake	wake	rank	yank
Rick	lick	mare	male	rate	wait	rot	yacht
wrong	long	more	mole	red	wed	rear	year
rye	lie	our	owl	ray	way	roar	you're
right	light	tire	tile	right	white		
read	lead			rent	went		
rock	lock			ring	wing		
				ripe	wipe		
				ride	wide		
				raced	waste		
				rest	west		
				round	wound		
				rake	wake		
				run	won		

It was a long *rain*.	The *ring* was broken.
It was a long *lane*.	The *wing* was broken.
She won the *race* at the county fair.	The athletes always *run*.
She won the *lace* at the county fair.	The athletes always *won*.
He walked to the *right*.	She didn't want to *rake* it up.
He walked to the *light*.	She didn't want to *wake* it up.
He *feels* the earthquake.	The *rot* was moldy and damp.
He *fears* the earthquake.	The *yacht* was moldy and damp.
Across the field ran a large *mare*.	*Roar* loud, he said.
Across the field ran a large *male*.	*You're* loud, he said.

because its features can be explained more easily. The choice of retroflexed or bunched [r] will depend on the client and the type of aberrant production presented.

Apico-Prepalatal Retroflexed Articulation. The client is instructed to elevate the front of the tongue so that the tongue tip is pointing behind the alveolar ridge. The tongue tip should come close to the area behind the alveolar ridge but should not touch it. The posterior edges of the tongue are in contact with the upper molars. First, instruct the client to glide the tongue, which is touching the alveolar ridge, forward and backward, "sweeping" the palatal area. Next, instruct the client to execute, with a slightly open-mouth posture, the same action but this time *without* touching the palatal area. If, at the same time, the back edges of the tongue are raised and voicing is added, an r-like quality might be heard when the client moves the tongue slowly backward from the alveolar ridge to the prepalatal palate. If the [r]-production seems close but not quite on target, it is important to remember the tension of the tongue. Clinicians will often have the child try to "tense" the tongue by pushing on the desk or pretending they are lifting something heavy. This slight tongue tension may be enough to change the quality to an acceptable sounding [r].

An additional consideration for the client using w/r substitutions is lip rounding. Although some degree of lip rounding is usually present during retroflexed [r]-productions, care needs to be taken that this rounding does not trigger [w]. In addition, if the client's productions continue to give a [w] impression, the clinician needs to make sure that the back portion of the tongue is not elevated. Under the condition of a fairly wide open-mouth posture, for example, it will be more difficult for the client to maintain a high-back tongue position.

For [j/r] substitutions, the elevated tongue tip becomes an important factor. [j] is characterized by a convex shape of the tongue with the midportion of the dorsum coming very close to the midportion of the palate. The retroflexed [r], on the other hand, is marked by a concave shape of the front and mediodorsal portions of the tongue with the tongue tip pointing into the direction of the prepalatal area.

When [l] is substituted for [r], two changes must be achieved for a norm [r]: (1) release the contact between the tongue tip and the alveolar ridge and (2) raise the lateral edges of the tongue so that airflow is directed medially.

Mediodorsal-Mediopalatal Bunched Placement. The bunched [r] is produced with the tongue tip down while central portions of the tongue's body are elevated. The characteristic rhotic resonance is created by a voiced medial-sagittal airflow over the relatively broad surface of the tongue. The client should be instructed to lower the tongue tip so that it rests on the top of the lower incisors. The client must also be aware that the lateral edges of the tongue need to touch the upper molars. A practice progression might start with the client articulating [d], noting how the back portions of the tongue touch the molars. Next, the tongue tip should be lowered, leaving the back of the tongue in the same position. Finally, the whole body of the tongue, including the tongue tip, must be moved backward, posteriorly. The necessary change could be aided by gently pushing back the tip of the tongue with a tongue depressor so that the mediodorsal portion of the dorsum becomes more elevated.

To move from [w] to a bunched [r], two steps need to be accomplished: (1) the lips need to be retracted slightly and (2) the elevation of the tongue's dorsum needs to be more anteriorly located. First, have the client try a "small smile" while saying [w]. Next, while prolonging this [w], have the client slowly move the whole body of the tongue forward. Because it is difficult to define production elements of "rhotic resonance," the clinician may need to experiment with varying tongue positions to attain an acceptable [r] quality.

If the client substitutes [j] for [r], organ and place of articulation remain the same; both are considered mediodorsal-mediopalatal consonants. However, the manner of articulation needs to be somewhat modified. When comparing [j] to [r] in this respect, the distance between organ and place of articulation is smaller for [j]. Therefore, for [r], the dorsum of the tongue must be lowered slightly. One could also achieve the larger distance between organ and place of articulation by lowering the jaw during the [j] production. In addition, the medial groove of the tongue is more pronounced for [r]. To achieve this, the client could roll the tongue after having lowered the tongue's dorsum.

If the [r] substitution is [l], the contact between the tip of the tongue and the alveolar ridge must first be released; that is, the tongue tip must be dropped. In addition, the lateral edges of the tongue must be slightly elevated to prevent lateral airflow. Finally, the dorsum of the tongue must be moved back.

Central Vowels with r-Coloring. The central tongue position is the primary articulatory feature of the vowels [ɝ] and [ɚ]. However, their important additional characteristic is r-coloring. This r-coloring is similar to the main feature of consonantal [r]; there are therefore two ways to achieve the r-quality for [ɝ] and [ɚ]: retroflexed or bunched tongue formations. If the vowels are perceived as lacking r-coloring, the individual does not realize either a retroflexed tongue position or an adequate bunching of the central portions of the tongue (Secord, 1981b). If the client is substituting [ɜ/ɝ] and [ə/ɚ], only this r-coloring needs to be added. During the respective vowel productions, the client should either (1) point the tongue tip in the direction of the prepalatal area or (2) push the tongue posteriorly, creating more of a bulge in the tongue's midsection. Instructions at the beginning of the phonetic placement techniques for the retroflexed and bunched [r] sounds may prove helpful.

Sound Modification Methods: [r] and Central Vowels with r-Coloring. Several of the following modification methods utilize sounds that were noted as substitutions for [r]. For example, a client may have a [j/r] substitution, and [j] is one of the sounds that can be modified

to an [r]. Substituting one of these sounds for [r] does not eliminate the possibility of modifying it to a norm [r] articulation. In fact, this may prove to be a relatively effective way to achieve a regular [r].

1. *[d]-[r] method.* With this sound modification method, the goal is a retroflexed r sound. The client is instructed to:

a. Produce [d] followed by the central vowel [ʌ]. Normally, the tongue tip drops straight down from the release of the [d] to the vowel.

b. Glide the tongue tip back, pointing into the direction of the prepalatal area. The tongue tip should not touch the palate but rather the movement should follow the release of the [d]; that is, the tongue tip should drop and then move back. The [d]-production as a point of departure for [r] also underlines the necessary contact of the posterior edges of the tongue with the molars. This will in turn aid the elevation of the lateral edges of the tongue, which reinforces the [r] resonance.

2. *[l]-[r] method.* The end product of this sound modification method is again a retroflexed [r]. The steps necessary to modify the articulation from [l] to [r] are outlined in the section on phonetic placement of the retroflexed [r] sound: [l/r] substitutions.

3. *[j]-[r] method.* A higher degree of phonetic similarity exists between [j] and the bunched r sound than between [j] and the retroflexed production. The steps needed to modify the articulation from [j] to [r] are outlined in the section on phonetic placement of the bunched [r] sound: [j/r] substitutions.

4. *[ɝ] or [ɚ]-[r] method.* Clients who have difficulty with [r] usually show problems with the r-colored central vowels as well. If, however, a clinician decides to work on the consonantal

[r] and the client does have acceptable productions of the central vowels with r-coloring, a transfer of this r-coloring would be the method of choice. If the client has [ɝ] and [ɚ] but not [r], a word could be specifically divided to elicit the [r] sound. For example, the client could begin with the word *purr*. Then, the client tries *purring*. Next, a pause is made in the word: *pu-rring*. Finally, the last syllable is isolated as *ring:* a consonantal [r] is achieved.

CLINICAL APPLICATION

When to Initiate Therapy with r Problems

A clinical decision must be made if the client has either the r-colored central vowels or the consonantal [r], but not both. Should the clinician initiate "r" therapy? The fact that the r-coloring is somehow present should make this an easy sound to remediate. Or should the clinician wait and watch? The underlying assumption is that if the r-coloring is present in one sound, it will probably generalize to other sounds as well. Do children in fact generalize r-coloring in such a manner? After reviewing the literature of sound generalization research, Elbert and Gierut (1986) established certain "predictions" that can be used by clinicians to reduce the number of sounds to be worked on in therapy. The idea is that if a specific sound is taught, certain features of the newly acquired sound might transfer without therapy to other sounds requiring the same features. One prediction is that if one allophone is acquired, [ɝ], for example, norm production of [r] and [ɚ] will probably be achieved without therapy. In this case, a wait-and-watch decision might be best. However, not every child is able to generalize features from one sound to another. In addition, there may be other factors that will impact our decision making, such as the age of the child, the intelligibility of the child, parental concerns, and peer pressure, to mention just a few.

Where to Begin Therapy? Certain clinical decisions will need to be made in respect to therapy. First, should therapy begin with the consonantal [r] or the central vowels with r-coloring? This choice will be based on stimulability probes and the perceptual saliency of the error sound. Perceptual saliency refers to the conspicuousness, the noticeability, of the error sound to listeners. Given a client with a [w/r] or a [j/r] substitution and derhotacization of central vowels, the substitutions will probably be more prominent perceptually. Dialect might also play a role in our decision making. If dialect features include derhotacization of central vowels, the consonantal [r] would be our only therapy choice. Second, which type of [r]-production, the bunched or the retroflexed [r], should be the goal of phonetic placement or sound modification techniques? Again, the stimulability of the client will play a role. Placement techniques for both can be implemented and the resulting [r] evaluated. If an acceptable [r]-production is achieved in isolation, probes can determine which vowels or words promote the accurate use of the newly acquired sound. The therapeutic goal will be to appraise the client's individual possibilities and determine the most efficient means of changing aberrant productions to acceptable articulations. Every client will present us with a different set of challenges.

Coarticulatory Conditions

The retroflexed [r] sound offers a challenge when the clinician is trying to determine which vowel sounds might present coarticulatory conditions that assist its production. There are no vowels in General American English with a tongue placement similar to the retroflexed [r] position. If the retroflexed [r] follows front vowels, especially high-front vowels, at least elevated frontal portions of the tongue are promoted. But combinations with these vowels would necessitate a quick movement from a concave retroflexed [r] to a convex "bunched" tongue shape for the front vowels. On the other hand, the back vowels, with their characteristic posterior elevation of the tongue, are clearly not supportive of any retroflexed articulation. The central vowels without r-coloring, especially if they are produced with an elevated mandibular position, offer perhaps the best possibility. Next, the front vowels would clearly be better in supporting retroflexed [r] than the back vowels.

Similar coarticulatory conditions would exist for the central vowels and the bunched r-production with its relative centralized elevation of the tongue's dorsum. However, the secondary feature of lip rounding, which often characterizes the bunched [r], is also characteristic of the back vowels. Therefore, if the goal is the bunched [r], the sequence of vowels might be central vowels, back vowels, and finally front vowels.

As noted previously, the articulatory features of [r] may change with the individual and with the context in which the sound occurs. Because of this, clinicians will need to concentrate on the client's possibilities and on the coarticulatory conditions that seem to foster the norm production of these sounds.

Word Examples. Keeping in mind that individual and contextual variations will often dramatically alter the production of [r], the following one-syllable words are given to exemplify one possible vowel sequence that could be used for a child with an [r] problem. This order is based on the retroflexed [r] as target. The vowel sequence is the one suggested at the beginning of this section. Word examples are given for both the consonantal [r] and central vowels with r-coloring.

Consonantal [r] Words

rub - rough - run - rut - rush - rug - rung
ram - rap - ran - rat - rag - rack - rang
red - wren - rent - wrench - wreck
Ray - rain - rail - raid - race - rake
rim - rib - rip - ridge - rig - Rick - ring
real - read - reach
raw - Ron - rod - rot - rock - wrong
row - robe - rope - roll - road - wrote
room - roof - rude - rule - root

Central Vowels with r-Coloring

Words with the central vowel with r-coloring - [ɝ]	Words with centering diphthongs
her - burr - purr - fur - sir - spur - stir	air - hair - mare - bear - pear*
earn - earth - urge	ear - fear - deer - near - cheer - gear
worm - burn - turn - word - hurt - learn	are - bar - far - jar - car - star
slurp - skirt	oar - more - bore - pour - door
	blur
	lure - tour

MISARTICULATIONS OF [θ] AND [ð]

[θ] and [ð] are among the latest sounds to develop in the speech of children. Often, difficulties in articulating them extend into the beginning school year. Common errors are the substitution of [t/θ] and [d/ð]. Other misarticulations include the substitution of the labiodental fricatives [f] and [v] for [θ] and [ð]. Clinicians should also be aware that variations in [θ] and [ð] productions can be a feature of African American Vernacular English. The realization of these features is conditioned by the position of [θ] and [ð] within the word. These dialectal features are not considered articulation errors.

> See the Dialect Speaker section of Chapter 6 for more information on the influence of word position on [θ] and [ð] variations.

---

*Pronunciation of the words with centering diphthongs may vary from speaker to speaker. Thus, the word *hair* might be pronounced [hɛɝ] or [heˈɚ]. These differences could have an influence on the sequencing of the words.

Phonetic Description

[θ] and [ð] can be produced in two ways: as interdental or as addental fricatives. For the interdental realization, the tongue tip is protruded slightly between the front incisors. For the addental articulation, which is phonetically described as apico-dental, the tongue tip approaches the inner surface of the front incisors. The friction that characterizes these sounds as fricatives is created by a restriction of the breath stream between the apex of the tongue and the backside of the upper front teeth. For the interdental productions, this friction occurs between the apex and the cutting edge of the front incisors. For both productions, the tongue remains relatively flat.

Linguistic Function

Frequency of Occurrence. On a frequency of occurrence list for General American English speech sounds, [θ] and [ð] are not neighbors. Whereas [ð] shows up slightly above the middle, occupying a rank order of approximately ten among twenty-four consonants, [θ] is among the last on the list, ranking number twenty-one out of a total of twenty-four (Carterette and Jones, 1974; Mines, Hanson, and Shoup, 1978). Only word-initial [θr] is considered a fairly frequent cluster in General American English (Mader, 1954; Dewey, 1923; French, Carter, and Koenig, 1930).

Phonotactics. Both [θ] and [ð] are found in word-initial and word-final positions. [ð] occurs primarily in word-initial positions, whereas [θ] occurs approximately half the time in word-initial positions, the other half fairly evenly split between word-medial and word-final positions (Mader, 1954). Table 8.17 lists examples of consonant clusters with [θ] and [ð].

Table 8.17 Consonant Clusters with [θ] and [ð]

Word-Initiating		Word-Terminating	
[θr]	thread, three	[tθ]	width, hundredth
		[lθ]	health, wealth
		[nθ]	ninth, month
		[ŋθ]	length, strength
		[ðd]	bathed, breathed
		[ðz]	bathes, breathes

Morphophonemic Function. Word-final clusters that end in [θ] or [ð] can signal (1) plurality, as in mo<u>nths</u> and mou<u>ths</u>; (2) third-person singular, as in ba<u>thes</u> and brea<u>thes</u>; and (3) past tense, as in ba<u>thed</u> and brea<u>thed</u>.

Minimal Pairs. Frequent sounds substituted for [θ] and [ð] include [s]-[z], [t]-[d], and [f]-[v]. Table 8.18 lists minimal pairs and sentences with these sounds.

Types of Misarticulation

1. *[t/θ] and [d/ð] substitutions.* Examples of these frequent substitutions are [tʌm] for *thumb* and [dɪs] for *this*. This misarticulation involves changes in both place and manner of articulation: The place of articulation is moved posteriorly to the alveolar ridge, while the manner of articulation is changed into a stop-plosive.

Phonetic transcription of the error: [t] or [d]

2. *[f/θ] and [v/ð] substitutions.* Examples are [fʌm] for *thumb* and [vɪs] for *this*. Although the fricative manner of articulation is similar for [f] and [v] and [θ] and [ð], both organ and place of articulation change. The constriction for the labiodentals [f] and [v] is established between the bottom lip and the upper incisors. The tongue does not play a role in their

Table 8.18 Minimal Pair Words and Sentences Contrasting [θ] and [ð] to [s] and [z], [t] and [d], and [f] and [v]

[θ] versus [s]		[θ] versus [s]		[ð] versus [z]		[ð] versus [z]	
thank	sank	Beth	Bess	then	Zen	clothe	close
thick	sick	faith	face			teethe	tease
thin	sin	path	pass			breathe	breeze
think	sink	mouth	mouse				
thinner	sinner	myth	miss				

[θ] versus [t]		[θ] versus [t]		[ð] versus [d]		[θ] versus [d]	
thank	tank	bath	bat	than	Dan	breathe	breed
thick	tick	Beth	bet	then	den	loathe	load
thin	tin	math	mat	though	dough		
thought	taught	tooth	toot	thine	dine		
		path	pat				

[θ] versus [f]		[ð] versus [v]	
thin	fin	than	van
		that	vat
		thine	vine

The fog was *thickening*.	They walked by the *clothing* store.
The fog was *sickening*.	They walked by the *closing* store.
It hurts when children *teethe*.	She couldn't *breathe* through the testing, so she left.
It hurts when children *tease*.	She couldn't *breeze* through the testing, so she left.

production. The necessary constriction for [θ] and [ð], though, does involve the tongue; either the tongue tip is protruded slightly between the teeth for the interdental or the tongue approximates the back of the upper incisors for the apico-dental [θ] and [ð].

Therapeutic Suggestions

Phonetic Placement

Interdental Productions. [θ] and [ð] are articulated with

1. the tongue tip *slightly* protruded between the upper and lower incisors,
2. the top of the tongue lightly touching the lower edges of the front teeth,
3. the underside of the tongue resting on the top edges of the lower incisors, and
4. the body of the tongue relatively flat.

The expiratory airflow should be directed over the surface of the tongue between tongue tip and the bottom edge of the front incisors. Specific tongue activities could be implemented prior to this placement. For example, the client could move the tip of the tongue forward and backward over the bottom edge of the front incisors. Next, with the tip of the tongue placed lightly on the bottom edge of the front incisors, the client lowers the tongue tip minimally during expiration. The goal is to create awareness of the airflow over the surface and tip of the tongue. Because the tip of the tongue is visible during the interdental production, a mirror will provide excellent feedback. Care should be taken that this placement is not established with excessive tongue protrusion. The tongue tip should barely be visible between the teeth.

Apico-Dental Productions. The tongue tip is placed touching the posterior surface of the front incisors. The body of the tongue should be relatively flat. During expiration, the client now glides the tongue back slightly until a friction noise is heard. The required posterior movement is minimal. For the client with a [t/θ] substitution, care must be taken that the posterior movement does not result in the tongue tip coming into contact with the alveolar ridge.

The substitutions [t/θ] and [f/θ] can be effectively influenced by employing sound modification methods. Therefore, the descriptions for changing the articulation from [t] and [f] to an interdental or addental [θ] and [ð] will be found in the following section.

Sound Modification Methods

1. *[t]-[θ] method.* These two sounds are distinguished by their place and manner of articulation. To move from [t] to [θ], the place of articulation must be moved anteriorly. Also, the manner of articulation changes from a stop to a fricative. The client should be instructed to:

   a. *Slowly* release [t]. This should result in a frictionlike sound.

   b. Maintain this frictionlike quality while moving the tongue forward until its tip comes very close to the back of the front incisors. If this constriction is continued, the client should feel the air

flowing over the tip of the tongue, forcing its way between the tongue and the back of the upper front teeth.

2. *[f]-[θ] method.* For this method, organ and place must be modified; the manner of articulation remains the same. The easiest articulation to achieve when modifying [f] to [θ] is the interdental one. Two different ways can be used:

   a. During the production of [f], the client pulls the bottom lip away from the upper incisors.

   b. The friction sound must continue during the placement of the tongue tip between the upper and lower incisors.

Or during the production of [f], the client is instructed to

   a. "Split the /f/ in half with his tongue by sticking his tongue between his teeth" (Secord, 1981b, p. 32). Here, the goal is the release of the labiodental placement when the client places the tongue between the incisors.

   b. The friction sound must continue during the placement of the tongue.

3. *[s]-[θ] method.* If the client has an acceptable [s], this seems to be the easiest sound modification method to use because the place of articulation is the only feature distinguishing the two sounds. The goal is an apico-dental [θ]. During the [s]-production,

   a. Glide the tongue forward until the tip almost touches the back of the upper incisors.

   b. Feel the air flowing between the tongue tip and the back of the teeth.

Coarticulatory Conditions

Due to the high-front position of the tongue during [θ] and [ð] realizations, high-front vowels offer perhaps the best coarticulatory conditions following these sounds. The back vowels with the positioning of the tongue toward the back of the mouth would not aid the production. Therefore, a possible vowel sequence is high-front, mid-front, low-front, followed by central vowels, and finally the back vowels moving from low- to mid- to the high-back vowels.

Compared to the voiceless [θ], the voiced [ð] has a much higher frequency of occurrence in General American English. This would suggest that practice with [ð] will be an important aspect of therapy.

Word Examples. The following one-syllable words are ordered from relatively easy to more difficult coarticulatory conditions for a child with [θ] and [ð] problems.

[θ] Words	[ð] Words
theme	thee - these
thin - thick - thing - think	this
	they
theft	them - then - their - there
thank - thanks	
thumb - thud - thug - thump	that - than - that's
	the
third - thirst	though - those
thaw - thought - thawed - thong	

The following sections describe phonetic errors that are less frequently encountered. These errors include voicing problems and difficulties with f-sounds, affricates, and consonant clusters.

*M*ISARTICULATIONS OF [f] AND [v]

[f] is one of the earliest fricatives to emerge in the speech of children, and it is usually mastered between 3 and 4 years of age. However, if sound mastery data are examined (see Chapter 5), the voiced [v] is consistently noted as being later in acquisition than its voiceless

cognate. When Sander (1972) reinterpreted the Wellman and colleagues (1931) and Templin (1957) data, he reported that 90 percent of the children had mastered [f] by age 4, compared to only 51 percent for [v]. It was not until age 8 that 90 percent of the children had mastered the voiced [v]. Therefore, approximately four years separate similar levels of competency for [f] versus [v].

What could account for this large difference in the age of acquisition? Although differences exist between the mastery ages of other consonant cognates as well, such large age variations are noted only for [f] and [v]. Perhaps the later acquisition of [v] reflects a much lower frequency of occurrence in General American English when compared to [f]. If it is not a frequent sound, children may simply not be utilizing it, thus, seemingly, extending the mastery age. However, frequency of occurrence data for children (Carterette and Jones, 1974; Mader, 1954) do not support this hypothesis. The frequency of occurrence for [f] and [v] is relatively similar. A second possibility is that it is not the quantity of different words but rather a limited number of highly frequent words with [v] that raise the frequency count. (A similar case can be made for the voiced [ð]. Its relative high frequency of occurrence can be attributed to a small number of very frequently used words, such as *the*.) Two studies (Denes and Pinson, 1973; Dewey, 1923) may support this hypothesis. These investigators found that *of* [ʌv] was among the ten most frequently used words in General American English. Such words as *have* and *give* would also seem to be fairly common words. The Mader (1954) study also adds some credibility to this hypothesis. If the frequency of occurrence according to the position in the word is examined for first-, second-, and third-grade children, the majority of the [v]-sounds occur in word-final positions. These are merely possibilities for explaining the differences between the reported ages of acquisition for [f] and [v]. Whatever the reason, the later age of acquisition for [v] may have clinical implications.

In the previous therapeutic discussions for phonetic errors, it has been assumed that one would proceed clinically from one consonant cognate to the other. Thus, therapy with [s] would closely coincide with [z] work. The acquisition information might cause us to question the validity of this procedure for [f] and [v]. These data suggest that therapy for [f] should be initiated prior to [v]. Depending on the age of the child, it may not be realistic to expect the same level of accuracy for [v]. One of the predictions established by Elbert and Gierut (1986) might be considered here. They stated that if one member of a cognate pair is achieved in therapy, improvement will occur with the other member. Interpreted in light of the acquisition data, therapy would most often begin with [f]. However, we might want to wait and watch to see if [v] would develop on its own. For many children, [v] acquisition appears to take place much later than the mastery of the voiceless [f].

Phonetic Description

[f] and [v] are labiodental fricatives. A constriction is created by bringing the inner edge of the lower lip into close contact with the edges of the upper incisors. If this contact is very light, the breath stream can pass between the inner edge of the lower lip and the cutting edge of the upper incisors. Firmer contact between the lower lip and upper teeth might cause the breath stream to flow around the incisors, some of the air being forced out in the region of the canine and premolar teeth. The upper lip remains inactive during [f] and [v] articulation.

Types of Misarticulation

1. *[p/f] and [b/v] substitutions.* Examples of these substitutions include [pɪŋgɚ] for *finger*

or [ʃʌbəl] for *shovel*. Place and manner of articulation have been modified for this substitution. The labiodental articulation is replaced by a bilabial one and the fricative is changed to a stop-plosive.

Phonetic transcription of the error: [p] or [b].

2. *Bilabial fricative substitution.* For this substitution, only the place of articulation has been altered from a labiodental to a bilabial production. The symbols [ɸ] and [β] are used to denote voiceless and voiced bilabial fricatives.

Phonetic transcription of the error: [ɸ] or [β].

Therapeutic Suggestions

Phonetic Placement.   To develop an awareness of the labiodental articulation, the client should "bite down" on the lower lip with the upper teeth. This will probably result in the client touching the outside edges of the lower lip. Because [f] is produced with the inside of the lower lip contacting the the upper incisors, the client should then glide the lower lip along the cutting edges of the upper teeth toward the inside of the lip, letting the lip "pop out" of the bite. When the upper incisors are lightly positioned on the inner edge of the lower lip, the client should blow, allowing air to escape between this narrow slit. If the labiodental contact is too firm, the jaw can be lowered *slightly*.

If the client realizes a [p/f] substitution, the presence of airflow should be targeted. Although the airflow for [f] is relatively weak, a light feather or a small piece of tissue placed in front of the mouth should show some movement during the entire [f] production. This could then be contrasted to the lack of movement during the stop phase of the [p] articulation. In isolation, producing [p] causes movement of the feather only at the very end, during the plosive portion of the articulation.

The labiodental contact is also an important aspect of the phonetic placement for the client who demonstrates a bilabial fricative ([ɸ] or [β]) substitution. Because the substitution and the target sound are both fricatives, if the labiodental positioning can be established, an acceptable [f] will result. A passive method may assist in this placement. During the bilabial fricative production, the bottom lip is pushed inward with the tip of the index finger. This should position the bottom lip approximately in the right spot for [f]. When a mirror is used, this passive method will allow the client visual feedback regarding the relative positioning of the lower lip and the upper incisors. In addition, auditory feedback is provided when the two different sound qualities are compared.

Sound Modification Methods

[p]-[f] Method.   During the stop phase of the [p]-production, the bottom lip is pushed inward with the tip of the index finger so that air can escape. The lower lip should be positioned in such a manner that its inner edge approximates the upper incisors. Initially, maintaining the position of the index finger can serve as an aid until the client is aware of the necessary articulatory placement.

Coarticulatory Conditions

Vowels with lip rounding, such as the back vowels (with the exception of [ɑ]), should be avoided when beginning syllable or word practice with a newly acquired [f]. Lip rounding is clearly an unfavorable coarticulatory condition. The central vowels with r-coloring, which are often produced with lip rounding, would not provide a beneficial coarticulatory condition either. When comparing the tongue placement and the relatively closed position of the jaw during normal [f] realizations, the sequence of vowels to be considered might be high-front, mid-front, low-front, followed by the central vowels without r-coloring. The final vowel sequence would start with the low-back vowels followed by the mid-, high-back, and central vowels with r-coloring.

Word Examples.   The following one-syllable words are ordered from relatively easy to more difficult coarticulatory conditions for a child with [f] difficulties. One-syllable words beginning with [v] are also included. However, it should be kept in mind that according to the Mader (1954) results, 96 percent of [v] sounds used by school-age children were in the medial and final word positions.

[f] Words	[v] Words
feet - feed - feel - field	
fit - fill - fin - fig - fish - fist	Vic - Vince
fade - fail - face - fake - faint	veil - vein - vase
fed - fell - fence	vet - vest
fat - fan - fast - fact	van - Val - vamp
fun - fudge	
fought - fall - fog - false	vault
phone - phones - fold	vote
foot - full	
food - fool	
fur - fern	Vern - verb

Affricate PROBLEMS

The affricates [tʃ] and [dʒ] develop relatively late in the speech of children. This may be due to the complexity of the production or possibly to their low frequency of occurrence in General American English. Several investigations (Carterette and Jones, 1974; Mader, 1954; Shriberg and Kwiatkowski, 1982a) that analyzed the continuous utterances of children and adults consistently rank both [tʃ] and [ʤ] as one of the least frequent consonants. This is further exemplified in Olmsted's (1971) study. In spontaneous speech, only one of the forty-eight children ranging from 36 to 54 months of age attempted [ʤ], and that child produced it in an aberrant manner. Although several of the acquisition studies did not test both [ʧ] and [ʤ], others (Arlt and Goodban, 1976; Prather et al., 1975; Templin, 1957) reported that there is a somewhat later age of acquisition for [ʤ] compared to [ʧ]. Sander's (1972) reinterpretation of the Wellman and colleagues (1931) and Templin (1957) data demonstrated similar mastery age levels for both the voiceless and voiced affricates. However, a relatively long time span separated the age when the majority of the children (51 percent of the children tested) versus most of the children (90 percent of the children tested) mastered the affricates. At age 3;6, 51 percent of the children had mastered both affricates, but it was not until age 7 that 90 percent of the children had reached comparable mastery levels.

Phonetic Description

Although some descriptions of affricates give the reader the idea that they are merely the stops [t] and [d] followed by the fricatives [ʃ] and [ʒ], this is not entirely accurate. Based on palatograms, Kantner and West (1960) reported two factors that differentiate isolated consonant sequences from affricate productions: (1) the initial position of the stop portion and (2) the nature of the movement from the stop to the fricative portion of the affricates. First, the initial stop portion of [ʧ] is articulated closer to the articulatory position for [ʃ]; therefore, it is produced more posteriorly than is normally the case with an isolated [t]. Second, movement from the stop to the fricative portion of the affricate is characterized by the front of the tongue dropping relatively

slowly, creating momentarily a constriction that is typical for the [ʃ]-sound. This is different from the release of an isolated [t], in which the tongue drops suddenly to a neutral position. The degree of lip rounding during the production of these affricates depends primarily on the speaker and the phonetic context.

As noted, then, an affricate is not merely a stop followed by a fricative production. Its realization varies in characteristic ways from the articulation of an isolated stop followed by a fricative. However, in an attempt to simplify the directions for their use with children, it will often sound as if our goal is merely to fuse the stop with the fricative. In addition, the previously reported differences between affricates versus stop plus fricative productions may prove helpful to clinicians if the resulting sound quality is perceptually still not acceptable.

Types of Misarticulation

1. *[t/ʧ] and [d/ʤ] substitutions.* These misarticulations are characterized by the substitution of a stop for the affricate production. Examples include [tɝt] for the word *church* or [pədɑməz] for *pajamas*. Because the substituted stop and the stop portion of the affricate are the same, only the slow release of the stop to [ʃ] distinguishes these two speech sounds.

Phonetic transcription of the error: [t] or [d].

2. *[ʃ/ʧ] and [ʒ/ʤ] substitutions.* A substitution of a fricative for the affricate is exemplified by [wɑʃ] for *watch* and [ʒʌmp] for *jump*. The lack of the initial stop portion of the affricate distinguishes this substitution from the affricate production.

Phonetic transcription of the error: [ʃ] or [ʒ].

3. *[s/ʧ] and [z/ʤ] substitutions.* Examples for these substitutions include [pis] for *peach* and [zæm] for *jam*. This realization does not have any initial stop portion, only a fricative element. In addition, the fricative segment is articulated more anteriorly than the normal fricative portion of the affricates.

Phonetic transcription of the error: [s] or [z].

Therapeutic Suggestions

Phonetic Placement. The tongue tip is placed on the posterior edge of the alveolar ridge in a manner similar to [t]. This [t] realization should be released *slowly*. It is important that the client be aware that during the release, the lateral edges of the tongue need to remain in contact with the premolars and molars, similar to a [ʃ]-production. In addition, the tongue glides slightly back during the release. The posterior movement of the tongue can be aided by pushing the tongue back with a tongue depressor during the slow release of [t].

One could also begin with [ʃ] to emphasize the tongue placement necessary for the release of the stop portion of the affricate. The client produces [ʃ] and, without moving the body of the tongue, "stops" or "blocks off" the airflow with the tip of the tongue. The resulting stop is then again slowly released.

Sound Modification Methods

1. *[t]-[ʧ] method.* The description for employing this method is similar to the one explained in the first paragraph of the previous section on phonetic placement. In order to achieve success with this method, it is important that the lateral edges of the tongue remain in contact with the premolars and first molars during the slow release of the [t]. If this is not the case, a [tʰʌ] quality will result rather than [ʧ].

Secord (1981b) suggests telling "the client to practice saying /t/-/ʃ/ slowly at first, then rapidly until they blend and become one sound" (p. 41).

2. *[ʃ]-[ʧ] method.* The description for utilizing this method is similar to the one explained in the second paragraph of the previous section on phonetic placement.

3. *[s]-[ʧ] method.* During [s]-production, the client should glide the tongue slightly back. When an acceptable [ʃ]-quality is achieved, proceed according to the instructions for the [ʃ]-[ʧ] method.

Coarticulatory Conditions

Because of the anterior placement of the tongue for both the stop and the fricative portions of the affricate, the front vowels would seem to offer more coarticulatory support than the back vowels. Consequently, a possible vowel sequence would be high-, mid-, low-front vowels followed by the central vowels and the back vowels. The back vowels, however, offer two advantages: (1) the lip rounding of especially the high-back vowels might provide coarticulatory support for the lip rounding noted in the [ʧ]-production and (2) the back positioning of the tongue for the back vowels might enhance the backward gliding movement of the tongue in its transition from stop-plosive to the fricative portion of the affricate. If this proves to aid the production of [ʧ] in a given case, the vowel sequence might be the high-, mid-, and low-back vowels followed by the central and the front vowels. Clinicians should use probes to determine which vowel sequence would be more beneficial for their particular client.

Word Examples. The following one-syllable words are ordered from relatively easy to more difficult coarticulatory conditions for a child with an affricate problem. In this case, affricate-vowel probes demonstrated that the series of back vowels offered better coarticulatory conditions than the front vowels.

[tʃ] Words	[dʒ] Words
chew - choose	June - juice
choke - chore - chose	Joe - joke - Joan
chalk - chop - chopped - chops	jaw - jog - jar - job - John - jaws
chirp - churn	jerk - germ
Chuck - chug - chum - chunk	jug - junk - jump - jumped
chat - champ - chance	Jack - jam - jab
check - chair	gem - jet - Jeff
chain - chase	jay - Jane
chick - chin - chill - chips	Jim - Jill
cheek - cheep - cheese - cheat - chief	gee - jeep - Gene - jeans

VOICING PROBLEMS

Voicing problems manifest themselves in the substitution of a voiced for a voiceless cognate, such as [du] for *two,* or a voiceless for a voiced cognate, such as when *ball* is pronounced as [pɑl]. Voicing has phonemic value in General American English. Different word meanings are established by the presence or absence of a voicing component. This can be exemplified by the minimal pairs *face* and *vase* and *tot* and *dot.* Because of its phonemic relevance, a voicing problem should trigger evaluation to determine whether a phonemic disorder exists.

Several authors (i.e., Ingram, 1989b; Grunwell, 1987; Smit and Bernthal, 1983; Smith, 1979) have noted that children still show difficulties with certain aspects of voicing at age 4. The most common pattern is the voiced production of normally voiceless stops, fricatives, and affricates initiating a syllable or word (prevocalic voicing). Thus, *toe* and *soup* may be pronounced as [doᵘ] and [zup]. In addition, voiceless cognates are substituted for their voiced counterparts terminating a word or syllable (postvocalic devoicing); that is, *cub* becomes [kʌp] and *dog* [dɑk]. *Context-sensitive voicing* is a term used to refer to these types of voicing errors (Grunwell, 1987). According to Grunwell (1987), context-sensitive voicing, especially postvocalic devoicing, may continue in some children beyond 3 years of age.

Specific factors that need to be appraised before implementing therapy for difficulties with consonant voicing–devoicing include the frequency of occurrence in the speech of the client and the contexts in which the voicing–devoicing occurs. First, the voicing–devoicing difficulties should occur at a relatively high frequency before therapy is implemented. Second, some specific contextual modifications resulting in devoicing are commonly heard in General American English; these modifications would not be considered misarticulations. For example, devoicing of final consonants and assimilations of voicelessness are common (Abercrombie, 1967). Devoicing of final consonants can be found most often before a pause. Therefore, devoicing of final consonants could be realized during an articulation test as well as on spontaneous speech samples. Personal clinical experience has shown that final devoicing often occurs on plurals that end in [əz]: *matches* is pronounced as [mætʃəs] and *dishes* as [dɪʃəs]. Assimilations of voicelessness can be either progressive or regressive. During an utterance, these assimilations can often be heard if a voiceless consonant precedes or follows a voiced stop, fricative, or affricate. For example, we pronounce *news* as [nuz]. However, *news* is typically pronounced [nus] in the word *newspaper.* This devoicing of [z] is a regressive assimilation influenced by the following voiceless [p]. Although these types of sound change in context are common, they must be evaluated in relationship to their frequency of occurrence for a particular client. If the frequency is so high that intelligibility is somehow affected, even these "normal" modifications may warrant therapy.

Therapeutic Suggestions

Probably all children use some voicing distinctions in their speech. The task is to create an awareness of voicing versus lack of voicing for a particular cognate pair. The following guidelines can be supplemented with auditory discrimination exercises in order to enhance the general awareness of voicing versus devoicing. Minimal pair words that target the particular voicing–devoicing cognate difficulty can also be employed.

This sequencing of auditory discrimination exercises is suggested:

1. General awareness of the presence or absence of voicing could be aided by having the client listen to two sounds—[s] and [z], for example—and identify which one is voiced. This could be combined with the tactile feedback method, which is explained in the following section.

2. The cognates could be placed in minimally paired words and the client asked to identify voiced versus voiceless sounds at the beginning or end of a word. Word pair discrimination exercises would utilize the particular consonant cognates and the position of these sounds in words that are problematic for the client. If the client has trouble with the devoicing of final stops, word pairs such as *cap* versus *cab* and *lock* versus *log* could be identified.

Tactile Feedback Method. This method develops the client's awareness of the vibratory sensation associated with voicing. This is then contrasted to the lack of vibration present during voiceless sounds. Clients place their fingers on or slightly above the thyroid cartilage during the production of a voiced sound. Attention should be directed to the vibration that is felt. For children, this vibration can be compared to a motor being "on" during voiced versus "off" during unvoiced consonants. This method works well with fricatives and affricates but is difficult to implement with stop-plosives. The natural tendency to add a vowel after the production of stop sounds can trigger the feeling of vibration on unvoiced stop sounds. Actually, the vibration for the vowel *follows* the stop production, but many children will not be able to discern this. If the clinician decides to implement the tactile feedback method for establishing an awareness of voiced versus voiceless stop-plosives, the child should be instructed to whisper the stop to attain a voiceless realization while saying the voiced cognate with a "big (loud) voice." This should eliminate the voicing influence of the following vowel on the voiceless stop.

Auditory Enhancement Method. This method enhances the humming effect heard during the production of voiced consonants. The client's hands are cupped and placed over the ears. During the production of voiced consonants, the client should hear a humming not present during the production of voiceless consonants. A similar effect can be achieved by plugging each ear with an index finger. Difficulties may arise when using this method to discriminate between voiced and voiceless stops; the instructions noted in the tactile feedback method should be followed here as well.

Whispering Method. If a child produces a voiced consonant and its voiceless cognate is the goal, the clinician can have the child whisper the sound. As with all the previously noted methods, this one is implemented only until the client understands the distinction between voiced and voiceless productions.

Singing Method.   This method is implemented for clients who can produce a voiceless consonant but the goal is its voiced cognate. Here, the client "sings" the voiceless consonant. A familiar melody such as "Happy Birthday" is sung with the voiceless consonant combined with the [ʌ] vowel replacing the words: [pʌpʌpʌpʌ pʌpʌ]. If the client actually continues to sing—that is, to produce continuous voicing—the voiceless consonant will become voiced. If this is accomplished, the client is made aware of the voiced production, which can then be isolated from the tune.

Developing Voiced Stop Productions.   This technique is actually a sound modification method. The voiced stop-plosives are modified from the nasals, [m], [n], and [ŋ]. Personal clinical experience has shown that this technique is often surprisingly effective if one of the previous methods has failed. During the nasal production, the nostrils are pinched closed. The client releases the air orally. If the voicing of the nasal continues, [b] should result from [m], [d] from [n], and [g] from [ŋ]. The success of this technique depends on the continuation of the voicing component of the nasal sounds.

CONSONANT CLUSTER PROBLEMS

For some children, the acquisition of consonant clusters may extend into the beginning school years. Weiss, Gordon, and Lillywhite, (1987) reported that it was not until children were 7 years of age that all consonant clusters were realized in a regular manner. Children also seem to go through certain stages in acquiring consonant clusters (see Chapter 5). Consonant cluster reduction and substitution are two processes that describe these stages. One of the earliest stages in a child's attempt to produce consonant clusters is consonant clus-

ter reduction. This is exemplifed by the production of [dʌm] for *drum*. Typically, though not always, the marked member of the cluster is the one that is deleted (Ingram, 1989b). According to Greenlee (1974), the next phase in acquiring clusters is consonant cluster substitution, which is demonstrated when [dwʌm] is realized for *drum*. The last phase is the norm articulation of the consonant cluster.

At the word level, most consonants of General American English can be phonotactically members of a consonant cluster. Consonant clusters at the end of a word are often used to signal certain linguistic functions such as plurality (exemplified by the word *dogs*), third-person singular tense (as in *kicks*), past tense (as in *kicked*), and possessives (as in *Jack's*). At the spontaneous speech level, any consonant cluster may occur. Therefore, the treatment of consonant clusters will often be one stage of a therapy program. In addition, children may be referred for therapy who can produce the individual sounds of a cluster but have difficulty with clusters containing those sounds. Depending on the number and type of consonant clusters affected, this may reduce the intelligibility of the child's speech considerably. The following guidelines are given to aid in the treatment of consonant clusters.

Therapeutic Suggestions

In General American English, consonant clusters consist of either two or three consonants in word-initial position and from two to four consonants in word-final position. Consonant clusters with only two consonants are typically easier to produce than those with three or four consonants. In addition, before therapy with consonant clusters begins, all members of the consonant cluster should be sounds that the child can produce accurately. For example, if a clinician is working on [k] clusters but the child cannot produce [r], then [kr] clusters should be avoided.

Production of Word-Initial Clusters

Epenthesis. During the acquisition of clusters, children often insert a schwa between the two consonants. This is a process referred to as epenthesis. The same process can also be used to aid a client's production of a cluster. If the cluster is [sk], as in the word *skate,* the client starts with [s-keᴵt]. At first, the word should be slowly pronounced so that the schwa is somewhat prolonged. After a period of practice, the client attempts to shorten the schwa vowel gradually. This can often be achieved by increasing the tempo of the entire word. The end result should be a smooth transition from the first to the second consonant.

Pausing. For this method, a pause is inserted between the first and second member of the consonant cluster. Using the previous example, [sk] becomes [s] (pause) [keᴵt]. After a period of practice, the client again shortens the pause between the two consonants. Personal clinical experience has shown that visual feedback in the form of a drawn line or gestures can often aid children in shortening this pause. For example, a long line is drawn that can be successively shortened, or the clinician can start with hands outspread moving them closer and closer together to indicate a shorter pause. Due to the natural pause that occurs between two syllables, this method is especially effective for consonant clusters that occur across syllable boundaries, such as [ns] in *answer* or *pencil.*

Production of Word-Final Clusters

Prolonging the First Sound. This method is best suited for clusters whose first element can be easily prolonged, such as the fricatives, affricates, nasals, or liquids. The first sound is prolonged for about two seconds and is then followed by the second element of the cluster, as in the word *nest,* "sssssssssss-t" for [st]. With repeated practice, the prolongation of the first sound is then successively shortened.

Pausing. This technique presents itself as a possibility if the first element of the consonant cluster is a stop-plosive. The instructions are similar to those described under initial consonant clusters.

Production of Word-Medial Clusters. Many word-medial clusters, especially two-consonant clusters, occur across syllable boundaries, as in *base-ball* or *an-swer.* Other clusters are to be found initiating a syllable, as in *ze-bra* or *A-pril.* Although common pronunciations do not syllabify these clusters between the two elements, for therapeutic purposes they could be artificially divided into *zeb-ra* or *Ap-ril.* The previously mentioned pausing method could be easily implemented by inserting a pause between the two syllables. This pause could first be lengthened and then shortened as the client gains stability of production.

Coarticulatory Conditions

Three variables should be considered when working on consonant clusters: (1) the length of the cluster, (2) the position of the cluster in the word, and (3) the coarticulation between the specific elements of the cluster.

The *length of the cluster* refers to how many individual consonants form the cluster. Typically, the fewer the consonants, the easier the cluster will be for the client. Therefore, consonant clusters with two elements should be attempted prior to three-element clusters.

The *position of the cluster* in the word refers to whether the cluster initiates the word, terminates it, or occurs somewhere in the middle. Although most clinicians will probably begin with clusters initiating the word, medial clusters offer some positive features. The "natural" pause between two syllables can be used to separate the cluster into two discrete elements: For example, the [ns] cluster in *pencil* is divided into *pen-cil.* Again, this pause is at first prolonged and later shortened. Such a procedure gives the client, within a relatively natural word situation, time to produce the transition between the elements of the cluster. Inserting a pause can also be used for clusters that typically are not syllabified between the two elements of the cluster. If the consonant cluster [st] is selected, practice could include *Eas-ter, toaster,* and *roos-ter,* for example. If the client can produce the cluster without a pause between the syllables, it can then be transferred to the word-initiating position. The client would be instructed to whisper the first part of the word, saying the last *ster* portion in a louder voice. This does necessitate that the syllable boundary is now changed from between the cluster, s-t, to initiating the cluster, st-. However, if the client can make this transition, the consonant cluster stands now at the beginning of a word, *stir.* A similar technique can be used to gain word-final consonant clusters. In this case, the last *er* portion of the word is whispered, which results in e*ast, toast,* and *roost* productions.

A disadvantage to using the clusters medially is that the client has to deal with a two-syllable rather than a one-syllable word. If more difficulty is noted when the client has to articulate a two-syllable word, this technique loses its appeal. Both word-initiating and -terminating consonant clusters should then be practiced in one-syllable word contexts, for [st] in words such as *star* and *stone* or *nest* and *lost,* for example. Here, word-initiating clusters would probably be easier than word-terminating clusters. As with all stages of therapy, the clinician needs to establish which sequence offers more favorable effects for each individual client.

The third factor that needs to be considered is the coarticulation between the elements of the cluster. Given a specific target sound within the cluster, certain sound combinations will be easier to produce than others. For example, if the target sound is [s], consider the consonant cluster [sk], as in *skate,* versus [sp], as in *spot.* For [sk], the tongue must move quickly from a front approximation of the articulators to a stop closure involving the back of the tongue. With [sp], on the other hand, the [p] element can be articulated with very little or no tongue movement from the [s] position. When the coarticulation features are considered, [sp] appears easier to articulate than [sk].

Certain consonant clusters might also need to be carefully evaluated based on the original misarticulation. For the child who originally demonstrated a lateral [s], clusters with [l], a lateral sound, might trigger the old misarticulation, for example. Or, for the child who originally had a [t] for [k] substitution, the word-final cluster [kt], as in *kicked* or *locked,* might prove troublesome.

In addition, specific techniques used to elicit the norm production may be reinforced by the selection of specific consonant clusters. If the [t]-[s] method was used to establish [s], the cluster [ts] used at the beginning of therapy might reinforce the [s]-production. Similarly, a clinician who has established an acceptable [r] realization by means of the [d]-[r] method might use the consonant cluster [dr] to aid in stabilizing [r] during the initial stages of therapy.

The preceding guidelines have been provided to guide, not dictate, clinical decision making. The choice of the cluster and the sequencing of clusters within the therapy program will depend on the needs and the articulatory possibilities of the individual client. However, one of the tasks of a clinician is to understand and consider the factors that could have a positive or negative influence on the production of a specific target sound. This understanding will increase the efficacy of therapy.

SUMMARY

This chapter dealt with the phonetic (traditional-motor) approach to the treatment of articulation disorders, which is based on placement of the articulators in such a manner as to achieve an acceptable articulation of the sound in question. First, a sequence for therapy was outlined, beginning at the sound level and systematically moving to more complex articulatory conditions. Dismissal criteria were also suggested in the first portion of this chapter.

Misarticulations of several consonants were discussed in detail in the second portion of this chapter. These consonants represented the most frequently misarticulated speech sounds: misarticulations of [s] and [z], [ʃ] and [ʒ], [k] and [g], [l], [r], the central vowels with r-coloring, and [θ] and [ð]. Other sound problems included misarticulations of [f] and [v], the affricates [tʃ] and [dʒ], voiced and voiceless substitution, and consonant clusters. When applicable, phonetic placement as well as sound modification techniques were described. In addition, effects of coarticulation were examined for each of the noted problems.

Any successful application of this approach to articulation therapy presupposes a firm knowledge base concerning not only the phonetic characteristics of the sound's norm realization but also the misarticulated sound. An attempt has been made to provide both within this chapter.

CASE STUDY

The following are results from the Arizona Articulatory Proficiency Scale for Lori, age 7;6.

1.	horse	[hoɚθ]	17.	bird	[bɝd]		
2.	wagon	[wægən]	18.	pig	[pɪg]		
3.	red	[rɛd]	19.	cup	[kʌp]		
4.	comb	[koᵘm]	20.	car	[kɑɚ]		
5.	fork	[foɚk]	21.	ear	[ɪɚ]		
6.	knife	[naɪf]	22.	swing	[θwɪŋ]		
7.	cow	[kaᵘ]	23.	table	[teɪbəl]		
8.	cake	[keɪk]	24.	cat	[kæt]		
9.	baby	[beɪbi]	25.	ladder	[læɾɚ]		
10.	bathtub	[bæθtəb]	26.	ball	[bɑl]		
11.	nine	[naɪn]	27.	airplane	[ɛɚpleɪn]		
12.	train	[treɪn]	28.	cold	[koᵘld]		
13.	gun	[gʌn]	29.	jumping	[dʌmpɪŋ]		
14.	dog	[dɑg]	30.	television	[tɛləvɪzən]		
15.	yellow	[jɛloᵘ]	31.	stove	[ʂtoᵘv]		
16.	doll	[dɑl]	32.	ring	[rɪŋ]		
33.	tree	[tri]	42.	fish	[fɪʃ]		
34.	green	[grin]	43.	zipper	[ðɪpɚ]		
35.	this	[ðɪθ]	44.	nose	[noᵘð]		
36.	whistle	[wɪθəl]	45.	sun	[θʌn]		
37.	chair	[tɛɚ]	46.	house	[haᵘθ]		
38.	watch	[wɑt]	47.	steps	[ʂtɛpθ]		
39.	thumb	[θʌm]	48.	nest	[nɛst]		
40.	mouth	[maᵘθ]	49.	carrots	[kɛɚəts]		
41.	shoe	[ʃu]	50.	books	[bʊkθ]		

Lori demonstrates difficulties with [s], [tʃ], and [dʒ]. If you analyze the patterns for [s]-production you find that she substitutes [θ] for [s] and [ð] for [z] in most words. However, she dentalizes [s] when it occurs at the beginning of a word together with [t] (see *steps* and *stove*). Facilitating contexts can be noted at the end of a word in which [s] is produced correctly in [s] + [t] or [t] + [s] blends in words such as *nest* and *carrots*. It seems as if the combination with

[t] produces coarticulatory conditions that are favorable for [s]. Although [s] is a later developing sound than [tʃ], or [dʒ], these facilitating contexts could be used to initially begin work on [s]. In addition, [s] is a sound that occurs frequently in American English.

THINK CRITICALLY

1. You are working with a 7-year-old child, Larry, who has a [θ] for [s] substitution (as well as a [ð] for [z] substitution). Larry seems unable to distinguish between [s] and [z] when used in minimal pairs with voiced and voiceless "th." Based on his errors and his lack of discrimination abilities, construct a sensory-perceptual training program using identification, isolation, stimulation, and discrimination. Try to be as specific as possible about the targets you would use for each of the phases.
2. Maureen, a 7;6-year-old child, shows evidence of consistent dentalized [s] and [z] productions for [s] and [z] in all contexts. You cannot find facilitating contexts and have decided to do phonetic placement with the child. De-

scribe the advantages and disadvantages of using an apico-alveolar (tongue tip up) versus a predorsal-alveolar (tongue tip down) production. Select one of the phonetic placement techniques and describe step-by-step how you would explain the tongue placement and what the child needs to do to achieve a correct [s]-production.
3. Molly has a [w] for [r] substitution. Describe in detail the steps you would go through to achieve an [r]-production using the phonetic placement technique for the apico-predorsal [r]. If you now have [r] in isolation, what CV nonsense syllables and simple words would you use to stabilize the [r]?

TEST YOURSELF

1. Which of the following is not a phase of sensory-perceptual training?
   a. identification
   b. production
   c. isolation
   d. stimulation
   e. discrimination
2. Instructing the client on how to position the articulators in order to produce a norm production describes the
   a. auditory stimulation/imitation procedure
   b. phonetic placement method
   c. sound modification method
   d. facilitating context of a sound
3. In the word phase of the traditional-motor approach, all of the following contribute to the articulatory complexity of a word, except
   a. the length of the word
   b. the position of the target sound in the word

   c. the type of word (nouns are more concrete and should be used first)
   d. the syllable structure
4. The transfer of behavior to conversational speech in various settings is referred to as
   a. coarticulatory assistance
   b. facilitating contexts
   c. a home program
   d. carryover
5. What percentage of accuracy during natural spontaneous speech was mentioned as a possible criterion for dismissal?
   a. 100%
   b. 80%
   c. 50%
   d. 60%
6. Which would be an appropriate progression of a therapy sequence?
   a. phrases/sentences, words, spontaneous speech, sensory-perceptual training

b. words, nonsense syllables, sounds in isolation, spontaneous speech
c. sounds in isolation, nonsense syllables,
   words, phrases/sentences
d. sensory-perceptual training, sounds in
   isolation, phrases/sentences, nonsense
   syllables

7. Which of the following is part of a clinical
   responsibility that helps ensure that therapy
   was successful and the client has generalized
   sound productions across situations?
   a. reevaluation
   b. dismissal
   c. screening
   d. intervention

8. All of the following are therapeutic suggestions for problems with voicing except
   a. phonetic placement method
   b. tactile feedback method
   c. auditory enhancement method
   d. whispering method

9. The child has a [t] for [k] substitution. Which
   one of the following words might be problematic when working at the simple word stage?
   a. *king*
   b. *coop*
   c. *comb*
   d. *coat*

10. If you are working primarily on lip rounding
    for a correct [ʃ] production, which one of the
    following words would be a good coarticula-
    tory context?
    a. *shop*
    b. *shed*
    c. *shook*
    d. *sheep*

WEBSITES

http://members.tripod.com/Caroline_Bowen/
wordlists.html

This website, created by Caroline Bowen, provides
an extensive list of minimal pairs. It provides over
40 different lists of contrasting pairs of words.

www.asha.org/public/speech/disorders/Orofacial-
Myofunctional-Disorders.htm

The American Speech-Language-Hearing Association provides a summary of orofacial-myofunc-
tional disorders (tongue thrust) on this website. It
contains information on definition, causes, and the
effects on speech.

http://members.tripod.com/Caroline_Bowen/
kb/phonetic-placement-shaping-exercises-
12-pages.pdf

This website is a link to a pdf file that can be downloaded. The twelve-page resource is written by
Ken Bleile and contains step-by-step directions
for teaching phonetic placement of many late acquired sounds. Some sounds included are [s], [z],
[l], [r], [θ], and [ʃ].

http://speech-language-therapy.com/target_
selection.htm

This website by Carol Bowen provides an overview of target selection for the traditional motor
approach as contrasted to the nontraditional approach. It also gives references for each of the approaches as well as a discussion on whether the
clinician should choose "stimulable" sounds or
those that are considered nonstimulable. Again,
references are given to document each approach.

www.bridges4kids.org/pdf/Luker/
SpeechTherapy.pdf

This site, created by Calvin and Tricia Luker, gives
a comprehensive family guide to terminology that
is used in speech therapy. It lists over ten pages of
terms that are explained in a fairly simple manner
that parents could understand.

FURTHER READINGS

Bleile, K. M. (1996). *Articulation and phonological disorders: A book of exercises for students* (2nd ed.). San Diego, CA: Singular Publishing.

Hoffman, P., Schuckers, G., & Daniloff, R. (1989). *Children's phonetic disorders: Theory and treatment.* Boston: Little, Brown.

Passy, J. (2003). *A handful of sounds: Cued articulation in practice.* Camberwell, Melbourne, Victoria: Australian Council for Educational Research ACER Press.

Secord, W. (1981). *C-PAC: Clinical probes of articulation consistency.* Sedona, AZ: Red Rock Education.

Secord, W. (1981). *Eliciting sounds: Techniques for clinicians.* San Antonio: Psychological Corporation.

Williams, A. L. (2006). *Sound contrasts in phonology (SCIP).* Eau Claire, WI: Thinking Publications.

9

Treatment of Phonemic Errors

LEARNING OBJECTIVES

When you have finished this chapter, you should be able to:

- Identify the three principles underlying most of the phonologically based approaches.
- Define minimal pair contrast therapy.
- Explain how targets are selected for minimal opposition contrast therapy.
- Differentiate between maximal opposition and minimal opposition contrast approaches.
- Describe the multiple oppositions approach.
- Explain the unique approach of "cycles training."
- Describe metaphon therapy.
- Identify ways to connect the treatment of phonological disorders to language intervention techniques.

This chapter focuses on phonologically based approaches to treatment. Fey (1992) lists three basic principles underlying most of these approaches:

1. *Groups of sounds* with similar patterns of errors are targeted. In direct contrast to treating individual sounds in a sequential order, patterns of errors are noted and selected targets are chosen for therapy.

2. *Phonological contrasts* that were previously neutralized are established. Many of the phonologically based treatment methods use minimal pairs to contrast phonemic oppositions. If these distinctions can be made, one assumes that the child will generalize this knowledge to other phonemic contrasts.

3. A *naturalistic communicative context* is emphasized. Work on individual sounds or nonsense syllables is, strictly speaking, not a part of phonologically based therapy techniques.

Several of these treatment approaches will be described in this chapter. Although each uses a somewhat different analysis system to describe the patterns of errors, most of them employ minimal pairs in their remediation program. These *minimal pair contrast therapies* have been grouped together; their differences, however, will be discussed. Other treatment techniques, such as *cycles training* and *metaphon therapy,* which incorporate different concepts into their methodology, will also be addressed. The last portion of this chapter contains some guidelines for combining phonologically based approaches with other treatment necessities. This includes their integration with language therapy, exemplified by the child with co-occurring phonemic and language disorders and the child with an emerging phonological system. Finally, phonologically based approaches will be discussed in relationship to *vowel therapy* in children with multiple vowel errors.

As discussed earlier, the production of speech sounds—the phonetic form—and the contrastive use of phonemes within the phonological system—the phoneme function—are closely related. In addition, the phonological system interacts with other language areas. Although phonologically based approaches emphasize the function of phonemes, both the production of speech sounds and the relationship of phonology to other language areas should not be overlooked. This chapter will integrate some of these factors with a discussion of intervention techniques for phonemic disorders.

TREATMENT PRINCIPLES

Several principles underly the treatment of phonemic errors in phonologically based approaches. First, the phoneme as a basic unit differentiating between word meanings is at the core of these therapies. Consequently, intervention begins at the word level. This differs considerably from the traditional or motor approach, which typically begins with the production of the respective sound(s) in isolation. In addition, word materials used to treat phonemic errors are structured in a very specific manner. Phonemes are usually arranged contrastively between words, resulting in "minimal pairs"—two distinct words that differ by only one phoneme value.

Second, treatment focuses on the phonological system of the child. An analysis of the child's phonology as an integrated system results in knowledge of (1) the inventory and distribution of speech sounds, (2) the syllable shapes and phonemic contrasts utilized, and (3) the error patterns displayed. All of these factors become important when the child's phonological system, not the individual speech sound, is at the center of the remediation process.

Third, groups of sounds or sound classes, rather than just individual speech sounds, are targeted. Children with phonemic disorders often have difficulties with several phonemes. Their aberrant realizations may extend to whole classes of sounds, such as fricatives, for example. This makes it impossible for the child to establish phonemic contrasts; neutralization of phonemic oppositions therefore occurs. Phoneme-based remediation focuses on more than one sound or perhaps on an entire class of sounds at the same time. Several sounds may be targeted simultaneously, as in the cycles training approach (Hodson and Paden, 1991), or two sounds may be used to demonstrate phonemic oppositions, as in minimal contrast therapy (Blache, 1982; Blache, Parsons, and Humphreys, 1981; Cooper, 1985; Ferrier and Davis, 1973; Fokes, 1982; Lowe, Mount-Weitz, and Schmidt, 1992; Weiner, 1981; Weiner and Ostrowski, 1979). With phonologically based therapies, it is assumed that generalization will occur to other sounds or sound classes.

There are important differences between the traditional-motor approach (which is often used to treat phonetic errors) and phonologically based remediation methods (which target phonemic errors). Traditional-motor approaches represent therapy for *speech form,* the production of speech sounds. In contrast, phonologically based remediation methods target *phonemic function,* the contrastive use of phonemes to establish meaning differences. However, in the actual therapy situation, it is often impossible to separate these two different approaches entirely. Form and function constitute an interactive unity that often work together in our treatment of children with phonemic difficulties.

*M*INIMAL PAIR CONTRAST THERAPY

Minimal pair contrast therapy refers to the therapeutic use of pairs of words that differ by one phoneme only. These minimal pairs are used to establish contrasts not present in the child's phonological system. For example, an analysis reveals that a child does not differentiate between stops and fricatives; that is, all fricatives are produced as homorganic stops (e.g., [s] → [t], [f] → [p]). One type of minimal pair therapy might use [f], representing the fricatives, and [p], exemplifying stops, in word pairs such as *fin* and *pin,* to establish this opposition. The underlying principle is that by establishing the contrast between [f] and [p], generalization will occur to other stops and fricatives.

Minimal Opposition Contrast Therapy

What Is Minimal Opposition Contrast Therapy?
Minimal opposition contrast therapy is a method in which minimal pairs are employed as the beginning unit of therapy. The selection of the sounds for the minimal pairs is based on the principle that the two sounds are selected with as many articulation similarities as possible. Articulatory similarities are typically measured according to the phonetic production features of place, manner, and voicing. In minimal opposition contrast therapy, the sounds chosen differ in only one or two production features.

Although minimal opposition contrast is considered a phonologically based approach, the parameters for establishing these contrasts are phonetic in nature: Differences between phonetic production features are employed to determine the minimal contrast. Both speech "form," exemplified by the phonetic production features, and "function," the utilization of phonemic contrasts, are united for this therapy approach.

When to Use Minimal Opposition Contrast Therapy.   Which clients seem to be good candidates for this remediation plan? The minimal opposition contrast procedure targets the substitution of one phoneme for another. Sound distortions and omissions cannot be adequately addressed using phonemic contrasts. Therefore, clients who display a large number of sound distortions and omissions would probably not benefit from this therapy.

Therefore, those who primarily display phonemic substitutions are the best choices for minimal opposition contrasts. In addition, Lowe (1994) states that "the minimal opposition procedure is most appropriate for clients who are stimulable for the target sound" (p. 190). Hodson (1992) supports this view and adds that it appears inappropriate to set up a potentially frustrating situation by requiring differential productions of word pairs until the child can spontaneously and effortlessly say the target sounds within the pairs.

Before considering the minimal opposition contrast approach, clinicians will want to know if any data document its successful therapeutic use. Saben and Ingham (1991) found that therapy based on minimal opposition contrasts alone produced little progress in two clients. However, these clients improved when a traditional-motor approach was implemented together with the minimal opposition contrasts. So, then, does minimal opposition contrast seem a viable therapy method? There is as yet not much information available to answer this question. Based on very limited data, one would have to conclude that this procedure might work better if combined with a traditional-motor approach.

How to Select Target Sounds for Minimal Opposition Contrast Therapy.

When establishing the target sounds for minimal pairs, the following principles should be kept in mind (Lowe, 1994):

1. Phonemic substitutions form the basis for target selection. The norm production and the substitution(s) should first be analyzed.

2. The place-manner-voicing features for both the target sound and the substitution should be considered and the differences

> Place-voice-manner analysis for the various consonants can be found on pages 224–228.

counted. For example, if the child demonstrates an [f/v] and a [d/v] substitution, the number of differences between the two substitutions should be listed. The production features that primarily distinguish [f] from [v] are voicing; those that differentiate between [d] and [v] are manner and place.

3. The sound substitutions chosen should reflect the least number of differences in production features. Therefore, [f] and [v] would be selected because they demonstrate only one production feature difference; [d] and [v] differ in two production features.

4. The age of the child and the developmental level of the child's phonemic system should be evaluated. Earlier sounds have priority. For example, when place, manner, and voicing characteristics are analyzed, both [t/s] and [p/

b] substitutions represent differences of one production feature. However, [b] is earlier than [s]. Therefore, the [p]-[b] contrast is probably the better choice. See Table 9.1 for an overview of early and later developing sounds.

5. Sound substitutions that affect the child's intelligibility the most should have priority over those with little negative effect on intelligibility. This choice is primarily related to the frequency of occurrence of the two sounds. Therefore, if two sound substitutions demonstrate an equal number of differences in production features, priority should be given to the sound that impacts the intelligibility of the child the most.

6. Stimulable sounds have priority over those that are not stimulable.

This procedure can be exemplified in the following manner. A 5;6-year-old child demonstrates the following substitutions: [w/r], [θ/s], [ð/z], [d/ʤ], [t/ʧ], and [w/ʃ]. The production differences are as follows:

Substitution	Main Production Differences		
w/r	w = labial	glide	voiced
	r = palatal	liquid	voiced
θ/s	θ = dental	fricative	voiceless
	s = alveolar	fricative	voiceless
ð/z	ð = dental	fricative	voiced
	z = alveolar	fricative	voiced
d/ʤ	d = alveolar	stop	voiced
	ʤ = postalveolar	affricate	voiced
t/ʧ	t = alveolar	stop	voiceless
	ʧ = postalveolar	affricate	voiceless
w/ʃ	w = labial	glide	voiced
	ʃ = postalveolar	fricative	voiceless

Based on the number of production differences, two possibilities exist for target sounds: [θ-s] or [ð-z]. Both sound pairs are acquired at about the same time. Given that both sounds are stimulable, the best selection of target sounds would probably be [θ] and [s] because

Table 9.1   Early to Late Sounds: Approximate Development

Early Sounds	
Nasals	Typically, [m] and [n] develop before [ŋ].
Stops and [h]	[p], [b], [t], and [d] are early stops; [k] and [g] later ones. The appearance of [k] and [g] may extend into the development of early fricatives. [h] appears around the time of early stop development.
Glides	[w] is usually earlier than [j].
Liquids	[l] develops earlier than [r]. For some children, [r] may be among the later developing sounds.
Fricatives	[f] is an early fricative, often appearing much earlier than [v].
Later Sounds	
Fricatives	The sibilants [s], [z], [ʃ], are late, while [ʒ], [θ], and [ð] often belong to the latest developing sounds.
Affricates	Typically [tʃ] and [ʤ] develop after, or approximately at the same time, the fricatives [ʃ] and [ʒ] appear.

Source: Summarized from Bauman-Waengler (1994a).

[s] has a higher frequency of occurrence and will therefore have more of an impact on the child's intelligibility.

How Is Minimal Opposition Contrast Therapy Used? The two target sounds selected are placed in minimal pair words with the chosen sounds at the beginning: *think-sink, thing-sing,* or *sick-thick,* for example. However, there are often few words that are appropriate for children. Therefore, it has been suggested that if meaningful minimal pairs cannot be found for contrastive phonemes, near-minimal pairs should be used (Elbert and Gierut, 1986). **Near-minimal pairs** are pairs of words that differ by more than one phoneme, and the vowel preceding or following the target sound remains constant in both words. For example, *sir-third* or *thorn-sore* would be considered near-minimal pairs.

Many of the treatment protocols of minimal opposition contrast therapy include discrimination, imitation, and spontaneous production of the word pairs. After minimal pairs are chosen, the following steps are suggested (Blache, 1989).

Step 1: Discussion of Words. The therapist must be certain that the concepts portrayed are known to the child. To confirm this, the child can be asked to point to the picture named and questions can be asked about it. For example, if the chosen word pair was *fig-pig,* the clinician could ask, "Which one is a fruit?" or "Which one is an animal?"

Step 2: Discrimination Testing and Training. In this phase, the client's discrimination between the two sounds is tested. The therapist repeats the two words in random order while the child is instructed to point to the respective picture. If the response is correct seven consecutive times, the therapist can be reasonably certain that the client is differentiating between the two sounds.

It is advised that if the criterion level of seven correct discriminations in a row cannot be reached, poor auditory discrimination or memory skills may be the cause. These skills will then need to be addressed before continuing with the program.

Step 3: Production Training. This phase is directed toward the elicitation of the minimal pair words. The child is instructed to be the teacher, saying the words while the therapist points to the correct picture. In the selection of the target sound for the minimal pairs, the child can produce one of the sounds chosen while the other is not in the child's inventory. If the target sound is stimulable, the child will probably be able to contrast the minimal pair. If the target sound is not stimulable, which is typically the case, the child will say one word of the pair incorrectly. For example, in the previous example, [f] and [p] were selected. The child could produce [p] but not [f]. If the child says [pɪn] for *pin* and [pɪn] for *fin,* the therapist will point to *pin* both times; that is, the therapist will point to a word not intended by the child. Blache (1989) states, "The therapist then uses traditional cues to elicit the distinctive feature property" (p. 368). If the child cannot articulate the sound correctly, a traditional or motor approach could be implemented to achieve the sound at the *word level.* The word level is emphasized as the minimal unit. Immediate reinforcement should follow the correct sound production.

Step 4: Carryover Training. Once the target word can be accurately articulated, the following sequence is suggested:

Model	Example
"a" + word	a pig, a fig
"the" + word	the pig, the fig
"Touch the" + word	Touch the pig, Touch the fig
"Point to the" + word	Point to the pig, Point to the fig
longer expressions + word	That is a big pig, That is a big fig

The following additional treatment suggestions are summarized from Lowe (1994).

Therapy is structured so that the child is placed in a situation in which the production of the sound substitution results in a communication breakdown. This breakdown focuses attention on the contrastive function of the phoneme in question. The child will probably attempt to repair the communicative situation by producing the intended target sound in an appropriate manner.

After having identified the substitution and minimal pairs appropriate to the age and interests of the child, the following procedure is implemented:

1. Familiarize the client with the minimal pair words by showing pictures of each word, describing the attributes of each concept, or actually providing concrete objects as examples.

2. Show several exemplars of each word. The client must pick up the picture named by the clinician. In the [θ-s] example with the minimal pair *thing-sing,* the clinician could show different types of "things" versus various people singing.

3. Reverse roles: The client must name one of the words and the clinician picks up the appropriate picture.

4. Substituted sounds result in the clinician picking up the picture actually named, not

the one the child intended. A communicative breakdown has occurred due to inaccurate realization of the target sound.

5. Opportunity is given for the child to make some form of repair (attempts somehow to produce the sound in a different manner). The clinician rewards the attempt by picking up the intended picture.

CLINICAL APPLICATION

Selecting a Target for Minimal Opposition Contrast Therapy

The following substitutions are noted in the speech of the child H. H.

Substitution	Main Production Differences
[tʃ] → [t]	place, manner
[dʒ] → [d]	place, manner
[k] → [t]	place
[g] → [d]	place
[f] → [b]	manner, voicing
[θ] → [b]	place, manner, voicing
[ð] → [d]	place, manner
[ʃ] → [d]	place, manner, voicing
[ʃ] → [s]	place
[s] → [t]	manner
[z] → [t]	manner, voicing
[r] → [w]	place, manner
[l] → [w]	place, manner

Four substitutions are candidates for this approach: [k-t], [g-d], [ʃ-s], and [s-t]. Stimulability of the sounds would need to be ascertained before target sounds could be selected. If all are stimulable, [k] and [t] would be a good choice because they are early developing sounds.

Maximal Oppositions Approach

What Is the Maximal Oppositions Approach?
This treatment method is similar to minimal opposition contrasts in that minimal word pairs are used as the beginning unit of training. However, in direct contrast to minimal opposition contrasts, in which target sounds that are productionally similar are selected, the maximal oppositions approach chooses sounds that are productionally very different. Differences in production were originally defined (Elbert and Gierut, 1986; Gierut, 1989) according to the number of variations in place, manner, or voicing between the two sounds. If possible, sounds were then selected that demonstrated differences in all three production features.

In the meantime, the conceptual framework for this therapy has changed somewhat. Currently, the term *maximal oppositions* refers to differences in distinctive features. These differences vary along two dimensions: (1) the number of unique features that differentiate between the two phonemes and (2) the nature of the features—that is, if differences are major or nonmajor class features. The Chomsky-Halle (1968) system, which defines major class features as consonantal, sonorant, and vocalic, is used.

The concept of maximal oppositions training was first introduced by Elbert and Gierut (1986) in response to their continuum of productive phonological knowledge (see Chapter 7). A series of investigations (Dinnsen and Elbert, 1984; Elbert, Dinnsen, and Powell, 1984; Gierut, 1985) examined the relationship between "most" and "least" phonological knowledge and the amount of generalization that occurred within the phonological system of children. In one of these studies, findings indicated that children treated in the order of least to most phonological knowledge showed generalization across the overall sound system (Gierut, 1985). In other words, if treatment focused first on sounds that the child could not produce (consistent "error" productions) and only later targeted sounds that appeared in some contexts (inconsistent "error" productions), the most generalization occurred. On the other hand, if the order of treatment proceeded from most to least phonological knowledge, generalization was very limited. These findings led to the development of the maximal oppositions approach.

When to Use the Maximal Oppositions Approach. Which clients benefit most from maximal oppositions training? By examining the children in the series of investigations conducted to demonstrate this method, (Gierut, 1990, 1992), most subjects had at least six sounds that were missing from their phonetic and phonemic inventories. This suggests that clients who would benefit the most from this intervention strategy would be those with moderate to severe phonological disorders.

The maximal oppositions technique has been described in several research investigations in which its efficacy has been tested on several children. Gierut (1989) reported that after three different word pairs contrasting maximal oppositions had been presented, the child learned sixteen word-initial consonants and restructured his phonological system. Other studies (Gierut, 1990, 1991, 1992; Gierut and Neumann, 1992) supported these findings. When minimal versus maximal oppositions approaches were therapeutically contrasted, more generalization occurred using maximal contrasts (Gierut, 1990). Other studies challenged one of the basic principles of minimal pair therapy, the selection of sounds based on the concept of "substitution" and "error" sounds (Gierut, 1991, 1992; Gierut and Neumann, 1992). If both sounds used to establish word pairs were *not* in the child's inventory, this proved to be as effective as, or at times even more effective than, teaching one sound versus its substitution. In the last of the series of investigations, word pairs comparing two previously unknown phonemes that differed by maximal and major class features were found to be the preferred way to change the phonological system of the child (Gierut, 1992). Research findings seem to support the efficacy of maximal oppositions therapy.

How to Select Target Sounds for the Maximal Oppositions Approach. Between the earlier and the later versions of maximal oppositions therapy, the procedure for target selection changed (Elbert and Gierut, 1986; Gierut, 1989, 1992). Only the later selection procedures will be outlined here.

Two sounds not in the child's inventory (i.e., two unknown sounds) are selected. In addition, these two sounds should be maximally different according to their distinctive features. Two parameters are used to determine the maximum distinctive feature differences: (1) the number of unique distinctive features that differentiate the two sounds (more distinctive feature differences = maximum feature distinction) and (2) the nature of the feature—that is, whether it is a major or nonmajor feature class (major class features = maximum feature distinction) (see Box 9.1). Major class features are:

[+ vocalic]   differentiates vowels and liquids

from

stops, fricatives, affricates, nasals, and [h]

[+ consonantal]   differentiates stops, fricatives, affricates, nasals, and liquids

from

vowels, glides, and [h]

[+ sonorant]   differentiates nasals, liquids, glides, and [h]

from

stops, fricatives, and affricates

BOX 9.1   Major Class Features

Sonorants	Consonantal	Vocalic
vowels +	stops +	vowels +
glides +	fricatives +	liquids +
nasals +	affricates +	stops –
liquids +	nasals+	fricatives –
[h] +	liquids +	affricates –
stops –	vowels –	nasals –
fricatives –	glides –	[h] –
affricates –	[h] –	

Distinctive Feature Differences
Number of Features Excluding Major Class Features

	p	b	t	d	k	g	f	v	s	z	ʃ	ʒ	θ	ð	tʃ	dʒ
r	4	3	3	2	5	4	4	3	3	2	3	2	2	1	5	4
l	4	3	3	2	7	6	4	3	3	2	5	4	2	1	7	6
w	6	5	7	6	3	2	6	5	7	6	5	4	6	5	7	6
j	4	3	5	4	3	2	4	3	5	4	3	2	4	3	5	4
h	3	4	4	5	4	5	3	4	4	5	4	5	3	4	6	7

The following example (Subject 11 from Gierut, 1992) is given to illustrate the selection process used in maximum feature distinctions.

Inventory	Sounds Not in Inventory	Major Class Difference
m, n, ŋ, w, j, h,	r, l	
p, b, t, d,	k, g	yes, between r, l versus k, g
f, v, tʃ, dʒ	s, z, ʃ, ʒ, θ, ð	yes, between r, l versus s, z, ʃ, ʒ, θ, ð

Major class differences are evidenced between /r/ and /l/ and several other phonemes. Because both /r/ and /l/ are [+ voice], the voiceless consonants [– voice] would demonstrate one more distinctive feature difference than the voiced consonants. When feature differences are counted between the noted voiceless consonants and /r/ and /l/, the following number of distinctive feature differences emerges:

[r] and [k] = 5	[l] and [k] = 7
[r] and [s] = 3	[l] and [s] = 3
[r] and [ʃ] = 3	[l] and [ʃ] = 5
[r] and [θ] = 2	[l] and [θ] = 2

Note: The categories sonorant, consonantal, and vocalic are not counted again when figuring the number of distinctive features.

Therefore, considering both major class distinctions and the differences in distinctive features, the target phonemes would be /l/ and /k/. These phonemes would then be utilized to form minimal pairs such as *lane-cane, leg-keg,* and *lamp-camp.*

How Is the Maximal Oppositions Contrast Approach Used?

The perception of, or discrimination between, the phonological contrast is not directly trained; rather, treatment includes two phases, *imitation* and *spontaneous production,* for each sound pair. However, it should be noted in this context that this treatment protocol originated from a research project comparing different word pairs and their impact on changes within the phonological systems of children. For clinical purposes, practitioners may want to implement additional activities to serve the needs of individual clients.

Imitation Phase.   Minimal pair picture cards are presented and the client asked to repeat the clinician's model of the pictures. Several different activities can be used to maintain interest, such as matching or sorting pictures during imitative production, moving a car around one space on a track each time the word is imitated, playing various card games with the pictures, and so on. This phase of treatment continues until 75 percent imitative accuracy over two to maximally seven consecutive sessions is achieved.

Spontaneous Phase.   Word pairs are now produced by the client without the clinician's model. Again, various activities can be found to keep the child's interest. This phase continues until 90 percent accurate production without a model over three to maximally twelve consecutive sessions is achieved.

CLINICAL APPLICATION

Selecting Target Sounds with the Maximal Oppositions Approach

The following results are provided for H. H.

Inventory	Sounds Not in Inventory	Major Class Difference
m, n, ŋ		
w, j, h	r, l	
p, b, t, d	k, g	yes, between r, l versus k, g
f, v, s*	tʃ, ʤ, z, ʃ, θ, ð	yes, between r, l versus z, ʃ, ʒ, tʃ, ʤ, θ, ð

Major class differences are evidenced between /r/ and /l/ and several other phonemes. Because both /r/ and /l/ are [+ voice], the voiceless consonants [– voice] would render more distinctive feature differences. When feature differences are counted between the noted voiceless consonants and /r/ and /l/, the highest number of feature differences exists between /l/–/k/ and /l/–/tʃ/ (seven different features). Therefore, previously noted word pairs for /l/ and /k/ or word pairs such as *lane* versus *chain* and *Lynn* versus *chin* could be used in this maximal oppositions approach.

*[f] and [v] were each produced correctly one time during the articulation test; [s] was used as a substitution for [ʃ].

Multiple Oppositions Approach

What Is the Multiple Oppositions Approach?

This treatment method, developed by Williams (1992, 2000a, 2000b), is an alternative approach to contrastive minimal pairs. The approach directly addresses the collapse of multiple phonemes. For the child with extensive phoneme collapses, homonymy results in which two or more words are pronounced alike but have different meanings. This has a negative effect on the intelligibility and thus communication breakdowns result. In the multiple oppositions approach, the child is confronted with several sounds simultaneously within one phoneme collapse. The supposition is that by treating a larger number of contrasts, several phonemic oppositions could be added to the child's system. This should result in a shortened length of treatment, improved intelligibility, and more efficient intervention.

When to Use the Multiple Oppositions Approach.
According to Williams (2000a), this approach is for the treatment of severe speech disorders in children. When evaluating the method in an efficacy study, the children included for treatment exhibited moderate-to-profound phonological impairments. This was defined as the exclusion of at least six sounds across three manner categories. Because this treatment protocol is specifically designed to treat the collapse of multiple phonemic contrasts, the children should definitely demonstrate a collapse of phonemic contrasts that incorporates several different sounds.

Children who were treated using this method all demonstrated documented improvement. Although children who were more severe required a longer time to reach the generalization stage, system-wide changes were especially noted in the children with the most severe disorders.

How to Select Target Sounds for the Multiple Oppositions Approach. Selection of treatment targets is based on phonemic factors. Both maximal distinctions and maximal classifications are used to guide target selection. Maximal distinctions, similar to the maximal oppositions method, are those that are maximally different from the child's error. Maximal classifications indicate that those targets selected differ maximally in respect to place, voice, and manner. In addition, the child's unique organizational structure is considered. Sounds that have the potential for the greatest impact on the child's phonological reorganization should be targeted.

For example, the following demonstrates one phonemic collapse noted in our case study child H. H.:

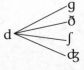

In this case [d] would be contrasted with [g], [ð], [ʃ], and [ʤ] in minimal pair sets (from the information supplied, it does not seem as though consonant clusters are targeted). These sounds would then be utilized to form minimal pairs such as *doe–go–though–show–Joe*.

How Is the Multiple Oppositions Approach Used? One treatment paradigm utilizing multiple oppositions with minimal contrast therapy demonstrated positive results (Williams, 2000a). A second study used a specific treatment paradigm (Williams, Epperly, Rodgers, and Feltes, 1999) that consisted of four treatment phases: (1) an imitative level until 70 percent accuracy across two consecutive treat-ment sets was obtained, (2) a spontaneous phase when accuracy reached 90 percent across two consecutive treatment sets, (3) spontaneous contrasts or generalization based on 90 percent accuracy of the target sound in untrained words, and (4) a conversation-based phase based on naturalistic intervention procedures. The author notes that some children required a broader-based intervention approach, such as a naturalistic approach, before generalization occurred.

Phonological Process Therapy

What Is Phonological Process Therapy? Phonological processes are often used to assess error patterns in the speech of children. As an assessment tool, its practical application is often traced back to David Ingram's (1976, 1989b) *Phonological Disability in Children.* Since that time, several assessment protocols and tests founded on the concept of phonological processes have been developed (e.g., Bankson and Bernthal, 1990; Dean, Howell, Hill, and Waters, 1990; Grunwell, 1985a; Hodson, 2004; Ingram, 1981; Khan and Lewis, 2002; Lowe, 1996; Shriberg and Kwiatkowski, 1980; Weiner, 1979). Although some therapy

It is fairly easy to construct minimal pairs with the substitution processes. For example, when treating velar fronting, minimal pairs contrasting /t/ and /k/ could be used. However, syllable structure processes are a bit more difficult. Final consonant deletion could be treated by contrasting words that contain a final consonant versus those that do not, for example, *bow* versus *boat*. Minimal pairs could also be constructed for consonant cluster reduction—*street* versus *treat*—and for unstressed syllable deletion—*before* versus *four*. On the other hand, reduplication does not seem to lend itself very effectively to the use of minimal pairs.

methods, such as cycles training or metaphon therapy, utilize phonological process *assessment* to determine training goals, a phonological process *therapy* as such does not exist. Typically, a phonological process is selected and minimal pair contrasts are then employed. If the child can produce the minimal pair distinctions, the phonological process has been suppressed.

In order to bridge the gap between the assessment of phonological errors (see Chapter 7) and their treatment, the following section will describe how minimal contrasts can be established when specific phonological processes have been selected as intervention targets.

When to Use Phonological Process Therapy. Which clients would benefit the most from specific phonological process therapies using minimal contrasts? For the young client whose phonological system is characterized primarily by the persistence of only a limited number of phonological processes, the phonological process therapy approach is probably a viable option. However, for the child who is unintelligible or who demonstrates a wide variety of phonological processes, other approaches that have been or will be discussed in the following sections (cycles train-

ing, maximal oppositions, metaphon therapy) may offer better possibilities.

As mentioned earlier, phonological processes are frequently used to assess patterns of phonemic errors. However, would minimal contrast therapy targeting specific phonological processes also influence their reduction? Weiner (1981) tested this hypothesis with two children using minimal contrast therapy in game activities. Accurate production was required or a breakdown in communication would occur. For example, in attempting to reduce the frequency of occurrence of final consonant deletion, *bow* and *boat* were contrasted. The child had to gather a certain number of pictures of *boat* from the clinician. If the child said *bow* although *boat* was intended, the clinician would pick up the picture of *bow*. A communicative breakdown had ensued. With this intervention method, a reduction of specific phonological processes was achieved, which generalized to nontrained words as well. Based on the results of this one study, phonological process therapy seems to enhance suppression of phonological processes. However, far more research is needed, especially in light of the newer developments multiple and maximal feature distinctions seem to offer.

How to Select Target Sounds with Phonological Process Therapy. Which phonological processes should be chosen for therapy, and how does this choice impact target selection? Phonological processes should be chosen based on

- their relative frequency of occurrence,
- the effect this process has on the client's intelligibility, and
- the age and phonological development of the child.

Good candidates for process selection are those that occur most often in the speech of the child because they will probably affect intelligibility to a higher degree. However, certain phonological processes will have more of an impact on intelligibility than others. For example, the process final consonant deletion affects many different sounds, whereas velar fronting is typically limited to a t/k substitution. Therefore, if a decision must be made between final consonant deletion or velar fronting, final consonant deletion would probably be the process to work on first. Finally, the age of the child must be considered. There are phonological processes that are normally suppressed at an early age, such as reduplication, and others that continue to operate until the end of the preschool years, such as stopping of /θ/ and /ð/. Therefore, earlier processes are typically targeted before later processes.

> For a list of the most common processes and the approximate age of suppression, see Chapters 4 and 5.

An example: A 4;6-year-old child demonstrates a high frequency of occurrence of final consonant deletion, consonant cluster reduction, gliding (/r/ → /w/), and stopping of /θ/ and /ð/. Based on his age and the impact on intelligibility, final consonant deletion would be a good choice for beginning therapy. The others are "late" processes that would probably not affect the intelligibility of a 4-year-old.

After an appropriate phonological process is selected, word pairs must be found for the beginning phase of minimal contrast training. The child's phonetic inventory and the stimulability of specific sounds will often guide the selection. Table 9.2 offers examples for a number of phonological processes.

How Are Minimal Pairs Used with Phonological Processes?

There are many ways these minimal pairs can be used in a therapy situation. Several of them have been discussed in the sections on distinctive feature therapy and minimal and maximal oppositions training.

These activities can be as varied as the clinician's imagination but should always incorporate the client's interest and level of ability. Also, communicative function should stand at the forefront of any activity.

CLINICAL APPLICATION

Selection of a Phonological Process

Consonant cluster reduction, final consonant deletion, and stopping are the most prevalent processes in H. H.'s speech. Consonant cluster reduction is a relatively late process and would therefore not be a good candidate for therapy selection. Final consonant deletion would probably impact the intelligibility of H. H.'s speech the most. Minimal pairs should be found that would contrast a word with a final consonant using a sound that H. H. can realize versus no final consonant. For example, [b] and [t] can be articulated in an acceptable manner but are deleted in word-final position. Selected minimal pairs would be exemplified by *meat* versus *me, boat* versus *bow,* or *tube* versus *two.*

CYCLES TRAINING

What Is Cycles Training?   This approach was developed by Hodson and Paden (1983, 1991). It is referred to as cycles training because the phonological patterns that are to be remediated are trained successively during specific time periods known as cycles. For example, certain patterns are trained for a given period of time in Cycle 1, others in Cycle 2.

This approach is unique for several reasons. First, there is no predetermined level of mastery for phonemes or phoneme patterns within each cycle. Therefore, clients do not have to reach 75 percent or 90 percent accuracy of any phoneme or pattern realization to move to the next cycle. The targeted patterns within the cycle are used to stimulate *emergence* of a specific sound or pattern, not *mastery* of it. The underlying premise for

Table 9.2 Examples for Constructing Minimal Pairs Using Phonological Processes

Substitution Processes	
Underlying Principle:	Construct word pairs with the target sound and the substitution. If the target sound is not stimulable, a traditional approach may be necessary to achieve correct production of the sound within a specific word context.
Velar Fronting	t/k and d/g substitutions: word pairs need to be found contrasting /t/ and /k/ and /d/ and /g/.
	Examples: *tea* versus *key, tape* versus *cape. Dumb* versus *gum, dull* versus *gull.*
Palatal Fronting	s/ʃ substitution: word pairs need to be found contrasting /s/ and /ʃ/.
	Examples: *sip* versus *ship, sell* versus *shell.*
Stopping of /s/ and /z/	t/s and d/z substitutions: word pairs need to be found contrasting /t/ and /s/ and /d/ and /z/.
	Examples: *toe* versus *sew, tee* versus *sea. D* versus *Z, do* versus *zoo.*
Gliding /r/ → /w/	w/r substitution: word pairs need to be found contrasting /w/ and /r/.
	Examples: *wed* versus *red, weed* versus *read.*

Unusual Processes	
Stops Replacing Glides /j/ → /d/	d/j substitution: word pairs need to be found contrasting /d/ and /j/.
	Examples: *yacht* versus *dot, yarn* versus *darn.*
Denasalization of /n/ → /d/	d/n substitution: word pairs need to be found contrasting /n/ and /d/.
	Examples: *knot* versus *dot, near* versus *deer.*

Processes Affecting Groups or Classes of Phonemes	
Underlying Principle:	Select contrast pairs containing sounds that the child can produce or are stimulable.
Final Consonant Deletion	Start with word pairs with and without final consonants, such as *bow* versus *boat.* If generalization does not occur, present word pairs contrasting another final consonant against no final consonant.
	Example: Child can produce [m, n, t, d, l, f, v, p, b] but not in word-final position. First, present contrasts such as *toe* versus *toad, low* versus *load.*
Consonant Cluster Reduction	Use singletons within the child's inventory to structure reduced consonant clusters contrasted to standard consonant clusters.
	Example: Cluster reductions are noted on several consonant blends. Child can produce [b], [p], [k], and [l] but says [kaʊn] for *clown,* [peɪ] for *play,* [bu] for *blue.* Begin with [pl] and contrast word pairs such as *plan* versus *pan, peas* versus *please.*
Stopping of Fricatives	Select a stimulable fricative, which is then contrasted with the homorganic stop.
	Example: Child is stimulable for [f] but uses p/f substitution in most contexts. Use word pairs such as *fig* versus *pig, fin* versus *pin.*

Unusual Processes	
Initial Consonant Deletion	Start with word pairs contrasting one initial consonant versus no initial consonant. If generalization does not occur, present word pairs with another initial consonant.
	Example: Child can produce [p, b, t, d, h, w, m, n] but inconsistently deletes these sounds at the beginning of a word. Use word pairs such as *beet* versus *eat*, *bee* versus *E*.
Sound Preference Substitutions	Select a stimulable sound and use it in a contrasting word pair with the sound preference.
	Child produces [s], [z], [ʃ], [tʃ], and [ʤ] as [t]. The child is stimulable for [ʃ]. Contrast word pairs such as *two* versus *shoe*, *top* versus *shop*.

this procedure is based on the known observation that phonological acquisition is gradual. The cycles approach is an attempt to approximate closely the way phonological development normally occurs, as a gradual process. Second, several sounds are targeted within one cycle. Although some of the patterns from Cycle 1 might be "recycled" in the next phase, new sound patterns are also introduced. Third, this approach targets very specific clients: It is explicitly designed for highly unintelligible children. The goal of cycles training is to increase intelligibility within a relatively short period of time. A by-product is the acquisition of certain sounds and patterns.

When to Use Cycles Training. Which clients benefit most from cycles training? This therapy targets highly unintelligible children. "This approach was *not* designed for children with mild speech disorders" (Hodson, 1989, p. 331). Although *highly unintelligible* is not explicitly defined, these children seem to be in the profound to severe range on the Assessment of Phonological Processes—Revised (Hodson, 2004). Utterances of the children in the profound category were characterized by extensive omissions, some phoneme sub-

stitutions, and a very restricted repertoire of consonants. Utterances of the children in the severe category had fewer omissions, but more substitutions and consonant classes were still limited (Hodson and Paden, 1991).

Is cycles training a viable therapy? According to the authors, it was developed, tested, and refined at experimental clinics in which this approach was utilized with over 200 clients (Hodson and Paden, 1991). Hodson (1992) further states that "most clients have been dismissed from our clinic as essentially intelligible in less than 1 year" (p. 252). This would seem to indicate that the cycles approach is an effective treatment method. However, enough research has not yet been conducted to confirm these statements. Bernthal and Bankson (2004) conclude by noting that the authors have a wealth of clinical experience to support this approach to intervention; however, published data, particularly of a comparative nature, are lacking. Further research is needed to verify the efficacy of this treatment approach.

How to Select Target Sounds with Cycles Training. The following are guidelines for potential target patterns or phonemes for Cycle 1

training: primary potential target patterns/
phonemes.

1. *Early developing phonological patterns.*
These patterns are typically present in
very young normally developing children.
Highly unintelligible children should be
assessed to determine their individual
abilities in the following categories. Deficiencies in the following categories would
be potential targets for Cycle 1 training.
   • *Syllableness.* Two- and three-syllable
   equal stress word combinations such
   as *cowboy* or *cowboy hat.* This category
   is evaluated according to whether the
   vowel nuclei exist, not in respect to the
   accurate production of all sounds.
   • *Word-initial singleton consonants.* Includes CV structures with the following
   phonemes: /m, n, p, b, t, d, w/.
   • *Word-final singleton consonants.* Includes VC structures with the following
   phonemes: /p, t/ and/or /k, m, n/.
   • *Other word structures.* Both CVC and VCV
   words are found in the child's speech.
2. *Posterior/anterior contrasts.* The child's
speech is examined to see whether either
alveolar or velar sounds are absent.
3. */s/ clusters.* The child's speech is examined
to see whether /s/ clusters are produced.
Based on clinical experience, the authors
have found that word-final /s/ clusters are
the most facilitating for these children.
Singleton /s/ is not targeted until a later
cycle.
4. *Liquids.* The child's speech is examined
to see whether /l/ and /r/ are produced. If
absent, these phonemes should be stimulated during each cycle.

If the child does not have one or more of
these patterns or phonemes, any of the aforementioned categories would be acceptable
targets for Cycle 1. Target selection of specific

phonemes also depends on the client's stimulability. The clinician should select the client's
most stimulable sounds or patterns so that
the child can experience immediate success.
Unacceptable targets include /ŋ/, /θ/, /ð/, the
syllabic /l/, and weak syllable deletion.

An example: A child demonstrates a high
frequency of occurrence of the following processes: final consonant deletion, consonant
cluster reduction, velar fronting, gliding (w/l
and w/r substitutions), and stridency deletion.
Going down the list of potential primary targets, the following emerge:

1. word-final singleton consonants
2. CVC structures
3. s-clusters
4. liquids
5. velars

Patterns Eliminated

1. Word-final singleton consonants were not
considered a Cycle 1 target because the
child did produce [p], [t], [m], and [n] in
the word-final position.
2. The child was not stimulable for
stridents.

Patterns Targeted

1. CVC structures to stimulate the understanding of final consonants
2. liquids
3. velars

Because the child was not stimulable for stridents, /s/ clusters, which would normally be
a primary target, were delayed until a later
cycle.

How Is Cycles Training Used?

Establishing a Cycle. Each phoneme within a
pattern should be targeted for *sixty minutes per*

cycle. If therapy is thirty minutes per session, two times a week, then the first phoneme would be targeted for one week of therapy. After completion of the first phoneme, a second one is initiated for the next sixty minutes. All remaining phonemes are presented consecutively for sixty minutes each. If the goal is a specific phonological pattern rather than an individual phoneme, at least two exemplars of the pattern should be presented in two consecutive sixty-minute time intervals before moving on to the next phoneme or pattern. For example, if the pattern targeted is CVC structures, then two different CVC word types should be utilized, CVCs with final voiced stops versus final nasals. Only one phonological pattern or phoneme should be targeted during any *one* session. In Cycle 1, all the patterns determined from the assessment are presented consecutively. Typically, this cycle contains between three and six different patterns or phonemes.

Preparing Word Cards for Therapy. Words are used as the minimal unit of production practice, and word cards that picture each of the chosen concepts are developed. Chosen words should be monosyllabic and incorporate facilitative phonetic environments. For example, words containing sounds that are produced at the same place of articulation as the substitute sound should be avoided. Thus, *cat, can, kite,* and *goat* should not be used if the child has a t/k substitution (Hodson, 1989). Object and action words are preferred. Obviously, the words should also be appropriate for the vocabulary level of the child.

Structuring the Remediation Session. The following format is given for each therapy session:

1. *Review.* The child reviews the preceding session's word cards.
2. *Auditory bombardment.* Amplified auditory stimulation is provided for one to two minutes while the clinician reads approximately twelve words that contain the target pattern for this session.
3. *Target word cards.* The client draws, colors, or pastes pictures of three to five target words on large index cards. During this phase, the child repeats the words modeled by the clinician.
4. *Production practice through experiential play.* During experiential play (e.g., fishing, bowling), clinician and child take turns naming the pictures. The clinician provides models and/or tactile cues (such as touching the upper lip of the child to indicate an alveolar sound or the throat to indicate a velar production) so that the child achieves 100 percent success on the target patterns. (This is why it is essential that target words are carefully selected.) Opportunities are also given to engage in conversation to determine whether the pattern is beginning to emerge spontaneously.
5. *Stimulability probes.* The child's stimulability is assessed for potential targets of the next session. For example, if /s/ clusters are prospects for the next session, the child is asked to model several words that contain different /s/ clusters. The most stimulable /s/ cluster is then targeted for the next session.
6. *Auditory bombardment.* Step 2 is repeated.
7. *Home program.* The parent or school aide participates in a two minutes per day home program that consists of reading the week's listening list (Step 2) and the child naming picture cards of the production practice words.

Metaphon Therapy

What Is Metaphon Therapy? Metaphon therapy orginated in the 1980s as a result of dissatisfaction with minimal pair management strategies for phonologically disordered children. In the experience of its developers, Janet Howell and Elizabeth Dean, the use of minimal pair contrasts was often not causing the necessary changes in the child's phonological system. This led to questioning the metaphonological skills of these children. In other words, what do children with phonological disorders know about sounds? The concept of metaphon therapy was born.

Similar to cycles training, metaphon therapy has evolved out of clinical experience and incorporates different approaches that are merged into two therapy phases. However, the framework established to guide therapy is obviously different from that proposed by cycles training. Metaphon therapy is based on metalinguistic awareness. **Metalinguistic awareness** is the ability to think about and reflect on the nature of language and how it functions (Pratt and Grieve, 1983). Specifically, metaphon therapy is structured to develop children's metaphonological skills. Metaphonology is defined as the ability to pay attention to, and reflect on, the phonological structure of language (Howell and Dean, 1991, 1994).

Is there evidence that supports the notion that children with phonological disorders have problems with metaphonological skills? Using different metaphonological tasks, several investigations have demonstrated that children with phonological disorders generally do not perform as well as normally developing children of a similar age (e.g., Bird and Bishop, 1992; Howell, 1989; Kamhi, Friemoth-Lee, and Nelson, 1985; Magnusson, 1983, 1991; Magnusson and Naucler, 1987; Stackhouse, 1985; Stackhouse and Snowling, 1983).

Metaphon therapy also assumes that phonologically disordered children fail to realize the communicative significance of the phonological rule system. Their difficulties do not pertain to producing speech sounds in a normal manner but to their failure to acquire the rules of the phonological system. Howell and Dean (1991, 1994) postulate that the best way to help these children change their rule systems is to provide them with information that will encourage them to make their own changes and thus impact their speech output. The phases of metaphon therapy are constructed in an attempt to provide this knowledge.

When to Use Metaphon Therapy. Which clients can benefit the most from metaphon therapy? Howell and Dean (1991, 1994) target preschool children because it is at this age that metaphonological knowledge is developing. The existing case studies have several features in common: Most of the children presented had very restricted phonetic inventories; all the children had unusual or idiosyncratic processes, such as initial consonant deletion; and all the children had a wide variety of phonological processes operating in their speech. Based on these results, one could conclude that metaphon therapy would be a good match for children who have moderate to severe phonological disorders and who have at least two or three processes that predominate their speech patterns.

Does metaphon therapy work? Both the first and second editions of Howell and Dean's book (1991, 1994) provide the results of an efficacy study that evaluated several aspects of metaphon therapy. Originally, thirteen children participated in the study; according to the second edition, the number of subjects now totals fifty. Preliminary results indicate that metaphon therapy does indeed work. First, the results indicate a reduction in the use of specific phonological processes pre- and posttreatment. Second, changes in the phonological system were accelerated beyond the expected level according to chronological development. Because the children in this study were not divided into treatment versus no-treatment groups, two different measures of language were used to verify whether treatment, not development, was actually responsible for the changes. Pre- and posttreatment scores for phonological processes were compared to those obtained from a second non-treated language area, which was measured by the British Picture Vocabulary Scale (Dunn, Dunn, Whetton, and Pintilie, 1982). Although significant differences could be verified between pre- and posttreatment phonological process scores, the scores from the British Picture Vocabulary Scale remained the same, verifying that treatment, not development, had caused the noted changes. Third, some subjects demonstrated a reduction in the targeted phonological processes, but for others the change was more generalized, causing a reduction in processes that were unrelated to those specifically targeted in treatment. Based on these results, metaphon therapy appears to be a viable therapeutic option, but more controlled studies are needed.

How to Select Target Sounds for Metaphon Therapy.

Dean and Howell (1991, 1994) use the *Metaphon Resource Pack* (Dean, Howell, Hill, and Waters, 1990) as the basis for their assessment procedure. Seventy words (forty-four monosyllabic and twenty-six multisyllabic) are elicited; thirteen different phonological processes are identified.

Howell and Dean provide the following general considerations that influence the choice among the processes to be treated:

1. Processes selected for treatment should not be those that are seen in normally developing children of the same age.
2. Variable use of a simplifying process, which may be evidence of spontaneous change in the child's phonological system, should be given priority in the selection process.

3. The effect the operation of the phonological process has on the intelligibility of the child is important. Processes that cause more disruption, such as stopping of fricatives or atypical processes, should be given priority.
4. The sounds available to the child, both spontaneously and on an imitative basis, play a role in the selection process; sounds that are not in the inventory but can be imitated are usually given priority.

An example: A child, age 4;4, demonstrates the following processes with an occurrence of over 50 percent:

Velar fronting	Word-initial and -final positions
Stopping of fricatives	All positions
Stopping of affricates	All positions
Initial consonant deletion	Limited to fricatives
Initial consonant cluster reduction/deletion	All contexts
Phonetic inventory:	[m, n, ŋ]
	[p, b, t, d, k, g]
	[w, j]
	[l]

Based on the child's age, velar fronting, stopping of fricatives, and initial fricative deletion were all potential target processes. Consonant cluster reduction could be seen as a consequence of the child's lack of fricatives and of the limited phonetic inventory. Velar fronting was chosen as the first target because the child did show evidence of suppression of this process in some contexts. Initial fricative deletion was selected as the second target on the grounds that the introduction of fricatives might generalize, eliminating the stopping of fricatives as well.

How Is Metaphon Therapy Used? There are two therapy phases. Phase 1 is designed to develop the awareness of the properties of sounds. This is done in a motivating setting where success is facilitated. Phase 1 is the most important phase because it forms the basis for the application to more realistic communicative settings emphasized in Phase 2.

Phase 1 Therapy: Developing Phonological Awareness. The primary aim of Phase 1 is to capture the child's interest in sounds and the entire sound system. Although this is a natural activity of normally developing preschoolers, Howell and Dean (1991, 1994) believe that such awareness has not been possible for the child with phonological disorders. The child and the clinician explore the properties of sounds together, how sounds differ from each other (i.e., place, manner, and voicing distinctions), and the importance of realizing these distinctions.

Phase 1 therapy is divided into four levels: concept level, sound level, phoneme level, and word level. Although the emphasis is somewhat different depending on whether the target selection is a substitution or a syllable structure process, each client moves through each of the levels with each process. Throughout Phase 1, the child remains a listener only.

Therapy for Substitution Processes

1. *Concept level.* During the discussion and exploration of sounds with the child, it is essential that there is a shared understanding of the vocabulary and concepts utilized. At the concept level, the child and the clinician play games that involve this vocabulary when talking about different classes of sounds. At this level, individual speech sounds are not contrasted; rather, some of their characteristics—such as long versus short, front versus back,

and noisy versus whisper—are considered. The child plays games such as matching long and short socks, ribbons, or strings; putting bricks at the front or back of the house; and growling noisily and in a whisper to identify the respective characteristics as a preparation for later place-manner-voicing comparisons of actual speech sounds. One hundred percent success should be achieved at this level. Therapy at this level may be brief, depending on the child's success.

2. *Sound level.* In this phase, the previous achievements are transferred to the description of sounds in general. Games might involve musical instruments, noisemaking rattles, shakers, and vocalizations made by the therapist and child, such as lions "roaring," people "singing," and cars "racing." The aim is to show that all sounds can be classified according to the dimensions specified in the concept level, that is, long–short, front–back, and noisy–whisper.

3. *Phoneme level.* After having achieved success at the first two levels, the client is now ready to move on to activities involving speech sounds. The child and clinician take turns producing a range of sounds that vary along the three dimensions previously indicated. Individual sounds are not yet the focus; rather, all sounds from one class are contrasted with sounds from another (e.g., different stops are contrasted with various fricatives). The respective speech sounds may be produced spontaneously or in response to a visual referent (a card with a mnemonic of the property in question). See Figure 9.1 for an example of Mr. Noisy and Mr. Whisper. At this level, speech sound activities can also be paired with those introduced at the concept level—for example, first the matching of long and short strings and then the identification of long and short sounds.

4. *Word level.* After the phoneme level, minimal pairs of words containing the targeted

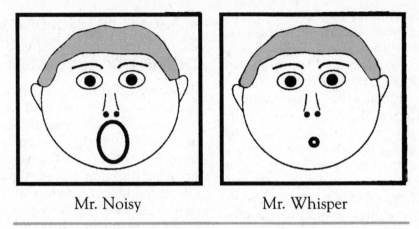

Mr. Noisy   Mr. Whisper

Figure 9.1 Examples of Mr. Noisy and Mr. Whisper

Source: Reproduced with permission from *Treating Phonological Disorders in Children: Metaphon-Theory to Practice* (p. 12), by Janet Howell and Elizabeth Dean, 1994, London: Whurr Publishers.

contrast are introduced. The client is asked to make a judgment about whether the sound is, for example, long or short, front or back, or noisy or whispered. Although the client is only a listener at this level, some discussion about the sound properties are included. For example, a noisy (voiced) sound is identified and then knowledge of other "noisy" sounds is questioned. Later, other minimal pair words may be introduced. In addition, visual referents used in previous levels may be placed on the back of the card to provide additional feedback about the target item.

Therapy for Syllable Structure Processes

1. *Concept level.* For syllable structure processes, such as initial or final consonant deletion, other concepts will be introduced, such as "beginning" and "end," for instance. These could be exemplified by the engine at the beginning of the train and the caboose at the end, or the nose of the alligator at the beginning and the tail at the end. If cluster simpli-

fication is the target, suitable contrasts could consist of the concepts of one horse in front of the wagon, two engines pulling the train, or three dogs pulling the sled.

2. *Syllable level/Word level.* At this stage, syllables representing the targeted contrast are utilized. For initial consonant deletion, for example, V and CV structures with nonsense syllables could be introduced with the analogy of a train with no engine versus one with an engine. Because it will not always be appropriate and motivating to stay with nonsense syllables, some words might be selected as well.

Phase 2 Therapy: Developing Phonological and Communicative Awareness. The link between Phases 1 and 2 is established by incorporating Phase 1 activities into Phase 2. Phonological awareness needs to be well developed before Phase 2 will be successful. Both Phase 1 and Phase 2 activities are essential for the core activity.

The core activity is structured so that the clinician and the client are taking turns in producing minimal pair words. If the child says the word pictured on the card accurately, positive feedback is given and expanded into a relevant discussion. For example: "Right, that was a noisy sound. I bet you know lots of other noisy sounds." If, however, the child produces one of the minimal pair words incorrectly, intending the other word, the clinician picks the word that was said, not the intended one. This may stimulate the child to produce a spontaneous repair. The clinician never comments directly on the child's inappropriate production of a particular word but draws the child's attention to the salient features of the contrast: "That was a noisy sound. Should it have been a whisper sound?" Phase 1 activities can be used prior to or after the core activity.

There are no instructions regarding the child who repeatedly does not produce the sound or sound pattern in question correctly. One assumes that one goes back to Phase 1 activities. Therefore, for children who are not stimulable for a particular sound and remain unstimulable throughout Phase 1, Phase 2 could prove to be frustrating. In a later portion of the text, Howell and Dean suggest, based on the child's increased metalinguistic awareness, a discussion of the reasons for the loss of contrast. "Referring to sounds in a way which allows children to discuss them allows specific exploration of the reasons why a child has failed to convey meaning" (Howell and Dean, 1994, p. 110).

The last phase moves the minimal word pairs into sentences such as "Put the picture of the pea/key in the box," and "Draw a picture of the pea/key on the board." Situations that facilitate communication and promote repairing communicative breakdowns are important variables. It is also stressed that a supportive environment is an essential ingredient of this therapy.

PHONEMIC DISORDERS WITH CONCURRENT LANGUAGE PROBLEMS: THERAPEUTIC SUGGESTIONS

Phonological disorders often co-occur with language disorders. Tyler and Watterson (1991) estimated a co-occurrence rate in preschoolers of between 60 and 80 percent. Based on data from 178 children with developmental phonological disorders, Shriberg and Kwiatkowski (1994) found that between 50 and 70 percent of these children had co-occurring expressive language problems, while 10 to 40 percent evidenced a delay in language comprehension as well. Other studies (Bishop and Edmundson, 1987; Shriberg, 1991; Shriberg, Kwiatkowski, Best, Hengst, and Terselic-Weber, 1986) support these statistics. Thus, most of the children seen clinically for a phonological disorder will also demonstrate other language problems.

The relationship between phonology and other areas of language is a complex one. A synergistic model of language (Schwartz, Leonard, Folger, and Wilcox, 1980; Shriner, Holloway, and Daniloff, 1969) proposes an intricate web of interdependencies between various aspects of language. This view has been tested by several investigations that examined specific remediation interactions between phonology and syntax in children with phonological disorders (Fey et al., 1994; Hoffman, Norris, and Monjure, 1990; Matheny and Panagos, 1978; Panagos, Quine, and Klich, 1979; Paul and Shriberg, 1982; Tyler and Watterson, 1991).

One hypothesis tested was whether treatment of one area, either phonology or syntax, would impact the other. Matheny and Panagos (1978) found a positive interaction between phonology and syntax; that is, instruction in either phonology or syntax resulted in gains in the other area also. With a slightly different conceptual basis, Hoffman, Norris, and

Monjure (1990) examined the impact of a whole language approach versus phonological instruction alone on the language abilities of two children. Language abilities were measured by a comprehensive language test, an articulation test, an index of phonological processes, and a narrative task. Both children's overall language skills increased. As might be expected, the child with a whole language approach showed greater improvement in expressive language skills (as measured by the narrative task), whereas the child with phonological instruction demonstrated more improvement in phonological skills (as measured by the articulation and phonological processes tests). These results seem to indicate that phonological intervention does impact other language areas and that language-based treatment might also have a positive influence on the child's phonological system.

However, other investigations have not supported these results (Fey et al., 1994; Tyler and Watterson, 1991). Based on their findings, Tyler and Watterson (1991) suggested that children with more severe deficits may not evidence generalization from one language area to another, whereas children with mild to moderate difficulties may benefit from therapy with either a phonological or a language-based approach. Fey and colleagues (1994), in a carefully controlled investigation with twenty-six children ages 44 to 70 months, examined the impact of two different types of language instruction on the phonological abilities of their subjects. Although the grammar of these children was affected by the training, there was no direct effect on the children's phonological skills. One of the conclusions of Fey and colleagues (1994) is that

> the strategy of trying to improve intelligibility by focusing intervention on grammar (or even broader discourse patterns) is not defensible at this time. . . . For most children who have impairments in both speech and language, we believe that some

> clinical attention must be focused directly on both areas. (p. 605)

Although more research is needed on the interaction of phonology with other language areas, it is currently safe to say that (1) most children with phonological disorders will also demonstrate language difficulties and (2) intervention will need to target both phonology and any additional deficient language areas. To achieve this, a specified amount of time could be allotted to each deficient area: phonology, morphosyntax, semantics, or pragmatics. It would, of course, be more time efficient if some language therapy goals could be unified. In the following section, some suggestions will be offered on how specific phonological remediation goals could be combined with noted morphosyntactic and semantic problems. Although divisions into morphosyntax and semantics, for example, are made to aid organization, it should always be kept in mind that a complex interaction exists between all language components. The next section addresses only some of the more common difficulties observed in children with language impairments.

Connecting Phonology to Morphosyntax

Various morphological problems in children with specific language impairment (SLI) have often been observed (e.g., Bishop, 1994; Eyer and Leonard, 1994; Johnston and Schery, 1976; Khan and James, 1983; Leonard, 1994; Leonard, McGregor, and Allen, 1992; Oetting and Horohov, 1997; Oetting and Rice, 1993; Paul and Shriberg, 1982; Rice and Oetting, 1993; Rice, Wexler, and Cleave, 1995). Based on findings of several of these investigations, Leonard, McGregor, and Allen (1992) summarized the grammatical morphemes that were used less frequently by SLI children. These results are listed in Table 9.3.

Table 9.3 Problematic Morphemes for Children with Specific Language Impairment

Grammatical Morpheme	Examples
Present progressive -ing*	swimming, eating
Plural -s	coats, shoes
Preposition on	on the table, on top
Possessive 's	Daddy's, dog's
Regular past tense -ed	walked, stopped
Irregular past tense	caught, drank
Regular third person -s	he hits, she throws
Articles a and the	a sweater, the man
Copula	He is tall, She's happy
Auxiliary be	They are singing, She's talking

Source: Adapted from Leonard, McGregor, and Allen (1992).

*This grammatical morpheme is least likely to reveal a difference between children with and without language disorders, although in some studies, children with language impairments also evidenced difficulty.

If this list of grammatical morphemes is examined according to their production difficulties, it becomes clear that phonologically disordered children might have problems actually producing some of them. Plurality, past tense -ed, possessive, and third-person singular, for example, very often result in word-final consonant clusters. If the child deletes final consonants or reduces consonant clusters, the grammatical function of these morphemes will be lost. Even for the child displaying primarily substitution processes, these morphemes may not be realized accurately. In order to preserve morphemic contrasts, attention must be given to final consonants and consonant clusters when working with the child with a phonological disorder.

Remediation Suggestions

1. If a therapy goal is final-consonant deletion, words that incorporate specific grammatical morphemes in contrasting word pairs could be targeted. The use of such pairs will depend on the sounds in the client's inventory and the targeted sound(s), but, whenever possible, aspects of morphology could be included, especially grammatical morphemes. The following are given as examples:

Grammatical morpheme	Examples
Plurality	toe-toes, key-keys, shoe-shoes
Possessive	Joe-Joe's, Ray-Ray's
Regular past tense	row-rowed, lay-laid, show-showed
3rd-person singular	I go–he goes, I do–he does

2. If a therapy goal pertains to consonant cluster reduction or deletion, contrastive word pairs like these incorporate grammatical morphemes:

Grammatical morpheme	Examples
Plurality	boat-boats, cup-cups, wheel-wheels
Possessive	cat-cat's, Dad-Dad's, dog-dog's
Regular past tense	walk-walked, kiss-kissed
3rd-person singular	I walk–he walks, I drink–he drinks
Irregular past tense	drink-drank, hold-held

3. In sentences that are more conversationally based, minimal pair words could be used systematically to represent other grammatical morphemes:

Grammatical morpheme	Examples
Copula	She is sad versus She is mad
	He is tall versus He is small
Auxiliary	He is shopping versus
	He is hopping
	She is kissing versus
	She is hissing
Preposition *on*	on the toe versus on the go
	on his hat versus on his bat

4. In sentences that are more conversationally based, subject and object pronouns could be systematically used:

	Examples
Subject pronouns	She is here versus He is here
	She opened the door versus Lee opened the door
	She has the tea versus She has the key
	He helped the man versus We helped the man
Object pronouns	Give it to Jim versus Give it to him
	The tea belongs to her versus The key belongs to her

5. Length and complexity of the utterance also needs to be considered as syntactical complexity has an effect on productional accuracy (Panagos, Quine, and Klich, 1979; Schmauch, Panagos, and Klich, 1978). The more complex the syntax, the more likely a child will demonstrate a breakdown in articulatory accuracy. Although one therapeutic goal may be to increase the length and complexity of a child's utterances, this should always be evaluated with respect to the interaction between production accuracy and syntactic complexity.

Connecting Phonology to Semantics

The majority of research on the semantic limitations in children with language impairments has focused on their use of nouns (Leonard, 1988; Rice, 1991). Such studies have found that language-impaired children are slow in using their first words, and subsequent vocabulary development occurs at a slower rate than in normally developing children. More recent literature has also examined the use of verbs in language-impaired children (Conti-Ramsden and Jones, 1997; Fletcher and Peters, 1984; King and Fletcher, 1993; Paul, 1993; Rice, 1994; Rice and Bode, 1993; Rice, Wexler, and Cleave, 1995; Watkins, Rice, and Moltz, 1993). These studies suggest that verbs and verb-related grammatical properties may be a particular problem for children with language impairments.

Remediation Suggestions

1. Although minimal pair words typically incorporate nouns ("things" are easier to picture), various verbs could also be targeted. These could be selected in accordance with the child's targeted sound or process. Some examples:

Velar fronting   [t/k] substitution
take-cake, tan-can, taught-caught

Stopping of fricatives   [t/s]
tea-see, toe-sew, tip-sip

Final consonant deletion
shoe-shoot, ray-rake, say-sail, go-goat

Initial consonant deletion
eat-beat, add-sad, add-mad

2. When targeted sounds emerge in the child's speech, expand vocabulary with new words containing the target. Research on the acquisition of newly acquired words in normally developing children (Leonard, Schwartz, Morris, and Chapman, 1981; Schwartz and Leonard, 1982) indicates that children appear to learn more easily and quickly new words that begin with consonants they have used previously in other words. Therefore, if a targeted sound is emerging in the child's speech, the clinician could try to utilize new practice words that also expand the vocabulary of the child.

THE CHILD WITH AN EMERGING PHONOLOGICAL SYSTEM: THERAPEUTIC SUGGESTIONS

As previously noted, the term *emerging phonological system* refers to a time period when sounds are beginning to be used to form conventional words—in other words, to the emergence of expressive language. By age 2, normally developing toddlers begin to combine single words into two-word utterances. However, this communicative development seems to lag behind in some 2-year-olds. Children whose comprehension abilities are considered normal but who fail to achieve a fifty-word vocabulary and two-word combinations by age 2 are referred to as "late talkers," toddlers with "slow expressive language development or delay" (Paul and Jennings, 1992; Reed, 1994; Rescorla and Schwartz, 1990), or as children with "specific expressive language impairment" (Paul, 1989; Rescorla and Ratner, 1996). It has been estimated that approximately 10 to 15 percent of the total 2-year-old population meet these criteria (Rescorla, 1989). Half of them seem to outgrow this delay; the other half will continue to demonstrate language problems at age 3 and beyond (Paul, 1991; Paul, Looney, and Dahm, 1991; Rescorla and Schwartz, 1990).

When children with slow expressive language development are compared to norm children of similar ages, their vocalizations occur less often (Paul and Jennings, 1992; Rescorla and Ratner, 1996). In addition, the phonetic profiles of these children show a reduced repertoire of consonants and syllable shapes (Paul and Jennings, 1992). Inventory constraints are especially notable in word-final positions (Rescorla and Ratner, 1996).

To evaluate the child's emerging phonological system, an independent analysis was suggested in Chapter 6. Such an analysis does examine the child's productions of individual words, but the utterances are not compared to the adult model. At this point in the child's development, it is far more important to note the child's actual usage of specific sounds within words. To this end, two types of data need to be collected: (1) the inventory of speech sounds and (2) the syllable shapes used.

General remediation strategies for children with slow emerging language development include developing expressive language skills, specifically expanding the number of vocabulary items, the consonant inventory, the syllable shapes, and finally the use of two-word utterances (Paul, 2007). At this stage of the child's development, therapy must represent a unified package. Therapy to promote phonological skills needs to be combined with increasing the child's lexicon. The use of specific syllable shapes will also be a consideration when selecting which words to target. Remediation for the child with an emerging language system must account for the interdependencies that exist between all language areas.

The following suggestions provide some points to consider when choosing the first words for children with small expressive vocabularies. The consonant inventory and the syllable shapes the child uses will be especially important variables in this selection process.

Combining Phonology with Semantics: Developing a Lexicon

1. First, the child's consonant inventory needs to be considered. Early vocabularies are influenced by the phonological composition of the word. Words that are easier for children to produce are more likely to be included in their early vocabularies (Leonard, Schwartz, Folger, Newhoff, and Wilcox, 1979; Stoel-Gammon and Cooper, 1984). In addition, children appear to learn more easily and quickly new words that begin with consonants they have used previously in other words (Leonard, Schwartz, Morris, and Chapman, 1981; Schwartz and Leonard, 1982). Therefore, new words that contain sounds already in the child's inventory should be targeted.

An example: The child's inventory contains the following sounds:

[m, n]
[p, b, t, d]
[h, j]

Depending on the child's present lexicon, the following might be good word choices:

me, no-no
puppy, baby, bye-bye, teddy, toe
happy, yes

2. The child's present use of syllable shapes needs to be considered. Early syllable shapes include V, CV, CVCV, and CVC. The therapist selects words with syllable shapes the child already uses, possibly including other early syllable shapes. In doing so, it should be kept in mind that the therapy goal is to *expand* the child's use of syllable shapes; therefore, early syllable shapes not in the child's repertoire should also be stimulated.

An example: If the child primarily realizes V, CV, and CVCV syllable shapes:

mama might be easier than *mom*
papa might be easier than *dad*
puppy or *doggie* might be easier than *dog*

kittie might be easier than *cat*
baby might be easier than *doll*

3. When expanding the child's consonant inventory, the normal developmental sequence should be the guiding principle. Children with slow emerging language seem to acquire consonants in the same order as normally developing children, only at a slower rate (Paul and Jennings, 1992). Therefore, early sounds that are not yet in the child's inventory should be targeted. For the child with only a few expressive words, Paul (2007) suggests introducing the sound by first using a babbling game activity rather than by putting it directly into words. The clinician begins by imitating the child's vocalizations. Once a reciprocal babbling exchange is established, the clinician introduces the new consonant into the babbling activity. Paul (2007) emphasizes that the goal of this activity is not to get the child to produce that particular sound but to increase the consonant inventory. Therefore, any new consonant, even if it is not the one modeled by the clinician, should be rewarded.

4. New words should be similar to those used first by normally developing children. These include, for example, names of important people in the child's environment, names for objects the child directly acts on, labels for objects that move and change, actions, games, and routines in which the child is an active participant (Owens, 2008; Pan and Gleason, 2005). Table 9.4 provides some examples of children's earliest words.

5. After having evaluated the child's inventory and use of syllable structures, words from a wide variety of grammatical classes should be selected. Although nouns dominate young children's early speech, children's vocabularies include words from a variety of grammatical classes from the beginning (Bloom, 1973; Nelson, 1973; Pan and Gleason, 2005).

Table 9.4 Children's Earliest Words: Examples from the Vocabularies of Children Younger than 20 Months

Sound effects
baa baa, meow, moo, ouch, uh-oh, woof, yum-yum

Food and drink
apple, banana, cookie, cheese, cracker, juice, milk, water

Animals
bear, bird, bunny, cat, cow, dog, duck, fish, kitty, horse, pig, piggy

Body parts and clothing
diaper, ear, eye, foot, hair, hand, hat, mouth, nose, shoe, toe, tooth

House and outdoors
blanket, chair, cup, door, flower, keys, outside, spoon, tree, TV

People
baby, daddy, gramma, grampa, mommy, [child's own name]

Toys and vehicles
ball, balloon, bike, boat, book, bubbles, plane, toy, truck

Actions
down, eat, go, sit, up

Games and routines
bath, bye, hi, night-night, no, peekaboo, please, shhh, thank you, yes

Adjectives and descriptives
allgone, cold, dirty, hot

Source: From "Semantic Development: Learning the Meanings of Words," by B. Pan and J. Berko Gleason, in *The Development of Language* (4th ed.) (p. 132), edited by J. Berko Gleason, 1997, Boston: Allyn & Bacon. Copyright © 1997 by Allyn & Bacon. Reprinted by permission.

Therefore, not only nouns should be targeted but also words that can be used to talk about the *relations* between objects. These relational words express more communicative functions and can be readily combined with other words into two-word utterances (Lahey, 1988; Lahey and Bloom, 1977). Table 9.5 lists some of the words Lahey and Bloom (1977) and Lahey (1988) proposed for a first lexicon. These one- or two-syllable words include both nouns and relational words as well as representing early syllable shapes.

At this stage in the child's development, articulation patterns will very often not mirror adult pronunciation. However, the therapy focus for these children is on expanding the use of consonants, syllable shapes, and words, not on norm production. Therefore, any word approximations produced by the child should be rewarded, not corrected. For example, if the word is *down* and the child says [daʊ] or [taʊ], this word approximation should be rewarded. Even if the child produces the final [n] in another word, that does not mean the child can produce [n] under different coarticulatory conditions in a new word. The goal during this phase of therapy is to stimulate word production, not articulatory "correctness."

TREATMENT OF MULTIPLE VOWEL ERRORS

There is an abundance of information available about children's difficulties with consonant articulation and their remediation. In contrast, vowel problems have not received the same degree of attention. This has been generally justified by the fact that vowels are mastered at an early age in the child's development. Therefore, children with phonological disorders will probably show few vowel errors. However, this assumption stands in contrast to the documented vowel errors that have been noted in many case studies and in the literature (e.g., Ball and Gibbon, 2002; Beebe, 1957;

Table 9.5   Words for a First Lexicon

Content Category	Relational Words		Substantive Words
	Relational words that are not object specific	Relational words that are more specific to objects but still relate to many objects	
Rejection	no		
Nonexistence or disappearance	no, all gone, away		
Cessation of action	stop, no		
Prohibition of action	no		
Recurrence of objects and actions on objects	more, again, another		
Noting the existence of or identifying objects	this, there, that		
Actions on objects		give, do, make, get, throw, eat, wash, kiss	
Actions involved in locating objects or self		put, up, down, sit, fall, go	
Attributes or descriptions of objects		big, hot, dirty, heavy	
Persons associated with objects (as in possession)			person names

Source: From "Planning a First Lexicon: Which Words to Teach First," by M. Lahey and L. Bloom, 1977, *Journal of Speech and Hearing Disorders, 42,* p. 350. Copyright © 1977 by the American Speech-Language-Hearing Association. Reprinted by permission.

Clark and Goldstein, 1996; Haas, 1963; Hargrove, 1982; Ingram, 1981; Khan, 1988; Leonard and Leonard, 1985; Pollock and Keiser, 1990; Pollock and Swanson, 1986; Renfrew, 1966; Reynolds, 1987, 1990; Stoel-Gammon and Herrington, 1990).

Although vowels are normally among the earliest sounds acquired, it appears that some phonologically disordered chil-dren demonstrate difficulties with regular vowel realizations. Using the Pollock and Keiser (1990) data as an estimate for the frequency of occurrence, one of their fifteen phonologically disordered children had distinct difficulties with vowel productions. This child's speech showed that approximately half of the vowels were in error. Vowel difficulties may well belong to the clinical profile of some children with phonological disorders.

When several studies containing vowel data from children with phonological disorders are reviewed, two patterns seem to emerge (Stoel-Gammon and Herrington, 1990). First, there are children with extremely limited vowel inventories. These children's vowel productions seem to resemble those of the babbling period with lax, nonhigh vowels predominating (Khan, 1988; Leonard and Leonard, 1985; Pollock and Swanson, 1986). A second group demonstrates relatively large vowel inventories but a high incidence of vowel errors—that is, a large number of vowel substitutions (Hargrove, 1982; Ingram, 1981; Stoel-Gammon and Herrington, 1990). The sequence of vowel acquisition in this group of children appeared to be similar to the one for younger normally developing children. In both groups of children with vowel problems, the vowels represented by the corners of the vowel quadrilateral were mastered earlier.

There is very little information available on deviant vowel systems. Although several authors state that some children with phonological disorders do have deviant vowel systems (e.g., Ball and Gibbon, 2002; Grunwell, 1987; Hodson and Paden, 1991; Lowe, 1994; Renfrew, 1966), neither assessment nor remediation procedures are described in these texts. However, more recently, Pollock (1991) described an assessment procedure for identifying vowel errors. In addition, Leonard and Leonard (1985) and Khan (1988) documented the gains that could be made when therapy focused on expanding the vowel inventory of children. Klein (1995) appears to be one of the first to describe therapy for vowel problems in some detail. If a child's vowel inventory is severely restricted or if the child's speech contains a high proportion of vowel substitutions, remediation focusing on vowel distinctions should be implemented.

How disordered should a vowel system be to warrant therapy? Three types of diagnostic information for vowel analysis are suggested: (1) the vowel inventory, (2) the accuracy of production, and (3) error patterns. Examination of the vowel inventory will determine whether the child has a limited or near normal inventory. Data on the accuracy of vowel production will be important when assessing children with a fairly complete vowel inventory but a high proportion of vowel substitutions. The third piece of diagnostic information, error patterns, will be especially valuable when planning therapy. Figure 9.2 is a matrix that can be used to record the vowel inventory of the child. The use of this matrix is similar to the consonant matrix presented in Chapter 7. Accurate and irregular vowel realizations can be recorded directly on the matrix. This will provide the inventory and the number of occurrences of accurate productions. Error patterns can also be identified by comparing the substitutions to the norm productions.

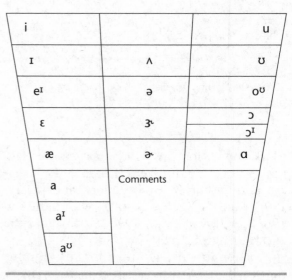

Figure 9.2 Vowel Matrix

The Child with a Very Limited Vowel Inventory: Therapeutic Suggestions

According to the rather limited data available, it appears that the vowel system of these children is characterized by only two or three vowels. These vowels are lax and nonhigh vowels such as [ɑ], [ɛ], [æ], or [ʌ]. Such lax, nonhigh vowels are typical for the babbling period. It can be assumed that the vowel development in these children parallels that of normally developing children. Stoel-Gammon and Herrington (1990) group vowel acquisition into three categories, which were determined after reviewing several studies in respect to the accuracy and the general order of acquisition of vowels in children (Hare, 1983; Irwin and Wong, 1983; Paschall, 1983; Wellman, Case, Mengert, and Bradbury, 1931):

Group 1

Vowels that are mastered relatively early	i, ɑ, u, o, ʌ

Group 2

Vowels acquired somewhere between early and late (some investigations reported early acquisition, others later)	æ, ʊ, ɔ, ə

Group 3

Vowels that are mastered relatively late	e, ɛ, ɪ, ɚ, ɝ

Using One Known and One Unknown Vowel in Minimal Pairs

1. *The child's vowel inventory needs to be compared to those vowels that are mastered relatively early.* A vowel from Group 1 that is productionally very different from one of the child's vowels is selected. For example, if the child has [ɑ], a lax, low-back vowel, the tense high-front vowel [i] would be a good candidate.

2. *The two vowels should be contrasted in minimal pairs.* Whenever possible, consonants from the child's inventory should be used. Examples:

Not in Inventory	In Inventory
me	ma
beet	bought
team	Tom
hee	haw

3. *Other early vowels in minimal contrasts with the original vowel are introduced.* Using the example with [ɑ], another productionally distinct vowel would be [u]. Examples:

Not in Inventory	In Inventory
moo	me, ma
boo	bee
moon	mean
new	knee

Using Two Unknown Vowels in Minimal Pairs

1. *This variation of maximal oppositions uses two unknown vowels in minimal pairs.* Two vowels that are not in the child's inventory should be chosen, if possible, from Group 1. The vowels should again be as productionally different as possible (a distinctive feature analysis could be used to determine the maximal feature distinctions). If the child's inventory includes [ɑ] and [ʌ], [i] and [o] might be selected. These sounds are placed in minimal pairs. Examples:

bean-bone

peek-poke

knee-no

eat-oat

2. *Two different unknown vowels are then targeted.* The selection process should consider the general order of vowel acquisition.

The Child with a High Proportion of Vowel Substitutions: Therapeutic Suggestions

Children with a high proportion of vowel substitutions usually show a relatively intact vowel inventory. An error pattern analysis can be helpful in selecting the target vowels.

This analysis procedure contrasts the target vowel to the substituted vowel. A list of all vowel substitutions together with their relative percentage of occurrence is generated. One possible target could be inconsistent vowel substitutions. For example, the following substitutions are noted:

ɛ/æ, frequency of occurrence = 30 percent

ɪ/æ, frequency of occurrence = 35 percent

correct production of [æ], frequency of occurrence = 35 percent

In this case, the [æ] would be selected as one vowel because of the demonstrated inconsistent substitutions. One of the substitutions for [æ] would be selected as the second vowel. In addition, the substitution chosen should be as productionally different as possible from the target. These two vowels would then be utilized as the vowel nuclei of minimally paired words. Using these criteria, [æ] and [ɪ] would be a good choice. These two vowels are then placed in minimal word pairs. Examples:

mat-mitt

bag-big

pan-pin

ham-him

A second possibility is to target a vowel that is used as a substitution for several different vowels. The following exemplifies this scenario:

Target Vowel	Substitution
i	ɪ
eᴵ	ɑ
ɛ	ɑ
æ	ɑ
ʊ	u

In this case, [ɑ] is used as a substitution for [eᴵ], [ɛ], and [æ]. Therefore, [ɑ] would be contrasted with either [eᴵ], [ɛ], or [æ]. Clear production differences should be given priority when selecting the targeted vowel. Contrasting [ɑ], a lax, low-back vowel to [eᴵ], a diphthong with a mid-high tense onglide, would provide such distinct differences. These two vowels would then be placed in minimal pairs. Examples:

tall-tail

cop-cape

top-tape

Therapy proceeds from vowels with dissimilar to more similar production features. In this example, [ɑ] and [ɛ] would be the next vowels targeted as the nuclei for minimal pairs.

SUMMARY

In this chapter, several different intervention approaches for the treatment of children with phonemic disorders have been described.

Some of these remediation programs use minimal pair contrasts as the beginning unit of remediation—for example, distinctive feature therapy, minimal opposition contrasts, maximum oppositions, maximum oppositions, multiple oppositions, and therapy designed to reduce the use of phonological processes. Other remediation techniques are unique, such as cycles training and metaphon therapy. These two therapy protocols, which have been developed and refined through actual clinical experience, forge together a combination of methods that can be effectively utilized to treat phonological disorders in children.

Discussion of the treatment approaches has been designed to answer specific questions. First: When should this therapy be chosen? Which clients could best be treated with this approach? Guidelines that broadly separate clients who might be better versus poorer candidates for each particular approach were given. Documented research on therapeutic efficacy of each model has also been provided. Second, selection of beginning targets and clinical applications have been supplied to exemplify the transition from assessment to intervention. Third, intervention methods have been outlined in some detail to indicate the utilization of each approach in a therapy setting.

The last portion of this chapter explored and suggested some special applications of phonological therapy. Phonological remediation principles with children displaying concurrent language difficulties and those with emerging phonological systems exemplified the merging of phonological intervention strategies with other language areas such as morphology and semantics. Finally, treatment principles for children with disordered vowel systems were presented to demonstrate how minimal pair contrasts can be structured within a remediation program.

Throughout this chapter, assessment results and their connection to therapy goals have been emphasized. Whenever possible, a direct link has been made between the assessment results outlined in Chapter 7 and the therapy procedures in this chapter. Several clinical applications have been provided to demonstrate the assessment–treatment connection, which is essential for professional speech-language services.

CASE STUDY

The following results are from the Hodson Assessment of Phonological Patterns (HAPP-3) (Hodson, 2004) for Andrew, age 5;6.

1. basket	[bætə]	
2. boats	[boʊ]	
3. candle	[tænə]	
4. chair	[teə]	
5. clouds	[jaʊd]	
6. cowboy hat	[taʊbo æt]	
7. feather	[pɛdə]	
8. fish	[pɪd]	
9. flower	[taʊə]	
10. fork	[pot]	
11. glasses	[jætət]	
12. glove	[dʌb]	
13. gum	[dʌm]	
14. hanger	[hændə]	
15. horse	[hoət]	
16. ice cubes	[aɪt jub]	
17. jumping	[dʌmp]	
18. leaf	[jif]	
19. mask	[mæt]	
20. music box	[mu ɪt bɑt]	
21. page	[peɪd]	

22.	plane	[peˈn]
23.	queen	[twin]
24.	rock	[wɑt]
25.	screwdriver	[dwu dwaˈvə]
26.	shoe	[du]
27.	slide	[jaˈd]
28.	smoke	[boʊt]
29.	snake	[deˈt]
30.	soap	[doʊp]
31.	spoon	[pun]
32.	square	[twɛə]
33.	star	[tɑə]
34.	string	[twɪn]
35.	swimming	[twɪmɪn]
36.	television	[tɛdəbɪdən]
37.	toothbrush	[tubət]
38.	truck	[twʌt]
39.	vase	[beˈd]
40.	watch	[wɑt]
41.	yoyo	[jʌjoʊ]
42.	zip	[jɪp]
43.	crayons	[tweˈən]
44.	black	[bæt]
45.	green	[dwin]
46.	yellow	[jɛjoʊ]
47.	three	[twi]
48.	thumb	[tʌm]
49.	nose	[noʊd]
50.	mouth	[maʊf]

We have decided to use the cycles approach. The following process is used to determine which patterns to target.

1. *Early developing phonological patterns:*
   Syllableness. The child seems to demonstrate evidence of this in words such as *cowboy hat* and *ice cubes.*

Word-initial singleton consonants. The child does use [m] *mouth,* [n] *nose,* [p] *page,* [b] *boats,* [t] *television,* [d] *snake* (although the pronunciation is incorrect, Andrew did use [d] initially), and [w] *watch.*

Word-final singleton consonants. Andrew uses [p] *soap,* [t] *truck* (he substitutes [t] for [k] but [t] is in word-final position), [m] *thumb,* and [n] *spoon.* No [k] is found in the word-final position.

Other word structures. Andrew can produce CVC structures (e.g., *mouth*) and CVCV structures (e.g., *yoyo, feather*)

2. *Posterior/anterior contrasts.* Although alveolar sounds are present, velar sounds are absent in Andrew's speech.

3. *[s] clusters.* Andrew does not seem to be able to produce [s] as a singleton nor in clusters.

4. *Liquids.* Andrew does not demonstrate that he can produce the liquids [l] and [r].

Patterns targeted: Based on stimulability, the following patterns could be targeted.

1. *Anterior–posterior contrasts.* Andrew has [t], therefore the velar [k] would be a target for the first cycle.

2. *[s] clusters.* Hodson and Paden (1991) recommend that word-final [s] clusters be targeted. The clinician would need to see which one(s) might be stimulable.

3. *Liquids.* Andrew does not produce any liquids. Stimulability should be probed on both [l] and [r]. One or both of these could be used in the first cycle.

THINK CRITICALLY

1. Based on the earlier case study from Andrew, age 5;6, we note that the following consonants are not in his inventory: [k], [g], [s], [z], [ʃ], [z], [θ], [ð], [ŋ], [l], and [r]. If you were going to use maximal oppositions, which two sounds would you target? First, find the sounds that have major class feature differences. Second, find the two sounds that have the most distinctive feature differences.

2. Based on the earlier case study from Andrew, age 5;6, note the collapse of phonemic contrasts. For example, the consonants [k], [s], [f] (one time in *flowers*), [ʃ], [tʃ], and [θ] are all collapsed to [t]. What other neutralization of phonemic contrasts can be noted in the articulation test results from Andrew? Use this information to establish treatment targets using the multiple oppositions approach.

TEST YOURSELF

1. Intervention using phonologically based approaches begins at
   a. teaching sounds in isolation
   b. teaching sounds in syllables
   c. the word level using any type of one-syllable words
   d. the word level using minimal pairs
2. Which one of the following pairs would be considered near minimal pairs?
   a. *bird-bad*
   b. *look-lake*
   c. *bird-sir*
   d. *rip-ship*
3. If meaningful minimal pairs cannot be found for contrastive phonemes, what should be used as the alternative?
   a. oral motor exercises
   b. near-minimal pairs
   c. a new set of contrastive phonemes
   d. cycles training
4. Cycles therapy was designed for a specific group of clients—those with
   a. highly unintelligible speech
   b. mild to moderate speech disorders
   c. phonetic errors
   d. [s] and [r] problems
5. How long should each phoneme within a pattern be targeted within the cycles approach?
   a. four sessions
   b. 30 minutes

   c. 60 minutes
   d. until 50 percent accuracy is achieved
6. The ability to think about and reflect on the nature of language and how it functions refers to
   a. cognition
   b. intelligence
   c. pragmatics
   d. metalinguistic awareness
7. Which one of the following therapy approaches utilizes metalinguistic awareness?
   a. cycles training
   b. metaphon therapy
   c. maximal oppositions
   d. multiple oppositions
8. Which one of the following therapy approaches contrasts two very different phonemes, both of which are not in the child's inventory?
   a. cycles training
   b. metaphon therapy
   c. maximal oppositions
   d. multiple oppositions
9. Which one of the following therapy approaches attempts to mirror the normal developmental process of a child's phonological system?
   a. cycles training
   b. metaphon therapy
   c. maximal oppositions
   d. multiple oppositions

10. If you are working at the word level on [s], which one of the following would represent combining work on phonology and morphology?
    a. working on third-person singular forms
    b. working on regular past tense
    c. working on new vocabulary words with [s] in the final position
    d. working on subject versus object pronouns *she* and *her*

WEBSITES

chhs.sdsu.edu/slhs/publications/barlow107.pdf

This website provides a link to a pdf article titled "Minimal Pair Approaches to Phonological Remediation." The article discusses the use of minimal pairs and then applies the information to a case study.

www.southalabama.edu/alliedhealth/speechandhearing/bbeverly/541phonemictx.pdf

This website is a link to a pdf file compiled at the University of South Alabama. The document includes a quick summary of phonemic treatment principles and each of the therapy techniques discussed in this chapter (minimal pairs, cycles approach, maximal oppositions, etc.).

http://academic.mu.edu/sppa/slong/sppa294-6.pdf

This is a PowerPoint presentation put together by an unknown source (maybe Stephen Long) at Marquette University. It is an overview of many of the topics that are covered in this chapter and provides a quick review and summary of each of the phonemic therapy methods.

www.latrobe.edu.au/hcs/projects/preschoolspeech
language/articphonol.html

This website was created by Brigita Balbata, Stephanie Barnes, Emily Bird, Cassandra Byers, Rebekah Kerr, and Emily Stevens in the School of Human Communication Sciences at La Trobe University, Melbourne, Australia, under the supervision of Dr. Beverly Joffe. The goal is to give readers an idea of what therapy approaches are available, the premise behind them, and who may benefit from them as evidenced in the literature. It summarizes several research articles that cover a wide variety of techniques such as the cycles approach, metaphon therapy, maximal oppositions, multiple oppositions, and nonlinear phonologies, to mention a few. This well-organized website is a good resource for students and clinicians.

FURTHER READINGS

Gierut, J. (1989). Maximal opposition approach to phonological treatment. *Journal of Speech and Hearing Disorders, 54*, 9–19.

Hodson, B., & Paden, E. (1991). *Targeting intelligible speech: A phonological approach to remediation.* San Diego: College-Hill Press.

Howell, J., & Dean, E. (1998). *Treating phonological disorders in children: Metaphon—theory to practice* (2nd ed.). London: Whurr Publishers.

Williams, A. (2000a). Multiple oppositions: Theoretical foundations for an alternative contrastive intervention approach. *American Journal of Speech-Language Pathology, 9*, 282–288.

Williams, A. (2000b). Multiple oppositions: Case studies of variable in phonological intervention. *American Journal of Speech-Language Pathology, 9*, 289–299.

Articulatory/Phonological Disorders in Selected Populations

LEARNING OBJECTIVES

When you have finished this chapter, you should be able to:

- Describe the articulatory/phonological characteristics, and treatment of childhood apraxia of speech.
- Name the three types of cerebral palsy, and the four areas that should be assessed in children with cerebral palsy.
- Describe the speech-related concerns and the therapeutic guidelines for treating the articulation problems of childhood cerebral palsy.
- Describe a cleft palate, including what structures may be involved and some of the typical errors noted in the speech of children with cleft palate.
- Differentiate between a "developmental error" and a "compensatory error" in a child with a cleft palate.
- Identify the four goals that should be kept in mind when treating children with a cleft palate.
- Define the three criteria that are important in establishing the definition of mental disability.
- Define hearing impairments according to kind and degree of hearing loss.
- Describe the common speech errors associated with an individual who has a moderate to severe hearing impairment.
- Identify guidelines for treating both the phonetic and the phonological skills of a child with hearing impairment.
- Describe the articulatory/phonological characteristics and treatment of acquired apraxia of speech in adults.
- Describe the types of dysarthrias that exist, the general characteristics of each, and the treatment guidelines for the dysarthric adult.

This chapter provides an overview of articulatory and phonological characteristics of selected populations. They represent a number of different disorders with specific speech problems as one of the hallmarks of their symptom complexes. Many comprehensive books have been written on each of these disorders. Therefore, the following synopsis represents only selected aspects of the main characteristics and the diagnostic-treatment principles for each of the disorders relating to articulatory and/or phonological impairment. Each individual discussion is organized into four sections: (1) definition and general features, (2) articulatory/phonological characteristics, (3) clinical diagnostics, and (4) therapeutic implications.

CHILDHOOD APRAXIA OF SPEECH: A DISORDER OF SPEECH MOTOR CONTROL

Definition and General Features

The term *developmental articulatory dyspraxia* was first used by Morley, Court, and Miller (1954) to describe a small group of children with articulation disorders that differed from other children with known speech sound realization difficulties. These children have subsequently been labeled as having *developmental apraxia of speech* (Rosenbek and Wertz, 1972), *congenital articulatory apraxia* (Eisenson, 1972), and *developmental verbal apraxia* (Edwards, 1973), to mention a few. Currently, the terms **developmental apraxia of speech (DAS)**, **developmental verbal dyspraxia (DVD)** and **childhood apraxia of speech (CAS)** are used to refer to children who evidence a lack of motor control of the oral mechanism for speech production that is not attributable to other problems of muscular

control (Hall, Jordan, and Robin, 1993). According to Velleman (2003), the preferred label is *childhood apraxia of speech* to distinguish this disorder from merely a "developmental" disorder that the child under normal circumstances could outgrow. This label will be used throughout this chapter. Difficulty in sequencing speech sounds is central to the disorder. **Sequencing errors** are defined as disruptions in the production of the correct ordering of speech sounds or syllables (Hall et al., 1993).

An exact delineation of symptoms of this disorder as well as the CAS concept itself are highly controversial. Early reports delineating the symptoms (Rosenbek and Wertz, 1972; Yoss and Darley, 1974a) were authored by individuals who had worked with acquired apraxia of speech in adults. They pointed out similarities and differences between the specific articulatory problems noted in adults with acquired apraxia of speech and children with so-called developmental apraxia of speech. The most important similarity between these two groups of clients pertains to the lack of sequential volitional control of the oral mechanism (Hall et al., 1993). However, the major difference is that a neurological basis for comparable speech symptoms could never be verified in children with developmental apraxia of speech (Aram, 1984; Ferry, Hall, and Hicks, 1975; Rosenbek and Wertz, 1972). Some authors (e.g., Aram, 1984; Hall et al., 1993) even argue against the assumption that an underlying neurological impairment is indeed the cause of childhood apraxia of speech.

Many have disputed the concept of, and supporting evidence for, childhood apraxia of speech. For example, after a complete review of the literature, Guyette and Diedrich (1981) state, "The diagnosis 'developmental apraxia of speech' is neither appropriate nor useful" (p. 44). Love (2000), on the other hand, believes that "despite the serious questions raised about etiology, pathology, and validity of the reported signs and symptoms of the CAS syndrome, it remains an appropriate and useful diagnostic category of childhood motor speech disability" (p. 95). Shriberg, Aram, and Kwiatkowski (1997a) state,

> *For clinical needs, CAS appears to provide a tentative explanatory label for children who have se-*vere, irregular, *and* persistent *speech disorders, in contrast to the* mild-to-severe, regular, *and typi-*cally self-limiting *error patterns of the common form of developmental phonological disorders. . . .* (p. 274)

This statement furnishes a good point of departure for further discussion. It exemplifies the tentative nature of the label while also suggesting the clinical necessity of differentiating the speech characteristics of CAS children from those evidenced by children with developmental phonological disorders. If one accepts the label CAS, both groups of children do have certain characteristics in common: The onset is early in the developmental period and the course is long term, often extending into adulthood (Shriberg et al., 1997a). Its estimated prevalence of occurrence is approximately 1 to 2 children per 1,000 (Shriberg et al., 1997a). Box 10.1 provides additional information on the demographics of childhood apraxia of speech.

Articulatory/Phonological Characteristics

Several studies have reported speech characteristics of children with suspected CAS. However, some of these reports refer to case studies describing only one or two children. Other investigations cannot be compared because uniform criteria were not used when selecting the subjects. Therefore, when interpreting the data, it should be remembered that methodological differences exist between the studies. With this in mind, the following speech char-

---

BOX 10.1   Childhood Apraxia of Speech: Demographics

- Over 80 percent of children with CAS have at least one family member with reported speech and/or language disorders (Velleman, 2003).
- CAS demonstrates higher rates of family history than other speech sound disorders, which suggests a genetic basis in at least some cases (Lewis et al., 2003).
- Up to 3 to 4 percent of children with speech delay are given the diagnosis of CAS (Delaney and Kent, 2004).
- Symptoms of CAS are common among children with Down syndrome (Kumin and Adams, 2000).
- Approximately 60 percent of children with autism spectrum disorder have speech problems; about 13 percent report primarily symptoms of apraxia of speech (Marili, Andrianopoulos, Velleman, and Foreman, 2004).

---

acteristics are offered for children with CAS (Hall et al., 1993).

1. *More errors made in the sound classes involving more complex oral gestures.* Thus, consonant clusters, fricatives, and affricates evidence a larger percentage of difficulty (Crary, 1984; Rosenbek and Wertz, 1972).

These same sound classes are also troublesome for children with developmental phonological disorders, although Jackson and Hall (1987) suggest that the CAS children may be acquiring these sounds at a much slower rate, only at older ages, and possibly only after intensive remediation procedures.

2. *Unusual errors not typically found in children with speech sound disorders.* These errors include sound additions, prolongations of vowels and consonants, repetitions of sounds and syllables (Rosenbek and Wertz, 1972; Yoss and Darley, 1974a), and unusual substitutions, such as glottal plosives and bilabial fricatives (Aram and Glasson, 1979).

3. *A large percentage of omission errors.* Several investigators have found that sound and syllable omissions are the most frequent type of errors noted in CAS children (LaVoi, 1986; Rosenbek and Wertz, 1972). However, Yoss and Darley (1974a) related the percentage of omissions to the complexity of the speech tasks. Polysyllabic words demonstrated more syllable omissions, whereas spontaneous speech included sound omissions. Other reports indicate that the high degree of omissions may be age-related, with younger children evidencing more and older children fewer omission errors (Aram and Glasson, 1979; Jackson and Hall, 1987).

4. *Difficulty producing and maintaining appropriate voicing.* CAS children may voice unvoiced sounds and devoice voiced sounds (Aram and Glasson, 1979; Lewis et al., 2004; Morley, 1959; Yoss and Darley, 1974a). These errors have also been verified by acoustic analyses (Robin, Hall, and Jordan, 1987).

5. *Vowel and diphthong errors.* Several studies have identified vowel and diphthong errors in CAS children (e.g., Davis, Marquardt, and Sussman, 1985; Rosenbek and Wertz, 1972). Pollock and Hall (1991) specifically describe the vowel errors of five school-age children with CAS. All of these children had difficulty with tense-lax vowel contrasts, and four of the five evidenced diphthong reduction.

6. *Difficulty sequencing speech sounds and syllables.* According to Hall, Jordan, and Robin (1993), sequencing problems are central to this disorder. Difficulty with sequencing seems to increase as the complexity and/or length of the utterance increases (e.g., Davis, Jakielski, and Marquardt, 1998; Ferry, Hall, and Hicks, 1975; Hardcastle, Morgan-Barry, and Clark, 1987). In addition, sound transpositions within a word, or metatheses, have been frequently cited in descriptions of CAS (Aram and Nation, 1982; Rosenbek and Wertz, 1972). It is not clear whether the frequency of metathetic errors is in fact higher for this population than for children with developmental phonological disorders (LaVoi, 1986; Parsons, 1984).

7. *Difficulties with nasality and nasal emission.* Conflicting reports exist as to whether problems with nasality and nasal emission constitute an error pattern noted in children suspected of CAS. Based on extensive clinical experience, Hall, Jordan, and Robin (1993) summarize by saying, "We find that, at some point, most children exhibiting CAS have problems with hypernasality, hyponasality, or nasal emissions. Sometimes this is quite subtle, in most instances, it is variable and inconsistent in occurrence" (p. 35).

8. *Groping behavior and silent posturing.* **Groping behavior** is an ongoing series of movements of the articulators in an attempt to find the desired articulatory position. **Silent posturing** refers to the positioning of the articulators for a specific articulation without sound production. Both groping behaviors and silent posturing have been noted in the speech of CAS children (e.g., Hall, 1989; Murdoch, Porter, Younger, and Ozanne, 1984). Hall, Jordan, and Robin (1993) state that silent posturing may be seen primarily in younger children while groping behavior is found later, in older children with CAS.

9. *Prosodic impairment.* General and more specific difficulties with prosody have often been reported in the speech of CAS children (e.g., Beutsen and Christman, 2002; Hall, 1989; Morley, 1972; Robin, Hall, Jordan, and Gordan, 1991). In a series of studies by Shriberg, Aram, and Kwiatkowski (1997a, 1997b, 1997c), inappropriate stress was found to be the only linguistic domain that differentiated CAS children from those with delayed speech development.

10. *Difficulty identifying rhymes and syllables.* Investigators (Marion, Sussman, and Marquardt, 1993; Marquardt, Sussman, Snow, and Jacks, 2002) have found that children with suspected CAS demonstrate problems with rhyming and syllabification. These disorders may be evidence of a more broad-based phonological or linguistic problem as opposed to just motor-based difficulties (Velleman, 2003).

Although all of these error patterns have been reported in the speech of children with CAS, not all of them occur in all CAS children. Inconsistency and variability of errors is probably the most frequent pattern characterizing this disorder. Children with CAS are often highly unintelligible. Another common feature is the lack of progress these children make in spite of a considerable amount of therapy over a longer period of time.

Clinical Implications: Diagnostics

Generally, a broad cluster of symptoms is assumed to represent CAS, including speech, nonspeech, and language deficits. But the all-important qualification is that "Not *all* symp-

> Studies seem to indicate that two groups of CAS children, which present similiar symptoms but different prognoses, exist (Fawcus, 1971; Milloy, 1985; Morley, 1972; Morley and Fox, 1969). One group consists of children with moderate or severe articulation disorders that do not resolve over time. The second group of children show comparable symptoms but develop mature articulatory skills by approximately age 10 (Milloy, 1985). Milloy (1985) used the term *immature articulatory praxis* (IAP) to describe the second condition, hypothesizing that this condition was a maturational disorder that resolved as the children grew older. IAP was found in many children with moderate learning disabilities, and a correlation existed between the degree of immaturity these children presented and the severity of their language deficit.

toms must be present; no *one* characteristic or symptom *must* be present; and the typically reported symptoms are not *exclusive* to [childhood] apraxia of speech. Compounding the problem is the observation that children change over time" (Jaffe, 1984, p. 170). Assessment, therefore, must be organized in a way that allows us to look at a wide range of symptoms.

The following assessment procedures are recommended for the child who is suspected of demonstrating CAS:

- hearing screening
- language testing
- thorough speech-motor assessment, including diadochokinetic rates
- articulation test
- language sample
- additional tests to examine the sequencing of sounds and syllables as well as their consistency

Hearing screening is a portion of every assessment; however, it should be evident that the child with suspected CAS does not have a hearing loss as the basis for the noted articulatory problems. Language testing is also an important dimension of the assessment process. Although some research studies have used the absence of receptive language problems as one of the criteria for inclusion in the group of children with suspected CAS, others report both expressive and receptive language difficulties co-occuring with CAS (e.g., Hall, Hardy, and LaVelle, 1990; Hall, Robin, and Jordan, 1986; Lewis et al., 2004; Lohr, 1978). Formal and informal assessment of language should always be used to gain a more complete understanding of the language proficiency of these children.

A speech-motor assessment needs to include sequential volitional movements of the oral muscles for both speech and nonspeech tasks. Oral diadochokinetic rates in nonspeech and speech activities should be evaluated as well (Haynes, 1985; Love, 2000; Love and Fitzgerald, 1984). Such information helps document the structural and neuromuscular adequacy of the oral peripheral mechanism. Its functional adequacy for nonspeech and speech tasks should be described and compared.

An articulation test and language sample can be used to appraise several speech parameters: types of errors, any unusual errors, voicing problems with consonants, vowel and diphthong errors, difficulties with nasality and nasal emission, and prosodic problems. Differences between productions of one-word responses and those requiring increased articulatory length or complexity need to be ascertained. Groping behavior and/or silent posturing are additional areas that require close observation.

There are tests and protocols specifically designed to assess CAS children. Examples include the Screening Test for Developmental Apraxia of Speech (Blakely, 2000), Verbal Motor Production Assessment for Children (Hayden and Square, 1999), the Apraxia Profile (Hickman, 1997), the Kaufman Speech Praxis Test for Children (Kaufman, 1995), the Milloy Assessment of Praxis (MAP) (Milloy, 1985), and Tests for Apraxia of Speech and Oral Apraxia-Children's Battery (Blakely, 1977). Velleman (2003) also offers a complete assessment protocol for various symptoms associated with childhood apraxia of speech.

Clinical Implications: Therapeutics

An established set of therapeutic approaches for the treatment of CAS does not exist. This is not surprising when one considers the limited understanding of the cause, nature, and differential diagnostic markers for this disorder. Even after a careful diagnostic evaluation of the appraisal data, only *suspected* CAS can nor-

mally be assumed. Based on this assumption, many different remediation approaches have been suggested. The following is a synopsis of the treatment suggested by Hall, Jordan, and Robin (1993). It is based on the analysis of outcome measures from many different remediation programs as well as their clinical experience.

1. *Intensive services are needed.* Children with suspected CAS require an extraordinarily high amount of intensive therapy carried out on an individual basis. The child, the child's caregivers, and the clinician must be dedicated to this concept. Hall, Jordan, and Robin (1993) recommend a summer program in which the children are in residence for six weeks, receiving four hours of therapy per day, five days a week.

2. *Remediation should progress systematically through hierarchies of task difficulty.* Where to begin with remediation and how to progress will depend on the assessment data from each individual child. Hall, Jordan, and Robin (1993) evaluate the child's strengths and progress in very small, carefully manipulated steps. They analyze what the child can do successfully and proceed from there. Therefore, the consonant inventory, distribution as well as syllable shapes, will provide important information when evaluating where to begin with therapy. Speech sounds that can be successfully articulated are combined into syllable structures already present in the child's speech. These are then gradually expanded to include a few monosyllabic words of high utility and, possibly, carrier phrases.

3. *Remediation stresses sequences of movements.* Careful incremental increases in sequencing movements and the "memory" for such movements are important. Articulation "memory" should be based on internalized tactile-kinesthetic-proprioceptive informa-

tion relating sounds that are heard to specific motor patterns. Chappell (1973) suggests increasing the demand for memory retention by interrupting the child between requests for response sequences.

4. *Many repetitions of speech movements are required in drill-oriented sessions.* Hall, Jordan, and Robin (1993) use three to ten repetitions of each stimulus. Stimuli range from CV utterances to multisyllabic words. Each set of repetitions is interrupted by the client returning to a neutral or resting position to reduce perseverative behavior.

5. *The clinician must determine the need for auditory discrimination tasks.* Not all children need enhancement of auditory discrimination skills. The clinician should determine whether, based on assessment data, the individual client needs work in this area.

6. *Remediation should emphasize self-monitoring.* Self-monitoring should be emphasized as early as possible within the remediation program (Yoss and Darley, 1974b). Some suggest that tactile and kinesthetic self-monitoring be trained (Weiss, Gordon, and Lillywhite, 1987).

7. *Input from multiple modalities is needed.* Multisensory input appears helpful to many children with suspected CAS. Various types of cueing have been introduced and can be utilized to meet the specific needs of these children. All of the cueing techniques represent visual and/or tactile cues used to help the child articulate certain sounds or sound sequences (see the following Clinical Application for sources).

8. *Remediation should include manipulation of prosodic features as an integral part of the total remedial program.* Whenever possible, rhythm, intonation, stress, and rate manipulation should be integrated into the therapy program from the beginning. The areas that specifically need to be targeted should be revealed by the diagnostic data. However, there are some children who do not seem capable of manipulating articulatory and prosodic features simultaneously. If this occurs, an articulatory goal is established first and prosody added later to articulation tasks that are relatively easy for the client.

9. *If necessary, the clinician should teach compensatory strategies.* Compensatory strategies include slowing the overall rate of speech, increasing the use of pauses between words and syllables, vowel prolongation, and the intrusion of a schwa vowel between consonants in a cluster. Hall, Jordan, and Robin (1993) state that compensatory strategies may be a necessary portion of therapeutic measures but should be generally seen as only a stage of remediation to facilitate a child's progress. When the compensatory strategies are no longer necessary, productions without them should become the goal.

10. *The clinician must provide successful experiences.* Treatment should begin at a level at which children can succeed. Therefore, it is important that the clinician understand the child's baseline level of articulatory functioning and the strengths that this individual demonstrates. Children with suspected CAS especially need success with speech goals to keep them motivated throughout the typically long and slow remediation process.

MOTOR SPEECH DISORDERS: CEREBRAL PALSY

Definition and General Features

Cerebral palsy (CP) is a nonprogressive disorder of motor control caused by damage to the developing brain during pre-, peri-, or early postnatal periods (Dillow, Dzienkowski, Smith, and Yucha, 1996; Hardy, 1994; Love, 2000). The condition results in a wide variety

Additional Therapeutic Techniques—Childhood Apraxia of Speech

The following additional therapy techniques have been used with children exhibiting developmental apraxia of speech.

Technique	Sources
Melodic intonation therapy	Albert, Sparks, and Helm (1973); Doszak, McNeil, and Jancosek (1981); Helfrich-Miller (1984); Krauss and Galloway (1982); Sparks, Helm, and Albert (1974).
Cueing techniques	
Touch-cue method	Bashir, Grahamjones, and Bostwick (1984).
Signed target phoneme	Shelton and Graves (1985).
Adapted cueing techniques	Klick (1984, 1994).
Cued speech	Cornett (1972).
Jordan's gestures	Jordan (1988, 1991).
Prompts for restructuring oral muscular phonetic targets	Hayden and Square (1994).
Multiple phonemic approach	Bradley (1989); Davis, Marquardt, and Sussman (1985); Marquardt and Sussman (1991); McCabe and Bradley (1975).
Sign/total communication	Air, Wood, and Neils (1989); Culp (1989); Ferry, Hall, and Hicks (1975); Harlan (1984); Jaffe (1984).
Dynamic motor approaches	Davis and Velleman (2000); Square (1999); Strand and Skinner (1999).
Rhythmic repetition	Velleman and Strand (1994, 1998).

of motor disabilities, dysarthria among them. Given that there are about 400,000 children living with cerebral palsy, this disorder constitutes the most common developmental motor impairment (Best, Bigge, and Sirvis, 1994; Kudrjavcev, Schoenberg, Kurland, and Groover, 1983; Love, 2000), occurring about 3 times in every 1,000 births (Bigge, 1991). The lack of volitional speech-motor control is among its central clinical features. However, cerebral palsy's symptom complex, characterized by a host of neurological malfunctions, is far more than disordered articulation. Rather, in addition to general movement and co-ordination problems, primarily caused by spastic conditions of muscles and increased

tendon reflexes, "these dysfunctions include disturbances in cognition, perception, sensation, language, hearing, emotional behavior, feeding, and seizure control" (Love, 2000, pp. 49–50).

The treatment of cerebral palsy requires a team approach to the problem, which is typically a cooperative effort of a physician specializing in these disorders, a physical and occupational therapist, a psychologist, a social worker, and a speech-language pathologist. Clinical management by the speech-language pathologist requires special considerations that differ considerably from those employed in the treatment of other children with articulatory/phonological disorders. Clinical management can be effective only if the complexity of the disabling condition is understood. This includes, among other important factors, being able to evaluate the intricate interrelationships between respiration, phonation, resonance, and articulation in normal individuals versus individuals with cerebral palsy.

Articulatory/Phonological Characteristics

Speech-related dysfunctions in cerebral palsy include respiratory, phonatory, articulatory, and prosodic abnormalities and velopharyngeal inadequacies (Bishop, Brown, and Robson, 1990; Dillow et al., 1996; Hardy, 1994; Love, 2000). Cerebral palsy encompasses many different types and degrees of speech-related problems. To facilitate an understanding of the various articulatory/phonatory characteristics, a distinction is usually made between three types of involvement commonly found in cerebral palsied individuals:

1. spasticity
2. dyskinesia
3. ataxia

Among cerebral palsied clients, spastic involvement is the most frequently found. Four major types of spastic involvement are recognized: spastic hemiplegia, spastic paraplegia, spastic diplegia, and spastic quadriplegia. With *spastic hemiplegia,* the arm and leg on one side of the body show signs of spastic paresis. *Spastic paraplegia,* which is relatively uncommon, is characterized by involvement of the legs only. In *spastic diplegia,* all four limbs are affected but the lower limbs show more involvement than the upper limbs. All four limbs are about equally involved in *spastic quadriplegia.* Spastic diplegics and quadriplegics are more likely to have speech disorders than are hemiplegics or paraplegics. Respiratory, phonatory, resonatory, and articulatory symptoms include the following:

Respiratory difficulties. Reduced vital capacity resulting in inadequate breath support for phonatory and articulatory purposes.

Laryngeal dysfunction. Responsible for harsh voices and, when coupled with respiratory aberrations, result in short phrasing and prosodic disturbances.

Velopharyngeal inadequacies. With the consequence of hypernasality.

Articulatory deficiencies. Affecting especially the production of fricatives and affricates as well as translating into an overall laborious, slow rate of speech. Muscle weakness, articulatory instability, and inaccuracy in finding target articulation points are also noted (Love, 2000).

Dyskinesias in cerebral palsy are best exemplified by athetoid conditions marked by unilateral or bilateral disturbances of posture, tonus, and motion. They have been reported to be far less frequent than spastic involvement within the cerebral palsied population (Erenberg, 1984; Love, 2000), but their effects on speech performance are often even more severe. More often than not, the degree of limb dysfunction mirrors the impairments of the speech mechanism. Many athetoid clients show dysfunction of every physiological component contributing to speech:

Respiratory difficulties. Breathing might be rapid and irregular (Davis, 1987), showing a lack of thoracic respiratory movement or even "reverse breathing," in which the sternum is flattened instead of lifted during inspiration.

Laryngeal dysfunction. General hypertonicity, which can immobilize the phonatory process altogether, can be more pronounced than in spastic involvement. If any voice results, it is commonly marked by an especially strained quality, hard glottal onset, and reduced intensity and prosody realizations.

Velopharyngeal inadequacies. Slow velar activity often results in hypernasal effects.

Articulatory deficiencies. Abnormally large jaw movements during articulation; tongue movements are restricted and for articulatory purposes highly dependent on jaw activity (Kent and Netsell, 1978). This results in distortions of consonant as well as vowel productions (positioning of the mandible during speech can somehow establish necessary differences in tongue height, but not in anterior-posterior tongue movements for the production of front versus back vowels).

Ataxia is infrequent among cerebral palsied clients (Hardy, 1983; Pharoah, Cooke, Rosenbloom, and Cooke, 1987). This is probably why systematic studies of the speech of ataxic dysarthric children have not been published (Love, 2000). The main symptom of ataxic involvement is incoordination of essentially hypotonic muscle action. Based on clinical observation, it appears that the speech characteristics of ataxic cerebral palsied individuals are very similar to those of adults with ataxic dysarthria (Love, 2000). The following characteristics are noted in children and adults with ataxia:

Respiratory difficulties. Shallow inspiration and lack of expiratory control.

Laryngeal dysfunction. Harsh voice productions, reduced range of prosodic feature realization.

Velopharyngeal inadequacies. Hypernasality is not typical.

Articulatory deficiencies. Imprecise consonants and vowel distortions, inconsistent sound substitutions and omissions, and

a general dysrhythmia (Darley, Aronson, and Brown, 1975; Ingram, 1966; Ingram and Barn, 1961).

Table 10.1 summarizes the three different types of cerebral palsy.

Several studies have verified that children with cerebral palsy demonstrate speech errors of temporal and motor control (Crary and Comeau, 1981; Farmer and Lencione, 1977; McMahon, Hodson, and Allen, 1983). Based on this evidence, Milloy and Morgan-Barry (1990) describe the following phonological processes that relate to these difficulties:

Phonological Processes

Related to temporal coordination. Voicing difficulties, including devoicing of initial consonants or voicing of unvoiced sounds, variable realizations of voiced-voiceless cognates, prevocalic voicing, consonant cluster reductions, final consonant deletions, stopping of fricatives or frication of stops, weak syllable deletions.

Related to motor control, errors of phonetic placement. Fronting, backing, stopping, gliding, lateral realization of apical and coronal fricatives, vowelization of [l] and [r], nasalization.

Clinical Implications: Diagnostics

The primary communicative impairment of children with cerebral palsy is clearly motor speech in nature. But these children present a variety of clinical pictures having to do with both the type and the severity of involvement. On the other hand, all children with cerebral palsy share some common factors that directly relate to basic functions subserving speech, namely problems with respiration, phonation, resonation, and articulation. It is important to assess kind and degree of nmary of Types of Cerebral Palsy

Site of Trauma	Muscular Involvement	Speech Disorder
Pyramidal tract monolateral lesion of fibers	Hypertonicity of upper and lower limbs on one side	Speech usually auditorily acceptable although there may be developmental delay
Uncertain, probably bilateral lesion	Hypertonicity of lower limbs; may extend to torso musculature	Possible problems of respiration and breath control for speech
Uncertain, probably bilateral lesion	All four limbs involved, lower limbs more severely affected; may extend to torso and neck muscles	Variable, depending on extent of neuromotor disability; may show dysprosody with problems of articulation
Bilateral lesion within pyramidal tract	Equal degree of spasticity in all four limbs	Articulatory problems and dysphonia in varying degrees of severity
Basal ganglia	Impairment of voluntary movements due to either extreme muscle tone or extreme flaccidity Involuntary continuous muscle movement occurs	Speech defects, very variable in severity, generally slow, with poor articulation, and problems of phonation, stress, and rhythm
Cerebellum	Incoordination of movement with inability to maintain posture and balance	Speech mainly defective; articulation problems and dysrhythmia evident

ental Neurological Disorders," by N. Milloy and R. Morgan-Barry, in *Developmental*), edited by P. Grunwell, 1990, Edinburgh: Churchill Livingstone. Reprinted by er Churchill Livingstone.

these systems may have on

espiration may lead to dif-
ng vocalization, difficul-
ocalization, variations in
hay affect word and sen-
ability to sustain vocal-
isyllabic words or longer
oss of expiratory support
ce.

Problems with *phonation* may result in interruptions in phonation, breathy voice, harsh voice, pitch and intensity variations, and problems in coordinating voicing and articulation.

Problems with *resonation* may result in various degrees of hypernasality, variations in nasality within an utterance, and lack of intelligibility due to nasality problems.

Problems with *articulation* may result in difficulties in achieving speech sound productions, sound distortions, and disorganized phonological systems, possibly leading to problems with language and learning to read.

When assessing the child with cerebral palsy, it is essential to remember that the smooth integration of all systems subserving speech is a real problem for these children. Therefore, the assessment and treatment of children with this disorder must account for far more than just speech sound production difficulties.

The high diversity of possible involvements requires an encompassing evaluation. In addition to respiratory, phonatory, resonatory, and articulatory limitations and possibilities, data from the following areas should be supplemented:

• cognitive skills
• sensory and perceptual abilities beginning with an audiological evaluation
• client's emotional behavior
• feeding/eating characteristics
• language competence

Often, the speech-language pathologist will become part of an early intervention team for infants who have been identified with cerebral palsy. As a member of this team, the speech-language pathologist will be asked to assess prespeech skills as prerequisites for the development of articulation skills. These prerequisites include:

1. Head control with stability of the neck and shoulder girdle. Such stability provides later control and mobility of oral structures.
2. A coordinated pattern of respiration and phonation.
3. A variety of feeding experiences to enhance normal feeding patterns.
4. Babbling practice (Air et al., 1989; Levin, 1999).

As one example, the Pre-Speech Assessment Scale (Morris, 1975) is a tool that can assist the speech-language pathologist in appraising prespeech behavior. This scale examines postural tone and movement, response to sensory stimuli, feeding, biting, chewing, sucking, swallowing, respiration, phonation, and sound play.

Clinical Implications: Therapeutics

As always, the selection of appropriate therapeutic measures to influence the communicative abilities of clients with cerebral palsy, especially to guide and improve development in young children, is a direct outgrowth of the specific diagnostic results. Established methods for the treatment of various "types" of cerebral palsy amount only to guidelines for elementary orientation.

There are, nevertheless, general principles that apply to all remediation efforts with young clients who have cerebral palsy. First, some prespeech prerequisites must be met, the afore-

Capute (1974) reports that about 50 to 60 percent of the cerebral palsied population show some degree of mental retardation, with the rest of these individuals demonstrating intelligence within normal limits. Impaired language development, learning difficulties, and academic problems often occur in children with cerebral palsy (Haynes and Pindzola, 1998). In addition, an audiological evaluation is a necessity for children with cerebral palsy. Athetotics in particular have higher auditory detection thresholds, poorer speech reception thresholds, and poorer speech discrimination than do children without cerebral palsy (DiCarlo 1974).

mentioned head control and the coordination of respiratory patterns with voice production, for example. The necessity of coordination between breathing and phonation for future articulation work is self-evident, but a certain degree of posture control is equally indispensable. Another, although controversial (Jaffe, 1984), prerequisite pertains to the inhibition of certain chewing and swallowing behaviors, specifically the chewing reflex, which might interfere with oral-motor activities for articulatory tasks. Neurodevelopmental therapy—for example, the so-called Bobath approach to the treatment of infants with cerebral palsy—heavily emphasizes the early reduction of abnormal oral reflexes within a prespeech program (Bobath, 1967; Bobath and Bobath, 1972).

The next therapeutic phase with young children who have cerebral palsy pertains to communication and speech-language stimulation. In infants, it might start with vocal play and babbling practice. Box 10.2 offers references that provide more detail in the areas of assessment and treatment of prespeech behaviors, speech-language stimulation, and feeding.

For the older child with cerebral palsy, a basic consideration is the facilitation of desired movements while inhibiting the abnormal reflex patterns. Before a speech-language clinician can address the coordination of respiration, phonation, resonation, and articulation, the child must be able to maintain some reflex-inhibiting postures that the physical therapist will recommend. Because this is usually one of the primary goals of the early intervention team, the child should already have developed some skills in this area. If the child

---

BOX 10.2   Selected References for the Assessment and Treatment of Prespeech Behaviors and the Assessment of Feeding

Assessing and Treating Prespeech Behaviors

Harding, C. G. (1983). Setting the stage for language acquisition: Communication development in the first year. In R. M. Golinkoff (Ed.), *Transition from prelinguistic to linguistic communication.* Hillsdale, NJ: Lawrence Erlbaum Associates.

Morris, S. (1987). Therapy for the child with cerebral palsy: Interacting frameworks. *Seminars in Speech and Language, 8,* 71–86.

Proctor, A. (1989). Stages of normal noncry vocal development in infancy: A protocol for assessment. *Topics in Language Disorders, 10*(1), 26–42.

Proctor, A., & Murnyack, T. (1995). Assessing communication, cognition, and vocalization in the prelinguistic period. *Infants and Young Children, 7*(4), 39–54.

Rosetti, L. (1994). *Communication intervention: Birth to three.* San Diego, CA: Singular.

Assessing and Therapy for Feeding

Alexander, R. (1987). Oral-motor treatment for infants and young children. *Seminars in Speech and Language, 8,* 87–100.

Alexander, R. (1987). Prespeech and feeding development. In E. McDonald (Ed.), *Treating cerebral palsy.* Austin, TX: PRO-ED.

Gisel, E., Schwartz, S., Petryk, A., Clarke, D., & Haberfellner, H. (2000). "Whole body" mobility after one year of intraoral appliance therapy in children with cerebral palsy and moderate eating impairment. *Dysphagia, 14,* 226–235.

Hall, S., Circello, N., Reed, P., & Hylton, J. (1987). *Considerations for feeding children who have a neuromuscular disorder.* Portland, OR: CARC Publications.

Jaffe, M. (1989). Feeding at-risk infants and toddlers. *Topics in Language Disorders, 10*(1), 13–25.

McGowan, J., & Kerwin, M. (1993). Oral motor and feeding problems. In K. Bleile (Ed.), *The care of children with long-term tracheostomies* (pp. 157–195). San Diego, CA: Singular.

can inhibit abnormal reflexes and realize certain movements required for speech, articulation training can be initiated.

Traditionally, therapy began with establishing temporal coordination and motor control of the speech musculature. Goals were to increase the speed, range, and accuracy of movement of the tongue, lips, and jaw (Gibbon and Wood, 2003; Westlake and Rutherford, 1961). These goals were then integrated with the maintenance of body and head tonus as well as with respiration, phonation, and resonation (Barlow and Farley, 1989). Oral exercises usually preceded phonetic placement. Selection of the target sound was guided by stimulability, consistency, and visibility and whether the sound was an early or late developing sound. Therefore, stimulable, visible sounds that were produced in some contexts accurately and were early to be acquired were normally given priority (Love, 2000).

However, there were those who felt that groups of sounds rather than a single sound should be treated (Hardy, 1983). Based on guidelines drawn up by Hardy (1983) and Crary (1993), the following procedures are offered:

1. *Consonants that are realized correctly in prevocalic positions but are misarticulated in postvocalic positions should be treated first.* Generally, postvocalic errors will be more easily remedied if the child can produce the sound in a prevocalic position.

2. *Distortions should be treated before substitutions,* especially those distortions that fall short of the target because of motor involvement. Prognosis should be better if the child can almost produce the sound, although distorted, rather than delete or use a substitute for the sound.

3. *Training articulatory omissions and substitutions that fall short of the target because of motor involvement should be delayed.* Compensatory articulatory efforts for sounds that are difficult to produce should be trained instead. The child will usually have already developed some type of compensatory sound realization. The duty of the clinician is to refine this production as much as possible.

4. *A multiple auditory-visual stimulation approach* is preferred over auditory stimulation alone.

5. *Voice–voiceless distinctions should be trained by slowing the speech process* and then concentrating on the production of the voicelessness of the sound. This is important because cerebral palsied children have a tendency to substitute voiced for voiceless consonants.

6. *It is important to remember that some cerebral palsied children cannot achieve "normal" articulation.* In these cases, *reasonable compensations* are the goal; they can be very efficient for communicative purposes.

Occasionally, the physical handicap is so severe that effective verbal communication cannot be achieved at all. If that is the case, *augmentative communication*—that is, the use of any means (gestural, boards with words or pictures, electronic devices) to promote meaningful communicative exchange—must be implemented (Beukelman, Yorkston, and Dowden, 1985).

CLINICAL APPLICATION

Communication Augmentation

Communication augmentation refers to any approach designed to support, enhance, or augment the communication of individuals who cannot use speech in all situations (Beukelman, Yorkson, and Dowden, 1985). Augmentative approaches have as a goal the expansion of the symbolic communication capabilities of nonspeaking individuals. Common types of augmentation include manual communication, communication boards, and electronic or computer-based aids. For individuals with motor involvement, such as children with cerebral palsy, the augmentation system must be chosen with special care. The American Speech-Language-Hearing Association Ad Hoc Committee on Communication Processes and Nonspeaking Persons (1980) identifies three components for the assessment of augmentative communication:

1. The appropriateness of augmentative communication must be appraised. Not all nonspeaking individuals can benefit from such a system (Bryen, Goldman, and Quinlisk-Gill, 1988; Owens and House, 1984). For the child with cerebral palsy, for example, cognitive and speech motor abilities will need to be weighed in relationship to augmentative means.
2. The appropriateness of the augmentative communication mode must be appraised. A decision must be made as to which type or types of augmentative system is appropriate for the individual. Of particular importance are the motoric abilities of the client (Shane and Wilbur, 1980; Silverman, 1980). Restricted motor skills often limit the types of system that can be utilized. This will be a major consideration when evaluating augmentative communication for the child with cerebral palsy.
3. The appropriate symbol system or systems must be found. Cognitive ability, visual acuity, and the receptiveness of the environment all need to be thoroughly assessed within this category (Chapman and Miller, 1980).

Although augmentative communication may prove to be the only possibility for some children with cerebral palsy, the selection and implementation of such a system for children with severe motoric limitations remain a challenge.

*C*LEFTING: CLEFT PALATE AND CLEFT LIP

Definition and General Features

Occurring in 1 of about 700 births (Brogan and Woodings, 1976), palatal and (upper) lip clefts are among the most frequent congenital anomalies (American Cleft Palate–Craniofacial Association and Cleft Palate Foundation, 1997). **Clefting** refers to a division of a continuous structure by a cleavage, a split prominently caused by a failure of the palate to fuse during fetal development (Shprintzen, 1995). Examples of clefting are cleft palate and cleft lip. Both the hard and soft palates and the lips form normally uninterrupted structures within their anatomical boundaries. If clefting occurs, a gap severs their unity, dividing the roof of the mouth (which also constitutes the floor of the nasal cavity) and/or the upper lip sagittally into separated left and right portions.

Palatal clefts have several etiologies that cause a failure of the regular median fusion of the embryo's oral-facial structures between the eighth and twelfth weeks of gestation. In addition, there is also the possibility of a rupture of already fused oral-facial elements (Kitamura, 1991). Contrary to common understanding, no single cause for clefting exists; "clefting is . . . a clinical outcome of many possible diseases" (Shprintzen, 1995, p. 5).

Although there are many classification systems, the recommendations by Harkins and colleagues (1960, 1962) from the American Cleft Palate Association (now the American Cleft Palate–Craniofacial Association) have been most frequently adopted (Bzoch, 1997).

1. Clefts of prepalate
- *Cleft lip:* unilateral, bilateral, median, prolabium (central segment of upper lip), congenital scar
- *Cleft of alveolar process:* unilateral, bilateral, median, submucous
- *Cleft of prepalate:* any combination of foregoing types, prepalate protrusion, prepalate rotation, prepalate arrest (median cleft)
2. Clefts of the palate
- *Clefts of soft palate:* extent, palatal shortness, submucous
- *Clefts of hard palate:* extent, vomer attachment, submucous

3. Clefts of prepalate and palate
4. Facial clefts other than prepalate and palate

Unilaterality or bilaterality of hard palate clefts refers to their presence on one or both sides of the hard palate, median clefts to their presence at the midline. These clefts are along a line where the lower edge of the nasal septum attaches to the palate. *Submucous clefts,* on the other hand, are characterized by an intact mucous membrane covering a cleft. This cleft may be separating muscular portions of the soft palate and/or a cleavage of the posterior bony portions of the hard palate. A V-shaped indentation in this area might be felt with the finger. Another sign of the probable existence of a submucous cleft is a divided uvula, a *bifid uvula.* Quite in contrast to unilateral and bilateral clefts, submucous clefts seldom cause feeding problems or abnormal speech.

Articulatory/Phonological Characteristics

Children with cleft palate may exhibit developmental and/or compensatory articulatory and phonological disorders (Bzoch, 1997; Lynch, 1986; Pamplona, Ysunza, Gonzalez, Ramirez, and Patino, 2000; Whitehall, Francis, & Ching, 2003). Developmental speech-language delays are similar to those found in children without clefts, but they occur more frequently in children with cleft palates (Schonweiler, Schonweiler, Schmelzeisen, and Ptok, 1995; Trost-Cardamone, 1990a). Therefore, children with developmental delays are characterized by articulatory and phonological skills that resemble those of younger normally developing children. Developmental delays cannot always be said to be completely independent from the underlying condition. Consonant cluster reductions, for example, a frequent occurrence in children with speech-language delays, can often be traced to placement or omission errors that are disorder-specific in children with palatal clefts.

Compensatory errors pertain to specific errors of organ/place of articulation that may occur in patients who have inadequate closure of the velopharyngeal valve or a cleft or fistula in the hard palate (Witzel, 1995). They have also been described as "compensatory adjustments" (Morley, 1970). These sound substitutions or distortions are produced more posteriorly and inferior in the vocal tract by posterior positioning of the tongue, associated true and false vocal fold adduction, or abnormal positioning of the arytenoid cartilage and epiglottis. Due to difficulties with velopharyngeal closure, these errors are thought to be a compensatory attempt to modify the airstream below the velopharyngeal valve. But compensatory errors are not always a direct result of velopharyngeal incompetence. Velopharyngeal incompetence may actually result from compensatory articulation due to limited movements of the velopharyngeal valve during productions of specific sounds. Table 10.2 lists the types of compensatory articulation errors (Trost, 1981; Witzel, 1995).

Although specific sound production difficulties have often been noted in the speech of cleft palate children, they may not be entirely phonetic in nature. Children with cleft palate may also evidence difficulties with the organization of phonemes within their language system; that is, they may demonstrate phonological disorders (Broen and Moller, 1993; Chapman, 1993; Chapman and Hardin, 1992; Chapman, Hardin-Jones, and Halter, 2003; Estrem and Broen, 1989). Early delays in phonological development were exemplified by a high frequency of deletion of final consonants, syllable reduction, and backing. How-

Table 10.2   Compensatory Articulation Errors

Compensatory Articulation	Production Characteristics	Substitution for:
Glottal stop	Adduction of true vocal folds; greater air pressure may even result in false vocal fold adduction.	Stop-plosives
Laryngeal stop	Abnormal positioning of epiglottis. Epiglottis comes in contact with pharynx.	Stop-plosives, consonants
Laryngeal fricative	Abnormal positioning of epiglottis. Epiglottis approaches pharynx.	Fricatives
Laryngeal affricate	Epiglottis briefly contacts pharynx, then constricts the airstream.	Affricates
Pharyngeal stop	Dorsum of tongue moves posteriorly, contacting the pharynx, causing a buildup and release of air.	Stop-plosives
Pharyngeal fricative	Dorsum of tongue moves posteriorly toward the pharynx; constricts airstream, causing frication.	Fricatives
Pharyngeal affricate	Dorsum of tongue briefly contacts pharynx; then constricts the airstream.	Affricates
Posterior nasal fricative	Posterior dorsum of tongue and soft palate are positioned to generate friction at VP valve; always accompanied by nasal air emission.	Fricatives
Posterior nasal affricate	Posterior dorsum of tongue and soft palate are positioned to create both stopping and friction; always accompanied by nasal air emission.	Affricates
Middorsum palatal stop	Middorsum of tongue contacts the hard palate at approximate place for [j].	[t], [d], [k], and [g]
Middorsum palatal fricative	Middorsum of tongue approaches the hard palate to create friction.	Fricatives
Middorsum palatal affricate	Middorsum of tongue contacts the hard palate followed by frication.	Affricates

ever, at the age of 4 to 5 years, these problems were less apparent.

Clinical Implications: Diagnostics

Obviously, the initial diagnosis of clefting in a newborn—its nature, site, and extent—is a medical task. So is the beginning of its man-

agement, typically involving at least a pediatrician, an orthodontist, and an otolaryngologist. But clefts are a matter of long-term care requiring a team of specialists for successful assessment and management. Speech-language pathologists are important members of this team. Their primary job is to assess the child's communicative status and development. This is a challenging task. Not only are all clefts different (including their various effects on verbal communication), but also the personalities of the children and their caregivers are very different in their ability to cope with the situation and its clinical consequences. However, the biggest diagnostic challenge might be the developmental aspects of the disorder, that is, the changing nature of the appraised findings. Today's status will differ from tomorrow's because of natural growth factors, the necessary corrective measures of medical intervention, and compensatory prospects. Diagnostics involving children with clefts is a truly ongoing process.

The areas of diagnostic concern again underline the necessity of a team approach to the clinical management of cleft palate children. For example, they are all prone to intermittent middle-ear infections and their concomitant conductive hearing loss. This means that an otolaryngologist and an audiologist need to be involved to closely monitor the condition and hearing ability of all children with palatal clefts. The findings are important for the speech-language clinician because "evidence indicates that children with recurrent middle ear problems are slower to acquire speech production skills" (Broen and Moller, 1993, p. 230).

The central diagnostic issue pertains to the velopharyngeal port incompetency (VPI)—to its phonatory, resonatory, and articulatory effects. VPI applies to both structural abnormalities and neuromuscular inadequacies. Whereas structural abnormalities will largely be corrected by surgical and/or prosthetic measures, some functional deficits in respect to speech often remain, resulting in hypernasal resonance, nasal air emission, sound distortions, and sound substitutions. The latter two are characterized by these children's tendency to *articulatory backing,* a compensatory measure of cleft palate children to produce speech sounds

more posteriorly in the oral cavity than is normally the case (Trost, 1981). Velopharyngeal incompetency impairs the intraoral pressure buildup necessary for the norm production of many speech sounds—primarily stops, sibilants, fricatives, and affricates, the so-called pressure consonants. Nasals and semivowels such as [w] and [j] remain relatively intact.

One of the most striking features characterizing the speech of children with cleft palates with velopharyngeal incompetence is the substitution of glottal stops for stop-plosives, a maladaptive compensatory articulatory behavior triggered by the impossibility of accumulating the intraoral pressure required for the regular production of these pressure consonants. During this substitution, the standard positioning of the articulators is sometimes retained. For example, for [p], the lips are closed and suddenly opened simultaneously with the release of the glottal stop. This often results in an impression of a slightly distorted yet acceptable [p]-production. In addition to the articulatory consequences of VPI, dental anomalies and problems with occlusion of the mandibular and maxillary arches often contribute to the aberrant articulation of children with cleft palate.

"The primary clinical task for the speech-language pathologist is to assess the child's phonological status and then infer the effects of structural deviations on the phonological behavior observed" (Trost-Cardamone and Bernthal, 1993, p. 317). Such a task will differ considerably from child to child, mostly according to age and linguistic/cognitive levels of the individual client, but it always involves:

1. speech sampling and analysis, including sound inventory and phonological pattern development
2. stimulability probes
3. intelligibility judgments
4. oral-facial examination

CLINICAL APPLICATION

Clinical Test Battery for Children with Cleft Palates

Bzoch (1997) recommends the following clinical test battery:

Language Testing:

Audiometric Evaluation

Nasal emission test	A simple airflow paddle held under the nose (Bzoch, 1979), a small mirrored surface, or a headset listening device is sufficient to enhance the auditory and visual perceptions of nasal airflow. Ten two-syllable words, each containing two [p] or [b] sounds, are used in this test.
Hypernasality test	This measure uses ten one-syllable words beginning with [b] and ending with [t]. The subject repeats each word twice. On the second repetition, the examiner pinches the nares closed. A perceptual judgment of hypernasality is indicated if words shift in quality between the first and second repetition.
Hyponasality test	This measure uses ten one-syllable words beginning with [m] and ending with [t]. The subject repeats each word twice; on the second repetition, the examiner pinches the nares closed. On this test, there *should be a shift in quality* between the first and second repetition.
Phonation test	[i], [ɑ], and [u] are prolonged for ten seconds. The examiner notes any aspirate or hoarse phonation. Also, if the client cannot sustain phonation for ten seconds, this would indicate a habituated breathy voice. This can be confirmed by the conversational speech sample.
Articulation test	Special tests examining typical errors noted in the speech of children with cleft palate are available. These include, for example, the Iowa Pressure Test (Morris, Spriestersbach, and Darley, 1961) and Bzoch Error Pattern Diagnostic Articulation Test (described in Bzoch, 1979).
Screening nasometer test	This test is used for children from 2 to 6 years of age. Procedures can be found in many sources. A few examples include Dalston (1997); Dalston, Warren, and Dalston (1991); Fletcher (1970); and Kay Elemetrics Corporation (1988).

Each of these assessment areas has been discussed previously in some detail (see Chapters 6 and 7). Procedures do not differ significantly with the cleft palate child.

One important aspect of the diagnosis with these children is to find, and distinguish between, error patterns that are developmental in nature and those that, as a result of the cleft, have a structural or physiological basis. Some patterns are sometimes seen in children with cleft palate but are not typical for children with structurally and functionally intact oral and pharyngeal mechanisms. The following list is provided by Trost-Cardamone and Bernthal (1993):

1. *Consonant distortions associated with nasal emissions.* There are three error patterns associated with nasal emission. It is important to distinguish between them because different interventions may be in order for each.

- *Nasal emission due to a persistence of velopharyngeal inadequacy.* This is characterized by nasal emission distortion during production of all pressure consonants and pervasive hypernasality accompanying production of vowels and the vocalic consonants [l], [r], [j], and [w].
- *Nasal emission due to oronasal fistulae.* An oronasal fistula is an opening between the oral and nasal cavity. Although some can be easily eliminated surgically, others are too large for successful closure. There is a relationship between the location of the fistula and the consonants affected. Posteriorly located fistulae (near the juncture between the hard and soft palate) affect primarily [k] and [g] with little influence on anteriorly produced consonants. When the fistula is anteriorly located, [t], [d], [s], [z], [p], and [b] are likely to be distorted.
- *Nasal emission that is speech sound specific.* This may occur in the absence of clefting or velopharyngeal impairment. It does not affect a class of sounds and is rarely associated with hypernasality. Nasal emission does not require surgical intervention; it is probably due to faulty learning and can usually be treated with speech therapy, if properly diagnosed.

2. *Vowel distortions secondary to hypernasality.* It is important for the clinician to differentiate between vowel distortions that may result from deviant articulatory placement and those that are deviations due to hypernasal resonance as the result of deficient velopharyngeal valving.

3. *Compensatory articulations.* Several types of compensatory articulations have been provided in Table 10.2. The clinician should differentiate between compensatory articulations that are used as substitutions and those that occur as coarticulations.

4. *Atypical backed articulation.* These articulations include back-velar substitutions for [l], [r], and [n]. The posterior shifts may result from attempting to capture airflow or use of the back of the tongue to help seal the velopharyngeal port. Such productions should be analyzed to determine whether they are part of a phonological pattern of backing or whether they represent selective articulatory substitutions.

Clinical Implications: Therapeutics

Many children with cleft palates undergo palate repair by the age of 18 months. They remain free of compensatory sound production errors such as glottal for oral stops and pharyngeal for oral fricatives (Hall and Golding-Kushner, 1989). Other children require therapeutic intervention. To implement therapy with cleft palate clients, four overall goals should be kept in mind:

1. Improve the placement of consonant productions by promoting a more forward place of articulation.
2. Improve velopharyngeal valve function and decrease hypernasal resonance quality.
3. Modify compensatory articulations.
4. If developmental phonological errors exist, improve the child's phonological system (Van Demark and Hardin, 1990).

Improving the placement of consonant productions and modifying compensatory articulations are usually accomplished by direct work on place of articulation—that is, motor placement techniques. Glottal stops can easily be eliminated by using maneuvers that keep the vocal folds apart, such as gentle whispering, overaspiration, or the use of a sustained [h] (Golding-Kushner, 1995). Slight overaspiration by using a sustained [h] usually breaks the glottal pattern because it requires an open glottis. Voiceless oral stops are first introduced at the end of a prolonged [h]. In addition, the voiceless stop itself is overaspirated. If the word were *pie,* the production would sound similar to a prolonged [h] + [p] + *high.* Trost (1981) reports that teaching voiceless homorganic oral fricatives before establishing oral stops is a good technique for breaking up compensatory coarticulations. Nasal occlusion and release help to eliminate nasal snorting and to establish stops and fricatives. By occluding the nares, clients quickly learn to direct the airstream orally.

Sometimes, even after surgery, the velopharyngeal mechanism is only marginally adequate for articulatory function; hypernasality may still persist to varying degrees. If further surgery and/or prosthodontic intervention is not indicated, improving velopharyngeal valve function and decreasing hypernasal resonance quality might then become a treatment goal. Several ways have been suggested to improve velopharyngeal valve function. The velum has been massaged, as well as electrically stimulated, and various devices have been used to improve the effectiveness of these exercises (Starr, 1993). Behavioral approaches that provide feedback to clients are attempts to enhance their awareness and control of the velopharyngeal mechanism. Perceptual and acoustic feedback, visual feedback, and airflow and air pressure feedback have been offered with varying degrees of success (see Starr, 1993, for a review of these techniques). However, due to lack of clinical studies, outcome measures for these techniques remain unclear.

Decreasing hypernasal resonance may be another important therapy goal for cleft palate clients. Hypernasal resonance may occur in individuals with adequate and inadequate velopharyngeal competency. One such technique, increased mouth opening or orality

(Boone and McFarlane, 1988; Waengler, 1981; Waengler and Bauman-Waengler, 1987b), will be described because of its overlap with previously mentioned articulatory principles.

Studies have shown (Waengler, 1981; Warren, 1979) that during sound articulation, varying degrees of velar activity occur. For example, stop-plosives require complete closure of the nasopharyngeal port for the necessary buildup of intraoral air pressure. Productions of [ɑ] or [w], on the other hand, do not demand the same degree of closure to prevent undue nasal resonance. Only during the production of stops and sounds with little articulatory possibility for oral air escape, sibilants and affricates, for example, is complete velopharyngeal closure necessary. With more "open" sounds, the same degree of closure is not required.

If "open" sounds require less velar activity to keep nasality effects from occurring, more open versions of the respective phoneme realizations should at least lessen, and possibly prevent, such consequences. Consider /i/ realizations as an example. They can be achieved in several ways, specifically with a more or less restricted oral passageway, without violating phonemic boundaries. Under otherwise comparable conditions, orally more open productions will put less demand on proper velar function than the orally more restricted ones and are, therefore, preferable for the purpose at hand.

Examples such as this illustrate the clinical practicalities of the principle to be applied: The task is to train the hypernasal child to utilize systematically the widest oral-articulatory posture that doesn't interfere with the phoneme value the sound represents for the production of the sound in question (Waengler and Bauman-Waengler, 1987b). This might necessitate some preliminary practice in the form of relaxation exercises for lips, tongue, and, especially, jaw.

Case Study JD

| In the United States, the trend for many years has been toward early closure of palatal clefts, typically between the ages of 6 and 18 months (Marsh and Lehman, 1988). | This case study is adapted from Albery and Russell (1990). JD was born with a cleft of the soft palate which was repaired relatively late at age 2;6.

According to the authors, progression through the early speech stages with an open cleft had influenced his artic- | ulatory development. His deviant and restricted inventory is not, therefore, typical but does exemplify some of the compensatory articulation errors noted in Table 10.2.

JD's speech was highly unintelligible as the inventory restrictions resulted in the loss of numerous phonemic contrasts. |

Phonetic Inventory:

[m], [n], [w], [j], [h]		Articulated in a regular manner in the prevocalic, intervocalic, and, where applicable, postvocalic word positions.
[ʔp], [ʔb]		A glottal component accompanied the bilabial productions in the prevocalic word positions.
[p], [b], [t], [d], [k], [g],	→ [ʔ]	Stop-plosive productions (including [p] and [b] in intervocalic and
[f], [v], [ʃ], [ʒ], [θ], [ð]	→ [ʔ]	postvocalic positions), most fricatives, and affricates were realized as
[ʧ], [ʤ],	→ [ʔ]	glottal stops.
[s]	→ [ħ]	[s] was realized as a voiceless pharyngeal fricative [ħ] in all word positions.
[z]	→ [ʕ]	[z] was realized as a voiced pharyngeal fricative [ʕ] in all word positions.
[l]	→ [ĩ]	[l] was nasalized in the postvocalic word position.
[r]	→ [w]	[r] was realized as [w].

Mental Disability

Definition and General Features

The various attempts to define mental disability reflect the different understanding of, and attitudes toward, the disorder at different times. At least nine different "official" definitions of mental retardation exist from 1921 to 1992. The 1992 definition by the American Association on Mental Retardation (AAMR), the successor organization of the former American Association for the

Study of the Feebleminded and the American Association on Mental Deficiency, is no exception:

Mental retardation refers to substantial limitations in present functioning. It is characterized by significantly subaverage intellectual functioning, existing concurrently with related limitations in two or more of the following adaptive skill areas: communication, self-care, home living, social skills, community use, self-direction, health and safety, functional academics, leisure, and work. Mental retardation manifests before age 18. (AAMR, 1992, p. 5)

In such a definition, three criteria stand out:

1. subaverage intellectual functioning
2. limitations in adaptive skills
3. manifestation before 18 years of age

Subaverage intellectual functioning refers in this definition to approximately two standard deviations below the mean on suitable standardized intelligence quotient tests, translating into a score of about 70 or below. *Adaptive skills* refers to functioning in two or more general areas of specified everyday living activities; limitations of such skills pertain essentially to restrictions in learning within the individual's own living circumstances. The manifestation of a mental disability before age 18 identifies such deficiencies as a developmental disorder beginning somewhere between the time of conception and official adulthood. This would eliminate individuals who in adulthood might show signs of dementia and demonstrate similar problems in adaptive behavior, for example.

The 1992 definition further states that an individual must show significant deficits in adaptive behavior relative to his or her own cultural group. This delineation is used to rule out linguistic and cultural differences that might limit the individual's functioning in a larger setting. Paul (2007) notes, "In the old days it sometimes happened that children were labeled retarded simply because they did not speak English as their first language and could not respond to testing or questions in the school language" (p. 117). By emphasizing adaptive behavior, these misdiagnoses are now, one hopes, eliminated.

Prevalence figures for this disorder depend, of course, on the definition of the disorder used. Because definitions changed in the past and will change in the future, these figures are notoriously unreliable. The President's Committee on Mental Retardation (1978) estimated the prevalence of this disorder to be about 3 percent of the population; however, other sources (Mercer, 1973; Tarjan, Wright, Eyman, and Keeran, 1973) support only a 1 percent prevalence.

For the first time in 1992, the AAMR definition eliminated severity classifications. When compared to former definitions, this amounts to a drastic change. However, many good reasons can be given for this change. Foremost, the widespread overrating of IQ scores and their possibly negative impact on aspects of care and education for individuals with mental disabilities are arguments against this system. Nevertheless, classification according to severity is still practically very much a part of the general understanding of this disorder. Therefore, severity subgroups are delineated here for orientation purposes. The percentage of persons with mental disability in each of the classification categories is from the President's Committee on Mental Retardation (1978).

Classification	IQ score	Percentage of persons with a mental disability
mild	69 to 55	89.0%
moderate	54 to 40	6.0%
severe	39 to 25	3.5%
profound	below 25	1.5%

Specific associated problems may also impact the communicative behavior of this population. Both sensorineural and conductive hearing losses as well as abnormal middle ear function are prevalent in these individuals. Estimates of middle-ear dysfunction range from 30 to 63 percent and seem to be especially high in individuals with severe retardation (Givens and Seidemann, 1977; Lloyd and Fulton, 1972). Nolan, McCartney, McArthur, and Rowson (1980) found that nearly half of the individuals with mental disabilities they tested had hearing impairments.

Articulatory/Phonological Characteristics

All subgroups of children with mental disabilities demonstrate a higher prevalence of speech problems. It has been estimated that 70 percent of these children have some form of speech production difficulty (Fristoe and Lloyd, 1979). Generally, their speech has been described as indistinct, slurred, and sluggish. They tend to lack articulatory precision and appropriate pauses and phrasing (Weiss, Gordon, and Lillywhite, 1987). The phonological characteristics of the population with mental disabilities can be summarized as follows (Kumin, 1998; Shriberg and Widder, 1990; Stoel-Gammon, 1998):

1. Speech sound errors are more common than in the nondisabled population.
2. Deletion of consonants is the most frequent error.
3. Errors are typically inconsistent.
4. Patterns are similar to children who are not mentally disabled but demonstrate a functional delay.

In general, individuals with mental disabilities demonstrate the same phonological processes as nonretarded children but with a higher frequency of occurrence (Klink, Gerstman, Raphael, Schlanger, and Newsome, 1986; Moran, Money, and Leonard, 1984). The most common phonological processes are the reduction of consonant clusters and final consonant deletion (e.g., Bleile and Schwartz, 1984; Klink et al., 1986; Sommers, Patterson, and Wildgren, 1988). Variable use of these processes is also noted in this population. It has been hypothesized that individuals with mental disabilities may use these processes for other reasons than

to simplify their speech. For example, Shriberg and Widder (1990) suggest that consonant deletions may reflect cognitive processing constraints in the motor assembly stage of speech production.

Clinical Implications: Diagnostics

Individuals who are mentally disabled are a diverse group of people. Not only are individuals with mental disabilities quite different among themselves but also the boundaries between mentally disabled and what is considered to be norm are rather indistinct: "Mental retardation is on a continuum with normalcy" (Ingalls, 1978, p. 2). That is not to say that individuals with mental disabilities are not different from individuals who are considered to be normal; they are. For example, although the cognitive development of children with mental disabilities is said to be generally similar to that of nondisabled children, only slower (Owens, 2002), and cognitive skills have been proven to keep on growing through adulthood (Berry, Groenweg, Gibson, and Brown, 1984), organizational and recall problems, as well as difficulties in recognizing the significant feature of a given situation, distinguish children with mental disabilities from their nondisabled peers (Das, Kirby, and Jarman, 1975; Meador, 1984).

With this group diversity in mind, assessment procedures will largely depend on the age of the individual and the level of speech and language functioning. Some individuals with mental disabilities will not have speech at all and alternative means of communication will need to be explored. For the very young child who is beginning to develop first words, an independent analysis can be used to examine the inventory of sounds the child is using. For older children

> An independent analysis for children with emerging phonological systems is discussed in Chapter 6.

and adults with more developed speech and language skills, the following assessment procedures could be used:

1. *Articulation test.* An articulation test will determine the consonant and vowel inventory. Phonological patterns can also be analyzed, as well as the intelligibility of the speech at the single-word level.

2. *Spontaneous speech sample.* This will determine the consonant and vowel inventory in conversational speech. Phonological patterns can be noted as well as the overall intelligibility in natural communicative situations. Differences in intelligibility between the spontaneous speech and the articulation test should be evaluated.

3. *Motor speech capabilities.* Speech structure and function should be assessed to determine the individual's motor capabilities.

4. *Hearing acuity and middle-ear function.* Due to the large percentage of hearing losses and problems with middle-ear function, it is important to have a complete understanding of the individual's current hearing realities.

5. *Language.* The language of the client should be assessed to determine the level of linguistic functioning.

6. *Assessment of the environment.* The environment in which the individual lives and works will determine communicative needs. One of the major roles of a clinician is to assess the communicative environment in which the individual resides. This should provide information about the circumstances demanding communication of some sort and how the client is currently communicating to express needs, wants, and desires.

Although the diagnostic assessment of the individual with mental disabilities is executed in a manner essentially similar to that used with nondisabled clients, specific factors need to be kept in mind. Individual differences such as age, level of cognitive functioning, level of speech and language functioning, and learning style will naturally alter the methods used.

Clinical Implications: Therapeutics

"Each child with mental retardation presents a unique pattern of communicative abilities and difficulties which must be identified as a result of a thorough individual assessment. There is, therefore, no intervention prescription for children with retardation" (Long and Long, 1994, p. 174). Some guiding principles for clinicians can nevertheless be suggested within an intervention framework. The following principles may be applicable to the treatment of articulatory/phonological disorders in the population with mental disabilities (Owens, 2002; Swift and Rosin, 1990; Weiss, Gordon, and Lillywhite, 1987):

1. Use overlearning and repetition.
2. Train in the natural environment.
3. Begin as early as possible.
4. Follow developmental guidelines.
5. Concentrate more on overall intelligibility rather than on training individual sounds.

One could also add to this list:

6. Enlist the help of the client's caregivers.
7. Direct all therapeutic activities to communication training serving the daily routine.
8. All intervention efforts should be commensurate with the client's ability to grasp and attend to the respective tasks. This typically translates into short, repetitive, reinforced activities "meaningful to the situation and [resulting] in real consequences" (Owens, 2002, p. 495).

With very few exceptions, traditional-motor approaches with these individuals have been of little value in the treatment of speech production problems (Sommers, 1969). Therefore, a sound-by-sound approach using placement techniques would probably not be a good choice. The cycles approach has been adapted for use with children with mental disabilities in classroom settings. In these cases, time allotments have been doubled for the children; thus, each phoneme or pattern is targeted for two hours rather than for sixty minutes (Hodson, 1989). A training period of three years or more may be required before substantial intelligibility gains are observed. Hodson (1989) summarizes by saying, "Mentally retarded children seem to be especially in need of a comprehensive, system-oriented phonological remediation approach because they lack the normal cognitive abilities requisite for integration of isolated phoneme parts" (p. 331).

Many of the treatment programs for children and adults with mental disabilities target the increase of overall functional language skills. Although intelligibility is an often noted problem with these individuals, there is very little information available on the treatment of the phonological systems. One possibility, developed by Swift and Rosin (1990), presents a remediation sequence for improving intelligibility of children with Down syndrome. Although this program was designed for a specific population of children, it could be adapted for other children with mental disabilities (in Swift and Rosin's study, the children were mildly and moderately retarded with little evidence of hypotonicity).

During the early linguistic stage, single words and early two-word utterances are emphasized. In structured sound play, the clinician selects objects and toys that should elicit intended sounds. For example, if bilabial sounds were targeted, *ball, baby, bye-bye,* and *moo* could be selected. Drill work is then used to increase the target behavior, attention, and syllable sequencing. The authors also use other techniques, such as melodic speech, visual cues, cued speech, auditory bombardment, and an auditory training unit. Overlearned phrases associated with frequently occurring situations (scripts) are trained as well. In addition, augmentative communication is recognized as a valid option within the oral language intervention program.

During the late linguistic stage, drill work and the learning of scripts continue. In addition, repair strategies are now taught that may aid overall speech intelligibility. Repair strategies include a listener's request for clarification when the message is not understood, for example. Repair strategies from a speaker's point of view include repeating, rewording, and adaptations of the prosodic features (e.g., slowing the rate, adjusting phrasing, and using stress and inflection to enhance the meaning). Throughout the program, communication should be as functional as possible.

The decision to use an augmentative or alternative system for communication with individuals with mental disabilities should be based on the same criteria used with any client. If the cognitive and language comprehension levels allow it, alternative/augmentative communication devices can certainly increase the potential for successful communication. The general advice is to try speech therapy first—for one year at least—before nonspeech communicative means are introduced, even if all requirements for their use are met (Long and Long, 1994; Owens and House, 1984).

CLINICAL APPLICATION

Speech Goals and Activities for Facilitating the Development of Speech and Improving Intelligibility

The following goals and suggestions are offered by Miller (1988). Although they were proposed for Down syndrome children, they could be used with other children with mental disabilities who are in the beginning stages of speech and language development.

Speech Goals for the Child

1. *Increase the ability to respond to people and objects.* The more this skill can be promoted, the greater the opportunity for enhancing communication.
2. *Increase the frequency of vocal and verbal productions.* The more output, the more opportunity for modifying the quality of speech.
3. *Increase production of sounds and the variety of sounds made.* This includes not only the actual production of speech sounds but also speaking rate, loudness, and intonation changes. These variables will add to the intelligibility of the child.
4. *Transition from babbling behavior to using words* to *represent objects and actions in the environment.* It appears that children who are mentally disabled are trying to say words earlier than they are recognized by the caregivers in the children's environments. Their speech is often difficult to understand and the words they use are simply labels and not descriptive.

Suggestions for Caregivers

1. Identify situations and activities throughout the day in which the child is most vocal. Make a list of these situations over a week or two, noting the situation, the length of time the situation continues, and how many times these situations occur during the day.
2. Document how much the child responds to people and things by looking, touching, or playing during a particular situation. Communication depends to a large degree on responsiveness.
3. Try to increase the time the child spends in these communication-enhancing situations (noted in speech goal number 1).
4. Introduce the children to music at an early age. Children frequently respond enthusiastically to this stimulation. The type of music will depend on the child.
5. Speech activities should be a natural part of the child's day. During ordinary caregiving tasks, talk to the child about the objects and the activities. Introduce interactive games such as "pat-a-cake," "peek-a-boo," and "so big." These activities promote vocalizations as well as develop responsiveness to turn taking and social interaction.

Based on a thorough assessment, the speech-language clinician can suggest sounds, sound patterns, and words that may be included in activities for the child's day. Suggestions offered in The Child with an Emerging Phonological System section of Chapter 9 could also be incorporated here.

HEARING IMPAIRMENT

Definition and General Features

Hearing loss (or hearing impairment) is a generic term for any diminished ability in normal sound reception. The different etiologies that can result in hearing loss are only indirectly part of this definition. Commonly, hearing loss is described by type and degree of the particular auditory dysfunction (Northern and Downs, 1984). As far as the types of hearing impairment are concerned, conductive, sensorineural, and mixed dysfunctions are distinguished. The degree of hearing loss is categorized by reference to decibel (dB) levels, indicating the increase in intensity needed to make sound audible for the individual in question.

Conductive hearing loss refers to transmission problems affecting the travel of air-conducted sound waves from the external auditory canal to the inner ear. This affects the mechanical transfer of sound waves. A prominent medical condition causing conductive hearing loss is otitis media. **Sensorineural hearing loss** occurs as a consequence of damage to the sensory end organ, the cochlear hair cells, or the auditory nerve. In these cases, air-conduction and bone-conduction thresholds are typically comparable. Mumps, among other medical conditions, can cause a sensorineural auditory dysfunction. If both a conductive and a sensorineural loss can be established, a *mixed hearing loss* exists.

> To determine hearing loss, a three-frequency average is typically used, which is the average for 500, 1,000, and 2,000 Hz in the better ear (Reed, 1994).

The different degrees of hearing loss indicate the severity of the problem and are calculated according to the (approximate) threshold findings obtained. (*HL* stands for "hearing level.")

26 to 40 dB HL = mild hearing loss

41 to 55 dB HL = moderate hearing loss

56 to 70 dB HL = moderately severe hearing loss

71 to 95 dB HL = severe hearing loss

96+ dB HL = profound loss (Bess and McConnell, 1981)

Severity levels of hearing loss, determined by objective audiometric means, are not necessarily reliable indicators of speech-language function. Individuals deal differently with losses of hearing ability, especially within the context of communication. A loss of 50 dB HL bilaterally in two children, for example, can have a notably different influence on their verbal communication. Such different effects of an objectively established hearing loss can become especially important when dealing with children in various phases of their speech-language development. Even relatively mild auditory dysfunctions with relatively minor communicative consequences for adult speakers/listeners might have lasting detrimental developmental effects in children. Nevertheless, the diminished ability to receive sound for comprehension is normally identified by the degree of hearing loss.

Articulatory/Phonological Characteristics

Speech production in the hearing impaired is affected by the degree of hearing impairment and the frequencies involved. Generally, the greater the hearing loss, the more likely errors will extend from consonant and vowel productions to errors in stress, pitch, and voicing (Hull, 2001; Osberger and McGarr, 1982). Most of the literature describing the speech characteristics of hearing impaired individuals has examined children with severe to profound hearing losses. Little seems to be available about specific speech characteristics of children with less severe losses. Keeping this in mind, the following consonant, vowel, and prosodic feature differences have been noted in the speech of hearing impaired children.

Consonant production in hearing impaired children is generally characterized by deletions and substitutions. Both initial and final consonant deletions occur; however, final consonant deletions are far more prevalent (Abraham, 1989). Frequently occurring substitutions include (1) confusion of voiced and voiceless cognates, (2) substitution of stops for fricatives and liquids, and (3) confusion between oral and nasal consonants (Levitt and Stromberg, 1983). Studies with children who are hard of hearing have reported that consonants produced with the blade of the tongue ([t, d, s, z, ʃ, ʒ, tʃ, dʒ]) are more likely to be in error. The affricates are ranked as most difficult for children who are profoundly hearing impaired as well as those who are hard of hearing (Markides, 1970; Smith, 1975). These findings are not, however, completely supported by an investigation by Abraham (1989). Based on the data obtained from thirteen children with severe and profound hearing impairments, she found that there was a marked difference in the accuracy of production word-initially versus word-finally. All sounds demonstrated a lower percentage of accuracy word-finally. Although the affricates were below 50 percent accuracy, consonants with even lower percentages of accuracy included [z] and [ð].

Children with hearing impairments have been found to use at least partially rule-governed phonological systems (Abraham, 1989; Dodd, 1976). They use phonological processes similar to those of young normally developing children, although they use these processes more frequently. The overall intelligibility of speech is often reduced, particularly as linguistic complexity increases (Radziewicz and Antonellis, 1997).

Vowels tend to be neutralized; therefore, front and back vowels have a tendency to sound like central vowels (Ling, 1976). Other vowel errors include tense for lax (and lax for tense) substitutions, especially the front vowels [i] and [ɪ]. Due to poor control of timing, diphthongs are often produced as monophthongs and vice versa (Levitt and Stromberg, 1983).

Prosodic features can also be affected, although more difficulties are evidenced in profoundly impaired than in the hard-of-hearing population. Problems include reduced speech rate, slow articulatory transitions with frequent pauses, poor coordination of breathing with syntactic phrasing, use of duration to create stress patterns, and distorted resonance (Dunn and Newton, 1994).

Clinical Implications: Diagnostics

In addition to audiometric results, the speech-language diagnostician assessing the impact of impaired hearing on the articulatory/phonological status of a client needs a host of appraisal data before any diagnostic conclusion can be reached. These include cause, age of onset, and identification of the impairment; its etiology and type; and length of previous intervention efforts. Speech intelligibility measures as well as results of formal and informal testing for language skills should also be included in the assessment data.

Finally, the client's and caregivers' attitudes toward the disorder and the need for intervention will give indications about the degree of motivation and possibly the impact of therapy.

Phonetic and phonological assessments need to be completed for the child with a hearing impairment. The following assessment procedures are outlined in Dunn and Newton (1994):

1. *Speech-motor assessment.* This is used to rule out any gross neurological or anatomical limitations that might interfere with speech sound production.

2. *Syllable imitation.* This tests the coordination of the speech mechanism during nonmeaningful speech.

3. *Administration of the Phonetic Level Evaluation (PLE)* (Ling, 1976). This instrument evaluates suprasegmental and segmental skills through the imitation of nonsense syllables. The test provides a systematic, comprehensive hierarchy for the assessment of syllables with varied phonetic contexts. However, the PLE has specific shortcomings (see Dunn and Newton, 1994, pp. 130–132) and should not be used as the only evaluative measure for the hearing impaired child.

4. *Spontaneous speech sample.* Depending on the age and developmental level of the child, this could be either single words or continuous speech. Ideally, the speech sample should include both.

5. *Analysis of the segmental and suprasegmental characteristics of the spontaneous speech sample.* Segmental analysis should include those procedures outlined in this text in Chapter 7 (i.e., consonant and vowel inventory and distribution, syllable shape, and phonological pattern analysis). A suprasegmental analysis determines whether the child uses rate, pauses, stress, and intonational patterns appropriately. This can be done informally, with the clinician marking appropriate and inappropriate patterns. Dunn and Newton (1994) suggest a more formal measure developed at the National Technical Institute for the Deaf (Subtelny, 1980). This procedure provides rating scales for a variety of suprasegmental characteristics.

Clinical Implications: Therapeutics

With clients who are hearing impaired, the speech-language clinician's remedial task is mainly directed to the improvement of the client's speech intelligibility. "The term '**speech intelligibility**' may be defined generically as that aspect of oral speech-language output that allows a listener to understand what a speaker is saying" (Carney, 1994, p. 109). Such a task involves, above all, structured work on principle articulation errors and the selection of a suitable phonetic treatment program. Both of these objectives depend on two prerequisites (Dunn and Newton, 1994):

1. the improvement of the residual hearing by speech signal amplification and the methodical habituation of its application
2. the maximal utilization of the level of residual hearing for speech perception through systematic articulatory training

The first prerequisite presupposes wearing an individualized hearing aid at all times and possibly using auditory trainers during clinical sessions. In addition, it involves step-by-step procedures so that the client fully recognizes the speech-related benefits of the amplification. A primary responsibility of the speech-language clinician called to improve a client's intelligibility level is, therefore, to ensure constant proper amplification, not just during therapy, and to facilitate the client's adjustment to the new hearing situation.

The maximal utilization of the client's level of residual hearing poses another challenge. Children with hearing impairments miss important information for the recognition of speech signals, which is the main reason for their lack of intelligibility. Essentially, they produce what they are able to hear, leaving out what they are unable to receive. In directing their attention systematically to specific oral/facial movements accompanying normal suprasegmental and segmental production, their residual hearing can be more effectively utilized which can, in turn, positively influence intelligibility. In connection with suitable amplification, these efforts should increase speech intelligibility, especially in respect to voice, suprasegmental realization, and vowel production—three especially conspicuous error areas of children who have hearing impairments.

However, children with hearing impairments will also need systematic training on the phonetic as well as the phonological level.

CLINICAL APPLICATION

Teaching Speech Sound Production to Individuals with Hearing Impairment

Several approaches have been implemented with hearing impaired individuals to teach speech sound production. Examples include the Auditory Global Approach (Calvert and Silverman, 1983) and multisensory approaches, prominent examples being Ling's program (1976) and Osberger's (1983) modification of the Ling approach. The multisensory approaches use a variety of sensory modalities to first achieve accurate imitative production at the syllabic level. When a certain level of accuracy is reached, instruction begins at the word level. These approaches train speech sound production; they do not provide hearing impaired children with a systematic means of developing their phonology.

Dunn and Newton (1994) suggest a program that simultaneously teaches phonetic and phonological skills. The training sequence is as follows:

1. *Establish a suprasegmental base.* This is initially achieved through coordination of pitch, duration, and intensity with babbling or vocal play. Once this suprasegmental base is established, it will carry over to the various other stages of treatment. Dunn and Newton (1994) state in this context that "Clinicians' eagerness to work on consonants before a suprasegmental base is established may result in many of the disordered patterns characteristic of deaf speech" (p. 140).

2. *Teach the segmental speech sounds.* This begins with basic vowel patterns. The patterns are first generated within any context the child can accurately produce, preferably a CV or VC syllable structure. Both Calvert and Silverman (1983) and Ling (1976) provide procedures and strategies for achieving a new sound with the hearing impaired population.

3. *Generalize a stable production by using different phonetic contexts and new syllable types.* Once a production is stable in one basic context, new contexts are selected. Productions move from various other syllable types to monosyllabic words and, finally, to two-syllable words. With one- and two-syllable words, the child is responsible only for accurate production of the target sound. For example, if the target sound is [b] and the selected word is *boat,* [bo] would be considered an accurate production. Two-syllable words begin with those containing reduplicated syllables such as *bye-bye* or *booboo.* In this phase, acceptable speech sound production is applied to meaningful words. In addition, prosodic variation is practiced with these words.

MOTOR SPEECH DISORDERS: ACQUIRED APRAXIA OF SPEECH

Definition and General Features

The general term *apraxia* refers to a disorder in the execution of purposeful movements; reflexive or automatic motor actions remain largely intact. For example, as soon as an otherwise reflexive action is intended—on request, for example, or by one's own volition—gross execution difficulties occur. *Acquired apraxia of speech,* therefore, is the impaired volitional production of articulation and prosody (Ballard, Granier, and Robin, 2000; Kent and Rosenbek, 1983). These articulatory and prosodic aberrations do not result from muscle weakness or slowness but from impairment to the central nervous system's programming of oral movements. Apraxia of speech represents an inability to program and sequence articulatory requirements for volitional speech (Darley, Aronson, and Brown, 1975; Johns and Darley, 1970). Thus, **apraxia of speech** is a disorder of expressive communication as a result of brain damage affecting the normal realization of speech sounds, sound sequences, and prosodic features representing speech. Auditory comprehension, in principle, remains intact (Ballard, Granier, and Robin, 2000; Darley et al., 1975).

Damage to two central nervous system areas is held responsible for the communication disorder found in apraxia of speech. The most common cause is injury to the dominant side of the brain's frontal lobe—more specifically its posterior inferolateral regions, otherwise known as *Broca's area.* However, lesions to several cortical and subcortical areas might be involved as well, specifically those of the supplemental motor cortex and the basal ganglia (Dworkin, 1991).

Apraxia of speech should be separated from the dysarthrias, another motor speech disorder that affects verbal expression. The following guidelines are given for differentiation between the two (Darley et al., 1975; LaPointe and Wertz, 1974; Shipley and McAfee, 1998; Wertz, LaPointe, and Rosenbek, 1984):

Apraxia of speech	Dysarthria
Absence of any muscular weakness, paralytic condition, or discoordination.	Presence of muscular weakness. Change in muscular tone secondary to neurologic involvement.
Speech process of articulation is primarily affected.	All processes for speech are affected: respiration, phonation, resonation, and articulation.
Speech errors result from disruption of the central nervous system's programming of oral movements.	Speech errors result from disruption of the central and peripheral nervous system's control of muscular movements.
Inconsistent articulatory errors.	Consistent, predictable articulatory errors.

Apraxia of speech differs from the aphasias by the language involvement of the latter. Such a differentiation appears quite clear as long as a comparison is made between apraxic speakers, on the one hand, and those afflicted with Wernicke's or sensory aphasia, on the other. A valid distinction between apraxic speakers and those with Broca's, that is, expressive or motor aphasia, is far less obvious and has triggered an ongoing discussion of long standing (Martin, 1974; Noll, 1983). Both apraxic speakers and Broca's aphasics have little, if any, language involvement and somewhat common problems with verbal output

(Benson, 1979; Luria and Hutton, 1977). Of course, statements like these depend largely on the definition of the term *language involvement*. When the syntactic realization of grammatical rules is taken into account, individuals with Broca's aphasia are dysgrammatic; apraxics are not. Thus, although some vagueness between the terms *Broca's aphasia* and *apraxia of speech* certainly remains, one can generally summarize that

> *Aphasia is a language disorder caused by injury to the dominant hemisphere responsible for processing the language code. Apraxia is a motor speech disorder resulting from damage to neural circuits of the dominant hemisphere responsible for programming speech movements. (Marquardt, 1982, p. 3)*

Apraxia of speech can, of course, co-occur with aphasia and does so frequently (Metter, 1985).

Apraxia of speech should also be distinguished from oral (nonverbal) apraxia. **Oral (nonverbal) apraxia** is a disturbance of the planning and execution of volitional *nonspeech* movements of oral structures, that is, those movements not representing speech production. For example, if a client is asked to lick his lips, he might blow instead (Johns, 1985). The same client might be perfectly able to drink some juice, swallow the sip, and lick a drop off his lips (Meitus and Weinberg, 1983). On request, though, he cannot perform the same motor action; attempts will probably result in a series of laborious, bizarre trials. As might be expected, clients with apraxia of speech often suffer from oral (nonverbal) apraxia as well.

Articulatory/Phonological Characteristics

The following characteristics of apraxia of speech have been noted (Bauman and Waengler, 1977; Croot, 2002; Darley, 1978;

Darley et al., 1975; Deal and Darley, 1972; Haley, Ohde, and Wertz, 2000; Johns and Darley, 1970; LaPointe and Johns, 1975; Shankweiler and Harris, 1966; Waengler and Bauman-Waengler, 1980, 1987a; Wertz, LaPointe, and Rosenbek, 1984):

1. *Effortful, trial-and-error groping of articulatory movements and attempts at self-correction.* This may result in equalization of syllabic stress patterns, slow rate of speech, and other prosodic alterations.
2. *Prosodic disturbances.*
3. *Difficulty initiating utterances.*
4. *Articulatory inconsistency on repeated production of the same utterance.* However, islands of clear, well-articulated speech exist.
5. *Sound substitution errors predominate.* Additions and prolongations also occur; distortions and omissions are less frequent.
6. *Sound or syllable transpositions may occur.*
7. *Occasionally, articulatory errors are complications rather than simplifications.* A consonant cluster may be substituted for a single consonant.
8. *Errors are typically phonetically related to one another.* Substitutions, for example, may be related in place or manner of articulation to the intended sound.
9. *More errors occur on consonants that require more precise articulatory adjustments*—for example, fricatives and affricates.
10. *Number of errors and articulatory struggle increase as the word increases in length.*
11. *Speech comprehension and word recognition abilities are often far better than speech production abilities.*
12. *Clients recognize their errors.* This may cause numerous retrials or self-correction attempts.
13. *Under otherwise comparable conditions, more sound production errors occur in stressed than in unstressed syllables.*

Clinical Implications: Diagnostics

A diagnosis of apraxia of speech may not have been made before a clinician sees the client. Therefore, the following areas should be included in a thorough evaluation of a client with suspected apraxia of speech (Haynes and Pindzola, 1998):

1. aphasia test
2. intelligence, cognitive, and memory tests, as needed
3. apraxia battery
4. speech-motor mechanism examination
5. articulation test
6. spontaneous speech sample

For the purposes at hand, this diagnostic section will concentrate on those testing procedures that involve only aspects of articulation and phonology—that is, on numbers 3 through 6 of the listed categories.

CLINICAL APPLICATION

Formal and Informal Tests for Apraxia of Speech in Adults

Test of oral and limb apraxia	DeRenzi, Pieczuro, and Vignolo, 1966
Oral apraxia test	Darley, Aronson, and Brown, 1975
Test of verbal, oral, and limb apraxia	Rosenbek and Wertz, 1976
Test of oral and limb apraxia	Helm-Estabrooks, 1996
Dworkin-Culatta Oral Mechanism Examination	Dworkin and Culatta, 1980
Apraxia Battery for Adults	Dabul, 2000
Oral movement battery	Moore, Rosenbek, and LaPointe, 1976
Tests of integrity and consistency of phoneme production	Johns and Darley, 1970
Motor Speech Evaluation	Wertz, LaPointe, and Rosenbek, 1984

Some of these tests can be used to evaluate the presence of oral and limb apraxia as well as specific characteristics of apraxia of speech. Others will give the clinician information about the client's abilities to sequence words of varying length and complexity.

The speech-motor assessment examines the structure and function of the articulators. Although the function of the articulators is often assessed with one of the apraxia batteries, the oral-mechanism examination can also be used to determine the presence of oral (nonverbal) apraxia. If the structure is intact but commands eliciting nonverbal movements such as "pucker your lips" or "stick out your tongue" result in laborious, bizarre movements, oral apraxia may be suspected.

Both the articulation test and the spontaneous speech sample should answer the following questions:

- *Does the client have difficulty initiating utterances?* Does this difficulty have a pattern? For example, is it better with words or sentences? Does the content of the message play a role?
- *Are there any islands of well-articulated speech?* These are usually automatic-reactive responses such as the days of the week or "I can't say that"; however, are there others?
- *Which sound errors occur?* Evaluate the differences between one-word articulation tests and spontaneous speech. Also note the errors that occur as the complexity of the word or utterance increases. Furthermore, register substitutions, additions, prolongations, transpositions, distortions, and omissions.
- *Do sound errors have a pattern?* Errors are typically related to the target sound. A place-manner-voice analysis could demonstrate which patterns are occurring.

Observations should include ascertaining difficulties with fricatives, affricates, and consonant clusters, all typical problems for the individual with apraxia of speech.
- *Which prosodic aberrations occur?* Stress realizations (stressed versus unstressed syllables), intonation, rate of speech, and pausing should be observed and analyzed.

Clinical Implications: Therapeutics

In apraxia of speech, the client's ability to program and sequence articulatory requirements for volitional speech is impaired. This impairment ranges from mild to severe, with each client demonstrating a different clinical picture. Some may have difficulty only in sequencing certain multisyllabic words or with specific clusters; others may have extreme problems sequencing a simple CV word. Obviously, such varying degrees of impairment will influence the selection of therapeutic measures. In addition, certain aspects of motor production affect the error patterns of apraxic speakers (Knock, Ballard, Robin, and Schmidt, 2000; Robin, Bean, and Folkins, 1989; Wambaugh, Martinez, McNeil, and Rogers, 1999; Wertz et al., 1984). These general guidelines can be utilized when structuring therapy.

1. *Articulatory accuracy is better for meaningful than for nonmeaningful utterances.* Therefore, avoid nonsense syllables; all treatment stimuli should be meaningful.

2. *Errors increase as words increase in length.* Determine the level at which the client demonstrates accurate production most of the time, then build on that level. For example, if the assessment reveals that the client can produce CV, CVC, and VC words fairly accurately, start with this level of functioning and slowly build to CVCV structures or "easier" two-syllable words.

3. *Errors increase as the distance between successive points of articulation increases.* Evaluate your word material. Organize it so that this factor is taken into consideration. If you are working on consonant clusters, [st] should be easier than [sk]. If you are structuring words, *toilet* should be easier than *shopping*.

4. *Errors increase on consonants that require more precise articulatory adjustments.* Fricatives, affricates, and consonant clusters are extremely difficult for some apraxics. Begin with other sound classes until more volitional control is achieved.

Darley, Aronson, and Brown (1975) advocate the *phonetic placement approach* to help the client relearn the positioning of the articulators for the standard realization of speech sounds. Cognition, sensory perception, and neuromuscular action are (by definition) essentially unimpaired. Therefore, the positioning of the articulators necessary for the realization of the sound in question should be relatively easy to achieve.

The *sound modification method* presupposes the presence of some regular sound realizations. Applying the knowledge of phonetic sound production features, the clinician attempts to derive the target sound out of elements of another sound the client can realize in a regular manner. For example, assume that a client with generally acceptable [d] sounds demonstrates difficulty with [t], especially when initiating a stressed syllable. The client may actually need to be instructed only that the main phonetic differences between [d] and [t] pertain to voicing and lenis versus fortis production—organ, place, and manner of articulation are in both cases directly comparable. Thus, any whispered [d] will automatically result in a weak [t], which a slightly increased production effort will normalize. The client will not have to learn [t]-productions "from scratch." The sound modification method might prove to be beneficial for individual clients.

CLINICAL APPLICATION

Apraxia of Speech: A Phonological Disorder?

According to popular contemporary definitions that subsume articulation difficulties under the category of phonological disorders (e.g., Elbert, 1997), apraxia of speech would be labeled a phonological disorder. The treatment for apraxia of speech has historically been phonetically based; that is, it followed traditional articulation principles. However, taking the apraxics' relatively preserved language, cognitive, and perceptual skills into account, a remediation program based on phonological principles could offer some additional advantages.

1. Articulatory accuracy is, as a rule, better for meaningful than for nonmeaningful utterances. A minimal pair approach, for example, would speak directly to this issue by focusing on meaningful and meaning-differentiating communication.
2. Many of the minimal pair approaches are based on communicative breakdown. For example, the child actually means *key* but says *tea* and therefore receives the wrong picture card. Apraxic clients are very aware of errors and communicative breakdowns that occur when production accuracy fails. Therefore, this method could in some cases be more motivating than imitating nonsense syllables.

Generally, though, a minimal pair approach falls short for the communicative needs of the apraxic individual. There are just not very many minimal pairs that are used contrastively in everyday communicative situations. Nevertheless, for certain clients, adding phonemic to phonetic principles of treatment might be beneficial. Phonetic principles such as awareness of the articulatory complexity of the utterance, the consonants it contains, and the helpful or hindering coarticulation features could be easily combined with meaningful, communicatively contrasting situations.

---

*M*OTOR SPEECH DISORDERS: THE DYSARTHRIAS

Definition and General Features

The word *articulation* has its origin in the Greek root *arthr-,* referring to the jointed connection between the many different parts of the speaking process. *Dys-arthr-ia,* therefore, literally means "disordered articulation." To be sure, in this context, "articulation" is to be understood in the broadest possible sense, that is—as signifying all articulated movements that result in speech. The technical term *dysarthria,* on the other hand, denotes a rather explicit group of articulation disorders, namely, those caused by neurogenic abnormalities, more specifically by the impairment of a single portion or several portions of the (central and/or peripheral) nervous system that control and coordinate speech. **Dysarthrias** are neuromuscular speech disorders (Marquardt, 1982).

Dysarthrias have many different causes. Accident-induced trauma, tumors, cerebrovascular accidents (strokes), congenital conditions, and infectious and degenerative neurogenetic diseases are prominent among them. All of these events can bring about more or less pronounced paralytic conditions and coordination impairments of the voluntary musculature required for speech production. The result: dysarthrias.

Articulatory/Phonological Characteristics

It is customary to classify the dysarthrias according to the locus of the damage and its neuropathic consequences into five main types:

1. spastic dysarthria
2. ataxic dysarthria
3. hypokinetic dysarthria
4. hyperkinetic dysarthria
5. flaccid dysarthria

In addition, any simultaneous occurrence of characteristics of several types is labeled:

6. mixed dysarthria

Every main type has its cluster of speech impairing phonetic/articulatory production features (Darley et al., 1975; Dworkin, 1991; Wertz, 1985). They are summarized in Table 10.3.

Summaries like these are helpful, but any division of dysarthric characteristics into just five subtypes suggests more group uniformity than is actually the case. Although some within-group similarities can probably serve as general guidelines, several across-group features overlap considerably, "thus challenging the usefulness of group classifications" (Dworkin, 1991, p. 6). Several of the deficiencies mentioned belong in some measure simply to the clinical picture of most dysarthrias. These include the following:

Respiration. Irregular, generally shallow breathing patterns might suddenly become interrupted by some deep breaths; rapid inspiration, incomplete expiration phases; waste of expiratory air during speaking; lack of respiratory support.

Phonation. Strained voice; deviations from suitable loudness levels (either too loud or too soft) and voice quality (either too harsh or too "breathy," aphonic).

Resonation. Hypernasality and nasal air emission as a consequence of incomplete velopharyngeal closure, distorting all speech sounds with the exception of nasals.

Articulation. Labored, indistinct sound articulation, especially of consonants, resulting in distortions or substitutions. Consonant errors might affect whole sound classes; stops, for example, might

Table 10.3 Summary of Features of the Various Types of Dysarthria

Types	Features
Spastic Dysarthria	
(Resulting from upper motor neuron system disorders. Example: Pseudobulbar palsy.)	
Respiration:	Low respiratory frequency with shallow inspiration and lack of expiratory control.
Phonation:	Strained, harsh, low-pitch voice; reduced pitch and loudness ranges.
Resonation:	Hypernasality; nasal air emission.
Articulation:	Slow, labored, imprecise phoneme realization, especially of consonants.
Ataxic Dysarthria	
(Resulting from cerebellar lesions. Example: Cerebellar ataxia.)	
Respiration:	Shallow inspiration and lack of expiratory control. Rapid, irregular, forced breathing patterns.
Phonation:	Forced, hoarse-breathy, trembling voice. Generally reduced (but sometimes excessive) use of pitch and loudness.
Resonation:	Normal.
Articulation:	Slow, imprecise phoneme realization, especially of consonants. Sound prolongations. Irregular pausing between words, syllables, and sounds.
Hypokinetic Dysarthria	
(Resulting from disorders of the extrapyramidal system. Example: Parkinsonism.)	
Respiration:	Frequent respirations with shallow inspiratory phases and lack of expiratory control.
Phonation:	Harsh, tremorous voice; reduced pitch and loudness levels.
Resonation:	Normal.
Articulation:	Fluctuating imprecise articulation. Articulatory bursts. Low intelligibility.
Hyperkinetic Dysarthria	
(Resulting from disorders of the extrapyramidal system. Examples: Athetosis, chorea.)	
Respiration:	Frequent respirations with shallow inspirations and incomplete expirations; lack of respiratory control.
Phonation:	Strained, tremorous voice. Uncontrolled but generally reduced ranges in the expressive use of pitch and loudness.
Resonation:	Alternating hypernasality.
Articulation:	Variable imprecision of phoneme, especially consonant, realization.
Flaccid Dysarthria	
(Resulting from lower motor neuron system disorders. Example: Bulbar palsy.)	
Respiration:	Shallow, audible inspirations. Uneven, incomplete expirations. Low respiratory frequency; low expiratory air pressure.
Phonation:	Breathy, hoarse voice lacking expressive pitch and loudness variation.
Resonation:	Marked hypernasality with nasal air emission.
Articulation:	Slow, imprecise phoneme realization, especially of consonants.

Source: Summarized from Darley et al. (1975); Dworkin (1991); and Waengler and Bauman-Waengler (1987a).

be realized as homorganic fricatives. Also, second and third elements of consonant clusters might be deleted; rate of speech is usually slower than normal (bradylalia), but bursts of fast speech (tachylalia) might occur as well; qualitative and quantitative misrepresentations of vowels.

Prosody. Narrow range of intonational configurations ("monopitch"); (often greatly) reduced variety of expressive loudness levels ("monoloudness"); this generally reduced range of prosodic elements is sometimes interrupted by exaggerated stress and intonation patterns (Darley et al., 1975; Dworkin, 1991; Patel, 2002; Waengler and Bauman-Waengler, 1987a).

The physiological basis for all of these characteristics is a striking imbalance in the constant and subtle changes between phases of (relative) muscular tension and relaxation leading to normal speech events. The delicate synergism between the interaction of individual muscles and whole muscle groups to produce speech is in all cases of dysarthria disturbed. Instead, a disproportionate influence of agonistic and antagonistic forces determines dysarthric speech motor activity, distorting its normally smooth flow into effortful, poorly controlled speech production.

Common characteristics such as these exist across and within the main groups of dysarthrias. However, individual clients medically diagnosed with a specific type of dysarthria often show significant deviations from the noted group features. These individual differences are especially important within the assessment and intervention process. The speech-language clinician will always need to find out the specific deviations from norm each individual client displays.

Clinical Implications: Diagnostics

Most dysarthric clients are referred to us by physicians or medical institutions. As a rule, an official diagnosis has already been established, usually down to the subtype the client belongs to medically—spastic dysarthria, for example. What, then, remains for speech-language pathologists to assess and evaluate? Actually, quite a bit.

Even in the appraisal section of our assessment process, we need to go far beyond the initial (mainly medical) information available to us. As mentioned earlier, dysarthric subtype characteristics are somewhat vague and indeterminate and therefore constitute little more than a point of departure for any appropriate collection of clinical data. They are both helpful and insufficient for our purposes. They are helpul because they indicate what to suspect and what to look for. They are insufficient because individual cases more often than not show considerable deviations from average, book-based descriptions. That is why *all* dysarthric symptoms contributing to abnormal voice and speech production need to be appraised as precisely as possible.

One possible aid to precise appraisal is the use of instrumentation. There is certainly no scarcity of instruments available to be used to objectify the data. The problem does not lie in a lack of suitable instrumentation but in their proper application to the task at hand. Many clinicians are not trained well enough in instrumentation to feel comfortable with its proper use or do not have easy access to instrumentation. Another reason for the rare use of instruments in a clinical setting is a time concern: Clinicians feel too pressed for time to engage in the utilization of instruments in order to make their appraisal data more objective and verifiable.

A second way to make the appraisal of dysarthric clients more comparable, reliable, and precise is the use of a suitable protocol. Such a protocol might look like that found in Figure 10.1.

CLINICAL APPLICATION

Protocols for the Appraisal of the Speech Characteristics of Clients with Dysarthria

Frenchay Dysarthria Assessment	Enderby, 1980, 1983
Dysarthria Examination Battery	Drummond, 1993
Point-Place System	Rosenbek and LaPointe, 1985
Motor Speech Evaluation	Wertz, LaPointe, and Rosenbek, 1984
Assessments of Intelligibility of Dysarthric Speech	Yorkston and Beukelman, 1981

Some of these assessment instruments give profiles for the various diagnostic categories, whereas others provide severity ratings.

After having identified kind and severity of the dysarthric disturbances within the main subsystems contributing to speech, the clinician is now ready to interpret and evaluate them in their totality; that is, the clinician may draw a composite picture of the problem at hand—diagnosis in the narrow sense of the term. Diagnoses lead directly into therapy planning. They form the very basis for the professional selection of appropriate intervention measures.

Clinical Implications: Therapeutics

The speech-language clinician's main therapeutic goal is the improvement of the dysarthric client's intelligibility. Because the established deficits are caused by central and/or peripheral nervous system damage, this is done primarily by searching for, and training, compensatory measures. The diagnostic results should provide the necessary information about the kind and degree of shortcomings in the various subsystems constituting normal speech production (i.e., respiration, phonation, resonation, and articulation). This information becomes the basis for therapy planning.

Most therapy plans are based on the principle of treating disordered facets of the subsystems contributing to speech thoroughly and methodically (Dworkin, 1991; Johns, 1985; McHenry, 2003; Rosenbek and LaPointe, 1985; Yorkston, 1996; Yorkston, Beukelman, and Bell, 1988). Because speech results from cumulative effects of secondary physiological functions, the primary functions of structures in which speech is rooted have to be considered as well. Thus, speech breathing has to evolve out of systematically modified breathing patterns for vital silent breathing; articulation out of natural conditions of lip, tongue, and jaw movements; and the voicing/unvoicing of sound segments and suitable intonation patterning out of previously normalized voice production. In this way, an elaborate system of suitable exercises is created and diligently practiced. If aspects of different subsystems need to be combined— as in the case of respiratory preconditions for specific voice effects such as changes in pitch, loudness, quality, and quantity, for example— matters can quickly become complicated. Superior planning and tenacity as well as flexibility during the implementation of the program are prerequisite ingredients for the successful treatment of practically all dysarthric clients. A general guideline for this task pertains to the observance of certain sequences. For example, postural adjustments precede every specific measure; respiratory and resonatory dysfunctions have to be addressed before phonatory, articulatory, and prosodic ones (Dworkin, 1991).

Figure 10.1 Protocol for Assessing Respiration, Phonation, Resonation, and Articulation of Dysarthric Speech

1. Rate the degree of normal, near normal, or abnormal behavior on a scale from 1 to 5 by marking the double line at the judged value.

	normal		→		abnormal
	1	2	3	4	5

Respiration
Silent breathing
Speech breathing
   Inspiration
   Expiration
   Breath support
   Shouting
   Shortness of breath

Resonation
Nasality
Quality of prolonged vowels
   Constant   check one   [   ]
   Intermittent   [   ]

Phonation
Voice
Pitch
Volume

Lips
Appearance in resting position
Lip protrusion
Movement during speaking

Jaw
Appearance in resting position
Movement during speaking

Tongue
Appearance in resting position
Protrusion
Elevating tip of tongue
Lowering tip of tongue
Lateral movements
During speaking
Strength

Articulation
Vowels
   Quality
   Duration
Consonants
Clusters

Prosody
Stress
Intonation
Tempo
Rhythm

2. Itemize the most salient characteristic in each of the categories with a rating of 3 or more.
3. Repeat the rating process at least one more time on a different day.

The following general treatment goals are summarized by Rosenbek and LaPointe (1985):

1. *Help the person become a productive patient.* Clinician and client have agreed on the necessity and value of treatment, what is to be accomplished, and the treatment procedures.
2. *Modify abnormalities of posture, tone, and strength.*
3. *Modify respiration.*
4. *Modify phonation.*
5. *Modify resonation.*
6. *Modify articulation.*
7. *Modify prosody.*
8. *If indicated, provide alternative or augmentative modes of communication.*

The ordering of these goals does not imply a certain progression with one exception: The patient must accept an active role in treatment before changes in speech are possible. Exercises for each of these treatment goals are listed in Rosenbek and LaPointe (1985).

Dworkin (1991) provides a procedure based on a specific order of speech subsystems. The first-order subsystems consist of resonation and respiration; the second order is phonation; and the third order consists of articulation and prosody. First-order subsystems are treated first; second-order subsystems second, and third-order subsystems are last in the treatment sequence. Inhibition and facilitation techniques will probably need to precede the specific subsystem treatments. Inhibition techniques are implemented for increased tone and any associated weakness and paresis, hyperactive reflexes, hyperkinesia, and hypersensitivity. On the other hand, facilitation techniques are introduced to improve functioning of any of the following abnormal features: decreased tone and any associated weakness and paresis, hypoactive reflexes, and hyposensitivity.

The following general treatment objectives are provided by Dworkin (1991):

1. Promote adequate orofacial postures.
2. Promote integration of orofacial reflexes.
3. Improve orofacial muscle tone and strength.
4. Improve range, speed, timing, and coordination of orofacial muscle activities.

These general goals must be seen in light of the treatment hierarchy that includes first-, second-, and third-order subsystems. Detailed exercises for each of the subsystems are included in Dworkin (1991).

CLINICAL APPLICATION

Resources for Treatment of the Adult Client with Dysarthria

The following selected references are given to aid the clinician in the treatment of adult clients with dysarthria:

Berry, W. R. (1983). *Clinical dysarthria.* San Diego: College-Hill.

Darley, F. L., Aronson, A. E., & Brown, J. R. (1975). *Motor speech disorders.* Philadelphia: W. B. Saunders.

Duffy, J. R. (2005). *Motor speech disorders: Substrates, differential diagnosis, and management* (2nd ed.). St. Louis, MO: Mosby Year Book.

Dworkin, J. P. (1991). *Motor speech disorders: A treatment guide.* St. Louis, MO: Mosby Year Book.

Farber, S. D. (1982). *Neurorehabilitation: A multisensory approach.* Philadelphia: W. B. Saunders.

Johns, D. F. (Ed.). (1985). *Clinical management of neurogenic communicative disorders* (2nd ed.). Boston: Little, Brown.

McNeil, M. R., Rosenbek, J. C., & Aronson, A. E. (Eds.). (1984). *The dysarthrias: Physiology, acoustics, perception, management.* San Diego, CA: College-Hill Press.

Moore, C., Yorkston, K., & Beukelman, D. (Eds.). (1991). *Dysarthria and apraxia of speech: Perspectives on management.* Baltimore: Paul H. Brooks.

SUMMARY

There are several communication disorders with articulatory/phonological deficits as one of their central characteristics. This chapter provided an overview of the most prominent among them. First, the childhood disorders developmental apraxia of speech, cerebral palsy, clefting, mental disability, and hearing impairment have been reviewed. Acquired communication disorders with articulatory deficits commonly occurring in adults were then represented by apraxia of speech and the dysarthrias. Each of these disorders has been defined and general characteristics have been listed. Such an outline served as a foundation for the subsequent discussion of specific articulatory and phonological problems that are found in these populations. Assessment principles for the respective speech problems noted have been pointed out followed by selected therapeutic measures for the treatment of individuals within the seven populations.

For each of the disorders mentioned, an impressive list of specialized literature exists. References have been given throughout the chapter to guide interested students and practitioners to more in-depth information. Each disorder represents a complex entity, including many important variables and involving several groups of professionals. This chapter briefly summarized basic considerations of articulatory and phonological features and their clinical intervention.

CASE STUDY

The following results are from the Hodson Assessment of Phonological Patterns (HAPP-3) (Hodson, 2004) for Les, age 5;6. Les has been diagnosed with childhood apraxia of speech.

1. basket	[bæ.ə]	14. hanger	[æn.ə]
2. boats	[boᵘ]	15. horse	[oət]
3. candle	[dæ.nə]	16. ice cubes	[aɪ.tu]
4. chair	[teə]	17. jumping	[dʌm]
5. clouds	[daᵘ]	18. leaf	[jit]
6. cowboy hat	[taᵘ·bə.æt]	19. mask	[mæt]
7. feather	[bɛ.də]	20. music box	[mu.ɪt bɑ]
8. fish	[bɪt]	21. page	[beɪt]
9. flower	[daᵘ·ə]	22. plane	[beɪn]
10. fork	[fot]	23. queen	[din]
11. glasses	[dæ.ət]	24. rock	[wɑ]
12. glove	[dʌb]	25. screwdriver	[du.daɪ.ə]
13. gum	[dʌm]	26. shoe	[du]
		27. slide	[daɪt]
		28. smoke	[moᵘt]
		29. snake	[deɪt]
		30. soap	[doᵘp]

31. spoon   [bun]
32. square   [dɛ.ə]
33. star   [dɑə]
34. string   [twɪn]
35. swimming   [tɪ.mɪn]
36. television (TV) [tɛ.bi]
37. toothbrush   [tubət]
38. truck   [tjʌk]
39. vase   [beᴵd]
40. watch   [wɑt]
41. yoyo   [joᵛjoᵛ]
42. zip   [jɪp]
43. crayons   [deᴵ.ə]

44. black   [bæt]
45. green   [din]
46. yellow   [jɛjoᵛ]
47. three   [ti]
48. thumb   [dʌm]
49. nose   [noᵛd]
50. mouth   [maᵛf]

Although Les appears to have a fairly complete vowel inventory, with the exception of central vowels with r-coloring, his consonant repertoire is extremely limited. There are no fricatives, affricates, lateral or central approximants represented in this sample. At age 5;6 Les was considered highly unintelligible.

THINK CRITICALLY

1. Refer to the case study of Les, age 5;6, that was presented earlier. Which consonants does Les have in the prevocalic, intervocalic, and postvocalic positions? Given the fact that most children demonstrate a much larger inventory of consonants in the prevocalic position, what comments could you make about Les's inventory?

2. Which syllable shapes are present in the speech sample from Les? Do you see any evidence of CC structures?

3. Note the collapse of phonemic contrasts in Les's speech. Do you see any sound preferences?

TEST YOURSELF

1. Although an exact delineation of symptoms to describe childhood apraxia of speech is controversial, what is considered to be central to the disorder?
   a. oral weakness
   b. sequencing errors
   c. a central nervous system disorder
   d. cognitive impairment
2. Speech-related respiratory, phonatory, articulatory, and prosodic abnormalities, as well as velopharyngeal inadequacies, are primarily associated with
   a. developmental apraxia of speech
   b. hearing losses
   c. cerebral palsy
   d. mental disability
3. A management plan for a child with a cleft palate usually involves
   a. long-term care with a team of specialists
   b. short-term care with only a surgeon
   c. long-term care with only a speech-language pathologist
   d. short-term care with a team of specialists
4. Compensatory strategies for stop production in children with cleft palate include which one of the following?

a. glottal and laryngeal stops
b. gliding of fricatives
c. fronting
d. deaffrication

5. It is estimated that 70 percent of this group of children have some form of speech difficulty.
   a. children with mild hearing losses
   b. children with a mental disability
   c. children with a language disorder
   d. all of the above

6. The phonological patterns of children with a mental disability can be summarized as
   a. each child having a similar communication difficulty
   b. deletion of consonants is the most frequent error
   c. error patterns are consistent
   d. having error patterns that are very different when compared to children who demonstrate a functional delay

7. The degree of speech production difficulty in individuals with a hearing impairment is related to the
   a. type of hearing aid
   b. the degree of hearing loss
   c. the type of hearing loss
   d. b. and c.

8. Children with a moderate to severe hearing loss need training with which one of the following?
   a. suprasegmental aspects of speech
   b. oral-motor movements
   c. velopharyngeal function
   d. swallowing

9. Which one of the following is associated with acquired apraxia of speech?
   a. presence of muscular weakness and changes in muscular tone
   b. absence of paralytic conditions
   c. speech errors resulting from the disruption of central and peripheral nervous systems' muscular movements
   d. consistent, predictable articulatory errors

10. In treating the adult with dysarthria, which one of the following is not a treatment goal?
    a. modifying respiration
    b. modifying prosodic aspects of speech
    c. modifying the backing of stop consonants
    d. modifying any abnormalities in phonation and resonation

WEBSITES

www.apraxia-kids.org

This website, sponsored by a national organization, CASANA, includes information for families and professionals (speech-language pathologists, physicians, educators, etc.) who work with children who have apraxia. The website includes an Apraxia Library where you can search for new articles/research on any aspect related to CAS. There is a large amount of information specifically for the speech-language professional that pertains to assessment and treatment of childhood apraxia of speech.

http://gait.aidi.udel.edu/res695/homepage/pd_ortho/clinics/c_palsy/cpweb.htm

This website is created by the Alfred I. Dupont Institute in Wilmington, Delaware. It provides an in-depth description of cerebral palsy (causes, diagnosis, types, prognosis, treatment, etc.).

www.samizdat.com/pp5.html

This website is written by Lenore Daniels Miller, a speech-language pathologist. The information is written specifically for parents of a support group (Prescription Parents) related to cleft palate. The article also explains the role of a speech-language pathologist and the speech and language characteristics related to cleft palate.

www.nsslha.org/public/hearing/disorders/

This site, hosted by the National Student Speech Language Hearing Association, has fifteen different links associated with hearing loss. Each link provides a quick article on a different aspect of hearing loss in simplified, easy-to-understand language.

www.asha.org/public/speech/disorders/dysarthria.htm

The American Speech-Language-Hearing Association provides a good summary of the symptoms and treatment for dysarthria. The site also gives tips for a person with dysarthria and for a person who is listening to dysarthric speech.

FURTHER READINGS

Caruso, A., & Strand, E. (1999). *Clinical management of motor speech disorders in children.* New York: Thieme.

Falzone, S., Cardamone, J., Karnell, M., & Jones, M. (2006). *The clinician's guide to treating cleft palate speech.* Cambridge, MA: Elsevier.

Hull, R. (2001). *Aural rehabilitation: Serving children and adults.* Clifton Park, NY: Thomson-Delmar Learning.

Velleman, S. (2003). *Childhood apraxia of speech: Resource guide.* Clifton Park, NY: Thomson-Delmar Learning.

Workinger, M. S. (2005). *Cerebral palsy: Resource guide for speech-language pathologists.* Clifton Park, NY: Thomson-Delmar Learning.

Glossary

acoustic phonetics The study of the transmission properties of speech.

addental [s] A frequent s-sound distortion marked by too close an approximation of the organ of articulation and the place of articulation causing the resulting s-sound to lose its regular stridency, giving a "dull" or "flat" sound impression.

affricate Manner of articulation marked by a homorganic release of a stop with the auditory effect of a stop + fricative sequence, e.g., [ʧ].

affrication The replacement of fricatives by homorganic affricates. Example: [ʧu] for *shoe*.

age appropriate In accordance with developmental norm values of a given age.

allophonic variation The phonetic realization of a phoneme; also called phonetic variation. *See:* speech sounds.

alveolar Alveolar ridge of upper (frontal) teeth as place of articulation for consonant production, e.g., [t].

alveolarization The change of nonalveolar sounds, mostly interdentals and labio-dentals, into alveolar sounds.

anticipatory assimilation *See:* regressive assimilation.

apical Tip of the tongue as organ of articulation for consonant production, e.g., [θ].

apico-alveolar Referring to the organ of articulation (apex of the tongue) and the place of articulation (alveolar ridge) for sound production.

appraisal Beginning phase of the assessment process. The collection of data to be interpreted and evaluated in the diagnostic phase.

approximant A speech sound marked by a much wider passage of air resulting in a smooth (as opposed to turbulent) air flow, e.g., [w], [j].

apraxia of speech A disorder of expressive communication as a result of brain damage affecting the normal realization of speech sounds, sound sequences, and prosodic features representing speech (Darley et al., 1975).

articulation The totality of motor processes involved in the planning and execution of smooth sequences of highly overlapping gestures that result in speech.

articulation disorder Refers to difficulties with the motor production aspects of speech, or an inability to produce certain speech sounds that results in aberrations in their form when compared to regular pronunciation. Articulation disorders are phonetic in nature. *See:* phonological disorder.

articulators Anatomical structures utilized to generate speech sounds: organs and places of articulation.

articulatory backing A compensatory measure of cleft palate children to produce speech sounds more posteriorly in the oral cavity than is normally the case (Trost, 1981).

articulatory phonetics Deals with the production features of speech sounds, their categorization and classification according to specific production parameters.

aspirate Referring to [h] as a speech sound consisting of an audible puff of breath.

assessment Clinical evaluation of a client's disorder.

assimilation Adaptive articulatory changes by which one speech sound becomes similar, sometimes identical, to a neighboring sound segment.

assimilatory process Describes changes in which a sound becomes similar to, or is influenced by, a neighboring sound of an utterance.

association lines Indicators for connections between autosegments on different tiers.

auditory phonetics The study of speech (sound) perception.

autosegmental phonology One of the nonlinear phonologies proposing to factor out changes within the boundary of a segment by putting them onto another "tier."

avoidance factor The avoidance of words that do not contain sounds within a child's inventory.

backing Refers to a substitution in which the organ and/or place of articulation is more posteriorly located than the intended sound.

393

bifid uvula A uvula medially divided into two portions, a split uvula (uvula bifida).

binary system A system using a plus (+) and minus (–) system to signal the presence (+) or absence (–) of certain features.

bunched "r" Referring to the "bunched" corpus of the tongue during an r-sound production.

canonical babbling Collective term for the reduplicated and nonreduplicated babbling stages.

categorical perception The tendency of listeners to perceive speech sounds varied along a continuum according to the phonemic categories of their native language.

centering diphthong A diphthong in which the offglide, or less prominent element of the diphthong, is the central vowel [ə] or [ɚ]. Examples: with [ə], care [kɛə], with [ɚ] bar [bɑɚ] or wear [wɛɚ].

cerebral palsy (CP) A nonprogressive disorder of motor control caused by damage to the developing brain during pre-, peri-, or early postnatal periods.

checked syllable See: closed syllable.

childhood apraxia of speech (CAS) See: developmental apraxia of speech.

chronological mismatch Persistence of early phonological processes together with processes characteristic of later stages of phonological development.

citation articulation test Examines speech sound articulation in selected isolated words.

citing A single-word test response, e.g., the naming of a picture.

clefting A division of a continuous structure by a cleavage, a split prominently caused by a failure of the palate to fuse during fetal development.

close Referring to the relative closeness between the dorsum of the tongue and the roof of the mouth during vowel production, e.g., [u] (when compared to [ʊ]).

closed syllable A syllable that has a coda, e.g., stop; a checked syllable.

coalescence See: total assimilation.

coarticulation The concept that the articulators are continually moving into position for other segments over a stretch of speech.

coda All the sound segments of a syllable following its peak.

code switching The ability to change back and forth between dialects, in this case, specifically between African American Vernacular English and Standard American English.

coding Translating stimuli from one form to another, for example, from auditory to written form or from written to auditory.

cognate Referring to the similarity between two sounds; Cognates may refer to similar vowels, [i] and [ɪ] are i-type vowels or consonants that differ only in voicing features, e.g., [p] and [b] are cognates.

communication augmentation Any approach designed to support, enhance, or augment the communication of individuals who cannot use speech in all situations.

complete assimilation See: total assimilation.

comprehensive evaluation A series of activities and tests that allows a more detailed and complete collection of data than do screenings.

conductive hearing loss Refers to transmission problems affecting the travel of air-conducted sound waves from the external auditory canal to the inner ear.

consonant A speech sound with a significant constriction within the vocal tract, mainly in the oral and pharyngeal cavities, foremost along the sagittal midline of the oral cavity.

contact assimilation Also contiguous assimilation. An assimilatory process modifying immediately adjacent sounds.

contiguous assimilation See: contact assimilation.

contoid Nonphonemic consonantlike sound production.

coronal Pertaining to the corona of the tongue as organ of articulation, i.e., its frontal and lateral edges forming a near three-quarter circle. Example: [d].

coronal place node In feature geometry, refers to articulation of both the tongue tip and the tongue blade segments.

cueing techniques Visual and/or tactile cues used to help the child articulate certain sounds or sound sequences.

culture A way of life developed by a group of individuals to meet psychosocial needs. It consists of values, norms, beliefs, attitudes, behavioral styles, and traditions.

deaffrication The realization of affricates as homorganic fricatives. Example: [ʃiz] for cheese.

denasalization The replacement of nasals by homorganic stops. Example: [dud] for noon.

dental   Upper teeth as place of articulation for consonant production, e.g., [f].

dentalization   Nonstandard articulatory variation in the production of nondental consonants: using the dental place of articulation for a nondental consonant, e.g., [s̪] for [s].

derhotacization   Loss of r-coloring during the production of [r] and rhotacized central vowels.

derivational morpheme   Any grammatically significant addition to the word stem by affixes (prefixes, infixes, suffixes).

developmental apraxia of speech (DAS)   Refers to children who evidence a lack of motor control of the oral mechanism for speech production that is not attributable to other problems of muscular control (Hall, Jordan, and Robin, 1993).

developmental verbal dyspraxia (DVD)   *See:* developmental apraxia of speech (DAS).

diacritics   Marks added to sound transcription symbols in order to give them a particular phonetic value.

diagnosis   The end result of studying and interpreting of data collected during appraisal.

dialect   A neutral label that refers to any variety of a language that is shared by a group of speakers.

diphthong   A vowel in which there is a change in quality during its duration.

distinctive features   Phonetic constituents that distinguish between phonemes.

distribution of speech sounds   Refers to where the norm and aberrant articulations occurred within a word.

dorsal place node   In feature geometry, refers to those segments (vowels and consonants) articulated with the dorsum of the tongue.

dorsum   Surface area of the tongue.

duration symbols   Diacritics to mark the length of speech sounds.

dysarthrias   Neuromuscular speech disorders.

emerging phonology   The time span during childhood in which conventional words begin to appear as a means of communication.

epenthesis   A syllable structure process marked by the insertion of a sound segment into a word, mostly (but not always) a schwa insertion between two consonants, e.g., [pəliz] for *please*.

ethnicity   Refers to commonalities such as religion, nationality, and region that may affect a dialect.

facilitating context   Phonetic aspects of neighboring speech sounds able to support sound features to be acquired.

feature geometry   A group of nonlinear phonological theories that have adopted the tiered representation of features used in autosegmental phonology. Feature geometry attempts to explain why some features are affected by assimilation processes (known as *spreading* or *linking* of features) while others are affected by neutralization or deletion processes (known as *delinking*).

final consonant deletion   A syllable structure process by which a CVC syllable is by the omission of the final consonant converted into a CV syllable. The omission of a syllable-arresting consonant.

first word   An entity of relatively stable phonetic form that is produced consistently by the child in a particular context and is recognizably related to the adultlike word form of a particular language.

formal Standard English   Applies primarily to written language and the most formal spoken language situations; tends to be based on the written language and is exemplified in guides of usage or grammar texts.

fortis   Refers to relatively more articulatory effort among consonant cognates. Voiceless stop-plosives are fortis.

fricative   A manner of articulation characterized by an audible friction noise established by forcing expiratory air through a constricted passage in the oral cavity. Example: [f]. Extensive constrictions cause the hissing noise of sibilants, a subcategory of fricatives. Examples: [s], [ʃ].

fronting   A substitution process marked by the "fronting" of organ and place of articulation for palatal sounds into the coronal-alveolar region (palatal fronting) or the change of velar consonants into either palatal or alveolar consonants (velar fronting). Example: t/k substitution.

generative phonology   The application of principles of generative (or transformational) grammar to phonology.

glide   Manner of articulation, a shifting movement of the articulators from a narrower to a wider consonantal constriction, e.g., [w]; also called semivowel, sonorant.

gliding   A substitution process characterized by the replacement of liquids with glides.

gliding of liquids/fricatives The replacement of liquids or fricatives by glides. Example: [wɛd] for *red*.

glossing Repeating with normal pronunciation what the client has just said for easier identification later.

groping behavior An ongoing series of movements of the articulators in an attempt to find the desired articulatory position.

harmony process *See:* assimilation process.

hearing loss A generic term for any diminished ability in normal sound reception.

holophrastic period The span of time during which the child uses one word to indicate a complete idea.

idiosyncratic (or unusual) error patterns Error patterns not (or infrequently) seen in the normal speech development of children.

idiosyncratic processes Phonological processes found only in the speech of individual children with disordered phonology.

independent analysis Takes only the client's productions into account; they are not compared to the adult norm model.

individual sound approach Traditional or motor approach referring to the treatment of individual speech sounds in sequence. *See:* motor approach.

informal Standard English Takes into account the assessment of the members of the American English speaking community as they judge the "standardness" of other speakers.

intelligibility Refers to a judgment made by a clinician based on how much of an utterance can be understood.

interdental "s" A frequent s-sound distortion marked by the visibility of the tongue tip between the upper and lower incisors. Interdental s-productions sound very much like [θ] and [ð], respectively.

intervocalic Consonants or consonant clusters occurring between two vowels, typically at the juncture of two syllables.

inventory of speech sounds A list of speech sounds that the client can articulate within normal limits.

item learning The acquisition of word forms as unanalyzed units, as productional wholes.

jargon stage Characterized by strings of babbled utterances that are modulated primarily by intonation, rhythm, and pausing.

juncture symbols Diacritics to mark juncture phenomena within an utterance, e.g., *a + nice man* versus *an + ice man*.

labial Organ of articulation (lower lip), place of articulation (upper lip), e.g., [m] (bilabial).

labial assimilation The change of a nonlabial into a labial sound under the influence of a neighboring labial sound.

labialization Consonant productions with lip rounding, e.g., [sʷup] for [sup]. Equivalent to rounding of (unrounded) vowels.

labial place node In feature geometry, designates the lip articulation of the rounded vowels and the consonants /w/, /p/, /b/, /m/, /f/, /v/, and possibly /r/ in General American English.

laryngeal node In feature geometry, designates the glottal characteristics of the segment.

lateral Manner of articulation in which a midline closure within the oral cavity lets the expiratory airstream pass laterally into the cheeks, e.g., [l]; together with the rhotics collectively referred to as liquids.

lateral "s" A nonstandard s-sound production characterized by (uni- or bilateral) air flow during /s/ realizations. The result is an unusual, openly conspicuous "slurping" noise component.

lax Referring to a lesser degree of muscular activity during vowel production, e.g., [ɪ] (when contrasted to [i].

lenis Refers to comparatively less articulatory effort among consonant cognates. Most voiced sounds are lenis.

limitation Occurs when differences between the child's and the adult's system become limited to only specific sounds, sound classes, or sound sequences.

limited English proficient Used for any individual between the ages of 3 and 21 who is enrolled or preparing to enroll in an elementary or secondary school, who was not born in the United States, or whose native language is a language other than English. Individuals who are Native Americans or Alaska Natives and come from an environment where a language other than English has had a significant impact on the individuals are also included in this definition. The difficulties in speaking, writing, or understanding the English language compromise the individual's ability to successfully achieve in classrooms, where the language of instruction is English, or to participate fully in society (PL107-110, The No Child Left Behind Act of 2001).

linear phonologies   Phonological theories characterized by an assumption that all meaning-distinguishing sound segments are serially arranged.

linkage condition   Any condition governing the association of units on each tier.

lip symbols   Diacritics to mark rounding or unrounding of the lips during normally unrounded or rounded consonant realizations, e.g., [tʷɪn] = labialized, rounded [t].

liquid   Group term for the consonant categories laterals and rhotics; different from the glides because liquids lack an audible articulatory movement. Together with the glides and nasals (as well as all vowels), the liquids fall under the cover term *sonorants*.

liquid assimilation   The articulatory influence of a liquid on a neighboring nonliquid sound.

manner of articulation   The type of constriction the organ and place of articulation produce for the realization of a particular consonant.

manner of articulation features   Specify in generative phonology the way organ and place of articulation cooperate to produce sound classes, signaling differences between stops and fricatives, for example.

markedness   (Of phonemes) refers to sounds that are relatively more difficult to produce and are found less frequently in languages.

mediodorsal   Central portion of the tongue as organ of articulation for consonant production, e.g., [j].

mediopalatal   Central portion of hard palate as place of articulation for consonant production, e.g., [j].

metalinguistic awareness   The ability to think about and reflect on the nature of language and how it functions.

metaphonology   Involves the child's conscious awareness of the sounds within that particular language.

metaphon therapy   A therapy approach marked by the systematic training of phonological

awareness, especially the awareness of sound properties.

metathesis   The transposition of sounds within an utterance.

metrical phonology   One of the nonlinear phonologies emphasizing stress by building metrical trees that reflect the syntactic structure of an utterance.

micrognathia   Referring to an unusually small mandible.

minimal pair   Words that differ in only one phoneme value among their sound constituents, e.g., *book* versus *cook*.

minimal pair contrast therapy   The therapeutic use of pairs of words that differ by one phoneme only.

monophthong   A vowel that remains qualitatively the same throughout its entire production; a pure vowel.

morphophonemic function   The role of phonemes to signal grammatical units. For example: /s/ is a phoneme of the English language, as demonstrable by the minimal pair *sick* versus *thick*. However, /s/ also signals plurality, *book* versus *books*, a morphological function.

morphophonology   The study of the different allomorphs of the morpheme and the rules governing their use.

motor approach   Referring to the treatment of individual sounds based on the placement of the articulators for normal speech sound production. *See:* individual sound approach.

motor-based problem   A phonetic disorder characterized by misarticulations seen as disruptions at a relatively peripheral level of the articulatory process involving inadequate motor learning.

multilinear phonologies   *See:* nonlinear phonologies.

multiple-sound approach   Attempts to influence several error sounds simultaneously.

nasal   Manner of articulation for consonants produced with the velum lowered so that the expiratory air can pass freely through the nasal cavity, e.g., [m].

nasal assimilation   The articulatory influence of a nasal on a neighboring nonnasal sound.

nasality symbols   Diacritics to mark passing/nonpassing of expiratory air through the nasal cavity. Only nonnasal sounds can be nasalized, only nasals denasalized.

nasal "s" Irregular s-productions marked by nasal airflow caused by organic or functional deficiencies of velar movement resulting in incomplete nasal-pharyngeal closure.

natural class Phonemes that share one or more features and usually have similar patterns within a language system (Grunwell, 1987). *See:* naturalness.

naturalness (Of phonemes) designates the sound aspects, (1) the relative simplicity of a sound production and (2) its high frequency of occurrence in languages.

natural phonology A theory that incorporates features of naturalness theories and was specifically designed to explain the development of the child's phonological system.

natural process A process common in the speech development of children across languages.

near-minimal pairs Pairs of words that differ by more than one phoneme; the vowel preceding or following the target sound remains constant in both words.

noncontiguous assimilation *See:* remote assimilation.

nonlinear phonologies A group of phonological theories understanding segments as governed by more complex linguistic dimensions.

nonphonemic diphthong A diphthong that can be realized in its initial vowel-like portion without a change in word meaning, e.g., [heɪ] or [he] for *hay*.

nonreduplicated babbling Demonstrates variation of both consonants and vowels from syllable to syllable. Also called variegated babbling.

obstruents Consonants characterized by a complete or narrow constriction between the articulators hindering the expiratory airstream; includes the stop-plosives, the fricatives, and the affricates.

offglide The end portion of a diphthong, e.g., [ɪ] in [eɪ].

onglide The beginning portion of a diphthong, e.g., [e] in [eɪ].

onset Consists of all sound segments of a syllable prior to its peak.

open Referring to the relative open space between the dorsum of the tongue and the roof of the mouth during vowel production, e.g., [ʊ] (when contrasted to [u]).

open syllable A syllable that does not contain a coda, e.g., *do;* an unchecked syllable.

optimality theory A constraint-based approach which is one nonlinear (multilinear) theory of phonology.

oral (nonverbal) apraxia A disturbance of the planning and execution of volitional *nonspeech* movements of oral structures.

oral stops Manner of articulation with obstruction of the oral cavity by free nasal passage of the airstream, e.g., nasals.

ordering Occurs when substitutions that appeared unordered and random become more organized.

organ of articulation The part within the vocal tract that actually moves to achieve the articulatory result; the active articulator.

palatal Hard palate as place of articulation for consonant production.

palatalization Irregular articulatory variation in the production of consonants. Using the palate as place of articulation for nonpalatal consonants.

palatal "s" Irregular s-production characterized by a palatal (rather than alveolar or predorsal) approximation of the organ toward the place of articulation. The result is an auditory impression of close to a voiceless sh-sound, transcribed as [sʲ].

partial assimilation Assimilatory influence of one sound segment on another by which only parts of the phonetic characteristics of the influencing sound are imposed on the influenced sound resulting in a higher degree of similarity between the respective sound segments.

peak The most prominent, acoustically most intense part of a syllable; usually a vowel.

perceptual constancy The ability to identify the same sound across different speakers, pitches, and other changing environmental conditions.

perseverative assimilation *See:* progressive assimilation.

persisting normal processes The use of certain phonological processes beyond their typical age limits.

phoneme The smallest linguistic unit that is able, when combined with other such units, to establish word meanings and distinguish between them; exemplified by minimal pairs, e.g., *seek* versus *peak*.

phonemic awareness   Refers only to the phoneme level and necessitates an understanding that words are comprised of individual sounds.

phonemic diphthong   A diphthong that cannot be produced in only its initial onglide portion without a change in word meaning, e.g., [mas] versus [maᵘs].

phonemic error   The consistent replacement of one (American English) phoneme with another.

phonemic inventory   The repertoire of phonemes used contrastively by an individual.

phonemic problem   Any misarticulation based on difficulties with the language-specific linguistic function of speech sounds, their phoneme values.

phonetically consistent form   *See:* proto-word, quasi-word, vocable.

phonetic approaches   Each error sound is treated individually, one after the other. Also referred to as traditional-motor approaches.

phonetic context   The segmental, suprasegmental, and phonotactic environment in which a given speech sound occurs.

phonetic inventory   The repertoire of speech sounds for a particular client, including all the characteristic production features the client utilizes.

phonetic placement method   The clinician instructs the client how to position the articulators in order to produce a norm production.

phonetic problem   Any misarticulation based on phonetic production difficulties.

phonetics   The study of speech emphasizing the description and classification of speech sounds according to their production, transmission, and perceptual features.

phonetic variability   Refers to the unstable pronunciations of the child's first fifty words.

phonetic variation   The phonetic realization of a phoneme; also called allophonic variation.

phonological awareness   The individual's awareness of the sound structure or phonological structure of a spoken word in contrast to written words.

phonological development   Refers to the acquisition of speech sound form and function within the language system.

phonological disorder   Refers to an impaired system of phonemes and phoneme patterns within the context of spoken language. Exemplified by the improper use of phonemes to signify linguistic meaning within a language. Phonological disorders are phonemic in nature. *See:* articulation disorder.

phonological idiom   Refers to accurate sound productions that are later replaced by inaccurate ones. Also called regression.

phonological process   "A mental operation that applies in speech to substitute for a class of sounds or sound sequences presenting a common difficulty to the speech capacity of the individual" (Stampe, 1979, p. 1).

phonological processing   The use of sounds of a language to process verbal information in oral or written form that requires working and long-term memory.

phonological rules   Used to demonstrate the relationship between the underlying (phonological) and the surface (phonetic) forms. In generative phonological analysis, also formalized statements about the patterns of sound substitutions and deletions.

phonology   The description of the systems and patterns of phonemes that occur in a language. Phonologists analyze the language-specific distinctive phonemes and the rule-governed nature of these systems.

phonotactics   The description of the allowed combinations of phonemes in a particular language.

place node   In feature geometry, groups together all the different places of articulation.

place of articulation   The area within the vocal tract that remains motionless during consonant articulation, that is, the passive articulator; the part that the organ of articulation approaches or contacts directly.

plosive   Manner of articulation resulting from a previous complete occlusion at some point of the vocal tract; the sudden release phase of a stop.

postalveolar   Posterior portion of the alveolar ridge as place of articulation.

postdorsal Posterior portion of the tongue as organ of articulation for consonant production, e.g., [k].

postpalatal Posterior portion of the hard palate as place of articulation for consonant production.

postvocalic Consonants or consonant clusters following a vowel, typically occurring at the end of a word or utterance.

predorsal Anterior portion of the dorsum as organ of articulation for consonant production, e.g., predorsal [z] realization.

predorsal-alveolar Referring to the organ of articulation (predorsal portion of the tongue) and the place of articulation (alveolar ridge) for the production of speech sounds.

prelinguistic behavior Refers to all vocalizations prior to the first actual words.

prepalatal Anterior portion of hard palate as place of articulation for consonant production, e.g., [ʒ].

presystematic stage The stage in the phonological development of children when contrastive word units (rather than contrastive sounds of phoneme value) are acquired.

prevocalic Consonants or consonant clusters preceding a vowel, typically occurring at the beginning of a word or utterance.

progressive assimilation The assimilatory influence of a preceding sound on a following sound segment. Also called perseverative assimilation.

prosodic features Larger linguistic units, elements that occur across segments, influencing what we say.

proto-word Vocalizations used consistently by a child in particular contexts but without a recognizable adult model. Also called vocables, phonetically consistent forms, and quasi-words.

quasi-word *See:* phonetically consistent form, proto-word, vocable.

race A biological label that is defined in terms of observable physical features (such as skin color, hair type and color, head shape and size) and biological characteristics (such as genetic composition).

raised tongue position Too high a tongue position for the production of the vowel in question.

reduplicated babbling Marked by similar strings of consonant–vowel productions.

reduplication A syllable structure process because the syllable in question is "simplified" by a mere repetition of the first, e.g., [baba] for *bottle*.

regional dialects Those dialects corresponding to various geographical locations.

regression *See:* phonological idiom.

regressive assimilation The change of a sound's phonetic production characteristics under the influence of a following consonant, e.g., [ɪʃi] for *is she*. Also called anticipatory assimilation.

remote assimilation Assimilatory process modifying a speech sound separated by at least one other segment, especially when both the influencing and the influenced sounds belong to two different syllables. Also called noncontiguous assimilation.

retroflexed Produced with the tip of the tongue "curled back," e.g., one form of standard [r] production.

retroflexed "r" Referring to the tip of the tongue curled upward and back during a specific type of [r]-production.

rhotic Manner of articulation characterized by r-coloring.

rhotic diphthong A diphthong in which the offglide is the central vowel with r-coloring [ɚ]. *See also* centering diphthong.

rhyme Cover term for nucleus (vowel) and coda (the arrest of the syllable).

rising diphthong During production of these diphthongs, portions of the tongue move from a lower onglide to a higher offglide position; thus, relative to the palate, the tongue moves in a rising motion.

root node In feature geometry, links the segment to the prosodic tiers.

salience factor A child's active selection in early word productions of words containing sounds that are important or remarkable (salient) to the child.

screening Activities or tests that identify individuals for further evaluation.

segmental Referring to the discrete, sequentially arranged speech segments, to vowels and consonants.

semivowels The sonorants, especially the glides among them, as productionally characterized by an articulatory movement from a sagittally more constricted to a sagittally more open oral cavity.

sensorineural hearing loss Occurs as a consequence of damage to the sensory end organ, the cochlear hair cells, or the auditory nerve.

sequencing errors Disruptions in the production of the correct ordering of speech sounds or syllables.

sibilant A fricative sound characterized by a sharper sound due to the presence of high-frequency components. Examples: [s], [ʃ].

silent posturing Refers to the positioning of the articulators for a specific articulation without sound production.

skeletal (or CV) tier A representation of a syllable and its hierarchically related components onset and rhyme.

social or **ethnic dialects** Those dialects that are generally related to socioeconomic status and/or ethnic background.

sonorant consonants Consonants produced with a relatively open expiratory passageway; include the nasals, glides, and liquids.

sonorants A group of vowels and specific consonants which demonstrate more sonority; more relative loudness in relationship to other sounds with the same length, stress, and pitch.

sonority The relative loudness of a sound relative to that of other sounds with the same length, stress, and pitch.

sound modification method Based on deriving the target sound from a phonetically similar sound that the client can accurately produce.

speech intelligibility "That aspect of oral speech-language output that allows a listener to understand what a speaker is saying" (Carney, 1994, p. 109).

speech sound development Refers primarily to the gradual articulatory mastery of speech sound forms within a given language.

speech sounds Represent physical sound realities; end products of articulatory motor processes.

stimulability testing Testing the client's ability to produce a misarticulated sound in an appropriate manner when "stimulated" by the clinician to do so.

stop Manner of articulation resulting from a complete occlusion at some point of the vocal tract brought about by the cooperation of an (active) organ of articulation and a (passive) place of articulation; the buildup of expiratory air-stream pressure behind this closure, e.g., [p].

stopping A substitution process. The substitution of stops for homorganic fricatives or the omission of the fricative portion of affricates.

stress markers Diacritics to indicate different levels of syllable prominence in an utterance.

strident [s] An irregular s-production named after the auditory impression it creates, i.e., a shrill, irritating, often whistlelike sound component.

substitution The replacement of one sound/phoneme with another.

substitution process Describes those sound changes in which one sound class is replaced by another.

suppression Refers to the abolishment of one or more phonological processes as children move from the innate speech patterns to the adult norm production.

suprasegmentals Intonation, stress, juncture, tempo, and rhythm as speech characteristics "added to" its segmental (speech sound) components.

syllabic A consonant that functions as a syllable nucleus.

syllabification (1) The division of a (spoken or written) word into syllables. (2) The shifting of the syllable nucleus from a vowel to the following consonant, [bʌtən] → [bʌtn̩].

syllable arresting sounds *See:* coda.

syllable constraint Refers to any restriction or limitation established in the production of syllable shapes.

syllable nucleus The "core" of a syllable carrying its highest intensity and prosodic features, typically a vowel.

syllable releasing sounds *See:* onset.

syllable shape Refers to the structure of the syllables within a word.

syllable shape reduction The reduction of a syllable shape usually by the deletion of one of its consonant members.

syllable structure process Describes those sound changes that affect the structure of the syllable.

system An orderly combination of parts forming a complex unity.

systematic sound preference Pertains to the use of a single phonetic realization for several different phonemes.

system learning The acquisition of phonemic principles that apply to the phonological system in question.

tense Referring to a higher degree of muscular activity during vowel production, e.g., [i] (when compared to [ɪ]).

tiers Separable and independent levels that represent a sequence of gestures or a unified set of acoustic features.

tone-unit An organizational unit imposed on prosodic data.

tongue symbols Diacritics to describe deviations from normal tongue placement for speech sound realizations, e.g., [d̪il] = dentalized [d].

tongue thrust Refers to excessive anterior tongue movement during swallowing and a more anterior tongue position during rest.

tongue thrust swallow Referring to excessive anterior tongue movement during swallowing and a more anterior tongue position during rest. *See:* tongue thrust.

total assimilation The assimilatory influence of a sound segment on another by which all the phonetic properties of the influenced sound are changed into the sound category of the influencing sound. Also called complete assimilation.

traditional-motor approaches *See:* phonetic approaches.

transfer Indicates the incorporation of language features into a nonnative language, based on the occurrence of similar features in the native language.

trill A sound produced by the vibratory action of an organ of articulation tapping rapidly against a place of articulation.

unchecked syllable *See:* open syllable.

underlying form A purely theoretical concept that is thought to represent a mental reality behind the way people use language.

unrounding Spreading of the lips during sound production, e.g., [i] (when compared to [u]).

unstressed syllable deletion A syllable structure process (also called weak syllable deletion) marked by the omission of the unstressed syllable of a multisyllable word.

variable use of processes Processes operating on one target sound in a certain context that are in other contexts already suppressed or different processes operating on the same target phoneme.

variegated babbling *See:* nonreduplicated babbling.

velar Soft palate as place of articulation for consonant production, e.g., [g] in [gup].

velar assimilation The change of a nonvelar sound into a velar one under the influence of a neighboring velar sound.

velar harmony A (regressive) assimilation process in which a postdorsal-velar stop-plosive causes a preceding coronal-alveolar stop-plosive to change its organ and place of articulation, e.g., [gɑg] for [dɑg].

velarization The change of a nonvelar consonant into a velar one under the influence of a neighboring velar sound. Example: [gɑg] for *dog*.

vernacular dialects Those varieties of spoken American English that are considered outside the continuum of Informal Standard English.

vocable *See:* phonetically consistent form, proto-word, quasi-word.

vocalization (vowelization) The replacement of syllabic liquids and nasals, foremost [l], [r], and [n], by vowels. Example: [lædʊ] for *ladder*.

vocoid Nonphonemic vowel-like sound production.

voice symbols Diacritics to mark the voicing of an unvoiced or the unvoicing of a voiced consonant.

voicing The presence or absence of simultaneous vibration of the vocal cords resulting in voiced or voiceless consonants.

vowel A speech sound that is formed without significant constriction of the oral and pharyngeal cavities, especially along the sagittal midline of the oral cavity; normally serving as syllable nucleus.

vowelization The replacement of syllabic liquids and nasals, foremost [l], [r], and [n], by vowels. Example: [lædʊ] for *ladder*.

weak syllable deletion A syllable structure process (also called unstressed syllable deletion) marked by the omission of the unstressed syllable of a multisyllable word.

References

Abercrombie, D. (1967). *Elements of general phonetics*. Chicago: Aldine.

Abkarian, G. G., & Dworkin, J. P. (1993). Treating severe motor speech disorders: Give speech a chance. *Journal of Medical Speech-Language Pathology, 1,* 258–287.

Abraham, S. (1989). Using a phonological framework to describe speech errors of orally trained, hearing-impaired school-agers. *Journal of Speech and Hearing Disorders, 54,* 600–609.

Adams, M., Foorman B., Lundberg, I., & Beeler, T. (1997). *Phonemic awareness in young children: A classroom curriculum.* Baltimore: Brookes.

Air, D. H., Wood, A. S., & Neils, J. R. (1989). Considerations for organic disorders. In N. Creaghead, P. W. Newman, & W. Secord (Eds.), *Assessment and remediation of articulatory and phonological disorders* (2nd ed.) (pp. 265–301). New York: Macmillan.

Albert, M., Sparks, R., & Helm, N. (1973). Melodic intonation therapy for aphasia. *Archives of Neurology, 29,* 130–131.

Albery, E., & Russell, J. (1990). Cleft palate and orofacial abnormalities. In P. Grunwell (Ed.), *Developmental speech disorders* (pp. 63–82). New York: Churchill Livingstone.

American Association on Mental Retardation. (1992). *Mental retardation: Definition, classification, and systems of support* (9th ed.). Washington, DC: Author.

American Cleft Palate–Craniofacial Association and Cleft Palate Foundation. (1997). *About cleft lip and cleft palate.* Chapel Hill, NC: Author.

American Speech-Language-Hearing Association. (1985). Guidelines for identification audiometry. *ASHA, 27,* 49–52.

American Speech-Language-Hearing Association. (1989). Report of the ad hoc committee on labial-lingual posturing function. *ASHA, 31,* 92–94.

American Speech-Language-Hearing Association. (1990). Guidelines for screening for hearing impairments and middle ear disorders. *ASHA, 32* (Suppl. 2), 17–24.

American Speech-Language-Hearing Association. (1991). The role of the speech-language pathologist in management of oral myofunctional disorders. *ASHA, 33* (Suppl. 5), 7.

American Speech-Language-Hearing Association Ad Hoc Committee on Communication Processes and Nonspeaking Persons. (1980). Nonspeech communication: A position paper. *ASHA, 22,* 267–272.

American Speech-Language-Hearing Association Audiologic Assessment Panel 1996. (1997). *Guidelines for audiologic screening.* Rockville, MD: Author.

Anderson, P. (1941). *The relationship of normal and defective articulation of the consonant [s] in various phonetic contexts to auditory discrimination between normal and defective [s] productions among children from kindergarten through fourth grade.* Master's thesis, State University of Iowa, Iowa City.

Andrews, N., & Fey, M. E. (1986). Analysis of the speech of phonologically impaired children in two sampling conditions. *Language, Speech, and Hearing Services in Schools, 17,* 187–198.

Aram, D. M. (1984). Preface. In W. H. Perkins & J. L. Northern (Eds.), *Seminars in speech and language.* New York: Thieme-Stratton.

Aram, D. M., & Glasson, C. (1979). *Developmental apraxia of speech.* Paper presented at the annual meeting of the American Speech-Language-Hearing Association, Atlanta, GA.

Aram, D. M., & Nation, J. E. (1982). *Child language disorders.* St. Louis, MO: C. V. Mosby.

Archangeli, D. (1988). Aspects of underspecification theory. *Phonology, 5,* 183–207.

Archangeli, D. (1998). Optimality theory: An introduction to linguistics in the 1990s. In D. Archangeli & D. T. Langendoen (Eds.), *Optimality theory: An overview* (pp. 1–32). Malden, MA: Blackwell Publishers.

Archangeli, D., & Langendoen, D. T. (1997). *Optimality theory: An overview.* Oxford: Blackwell.

Archangeli, D., & Pulleyblank, D. (1994). *Grounded phonology.* Cambridge, MA: MIT Press.

Arlt, P. B., & Goodban, M. T. (1976). A comparative study of articulatory acquisition as based on a study of 240 normals, aged three to six. *Language, Speech, and Hearing Services in Schools, 7,* 173–180.

Arnold, G. E. (1943). Die nasalen Sigmatismen. *Archives für Ohren-, Hals- und Nasenheilkunde, 153,* 57.

Arnold. G. E. (1954). Nasal sigmatisms. *Talk, 35,* 2.

Atkinson-King, K. (1973). Children's acquisition of phonological stress contrasts. *UCLA Working Papers in Phonetics, 25,* 184–191.

Aungst, L., & Frick, J. (1964). Auditory discrimination ability and consistency of articulation of /r/. *Journal of Speech and Hearing Disorders, 29,* 76–85.

Baker, R. D., & Ryan, B. P. (1971). *Programmed conditioning for articulation.* Monterey, CA: Monterey Learning Systems.

Ball, M. J. (2002). Clinical phonology of vowel disorders. In M. J. Ball & F. E. Gibbon (Eds.), *Vowel disorders* (pp. 187–216). Boston: Butterworth-Heinemann.

Ball, M. J., & Gibbon, F. E. (2002). *Vowel disorders.* Boston: Butterworth-Heinemann.

Ball, M. J., & Kent, R. D. (1997). *The new phonologies: Developments in clinical linguistics.* San Diego, CA: Singular.

Ball, M. J., & Rahilly, J. (1999). *Phonetics: The science of speech.* London: Arnold.

Ballard, K., Granier, J., & Robin, D. (2000). Understanding the nature of apraxia of speech: Theory, analysis, & treatment. *Aphasiology, 14,* 969–995.

Bally, S. J. (1996). Communication strategies for adults with hearing loss. In M. J. Moseley & S. J. Balley (Eds.), *Communication therapy. An integrated approach to aural rehabilitation with deaf and hard of hearing adolescents and adults.* Washington, DC: Gallaudet University Press.

Bankson, N. W., & Bernthal, J. E. (1990). *Bankson-Bernthal test of phonology.* Chicago: Riverside Press.

Bardach, J., & Morris, H. L. (Eds.). (1990). *Multidisciplinary management of cleft lip and palate.* Philadelphia: W. B. Saunders.

Barlow, J. (2002). Resent advances in phonological theory and treatment: Part II. *Language, Speech, and Hearing Services in Schools, 33,* 4–8.

Barlow, J. A. (2001). Case study: Optimality theory and the assessment and treatment of phonological disorders. *Language, Speech, and Hearing Services in Schools, 32,* 242–256.

Barlow, S., & Farley, G. (1989). Neurophysiology of speech. In D. P. Kuehn, M. L. Lemme, & J. M. Baumgartner (Eds.), *Neural bases of speech, hearing, and language* (pp. 146–200). Boston: Little, Brown.

Barton, D. P. (1976). *The role of perception in the acquisition of speech.* Unpublished doctoral dissertation, University of London.

Barton, D. P. (1980). Phonemic perception in children. In G. Yeni-Komshian, J. Kavanagh, & C. A. Ferguson (Eds.), *Child phonology: Volume 2. Perception* (pp. 97–116). New York: Academic Press.

Bashir, A. S., Grahamjones, F., & Bostwick, R. Y. (1984). A touch-cue method of therapy for developmental verbal apraxia. In W. H. Perkins & J. L. Northern (Eds.), *Seminars in speech and language* (pp. 127–137). New York: Thieme-Stratton.

Battle, D. (1993). *Communication disorders in multicultural populations.* Boston: Andover Medical Publishers.

Baudouin de Courtenay, J. (1895). Versuch einer Theory phonetischer Alternationen: Ein Capitel aus der Psychophonetik. Translation in E. Stankiewicz (Ed.), *Selected writings of Baudouin de Courtenay.* Bloomington: Indiana University Press.

Bauer, H. R. (1988). The ethologic model of phonetic development: I. *Clinical Linguistics and Phonetics, 2,* 347–380.

Bauer, H. R., & Robb, M. P. (1989). *Phonetic development between infancy and toddlerhood: The phonetic product estimator.* Paper presented at the national convention of the American Speech-Language-Hearing Association, St. Louis.

Bauman, J. A., & Waengler, H.-H. (1977). Measurements of sound durations in the speech of apraxic adults. *Hamburger Phonetische Beiträge,* Monograph 23. Hamburg: H. Buske Verlag.

Bauman-Waengler, J. A. (1987). Experimental-phonetic analysis of duration in the speech of Parkinson's patients. *Beiträge zur Phonetik und Linguistik, 52, Festschrift H.-H. Waengler.* Hamburg: Helmut Buske Verlag.

Bauman-Waengler, J. A. (1991). Phonological processes in three groups of preschool children: A longitudinal study. *Proceedings from the XII International Congress of Phonetic Sciences, Aix-en-Provence, 3,* 354–357.

Bauman-Waengler, J. A. (1993a). *Dialect versus disorder: Articulation errors in African American preschool children.* Presentation at the state convention of the Pennsylvania Speech-Language-Hearing Association, Harrisburg, PA.

Bauman-Waengler, J. A. (1993b). *Language testing of African American children: Assessing assessment instruments.* Seminar presented at the state convention of the Pennsylvania Speech-Language-Hearing Association, Harrisburg, PA.

Bauman-Waengler, J. A. (1994a). Normal phonological development. In R. Lowe (Ed.), *Phonology: Assessment and intervention applications in speech pathology* (pp. 35–72). Baltimore: Williams & Wilkins.

Bauman-Waengler, J. A. (1994b). *Phonetic-phonological features in the speech of African American preschoolers.* Paper presented at the national convention of the American Speech-Language-Hearing Association, New Orleans, LA.

Bauman-Waengler, J. A. (1995). *Articulatory differences between two groups of African American preschoolers.* Paper presented at the national convention of the Canadian Association of Speech-Language Pathologists and Audiologists, Ottawa, Canada.

Bauman-Waengler, J. A. (1996). *Problems in assessing African American children with phonological disorders.* Seminar presented at the national convention of the Black American Speech-Language-Hearing Association, Milwaukee, WI.

Bauman-Waengler, J. A. (2002a). Segmental timing of phonologically disordered children: A developmental perspective. *Beihefte zur Zeitschrift fuer Dialektologie und Linguistik,* Steiner Verlag Wiesbaden, Stuttgart, Germany.

Bauman-Waengler, J. A. (2002b). *Segmental timing of sound errors in the speech of children with phonological disorders.* International Child Phonology Conference, Wichita, KS.

Bauman-Waengler, J. A., & Waengler, H.-H. (1980). Sound duration: Comparison between performances of subjects with central nervous disorders and normal speakers. *Proc. XVIII. Congress of the International Association of Logopedics and Phoniatrics, I,* 67–72.

Bauman-Waengler, J. A., & Waengler, H.-H. (1988). *Phonological process analysis in three groups of preschool children.* Paper presented at the national convention of the American Speech-Language-Hearing Association, Boston.

Bauman-Waengler, J. A., & Waengler, H.-H. (1990). *Individual variation in phonologically disordered preschoolers: A longitudinal study.* Paper presented at the national convention of the American Speech-Language-Hearing Association, Seattle.

Beebe, H. (1957). Dyslalia in a pair of twin girls. *Folia Phoniatrica, 9,* 91–95.

Bell, A. M. (1867). *Visible speech: The science of universal alphabetics.* London: Simpkin, Marshall.

Benson, D. F. (1979). Aphasia rehabilitation. *Archives of Neurology, 36,* 187–189.

Bernhardt, B. (1990). *Application of nonlinear phonological theory to intervention with six phonologically disordered children.* Unpublished Ph.D. dissertation. University of British Columbia.

Bernhardt, B. (1992a). The application of nonlinear phonological theory to intervention with one phonologically disordered child. *Clinical Linguistics and Phonetics, 6,* 283–316.

Bernhardt, B. (1992b). Developmental implications of nonlinear phonological theory. *Clinical Linguistics and Phonetics, 6,* 259–281.

Bernhardt, B. (1994). The prosodic tier and phonological disorders. In M. Yavaş (Ed.), *First and second language phonology* (pp. 149–172). San Diego, CA: Singular.

Bernhardt, B., & Gilbert, J. (1992). Applying linguistic theory to speech-language pathology: The case for nonlinear phonology. *Clinical Linguistics and Phonetics, 6,* 123–145.

Bernhardt, B. H., & Holdgrafer, G. (2001a). Beyond the basics I: The need for strategic sampling for in-depth phonological analysis. *Language, Speech, and Hearing Services in Schools, 32,* 18–27.

Bernhardt, B. H., & Holdgrafer, G. (2001b). Beyond the basics II: Supplemental sampling for in-depth phonological analysis. *Language, Speech, and Hearing Services in Schools, 32,* 28–37.

Bernhardt, B., & Stemberger, J. P. (1998). *Handbook of phonological development from the perspective of constraint-based nonlinear phonology.* San Diego, CA: Academic Press.

Bernhardt, B., & Stoel-Gammon, C. (1994). Nonlinear phonology: Introduction and clinical application: Tutorial. *Journal of Speech and Hearing Research, 37,* 123–143.

Bernthal, J. E., & Bankson, N. W. (2004). *Articulation and phonological disorders* (5th ed.). Boston: Allyn & Bacon.

Berry, P., Groenweg, G., Gibson, D., & Brown, R. (1984). Mental development of adults with Down syndrome. *American Journal of Mental Deficiency, 89,* 252–256.

Bertoncini, J., Morais, J., Bijeljac-Babic, R., McAdams, S., Peretz, I., & Mehler, J. (1989). Dichotic perception and laterality in neonates. *Brain and Language, 37,* 591–605.

Bess, F., & McConnell, F. (1981). *Audiology, education and the hearing impaired child.* St. Louis, MO: Mosby.

Best, C., & McRoberts, G. (2003). Infant perception of non-native consonant constrasts that adults assimilate in different ways. *Language and Speech, 3,* 183–216.

Best, C., McRoberts, G., & Goodell, E. (2001). Discrimination of non-native consonant contrasts varying in perceptual assimilation to the listener's native phonological system. *Journal of the Acoustic Society of America, 109,* 775–794.

Best, S., Bigge, J., & Sirvis, B. (1994). Physical and health impairments. In N. Haring, L. McCormick, & T. Haring (Eds.), *Exceptional children and youth: An introduction to special education* (pp. 300–341). New York: Merrill.

Beukelman, D. R., Yorkston, K. M., & Dowden, P. A. (1985). *Communication augmentation: A casebook of clinical management.* San Diego, CA: College-Hill Press.

Bigge, J. (1991). *Teaching individuals with physical and multiple disabilities* (3rd ed.). New York: Merrill.

Bird, J., & Bishop, D. V. (1992). Perception and awareness of phonemes in phonologically impaired children. *European Journal of Disorders of Communication, 27,* 289–311.

Bird, J., Bishop, D. V., & Freeman, N. H. (1995). Phonological awareness and literacy development in children with expressive phonological impairments. *Journal of Speech and Hearing Research, 38,* 446–462.

Birnholz, J. C., & Benacerraf, B. R. (1983). The development of human fetal hearing. *Science, 222,* 516–518.

Bishop, D. (1994). Grammatical errors in specific language impairment: Competence or performance limitations. *Applied Psycholinguistics, 15,* 507–550.

Bishop, D., & Adams, C. (1990). A prospective study of the relationship between specific language impairment, phonological disorders and reading retardation. *Journal of Child Psychology and Psychiatry, 31,* 1027–1050.

Bishop, D., Brown, B., & Robson, J. (1990). The relationship between phoneme discrimination, speech production, and language comprehension in cerebral-palsied individuals, *Journal of Speech and Hearing Research, 33,* 210–219.

Bishop, D., & Edmundson, A. (1987). Language-impaired four year olds: Distinguishing transient from persistent impairment. *Journal of Speech and Hearing Disorders, 52,* 156–173.

Bishop, D., & Robson, J. (1989). Unimpaired short-term memory and rhyme judgment in congenitally speechless individuals: Implications for the notion of "articulatory coding." *Quarterly Journal of Experimental Psychology, 41A,* 123–140.

Blache, S. (1978). *The acquisition of distinctive features.* Baltimore: University Park Press.

Blache, S. (1982). Minimal word-pairs and distinctive feature training. In M. A. Crary & D. Ingram (Eds.), *Phonological intervention: Concepts and procedures* (pp. 61–96). San Diego, CA: College-Hill Press.

Blache, S. (1989). A distinctive feature approach. In N. Creaghead, P. Newman, & W. Secord (Eds.), *Assessment and remediation of articulatory and phonological disorders* (2nd ed.) (pp. 361–382). New York: Macmillan.

Blache, S., Parsons, C., & Humphreys, J. (1981). A minimal-word-pair model for teaching the linguistic significance of distinctive feature properties. *Journal of Speech and Hearing Disorders, 46,* 291–296.

Blakeley, R. W. (1977). *Tests for apraxia of speech and oral apraxia—Children's battery.* Rochester, MN: Mayo Clinic.

Blakeley, R. W. (2000). *Screening test for developmental apraxia of speech* (2nd ed.). Tigard, OR: C. C. Publications.

Bleile, K. (2002). Evaluating articulation and phonological disorders when the clock is running. *American Journal of Speech-Language Pathology, 11,* 243–249.

Bleile, K., & Schwarz, I. (1984). Three perspectives on the speech of children with Down's syndrome. *Journal of Communication Disorders, 17,* 87–94.

Blockcolsky, V., Frazer, J., & Frazer, D. (1987). *40,000 selected words.* Tucson, AZ: Communication Skill Builders.

Bloom, L. (1973). *One word at a time: The use of single word utterances before syntax.* The Hague: Mouton.

Blumstein, S. (1973). *A phonological investigation of aphasic speech.* The Hague: Mouton.

Bobath, B. (1967). The very early treatment of cerebral palsy. *Developmental Medicine and Childhood Neurology, 9,* 373–390.

Bobath, K., & Bobath, B. (1972). Cerebral palsy, Part II: The neurodevelopmental approach to treatment. In P. H. Pearson & C. E. Williams (Eds.), *Physical therapy services in the developmental disabilities* (pp. 114–185). Springfield, IL: Charles C. Thomas.

Bogliotti, C. (2003). *Relation between categorical perception of speech and reading acquisition.* Proceedings of the 15th International Congress of Phonetic Sciences, Barcelona, Spain.

Bonvillian, J., Raeburn, V., & Horan, E. (1979). Talking to children—The effect of rate, intonation and length on children's sentence imitation. *Journal of Child Language, 6,* 459–467.

Boone, D. R., & McFarlane, S. C. (1988). *The voice and voice therapy.* Englewood Cliffs, NJ: Prentice-Hall.

Boothroyd, A. (1988). Perception of speech pattern contrasts from auditory presentation of voice fundamental frequency. *Ear and Hearing, 9,* 313–321.

Bosma, J. F. (1975). Anatomic and physiologic development of the speech apparatus. In E. L. Eagles (Ed.), *Human communication and its disorders* (Vol. 3) (pp. 469–481). New York: Raven Press.

Boutsen, F., & Christman, S. (2002). Prosody in apraxia of speech. *Seminars in Speech and Language, 23,* 245–255.

Boysson-Bardies, B., de (2001). *How language comes to children: From birth to two years* (M. DeBevoise, Trans.). Cambridge, MA: NET Press.

Boysson-Bardies, B., de, & Vihman, M. (1991). Adaptation to language. *Language, 67,* 297–339.

Bradley, D. P. (1989). A systematic multiple-phoneme approach. In. N. A. Creaghead, P. W. Newman, & A. Secord (Eds.), *Assessment and remediation of articulatory and phonological disorders* (2nd ed.) (pp. 305–322). Columbus, OH: Merrill.

Bradley, L., & Bryant, P. (1983). Categorizing sounds and learning to read: A causal connection. *Nature, 301,* 419–421.

Brady, N., Marquis, J., Fleming, K., & McLean, L. (2004). Prelinguistic predictors of language growth in children with developmental disabilities. *Journal of Speech, Language, and Hearing Research, 47,* 663–677.

Brady, S. (1986). Short-term memory, phonological processing and reading ability. *Annals of Dyslexia, 36,* 138–153.

Brady, S., & Fowler, A. E. (1988). Phonological precursors to reading acquisition. In R. L. Masland & M. W. Masland (Eds.), *Preschool prevention of reading failure* (pp. 204–215). Parkton, MD: York Press.

Briere, E. (1966). An investigation of phonological interference. *Language, 42,* 768–796.

Broen, P. A., & Moller, K. T. (1993). Early phonological development and the child with cleft palate. In K. T. Moller & C. D. Starr (Eds.), *Cleft palate. Interdisciplin-*

ary issues and treatment (pp. 219–249). Austin, TX: PRO-ED.

Brogan, W. J., & Woodings, T. L. (1976). A decline in the incidence of cleft lip and palate deformities in humans. *Clinics in Plastic Surgery, 3,* 647.

Bronstein, A. J. (1960). *The pronunciation of American English. An introduction to phonetics.* New York: Appleton-Century-Crofts.

Bross, R. (1992). An application of structual linguistics to intelligibility measurements of impaired speakers of English. In R. D. Kent (Ed.), *Intelligibility in speech disorders: Theory, measurement, and management* (pp. 35–65). Amsterdam: John Benjamins.

Brown, R. (1973). *A first language: The early stages.* Cambridge, MA: Harvard University Press.

Bruner, J. (1975). The ontogenesis of speech acts. *Journal of Child Language, 2,* 1–19.

Bryen, D., Goldman, A., & Quinlisk-Gill, S. (1988). Sign language with students with severe/profound mental retardation: How effective is it? *Education and Training in Mental Retardation, 23,* 129–137.

Butcher, A. (1990). The uses and abuses of phonological assessment. *Child Language Teaching and Therapy, 6,* 262–276.

Bzoch, K. (1979). Measurement and assessment of categorical aspects of cleft palate speech. In K. R. Bzoch (Ed.), *Communicative disorders related to cleft lip and palate* (2nd ed.) (pp. 161–191). Boston: Little, Brown.

Bzoch, K. (1997). Clinical assessment, evaluation, and management of 11 categorical aspects of cleft palate speech disorders. In K. R. Bzoch (Ed.), *Communication disorders related to cleft lip and palate* (4th ed.) (pp. 261–311). Austin, TX: PRO-ED.

Calvert, D. R., & Silverman, S. R. (1983). *Speech and deafness: A text for learning and teaching* (rev. ed.). Washington, DC: Alexander Graham Bell Association for the Deaf.

Camp, B., Burgess, D., Morgan, L., & Zerbe, G. (1987). A longitudinal study of infant vocalizations in the first year. *Journal of Pediatric Psychology, 12,* 321–331.

Campbell, T., & Shriberg, L. (1982). Associations among pragmatic functions, linguistic stress, and natural phonological processes in speech-delayed children. *Journal of Speech and Hearing Research, 25,* 547–553.

Capute, A. J. (1974). Developmental disabilities: An overview. *Dental Clinics of North America, 18,* 557–577.

Carney, A. E. (1994). Understanding speech intelligibility in the hearing impaired. In K. G. Butler (Ed.), *Hearing impairment and language disorders* (pp. 109–121). Gaithersburg, MD: Aspen.

Carney, E. (1979). Inappropriate abstraction in speech assessment procedures. *British Journal of Disorders of Communication, 14,* 123–135.

Carr, P. (1999). *English phonetics and phonology: An introduction.* Malden, MA: Blackwell.

Carrell, J., & Tiffany, W. R. (1960). *Phonetics: Theory and application to speech improvement.* New York: McGraw-Hill.

Carterette, E., & Jones, M. (1974). *Informal speech: Alphabetic and phonemic texts with statistical analyses and tables.* Berkeley: University of California Press.

Carver, C. M. (1987). Dialects. In S. Flexner & L. C. Hauck (Eds.), *The Random House dictionary of the English language* (2nd ed.) (pp. xxv–xxvi). New York: Random House.

Catts, H. (1993). The relationship between speech-language impairments and reading disabilities. *Journal of Speech and Hearing Research, 36,* 948–958.

Catts, H., Fey, M., & Zhang, X. (2001). Estimating the risk of future reading difficulties in kindergarten children: A research-based model and its clinical implementation. *Language, Speech, and Hearing Services in Schools, 32,* 38–50.

Catts, H., & Kamhi, A. (1999). Causes of reading disabilities. In H. Catts & A. Kamhi (Eds.), *Language and reading disabilities* (pp. 95–127). Boston: Allyn & Bacon.

Chan, A., & Li, D. (2000). English and Cantonese phonology in contrast: Explaining Cantonese ESL learners' English pronunciation problems. *Language, Culture, and Curriculum, 13*(1), 67–85.

Chaney, C. (1992). Language development, metalinguistic skills, and print knowledge in 3-year-old children. *Applied Psycholinguistics, 13,* 485–514.

Chapman, K. L. (1993). Phonological processes in children with cleft palate. *Cleft Palate-Craniofacial Journal, 30,* 64–71.

Chapman, K. L., & Hardin, M. A. (1992). Phonetic and phonologic skills of two year olds with cleft palate. *Cleft Palate-Craniofacial Journal, 29,* 435–443.

Chapman, K. L., Hardin-Jones, M., & Halter, K. (2003). The relationship between early speech and later speech and language performance for children with cleft lip and palate. *Clinical Linguistics & Phonetics, 17,* 173–197.

Chapman, R. S., & Miller, J. (1980). Analyzing language and communication in the child. In R. Schiefelbusch (Ed.), *Nonspeech language and communication: Analysis and intervention* (pp. 159–196). Baltimore: University Park Press.

Chappell, G. E. (1973). Childhood verbal apraxia and its treatment. *Journal of Speech and Hearing Disorders, 38,* 362–368.

Chen, H. P., & Irwin, O. C. (1946). Infant speech: Vowel and consonant types. *Journal of Speech Disorders, 11,* 27–29.

Cheng, L. L. (1991). *Assessing Asian language performance: Guidelines for evaluating limited-English proficient students* (2nd ed.). Oceanside, CA: Academic Communication Associates.

Cheng, L. L. (1993). Asian-American cultures. In D. Battle (Ed.), *Communication disorders in multicultural populations* (pp. 38–77). Boston: Andover Medical.

Cheng, L. L. (1994). Asian/Pacific students and the learning of English. In J. Bernthal & N. Bankson (Eds.), *Child phonology: Characteristics, assessment, and intervention with special populations* (pp. 255–274). New York: Thieme.

Chin, S. B., & Dinnsen, D. A. (1991). Feature geometry in disordered phonologies. *Clinical Linguistics and Phonetics, 5,* 329–337.

Chomsky, C. (1971). *Linguistic development in children from 6 to 10.* Office of Education: Final Report.

Chomsky, N. (1957). *Syntactic structures.* The Hague: Mouton.

Chomsky, N. (1967). Some general properties of phonological rules. *Language, 43,* 102–128.

Chomsky, N. (1982). *Lectures on government and binding.* New York: Foris.

Chomsky, N. (1988). *Language and problems of knowledge.* Cambridge, MA: MIT Press.

Chomsky, N., & Halle, M. (1968). *The sound pattern of English.* New York: Harper & Row.

Christensen, M., & Hanson, M. (1981). An investigation of the efficacy of oral myofunctional therapy as a precursor to articulation therapy for pre-first-grade children. *Journal of Speech and Hearing Disorders, 46,* 160–165.

Christian, D., Wolfram, W., & Nube, N. (1988). *Variation and change in geographically isolated communities: Appalachian English and Ozark English.* Tuscaloosa, AL: University of Alabama Press.

Clark, M. C., & Goldstein, B. (1996). *Analysis of vowel error patterns in children with phonological disorders.* Paper presented at the annual convention of the American Speech-Language-Hearing Association, Seattle, WA.

Clarke-Klein, S., & Hodson, B. (1995). A phonologically based analysis of misspellings by third graders with disordered-phonology histories. *Journal of Speech and Hearing Research, 38,* 839–849.

Clements, G. (1985). The geometry of phonological features. *Phonology Yearbook, 2,* 225–252.

Cohen, J., & Diehl, C. (1963). Relation of speech sound discrimination ability to articulation-type speech defects. *Journal of Speech and Hearing Disorders, 28,* 187–190.

Cohen, L. (2003). Commentary on part 1: Unresolved issues in infant categorization. In D. Rakison & L. Oakes (Eds.), *Early category and concept development* (pp. 193–212). New York: Oxford University Press.

Cohen, L., & Cashon, C. (2003). Infant perception and cognition. In R. Lerner, M. Easterbooks, & J. Mistry (Eds.), *Comprehensive handbook of psychology. Volume 6: Developmental psychology* (pp. 65–90), Hoboken, NJ: John Wiley and Sons.

Cole, R. A., & Perfetti, C. A. (1980). Listening for mispronunciations in a children's story: The use of context by children and adults. *Journal of Verbal Learning and Verbal Behavior, 19,* 297–315.

Compton, A. J. (1970). Generative studies of children's phonological disorders. *Journal of Speech and Hearing Disorders, 35,* 315–339.

Compton, A. J. (1975). Generative studies of children's phonological disorders: A strategy for therapy. In S. Singh (Ed.), *Measurement procedures in speech, hearing, and language* (pp. 55–90). Baltimore: University Park Press.

Compton, A. J. (1976). Generative studies of children's phonological disorders: Clinical ramifications. In D. Morehead & A. Morehead (Eds.), *Normal and deficient child language* (pp. 61–96). Baltimore: University Park Press.

Conly, U., Bauman-Waengler, J. A., & Waengler, H.-H. (1989). *Aberrant phonology in Japanese learners of American-English: Assessment and Intervention.* Paper presented at the National Convention of the American Speech-Language-Hearing Association, New Orleans, LA.

Connolly, J. H. (1986). Intelligibility: A linguistic view. *British Journal of Disorders of Communication, 21,* 371–376.

Conti-Ramsden, G., & Jones, M. (1997). Verb use in specific language impairment. *Journal of Speech and Hearing Research, 40,* 1298–1313.

Cooper, E. (1985). The method of meaningful contrasts. In P. Newman, N. Creaghead, & W. Secord (Eds.), *Assessment and remediation of articulatory and phonological disorders* (pp. 369–382). Columbus, OH: Merrill.

Copenhagen Conference. (1925). Association Phonétique Internationale, Copenhagen, Denmark.

Cornett, R. (1972). *Cued speech parent training and follow-up program.* Final report. Washington, DC: Bureau of Education for the Handicapped, DHEW, 96.

Cornwall, A. (1992). The relationship of phonological awareness, rapid naming and verbal memory to severe reading and spelling disability. *Journal of Learning Disabilities, 25,* 532–538.

Costello, J. (1975). Articulation instruction based on distinctive features theory. *Language, Speech, and Hearing Services in Schools, 6,* 61–71.

Crary, M. A. (1983). Phonological process analysis from spontaneous speech: The influence of sample size. *Journal of Communication Disorders, 16,* 133–141.

Crary, M. A. (1984). Phonological characteristics of developmental verbal dyspraxia. In W. H. Perkins & J. L. Northern (Eds.), *Seminars in speech and language* (pp. 71–83). New York: Thieme-Stratton.

Crary, M. A. (1993). *Developmental motor speech disorders.* San Diego, CA: Singular.

Crary, M. A., & Comeau, S. (1981). Phonologically based assessment and intervention in spastic cerebral palsy: A case analysis. *South African Journal of Communication Disorders, 28,* 31–36.

Creaghead, N., & Newman, P. (1989). Articulatory phonetics and phonology. In N. Creaghead, P. Newman, & W. Secord (Eds.), *Assessment and remediation of articulatory and phonological disorders* (2nd ed.) (pp. 9–32). New York: Macmillan.

Creaghead, N. A., Newman, P. W., & Secord, W. A. (Eds.). (1989). *Assessment and remediation of articulatory and phonological disorders* (2nd ed.). New York: Macmillan.

Croot, K. (2002). Diagnosis of AOS: Definition and criteria. *Seminar in Speech and Language, 23,* 267–280.

Cruttenden, A. (1981). Item-learning and system-learning. *Journal of Psycholinguistic Research, 10,* 79–88.

Cruttenden, A. (1985). Intonation comprehension in 10-year-olds. *Journal of Child Language, 12,* 643–661.

Crystal, D. (1981). *Clinical linguistics.* New York: Springer-Verlag.

Crystal, D. (1986). Prosodic development. In P. Fletcher & M. Garman (Eds.), *Language acquisition* (2nd ed.) (pp. 174–197). Cambridge: Cambridge University Press.

Crystal, D. (1987). *The Cambridge encyclopedia of language.* Cambridge: Cambridge University Press.

Culatta, R., Page, J. L., & Wilson, L. (1987). *Speech rates of normally communicative children.* Paper presented at the annual convention of the American Speech-Language-Hearing Association, New Orleans, LA.

Culp, D. M. (1989). Developmental apraxia and augmentative or alternative communication—A case study. In International Society for Augmentative and Alternative Communication, *AAC augmentative and alternative communication* (pp. 27–34). Baltimore: Williams & Wilkins.

Dabul, B. (2000). *Apraxia battery for adults* (2nd ed.). Tigard, OR: C. C. Publications.

Dalston, R. (1997). The use of nasometry in the assessment and remediation of velopharyngeal inadequacy. In K. R. Bzoch (Ed.), *Communication disorders related to cleft lip and palate* (4th ed.) (pp. 331–346). Austin, TX: PRO-ED.

Dalston, R., Warren, D., & Dalston, E. (1991). Use of nasometry as a diagnostic tool for identifying patients with velopharyngeal impairment. *Cleft Palate-Craniofacial Journal, 28,* 184–189.

Darley, F. (1978). Differential diagnosis of acquired motor speech disorders. In F. Darley & D. C. Spriestersbach (Eds.), *Diagnostic methods in speech pathology* (2nd ed.) (pp. 492–513). New York: Harper & Row.

Darley, F. (Ed.). (1979). *Evaluation and appraisal in speech and language disorders.* Reading, MA: Addison-Wesley.

Darley, F. (1984). Apraxia of speech: A neurogenic articulation disorder. In H. Winitz (Ed.), *Treating articulation disorders: For clinicians by clinicians* (pp. 289–305). Baltimore: University Park Press.

Darley, F. (1991). A philosophy of appraisal and diagnosis. In F. Darley & D. C. Spriestersbach (Eds.), *Diagnostic methods in speech pathology* (2nd ed.) (pp. 1–23). New York: Harper & Row.

Darley, F. L., Aronson, A. E., & Brown, J. R. (1975). *Motor speech disorders.* Philadelphia: W. B. Saunders.

Das, J., Kirby, J., & Jarman, R. (1975). Simultaneous and successive synthesis: An alternative model for cognitive abilities. *Psychological Bulletin, 82,* 87–103.

Davis, B., Jakielski, K., & Marquardt, T. (1998). Developmental apraxia of speech: Determiners of differential diagnosis. *Clinical Linguistics and Phonetics, 12,* 25–45.

Davis, B., Marquardt, T. P., & Sussman, H. M. (1985). *Developmental apraxia of speech: Case study.* Paper presented at the annual meeting of the American Speech-Language-Hearing Association, Washington, DC.

Davis, B. L., & MacNeilage, P. F. (1990). Acquisition of correct vowel production: A quantitative case study. *Journal of Speech and Hearing Research, 33,* 16–27.

Davis, B. L., & Velleman, S. (2000). Differential diagnosis and treatment of developmental apraxia of speech in infants and toddlers. *Infant–Toddler Intervention, 10,* 177–192.

Davis, L. F. (1987). Respiration and phonation in cerebral palsy: A developmental model. *Seminars in Speech and Language, 8,* 101–106.

Deal, J., & Darley, F. (1972). The influence of linguistic and situational variables on phonemic accuracy in apraxia of speech. *Journal of Speech and Hearing Research, 15,* 639–653.

Dean, E., Howell, J., Hill, A., & Waters, D. (1990). *Metaphon resource pack.* Windsor, UK: NFER Nelson.

DeCasper, A., & Fifer, W. P. (1980). On human bonding: Newborns prefer their mothers' voices. *Science, 208,* 1174–1176.

Delack, J. B., & Fowlow, P. J. (1978). The ontogenesis of differential vocalization: Development of prosodic contrastivity during the first year of life. In N. Waterson & C. Snow (Eds.), *The development of communication* (pp. 93–110). New York: John Wiley.

Delaney, A., & Kent, R. (2004). *Developmental profiles of children diagnosed with apraxia of speech.* Paper presented at the annual meeting of the American Speech-Language-Hearing Association, Philadelphia.

Denes, P. B., & Pinson, E. N. (1963). *The speech chain: The physics and biology of spoken language.* Garden City, NY: Anchor Press/Doubleday.

Denes, P. B., & Pinson, E. N. (1973). *The speech chain.* Garden City, NY: Anchor Press.

DeRenzi, E., Pieczuro, A., & Vignolo, L. A. (1966). Oral apraxia and aphasia. *Cortex, 2,* 50–73.

de Saussure, F. (1959). *A course in general linguistics.* (J. Cantineau, Trans.). London: Owen. (Original work published 1916).

de Villiers, P., & de Villiers, J. (1972). Early judgements of syntactic and symantic acceptability by children. *Journal of Psycholinguistic Research, 1,* 299–310.

Dewey, G. (1923). *Relative frequency of English speech sounds.* Cambridge, MA: Harvard University Press.

DiCarlo, L. M. (1974). Communication therapy for problems associated with cerebral palsy. In S. Dickson (Ed.), *Communication disorders: Remedial principles and practices* (2nd ed.) (pp. 358–397). Glenview, IL: Scott, Foresman.

Dickson, S. (1962). Differences between children who spontaneously outgrow and children who retain functional articulation errors. *Journal of Speech and Hearing Research, 5,* 263–271.

Diedrich, W. (1983). Stimulability and articulation disorders. In J. Locke (Ed.), *Assessing and treating phonological disorders: Current approaches. Seminars in Speech and Language, 4.* New York: Thieme-Stratton.

Dillow, K. A., Dzienkowski, R. C., Smith, K. K., & Yucha, C. B. (1996). Cerebral palsy: A comprehensive review. *The Nurse Practitioner, 21,* 45–61.

Dinnsen, D. A. (1984). Methods and empirical issues in analyzing functional misarticulations. In M. Elbert, D. A. Dinnsen, & G. Weismer (Eds.), *Phonological theory and the misarticulating child, ASHA Monograph No. 22* (pp. 1–4). Rockville, MD: ASHA.

Dinnsen, D. A. (1996). Context-sensitive underspecification and the acquisition of phonemic contrasts. *Journal of Child Language, 23,* 57–79.

Dinnsen, D. A. (1997). Nonsegmental phonologies. In M. J. Ball & R. D. Kent (Eds.), *The new phonologies* (pp. 77–125). San Diego, CA: Singular.

Dinnsen, D. A., & O'Connor, K. M. (2001). Implicationally related error patterns and the selection of treatment targets. *Language, Speech, and Hearing Services in the Schools, 32,* 257–270.

Dinnsen, D. A., & Chin, S. B. (1993). Individual differences in phonological disorders and implications for a theory of acquisition. In F. R. Eckman (Ed.), *Confluence: Linguistics, L2 acquisition, and speech pathology* (pp. 137–152). Amsterdam: John Benjamins.

Dinnsen, D. A., & Elbert, M. (1984). On the relationship between phonology and learning. In M. Elbert, D. Dinnsen, & G. Weismer (Eds.), *Phonological theory and the misarticulating child, ASHA Monograph, 22* (pp. 59–68). Rockville, MD: ASHA.

Dodd, B. (1976). The phonological systems of deaf children. *Journal of Speech and Hearing Disorders, 41,* 185–198.

Dodd, B. (1995). *Differential diagnosis and treatment of children with speech disorder.* London: Whurr.

Dodd, B., Gillon, G., Oerlemans, R., Russell, T., Syrmis, M., & Wilson, H. (1995). Phonological disorder and the acquisition of literacy. In B. Dodd (Ed.), *Differential diagnosis and treatment of children with speech disorder* (pp. 125–146). London: Whurr.

Dodd, B., & Iacano, T. (1989). Phonological disorders in children: Changes in phonological process use during treatment. *British Journal of Disorders of Communication, 24,* 333–351.

Donegan, P. J., & Stampe, D. (1979). The study of natural phonology. In D. A. Dinnsen (Ed.), *Current approaches to phonological theory* (pp. 126–173). Bloomington, IN: Indiana University Press.

Dore, J. (1975). Holophrases, speech acts and language universals. *Journal of Child Language, 3,* 22–39.

Dore, J., Franklin, M. B., Miller, R. T., & Ramer, A. L. (1976). Transitional phenomena in early language acquisition. *Journal of Child Language, 3,* 13–29.

Doszak, A. L., McNeil, M. R., & Jancosek, E. (1981). *Efficacy of melodic intonation therapy with developmental apraxia of speech.* Paper presented at the national convention of the American Speech-Language-Hearing Association, Los Angeles.

Drummond, S. S. (1993). *Dysarthria examination battery.* Austin, TX: PRO-ED.

DuBois, E., & Bernthal, J. E. (1978). A comparison of three methods for obtaining articulatory responses. *Journal of Speech and Hearing Disorders, 43,* 295–305.

Duffy, J. R. (1995). *Motor speech disorders: Substrates, differential diagnosis, and management.* St. Louis, MO: Mosby Year Book.

Duncan, L., & Johnston, R. (1999). How does phonological awareness relate to nonword reading amongst poor readers? *Reading and Writing: An Interdisciplinary Journal, 11,* 405–439.

Dunn, C., & Newton, L. (1994). A comprehensive model for speech development in hearing-impaired children. In K. G. Butler (Ed.), *Hearing impairment and language disorders* (pp. 122–143). *Topics in language disorders series.* Gaithersburg, MD: Aspen.

Dunn, L. M., Dunn, L., Whetton, C., & Pintilie, D. (1982). *British picture vocabulary scales.* Windsor: NFER Nelson.

Dworkin, J. P. (1991). *Motor speech disorders: A treatment guide.* St. Louis, MO: Mosby Year Book.

Dworkin, J. P., & Culatta, R. A. (1980). *Dworkin-Culatta oral mechanism examination.* Nicholasville, KY: Edgewood Press.

Edwards, J., Fox, R., & Rogers, C. (2002). Final consonant discrimination in children: Effects of phonological disorder, vocabulary size, and articulatory accuracy. *Journal of Speech, Language, and Hearing Research, 45,* 231–242.

Edwards, H. T. (2003). *Applied phonetics: The sounds of American English* (3rd ed.). San Diego: Singular.

Edwards, M. (1973). Developmental verbal dyspraxia. *British Journal of Disorders of Communication, 8,* 64–70.

Edwards, M. L. (1992). Clinical forum: Phonological assessment and treatment. In support of phonological processes. *Language, Speech, and Hearing Services in Schools, 23,* 233–240.

Eilers, R. E. (1980). Infant speech perception: History and mystery. In G. Yeni-Komshian, J. Kavanagh, & C. A. Ferguson (Eds.), *Child phonology: Volume 2. Perception* (pp. 23–39). New York: Academic Press.

Eimas, P. D., Siqueland, E. R., Jusczyk, P., & Vigorito, J. (1971). Speech perception in infants. *Science, 171,* 303–306.

Eisenson, J. (1972). *Aphasia in children* (pp. 189–202). New York: Harper & Row.

Elbers, L. (1982). Operating principles in repetitive babbling: A cognitive approach. *Cognition, 12,* 45–63.

Elbert, M. (1992). Clinical forum: Phonological assessment and treatment. Consideration of error types: A response to Fey. *Language, Speech, and Hearing Services in Schools, 23,* 241–246.

Elbert, M. (1997). From articulation to phonology: The challenge of change. In B. W. Hodson & M. L. Edwards (Eds.), *Perspectives in applied phonology* (pp. 43–60). Gaithersburg, MD: Aspen.

Elbert, M., Dinnsen, D., & Powell, T. (1984). On the prediction of phonologic generalization learning patterns. *Journal of Speech and Hearing Disorders, 49,* 309–317.

Elbert, M., & Gierut, J. (1986). *Handbook of clinical phonology: Approaches to assessment and treatment.* San Diego, CA: College-Hill Press.

Elliott, L. L. (1979). Performance of children aged 9–17 years on a test of speech intelligibility in noise using sentence material with controlled word predictability. *Journal of the Acoustical Society of America, 66,* 651–653.

Elliott, L. L., Connors, S., Kille, E., Levin, S., Ball, K., & Katz, D. (1979). Children's understanding of monosyllabic nouns in quiet and in noise. *Journal of the Acoustical Society of America, 66,* 12–21.

Emerick, L. L., & Haynes, W. O. (1986). *Diagnosis and evaluation in speech pathology* (3rd ed.). Englewood Cliffs, NJ: Prentice-Hall.

Enderby, P. (1980). Frenchay dysarthria assessment. *British Journal of Disorders of Communication, 15,* 165–173.

Enderby, P. (1983). The standardized assessment of dysarthria is possible. In W. R. Berry (Ed.), *Clinical dysarthria* (pp. 109–119). San Diego, CA: College-Hill Press.

Erenberg, G. (1984). Cerebral palsy. Current understanding of a complex problem. *Postgraduate Medicine, 75,* 87–93.

Estrem, T., & Broen, P. A. (1989). Early speech productions of children with cleft palate. *Journal of Speech and Hearing Research, 32,* 12–23.

Eyer, J., & Leonard, L. (1994). Learning past tense morphology with specific language impairment: A case study. *Child Language Teaching and Therapy, 10,* 127–138.

Faircloth, M. A., & Faircloth, S. R. (1970). An analysis of the articulatory behavior of a speech-defective child in connected speech and in isolated-word responses. *Journal of Speech and Hearing Disorders, 35,* 51–61.

Faircloth, S. R., & Faircloth, M. A. (1973). *Phonetic science: A program of instruction.* Englewood Cliffs, NJ: Prentice-Hall.

Farmer, A., & Lencione, R. (1977). An extraneous vocal behavior in cerebral palsied speakers. *British Journal of Communication Disorders, 12,* 109–118.

Farwell, C. B. (1976). Some strategies in the early production of fricatives. *Papers and Reports on Child Language Development, 12,* 97–104.

Fasold, R., & Wolfram, W. (1975). Some linguistic features of Negro dialect. In P. Stoller (Ed.), *Black American English* (pp. 49–87). New York: Deli.

Fawcus, R. (1971). Features of a psychological and physiological study of articulatory performance. *British Journal of Disorders of Communication, 6,* 99–106.

Ferguson, C. A. (1976). Learning to pronounce: The earliest stages of phonological development in the child. In F. D. Minifie & L. L. Floyd (Eds.), *Communicative and cognitive abilities: Early behavioral assessment* (pp. 273–297). Baltimore: University Park Press.

Ferguson, C. A., & Farwell, C. (1975). Words and sounds in early language acquisition: English initial consonants in the first fifty words. *Language, 51,* 419–439.

Ferguson, C. A., & Garnica, O. (1975). Theories of phonological development. In E. Lenneberg & E. Lenneberg (Eds.), *Foundation of language development* (Vol. 1) (pp. 153–180). New York: Academic Press.

Fernald, A., Taeschner, T., Dunn, J., Papousek, M., de Boysson-Bardies, B., & Fukui, I. (1989). A cross-language study of prosodic modification in mother's and father's speech to preverbal infants. *Journal of Child Language, 16,* 477–503.

Ferrier, E., & Davis, M. (1973). A lexical approach to the remediation of final sound omissions. *Journal of Speech and Hearing Disorders, 38,* 126–131.

Ferry, P. C., Hall, S. M., & Hicks, J. L. (1975). "Dilapidated" speech: Developmental verbal dyspraxia. *Developmental Medicine and Child Neurology, 17,* 749–756.

Fey, M. E. (1992). Clinical forum: Phonological assessment and treatment. Articulation and phonology: Inextricable constructs in speech pathology. *Language, Speech, and Hearing Services in Schools, 23,* 225–232. (Reprinted from *Human Communication Canada, 1985, 9,* 7–16.)

Fey, M. E., Cleave, P., Ravida, I., Long, S., Dejmal, A., & Easton, D. (1994). Effects of grammar facilitation on the phonological performance of children with speech and language impairments. *Journal of Speech and Hearing Research, 37,* 594–607.

Firth, J. R. (1948). Sounds and prosodies. *Transactions of the Philological Society.* Oxford: Blackwell.

Fisher, H. B., & Logemann, J. A. (1971). *The Fisher-Logemann test of articulation competence.* Boston: Houghton Mifflin.

Fisichelli, R. M. (1950). *An experimental study of the prelinguistic speech development of institutionalized infants.* Unpublished doctoral dissertation, Fordham University.

Fleming, K. (1971). Guidelines for choosing appropriate phonetic contexts for speech-sound recognition and production practice. *Journal of Speech and Hearing Disorders, 36,* 356–367.

Fletcher, P., & Peters, J. (1984). Characterizing language impairment in children: An exploratory study. *Language Testing, 1,* 33–49.

Fletcher, S. G. (1970). Theory and instrumentation for quantitative measurement of nasality. *Cleft Palate Journal, 7,* 601–609.

Fletcher, S. G. (1992). *Articulation. A physiological approach.* San Diego, CA: Singular.

Fletcher, S. G., Casteel, R., & Bradley, D. (1961). Tongue-thrust swallow, speech articulation, and age. *Journal of Speech and Hearing Disorders, 26,* 201–208.

Fletcher, S. G., & Newman, D. G. (1991). /s/ and /ʃ/ as a function of lingua-palatal contact place and sibilant groove width. *Journal of the Acoustical Society of America, 89,* 850–858.

Flexner, S. B. (Ed.). (1987). *The Random House dictionary of the English language* (2nd ed.). New York: Random House.

Fokes, J. (1982). Problems confronting the theorist and practitioner in child phonology. In M. Crary & D. Ingram (Eds.), *Phonological intervention: Concepts and procedures* (pp. 13–34). San Diego, CA: College-Hill Press.

Foster, D., Riley, K., & Parker, F. (1985). Some problems in the clinical application of phonological theory. *Journal of Speech and Hearing Disorders, 50,* 294–297.

Fourcin, A. J. (1978). Acoustic patterns and speech acquisition. In N. Waterson & C. Snow (Eds.), *Development of communication* (pp. 47–72). New York: John Wiley.

Fox, B., & Routh, D. K. (1975). Analyzing spoken language into words, syllables, and phonemes: A developmental study. *Journal of Psycholinguistic Research, 4,* 331–342.

French, A. (1988). What shall we do with 'medial' sounds? *British Journal of Disorders of Communication, 23,* 41–50.

French, A. (1989). The systematic acquisition of word forms by a child during the first-fifty-word stage. *Journal of Child Language, 16,* 69–90.

French, N., Carter, C., & Koenig, W. (1930). The words and sounds of telephone conversations. *Bell System Technical Journal, 9,* 290–324.

Fristoe, M., & Lloyd, L. (1979). Nonspeech communication. In N. R. Ellis (Ed.), *Handbook of mental deficiency, psychological theory and research* (2nd ed.) (pp. 401–430). Hillsdale, NJ: Erlbaum Associates.

Froeschels, E. (1931). *Lehrbuch der Sprachheilkunde* (3rd ed.). Leipzig-Vienna: Deuticke.

Froeschels, E. (1937). Uber das Wesen der multiplen Interdentalitat. *Acta oto-laryngol., 25,* 341.

Froeschels, E. (1952). *Dysarthric speech: Speech in cerebral palsy.* Magnolia, MA: Expression Co.

Fudala, J., & Reynolds, W. (2000). *Arizona articulation proficiency scale* (3rd ed.). Los Angeles: Western Psychological Services.

Garnica, O. (1973). The development of phonemic speech perception. In T. Moore (Ed.), *Cognitive development and the acquisition of language* (pp. 215–222). New York: Academic Press.

Gerken, L. (2005). Thirty years of research on infant speech perception: The legacy of Peter W. Jusczyk, *Language Learning and Development, 1,* 5–21.

Gesell, A., & Thompson, H. (1934). *Infant behavior: Its genesis and growth.* New York: McGraw-Hill.

Gibbon, F. (2002). Personal correspondence.

Gibbon, F., Shockey, L., & Reid, J. (1992). Description and treatment of abnormal vowels in a phonologically disordered child. *Child Language Teaching and Therapy, 8,* 30–59.

Gibbon, F., & Wood, S. (2003). Using electropalatography (EPG) to diagnose and treat articulation disorders associated with mild cerebral palsy: A case study. *Clinical Linguistics and Phonetics, 17,* 365–374.

Gierut, J. (1985). *On the relationship between phonological knowledge and generalization learning in misarticulating children.* Bloomington: Indiana University Linguistics Club.

Gierut, J. (1989). Maximal opposition approach to phonological treatment. *Journal of Speech and Hearing Disorders, 54,* 9–19.

Gierut, J. (1990). Differential learning of phonological oppositions. *Journal of Speech and Hearing Research, 33,* 540–549.

Gierut, J. (1991). Homonymy in phonological change. *Clinical Linguistics and Phonetics, 5,* 119–137.

Gierut, J. (1992). The conditions and course of clinically induced phonological change. *Journal of Speech and Hearing Research, 35,* 1049–1063.

Gierut, J. (1998). Treatment efficacy: Functional phonological disorders in children. *Journal of Speech, Language, and Hearing Research, 41,* S85–S100.

Gierut, J., & Morrisette, M. (2005). The clinical significance of optimality theory for phonological disorders. *Topics in Language Disorders, 25,* 266–280.

Gierut, J., & Neumann, H. (1992). Teaching and learning /θ/: A nonconfound. *Clinical Linguistics and Phonetics, 6,* 191–200.

Gilbert, J. H., & Purves, B. A. (1977). Temporal constraints on consonant clusters in child speech production. *Journal of Child Language, 4,* 417–432.

Giles, S. B. (1971). *A study of articulatory characteristics of /l/ allophones in English.* Unpublished doctoral dissertation, University of Iowa.

Gillon, G. (2000). The efficacy of phonological awareness intervention for children with spoken language impairment. *Language, Speech, and Hearing Services in Schools, 31,* 126–141.

Gillon, G. (2002). Follow-up study investigating benefits of phonological awareness intervention for children with spoken language impairment. *International Journal of Language and Communication Disorders, 37,* 381–400.

Gillon, G. (2004). *Phonological awareness: From research to practice.* New York: Guilford.

Givens, G., & Seidemann, M. (1977). Middle ear measurements in a difficult to test mentally retarded population. *Mental Retardation, 15,* 40–42.

Goguillot, L. (1889). Comment on fait parler les sounds-muets. Paris: G. Masson.

Golding-Kushner, K. J. (1995). Treatment of articulation and resonance disorders associated with cleft palate and VPI. In R. J. Shprintzen & J. Bardach (Eds.), *Cleft palate speech management. A multidisciplinary approach* (pp. 327–351). St. Louis, MO: Mosby Year Book.

Goldman, R., & Fristoe, M. (2000). *Goldman-Fristoe test of articulation* (2nd ed.). Circle Pines, MN: American Guidance Service.

Goldman, R., Fristoe, M., & Woodcock, R. (1970). *Goldman-Fristoe-Woodcock test of auditory discrimination.* Circle Pines, MN: American Guidance Service.

Goldsmith, J. A. (1976). *Autosegmental phonology.* Bloomington, IN: Indiana University Linguistics Club.

Goldsmith, J. A. (1990). *Autosegmental and metrical phonology.* Cambridge, MA: Basil Blackwell.

Goldstein, B. (1995). Spanish phonological development. In H. Kayser (Ed.), *Bilingual speech-language pathology: An Hispanic focus* (pp. 17–38). San Diego, CA: Singular.

González, G. (1988). Chicano English. In D. Bixler-Marquez & J. Ornstein-Galicia (Eds.), *Chicano speech in the bilingual classroom. Series VI, Vol. 6* (pp. 71–89). New York: Lang.

Gordon-Brannan, M. (1994). Assessing intelligibility: Children's expressive phonologies. In K. Butler & B. Hodson (Eds.), *Topics in Language Disorders, 14,* 17–25.

Gordon-Brannan, M., & Hodson, B. W. (2000). Intelligibility/severity measurements of prekindergarten children's speech. *American Journal of Speech-Language Pathology, 9,* 141–150.

Goswami, U., & Bryant, P. E. (1990). *Phonological skills and learning to read.* Hillsdale, NJ: Lawrence Erlbaum.

Greenlee, M. (1974). Interacting processes in the child's acquisition of stop-liquid clusters. *Papers and Reports on Child Language Development* (Stanford University), *7,* 85–100.

Grunwell, P. (1975). The phonological analysis of articulation disorders. *British Journal of Disorders of Communication, 10,* 31–42.

Grunwell, P. (1981). The development of phonology: A descriptive profile. *First Language, 2,* 161–191.

Grunwell, P. (1985a). *Phonological assessment of child speech.* San Diego, CA: College-Hill Press.

Grunwell, P. (1985b). Forum: Phonetic and phonological features. Comment on the terms "phonetics" and "phonology" as applied in the investigation of speech disorders. *British Journal of Disorders of Communication, 20,* 165–170.

Grunwell, P. (1986). Aspects of phonological development in later childhood. In K. Durkin (Ed.), *Language development in the school years* (pp. 34–56). London: Croom Helm.

Grunwell, P. (1987). *Clinical phonology* (2nd ed.). Baltimore: Williams & Wilkins.

Grunwell, P. (Ed.). (1990). *Developmental speech disorders: Clinical issues and practical implications.* New York: Churchill Livingstone.

Grunwell, P. (1997). Developmental phonological disability: Order in disorder. In B. W. Hodson & M. L. Edwards (Eds.), *Perspectives in applied phonology* (pp. 61–104). Gaithersburg, MD: Aspen.

Gutzmann, A. (1895). *Die Gesundheitspflege der Sprache.* Breslau: F. Hirt.

Gutzmann, H. (1912). *Sprachheilkunde: Vorlesungen über die Störungen der Sprache mit besondere Berücksichtigung der Therapie.* Berlin: Kornfeld.

Guyette, T. W., & Diedrich, W. M. (1981). A critical review of developmental apraxia of speech. In N. J. Lass (Ed.), *Speech and language: Advances in basic research and practice* (Vol. 5) (pp. 1–49). New York: Academic Press.

Haas, W. (1963). Phonological analysis of a case of dyslalia. *Journal of Speech and Hearing Disorders, 28,* 239–246.

Haelsig, P. C., & Madison, C. L. (1986). A study of phonological processes exhibited by 3-, 4-, and 5-year-old children. *Language, Speech, and Hearing Services in Schools, 17,* 107–114.

Hakes, D. T. (1982). The development of metalinguistic abilities: What develops. In S. Kuczaj (Ed.), *Language development* (Vol. II) (pp. 163–210). Hillsdale, NJ: Lawrence Erlbaum.

Haley, K., Ohde, R., & Wertz, R. (2000). Precision of fricative production in aphasia and apraxia of speech: A perceptual and acoustic study. *Aphasiology, 14,* 619–634.

Hall, C., & Golding-Kushner, K. J. (1989). *Long-term follow-up of 500 patients after palate repair performed prior to 18 months of age.* Presented at the Sixth International Congress on Cleft Palate and Related Craniofacial Anomalies, Israel.

Hall, M. (1938). Auditory factors in functional articulatory speech defects. *Journal of Experimental Education, 7,* 110–132.

Hall, P. K. (1989). The occurrence of developmental apraxia of speech in a mild articulation disorder: A case study. *Journal of Communication Disorders, 22,* 265–276.

Hall, P. K., Hardy, J. C., & LaVelle, W. E. (1990). A child with signs of developmental apraxia of speech with whom a palatal lift prosthesis was used to manage palatal dysfunction. *Journal of Speech and Hearing Disorders, 55,* 454–460.

Hall, P. K., Jordan, L. S., & Robin, D. A. (1993). *Developmental apraxia of speech: Theory and clinical practice.* Austin, TX: PRO-ED.

Hall, P. K., Robin, D. A., & Jordan, L. S. (1986). *The presence of word-retrieval deficits in developmental verbal apraxia.* Paper presented at the annual meeting of the American Speech-Language-Hearing Association, Detroit, MI.

Halle, M. (1962). Phonology in generative grammar. *Word, 18,* 54–72.

Hallé, P. A., de Boysson-Bardies, B., & Vihman, M. (1991). Beginnings of prosodic organization: Intonation and duration patterns of disyllables produced by Japanese and French infants. *Language and Speech, 34,* 299–318.

Halliday, M. A. (1975). *Learning how to mean: Explorations in the development of language.* New York: Elsevier.

Hanson, M. L. (1988). Orofacial myofunctional therapy: Guidelines for assessment and treatment. *International Journal of Orofacial Myology, 14,* 27–32.

Hanson, M. L. (1994). Oral myofunctional disorders and articulatory patterns. In J. E. Bernthal & N. W. Bankson (Eds.), *Child phonology: Characteristics, assessment, and intervention with special populations* (pp. 29–53). New York: Thieme.

Hanson, M. L., & Barrett, R. H. (1988). *Fundamentals of orofacial myology.* Springfield, IL: Charles C. Thomas.

Hardcastle, W. J., Morgan-Barry, R. A., & Clark, C. J. (1987). Articulatory and voicing characteristics of adult dysarthric and verbal dyspraxic speakers: An instrumental study. *British Journal of Disorders of Communication, 20,* 249–270.

Hardy, J. C. (1983). *Cerebral palsy.* Englewood Cliffs, NJ: Prentice-Hall.

Hardy, J. C. (1994). Cerebral palsy. In W. A. Secord, G. H. Shames, & E. Wiig (Eds.), *Human communication disorders: An introduction* (4th ed.) (pp. 562–604). New York: Merrill.

Hare, G. (1983). Development at 2 years. In J. V. Irwin & S. P. Wong (Eds.), *Phonological development in children: 18–72 months* (pp. 55–85). Carbondale, IL: Southern Illinois University Press.

Hargrove, P. (1982). Misarticulated vowels: A case study. *Language, Speech, and Hearing Services in Schools, 13,* 86–95.

Harkins, C. S., Berlin, A., Harding, R., Longacre, J., & Snodgrass, R. (1960). Report of the nomenclature committee. *Cleft Palate Bulletin, 10,* 11.

Harkins, C. S., Berlin, A., Harding, R., Longacre, J., & Snodgrass, R. (1962). A classification of cleft lip and palate. *Plastic and Reconstructive Surgery, 29,* 31.

Harlan, N. T. (1984). Treatment approach for a young child evidencing developmental verbal apraxia. *Australian Journal of Human Communication Disorders, 12,* 121–127.

Hawkins, S. (1979). Temporal coordination of consonants in the speech of children: Further data. *Journal of Phonetics, 13,* 235–267.

Hayden, D., & Square, P. (1994). Motor speech treatment hierarchy: A systems approach. *Clinics in Communication Disorders, 4,* 162–174.

Hayden, D., & Square, P. (1999). *Verbal motor production assessment for children (VMPAC).* San Antonio, TX: Psychological Corporation.

Haynes, S. (1985). Developmental apraxia of speech: Symptoms and treatment. In D. F. Johns (Ed.), *Clinical management of neurogenic communication disorders* (2nd ed.) (pp. 259–266). Boston: Little, Brown.

Haynes, W., & Moran, M. (1989). A cross-sectional developmental study of final consonant production in southern Black children from preschool through third grade. *Language, Speech, and Hearing Services in Schools, 20,* 400–406.

Haynes, W. O., & Pindzola, R. H. (1998). *Diagnosis and evaluation in speech pathology* (5th ed.). Boston: Allyn & Bacon.

Haynes, W. O., Pindzola, R. H., & Emerick, L. L. (1992). *Diagnosis and evaluation in speech pathology* (4th ed.). Englewood Cliffs, NJ: Prentice-Hall.

Healy, T. J., & Madison, C. L. (1987). Articulation error migration: A comparison of single word and connected speech samples. *Journal of Communication Disorders, 20,* 129–136.

Hecht, S., Burgess, S., Torgesen, J., Wagner, R., & Rashotte, C. (2000). Explaining social class differences in growth of reading skills from beginning kindergarten through fourth-grade: The role of phonological awareness, rate of access, and print knowledge. *Journal of Reading and Writing, 12,* 99–128.

Heffner, R-M. S. (1975). *General phonetics.* Madison, WI: University of Wisconsin Press.

Helfrich-Miller, K. R. (1984). Melodic intonation therapy with developmentally apraxic children. In W. H. Perkins & J. L. Northern (Eds.), *Seminars in speech and language* (pp. 119–125). New York: Thieme-Stratton.

Helm-Estabrooks, N. (1996). *Test of oral and limb apraxia (TOLA).* Chicago: Applied Symbols.

Hickman, L. A., (1997). *The apraxia profile.* San Antonio, TX: Psychological Corporation.

Hidalgo, M. (1987). On the question of "standard" versus "dialect": Implications for teaching Hispanic college students. *Hispanic Journal of Behavioral Sciences, 9,* 375–395.

Hilton, L. (1984). Treatment of deviant phonological systems: Tongue thrust. In W. Perkins (Ed.), *Phonological-articulatory disorders* (pp. 47–54). New York: Thieme-Stratton.

Hislop, A., Wigglesworth, J., & Desai, R. (1986). Alveolar development in the human fetus and infant. *Early Human Development, 13,* 1–11.

Hodson, B. W. (1984). Facilitating phonological development in children with severe speech disorders. In H. Winitz (Ed.), *Treating articulation disorders. For clinicians by clinicians* (pp. 75–89). Baltimore: University Park Press.

Hodson, B. W. (2004). *Hodson assessment of phonological patterns (HAPP-3).* Greenville, SC: Super Duper.

Hodson, B. W. (1989). Phonological remediation: A cycles approach. In N. A. Creaghead, P. W. Newman, & W. A. Secord (Eds.), *Assessment and remediation of articulatory and phonological disorders* (2nd ed.) (pp. 323–333). New York: Macmillan.

Hodson, B. W. (1992). Clinical forum: Phonological assessment and treatment, applied phonology: Constructs, contributions, and issues. *Language, Speech, and Hearing Services in Schools, 23,* 247–253.

Hodson, B. W. (1994). Helping individuals become intelligible, literate, and articulate: The role of phonology. *Topics in Language Disorders, 14*(2), 1–16.

Hodson, B. W., & Paden, E. P. (1981). Phonological processes which characterize unintelligible and intelligible speech in early childhood. *Journal of Speech and Hearing Disorders, 46,* 369–373.

Hodson, B. W., & Paden, E. P. (1983). *Targeting intelligible speech: A phonological approach to remediation.* San Diego, CA: College-Hill Press.

Hodson, B. W., & Paden, E. P. (1991). *Targeting intelligible speech: A phonological approach to remediation* (2nd ed.). San Diego, CA: College-Hill Press.

Hodson, B. W., Scherz, J. A., & Strattman, K. H. (2002). Evaluating communicative abilities of a highly unintelligible preschooler. *American Journal of Speech-Language Pathology, 11,* 236–242.

Hoek, D., Ingram, D., & Gibson, D. (1986). Some possible causes of children's early word extensions. *Journal of Child Language, 13,* 477–494.

Hoffman, P. (1990). Spelling, phonology, and the speech-language pathologist: A whole language perspective. *Language, Speech, and Hearing Services in Schools, 21,* 238–243.

Hoffman, P., Norris, J., & Monjure, J. (1990). Comparison of process targeting and whole language treatments for phonologically delayed preschool children. *Language, Speech, and Hearing Services in Schools, 21,* 102–109.

Hoffman, P., Schuckers, G., & Daniloff, R. (1989). *Children's phonetic disorders: Theory and treatment.* Boston: Little, Brown.

Hogg, R., & McCully, C. B. (1989). *Metrical phonology: A course book.* Cambridge: Cambridge University Press.

Holmgren, K., Lindblom, B., Aurelius, G., Jalling, B., & Zetterstrom, R. (1986). On the phonetics of infant vocalization. In B. Lindblom & R. Zetterstrom (Eds.), *Precursors of early speech* (pp. 51–63). New York: Stockton Press.

Hornby, P. A., & Hass, W. A. (1970). Use of contrastive stress by preschool children. *Journal of Speech and Hearing Research, 13,* 395–399.

Houston, D. M., & Jusczyk, P. W. (2000). The role of talker-specific information in word segmentation by infants. *Journal of Experimental Psychology, 26,* 1570–1582.

Howell, J. (1989). *The metalinguistic awareness of phonologically disordered and normally developing children: A comparative study.* Unpublished doctoral dissertation, University of Newcastle Upon Tyne, Great Britain.

Howell, J., & Dean, E. (1991). *Treating phonological disorders in children: Metaphon-theory to practice.* San Diego, CA: Singular.

Howell, J., & Dean, E. (1994). *Treating phonological disorders in children: Metaphon-theory to practice* (2nd ed.). London: Whurr.

Hsu, H. C., & Fogel, A. (2001). Infant vocal development in a dynamic mother–infant communication system. *Infancy, 2,* 87–109.

Hull, R. (2001). *Aural rehabilitation, serving children and adults* (4th ed.). Clifton Park, NY: Thomson-Delmar.

Hulme, C., & Snowling, M. (1992). Deficits in output phonology: An explanation of reading failure? *Cognitive Neuropsychology, 9,* 47–72.

Hurford, D., Darrow, L., Edwards, T., Howerton, C., Mote, C., Schauf, J., & Coffey, P. (1993). An examination of phonemic processing abilities in children during their first-grade year. *Journal of Learning Disabilities, 26,* 167–177.

Hutchinson, B. B., Hanson, M. L., & Mecham, M. J. (Eds.). (1979). *Diagnostic handbook of speech pathology.* Baltimore: Williams & Wilkins.

Hyman, L. (1975). *Phonology: Theory and analysis.* New York: Holt, Rinehart and Winston.

Ianucci, D., & Dodd, D. (1980). The development of some aspects of quantifier negation. *Papers & Reports on Child Language Development, 19,* 88–94.

Iglesias, A., & Anderson, N. (1995). Dialectal variations. In J. E. Bernthal & N. W. Bankson (Eds.), *Articulation and phonological disorders* (3rd ed.) (pp. 147–161). Boston: Allyn & Bacon.

Iglesias, A., & Goldstein, B. (1998). Language and dialectal variations. In J. Bernthal & N. Bankson, *Articulation and phonological disorders* (4th ed.) (pp. 148–171). Boston: Allyn & Bacon.

Ingalls, R. P. (1978). *Mental retardation: The changing outlook.* New York: John Wiley.

Ingram, D. (1974). Phonological rules in young children. *Journal of Child Language, 1,* 49–64.

Ingram, D. (1976). *Phonological disability in children.* New York: Elsevier.

Ingram, D. (1979). Phonological development: Production. In P. Fletcher & M. Garman (Eds.), *Language acquisition* (2nd ed.) (pp. 223–239). Cambridge: Cambridge University Press.

Ingram, D. (1981). *Procedures for the phonological analysis of children's language.* Baltimore: University Park Press.

Ingram, D. (1989a). *First language acquisition: Method, description, and explanation.* Cambridge: Cambridge University Press.

Ingram, D. (1989b). *Phonological disability in children: Studies in disorders of communication* (2nd ed.). London: Cole & Whurr.

Ingram, D., Christensen, L., Veach, S., & Webster, B. (1980). The acquisition of word-initial fricatives and affricates in English by children between 2 and 6 years. In G. H. Yeni-Komshian, J. F. Kavanagh, & C. A. Ferguson (Eds.), *Child phonology: Vol. I. Production* (pp. 169–192). New York: Academic Press.

Ingram, D., & Ingram, K. (2001). A whole-word approach to phonological analysis and intervention. *Language, Speech, and Hearing Services in Schools, 32,* 271–283.

Ingram, T. T. S. (1966). The neurology of cerebral palsy. *Archives of Diseases of Childhood, 41,* 337–357.

Ingram, T. T. S., & Barn, J. (1961). A description and classification of common speech disorders associated with cerebral palsy. *Cerebral Palsy Bulletin, 3,* 57–69.

International Phonetic Alphabet (revised 1993, updated 1996). *Association Phonétique Internationale.* Victoria, BC (University of Victoria), Canada.

Irwin, J. V., & Wong, S. P. (Eds.). (1983). *Phonological development in children 18 to 72 months.* Carbondale, IL: Southern Illinois University Press.

Irwin, O. C. (1945). Reliability of infant speech sound data. *Journal of Speech Disorders, 10,* 227–235.

Irwin, O. C. (1946). Infant speech: Equations for consonant-vowel ratios. *Journal of Speech Disorders, 11,* 177–180.

Irwin, O. C. (1947a). Infant speech: Consonant sounds according to place of articulation. *Journal of Speech and Hearing Disorders, 12,* 397–401.

Irwin, O. C. (1947b). Infant speech: Consonant sounds according to manner of articulation. *Journal of Speech and Hearing Disorders, 12,* 402–404.

Irwin, O. C. (1948). Infant speech: Development of vowel sounds. *Journal of Speech and Hearing Disorders, 13,* 31–34.

Irwin, O. C. (1951). Infant speech: Consonantal position. *Journal of Speech and Hearing Disorders, 16,* 159–161.

Irwin, O. C. (1965). *Speech and hearing therapy.* Pittsburgh, PA: Stanwix House.

Irwin, O. C., & Chen, H. P. (1946). Infant speech: Vowel and consonant frequency. *Journal of Speech and Hearing Disorders, 11,* 123–125.

Ivimey, G. P. (1975). The development of English morphology: An acquisition model. *Language and Speech, 18,* 120–144.

Jackson, M. R., & Hall, P. K. (1987). *A longitudinal study of articulation characteristics in developmental verbal apraxia.* Paper presented at the annual meeting of the American Speech-Language-Hearing Association, New Orleans, LA.

Jacobson, J., Boersma, D., Fields, R., & Olson, K. (1983). Paralinguistic features of adult speech to infants and small children. *Child Development, 54,* 436–442.

Jaffe, M. (1989). Feeding at-risk infants and toddlers. *Topics in Language Disorders, 10* (1), 13–25.

Jaffe, M. B. (1984). Neurological impairment of speech production: Assessment and treatment. In A. Holland & J. M. Costello (Eds.), *Handbook of speech and language disorders* (pp. 157–186). San Diego, CA: College-Hill Press.

Jakobson, R. (1949). On the identification of phonemic entities. *Travaux du Cercle Linguistique de Prague, 5,* 205–213.

Jakobson, R. (1962). Zur Struktur des Phonems (pp. 280–310). *Selected Writings I. Vol. 1, Phonological studies.* The Hague: Mouton.

Jakobson, R. (1968). *Child language, aphasia and phonological universals.* The Hague: Mouton. (Original work published 1942)

Jakobson, R., Fant, G., & Halle, M. (1952). *Preliminaries to speech analysis: The distinctive features and their correlates.* Cambridge, MA: MIT Press.

Jakobson, R., & Halle, M. (1956). *Fundamentals of language.* The Hague: Mouton.

Jakobson, R., & Halle, M. (1971). *Fundamentals of language* (2nd ed.). The Hague: Mouton.

Jakobson, R., & Lotz, J. (1949). Notes on the French phonemic pattern. In *R. Jakobson's Selected Writings I* (1962, pp. 426–434). The Hague: Mouton.

Jensen, T. S., Boggild-Andersen, B., Schmidt, J., Ankerhus, J., & Hansen, E. (1988). Perinatal risk factors and first-year vocalizations: Influence on preschool language and motor performance. *Developmental Medicine and Child Neurology, 30,* 153–161.

Jespersen, O. (1889). *The articulation of speech sounds.* Marburg: Elwert Verlag.

Jespersen, O. (1913). *Lehrbuch der Phonetik.* Leipzig: Teubner.

Johns, D. F. (Ed.). (1985). *Clinical management of neurogenic communication disorders* (2nd ed.). Boston: Little, Brown.

Johns, D. F., & Darley, F. L. (1970). Phonemic variability in apraxia of speech. *Journal of Speech and Hearing Research, 13,* 556–583.

Johnston, J. (1982). Interpreting the Leiter IQ: Performance profiles of young normal and language-disordered children. *Journal of Speech and Hearing Research, 25,* 291–296.

Johnston, J., & Schery, T. (1976). The use of grammatical morphemes by children with communication disorders. In D. Morehead & A. Morehead (Eds.), *Normal and deficient child language* (pp. 239–258). Baltimore: University Park Press.

Jones, C. L., & Lorman, J. S. (1986). *Apraxia: A guide for the patient and family.* Stow, OH: Interactive Therapeutics.

Jones, D. (1938). Concrete and abstract sounds. *Proceedings of the 3rd International Congress of Phonetic Sciences.* Ghent: Belgium.

Jones, D. (1950). *The phoneme: Its nature and use.* Cambridge: Heffer.

Jordan, L. S. (1988). *Gestures for cuing phonemes in verbal apraxia: A case study.* Paper presented at the annual meeting of the American Speech-Language-Hearing Association, Boston.

Jordan, L. S. (1991). *Treating apraxia of speech.* Paper presented at the Midwest Aphasiology Conference, Iowa City, IA.

Jusczyk, P., & Luce, P. (2002). Speech perception and spoken word recognition: Past and present. *Ear and Hearing, 23,* 2–40.

Jusczyk, P. W. (1992). Developing phonological categories from the speech signal. In C. A. Ferguson, L. Menn, & C. Stoel-Gammon (Eds.), *Phonological development: Models, research, implications* (pp. 17–64). Parkton, MD: York Press.

Kagan, J. (1971). *Change and continuity in infancy.* New York: John Wiley.

Kamhi, A. G. (1992). Clinical forum: Phonological assessment and treatment. The need for a broad-based model of phonological disorders. *Language, Speech, and Hearing Services in Schools, 23,* 261–268.

Kamhi, A. G., Friemoth-Lee, R., & Nelson, L. (1985). Word, syllable and sound awareness in language disordered children. *Journal of Speech and Hearing Disorders, 50,* 207–212.

Kamhi, A. G., Minor, J. S., & Mauer, D. (1990). Content analysis and intratest performance profiles on the Columbia and the TONI. *Journal of Speech and Hearing Research, 33,* 375–379.

Kantner, C., & West, R. (1960). *Phonetics* (rev. ed.). New York: Harper & Brothers.

Kaufman, N. (1995). *Kaufman speech praxis test for children.* Detroit: Wayne State University Press.

Kay Elemetrics Corporation (1988). *Instruction manual for the nasometer, Model 6200.* Pine Brooks, NJ: Author.

Keating, D., Turrell, G., & Ozanne, A. (2001). Childhood speech disorders: Reported prevalence, comordity, and socioeconomic profile. *Journal of Pediatric and Child Health, 37,* 149–171.

Kehoe, M. M. (2001). Prosodic patterns in children's multisyllabic word productions. *Language, Speech, and Hearing Services in Schools, 32,* 284–294.

Kenney, K. W., & Prather, E. M. (1986). Articulation development in preschool children: Consistency of productions. *Journal of Speech and Hearing Research, 29,* 29–36.

Kent, R. (1982). Contextual facilitation of correct sound production. *Language, Speech, and Hearing Services in Schools, 13,* 66–76.

Kent, R. D. (1997). *The speech sciences.* San Diego, CA: Singular.

Kent, R. D. (1998). Normal aspects of articulation. In J. E. Bernthal & N. W. Bankson (Eds.), *Articulation and phonological disorders* (4th ed.) (pp. 1–62). Boston: Allyn & Bacon.

Kent, R. D., & Bauer, H. R. (1985). Vocalizations of one-year-olds. *Journal of Child Language, 13,* 491–526.

Kent, R. D., Miolo, G., & Bloedel, S. (1994). The intelligibility of children's speech: A review of evaluation procedures. *American Journal of Speech-Language Pathology, 3*(2), 81–95.

Kent, R. D., & Murray, A. D. (1982). Acoustic features of infant vocalic utterances at 3, 6, and 9 months. *Journal of the Acoustical Society of America, 72,* 353–365.

Kent, R. D., & Netsell, R. (1978). Articulatory abnormalities in athetoid cerebral palsy. *Journal of Speech and Hearing Disorders, 43,* 353–373.

Kent, R. D., & Rosenbek, J. C. (1982). Prosodic disturbance and neurologic lesion. *Brain and Language, 15,* 259–291.

Kent, R. D., & Rosenbek, J. C. (1983). Acoustic patterns in apraxia of speech. *Journal of Speech and Hearing Disorders, 26,* 231–248.

Kercher, M. B., & Bauman-Waengler, J. (1992). *Performances of Black English speaking children on standardized language tests.* Presentation at the national convention of the American Speech-Language-Hearing Association, San Antonio, TX.

Kertesz, A. (1980). *Western aphasia battery.* London, Ontario: University of Western Ontario.

Khan, L. (1988). *Vowel remediation: A case study.* Paper presented at the national convention of the American Speech-Language-Hearing Association, Boston.

Khan, L. M. (2002). The sixth view: Assessing preschoolers' articulation and phonology from the trenches. *American Journal of Speech-Language Pathology, 11,* 250–254.

Khan, L., & James, S. (1983). Grammatical morpheme development in three language disordered children. *Journal of Childhood Communication Disorders, 6,* 85–100.

Khan, L., & Lewis, N. (2002). *Khan-Lewis phonological analysis* (2nd ed.). Circle Pines, MN: American Guidance Service.

King, G., & Fletcher, P. (1993). Grammatical problems in school-age children with specific language impairment. *Clinical Linguistics and Phonetics, 7,* 339–352.

Kiparsky, P. (1982). From cyclic phonology to lexical phonology. In H. van der Hulst & H. Smith (Eds.), *The structure of phonological representations* (Vol. II) (pp. 131–176). Dordrecht: Foris.

Kiparsky, P., & Menn, L. (1977). On the acquisition of phonology. In J. Macnamara (Ed.), *Language learning and thought* (pp. 47–78). New York: Academic Press.

Kitamura, H. (1991). Evidence for cleft palate as a postfusion phenomenon. *Cleft Palate Journal, 28,* 195–211.

Klein, E. S. (1996). *Clinical phonology: Assessment and treatment of articulation disorders in children and adults.* San Diego, CA: Singular.

Klein, H. B. (1984). Procedure for maximizing phonological information from single-word responses. *Language, Speech, and Hearing Services in Schools, 15,* 267–274.

Klein, H. B., Lederer, S. H., & Cortese, E. E. (1991). Children's knowledge of auditory/articulatory correspondences: Phonologic and metaphonologic. *Journal of Speech and Hearing Research, 34,* 559–564.

Klich, R. J., Ireland, J. V., & Weidner, W. E. (1979). Articulatory and phonological aspects of consonant substitutions in apraxia of speech. *Cortex, 15,* 451–470.

Klick, S. L. (1984). Adapted cueing technique for use in treatment of dyspraxia. *Language, Speech, and Hearing Services in Schools, 16,* 256–259.

Klick, S. L. (1994). Adapted cueing technique: Facilitating sequential phoneme production. *Clinics in Communication Disorders, 4,* 183–189.

Klink, M., Gerstman, L., Raphael, L., Schlanger, B., & Newsome, L. (1986). Phonological process usage by young EMR children and nonretarded preschool children. *American Journal of Mental Deficiency, 91,* 190–195.

Knock, T., Ballard, K., Robin, D., & Schmidt, R. (2000). Influence or order of stimulus presentation on speech motor learning: A principled approach to treatment for apraxia of speech, *Aphasiology, 14,* 653–668.

Kramer, J. (1939). *Der Sigmatismus, seine Bedingungen und seine Behandlung.* Solothurn: St. Antonius-Verlag.

Krauss, T., & Galloway, H. (1982). Melodic intonation therapy with language delayed apraxic children. *Journal of Music Therapy, 19,* 102–113.

Krech, H. (1969). *Die Behandlung gestörter s-Laute.* Berlin: VEB Verlag Volk und Gesundheit.

Kronvall, E., & Diehl, C. (1954). The relationship of auditory discrimination to articulatory defects of children with no known organic impairment. *Journal of Speech and Hearing Disorders, 19,* 335–338.

Kruszewski, N. (1881). *Über Lautabwechslung.* Kasan': Universitätsbuchdruckerei.

Kudrjavcev, T., Schoenberg, B. S., Kurland, L. T., & Groover, R. V. (1983). Cerebral palsy—trends in incidence and changes in concurrent mortality: Rochester, MN, 1950–1976. *Neurology, 33,* 1433–1438.

Kuhl, P., Conboy, B., Padden, D., Nelson, T., & Pruitt, J. (2005). Early speech perception and later language development: Implications for the "critical period." *Language Learning and Development, 1,* 237–264.

Kuhl, P., Stevens, E., Hayashi, A., Deguchi, T., Kiritani, S., & Iverson, P. (2006). Infants show a facilitation effect for native language phonetic perception between 6 and 12 months. *Developmental Science, 9,* F13–F21.

Kuhl, P. K. (1980). Perceptual constancy for speech sound categories in early infancy. In G. Yeni-Komshian, J. Kavanagh, & C. A. Ferguson (Eds.), *Child phonology: Volume 2. Perception* (pp. 41–66). New York: Academic Press.

Kuhl, P. K. (1987). Perception of speech and sound in early infancy. In P. Salapatek & L. Cohen (Eds.), *Handbook of infant perception: Volume 2. From perception to cognition* (pp. 275–382). New York: Academic Press.

Kumin, L. (1998). Speech and language skills in children with Down syndrome, *Mental Retardation and Developmental Disabilities Research Reviews, 2,* 109–115.

Kumin, L., & Adams, J. (2000). Developmental apraxia of speech and intelligibility in children with Down syndrome. *Down Syndrome Quarterly, 5,* 1–6.

Kussmaul, A. (1885). Die Störungen der Sprache. In H. V. Ziemsson (Ed.), *Handbuch der Speciellen Pathologie und Therapie: Volume 12* (pp. 1–299). Leipzig: F. C. W. Vogel.

Labov, W. (1991). The three dialects of English. In P. Eckert (Ed.), *New ways of analyzing sound change* (pp. 1–44). New York: Academic Press.

Labov, W. (1994). *Principles of linguistic change. Volume 1: Internal factors.* Oxford: Blackwell.

Labov, W. (1996). *The phonological atlas of North America.* Philadelphia: Linguistics Laboratory of the University of Pennsylvania.

Labov, W., Ash, S., & Boberg, C. (2005). *Atlas of North American English.* Berlin: Mouton de Gruyter.

Labov, W., Yaeger, M., & Steiner, R. (1972). *A quantitative study of sound change in progress.* Philadelphia: U.S. Regional Survey.

Ladefoged, P. (1971). *Preliminaries to linguistic phonetics.* Chicago: University of Chicago Press.

Ladefoged, P. (1982). *A course in phonetics* (2nd ed.). New York: Harcourt Brace Jovanovich.

Ladefoged, P. (1993). *A course in phonetics* (3rd ed.). New York: Harcourt Brace Jovanovich.

Ladefoged, P. (2006). *A course in phonetics* (5th ed.). Boston: Thomson Wadsworth.

Ladefoged, P., & Maddieson, I. (1996). *The sounds of the world's languages.* Oxford: Blackwell.

Lahey, M. (1988). *Language disorders and language development.* New York: Macmillan.

Lahey, M., & Bloom, L. (1977). Planning a first lexicon: Which words to teach first. *Journal of Speech and Hearing Disorders, 42,* 340–350.

Lapko, L., & Bankson, N. (1975). Relationship between auditory discrimination, articulation stimulability and consistency of misarticulation. *Perceptual and Motor Skills, 40,* 171–177.

LaPointe, L. L., & Johns, D. F. (1975). Some phonemic characteristics in apraxia of speech. *Journal of Communication Disorders, 8,* 259–269.

LaPointe, L. L., & Wertz, R. T. (1974). Oral-movement abilities and articulatory characteristics of brain-injured adults. *Perceptual Motor Skills, 39,* 39–43.

Larrivee, L., & Catts, H. (1999). Early reading achievement in children with expressive phonological disorders. *American Journal of Speech Language Pathology, 8,* 137–148.

LaVoi, G. W. (1986). *A comparative analysis of selected variables in apraxic and nonapraxic children.* Paper presented at the annual meeting of the American Speech-Language-Hearing Association, Detroit, MI.

Leafstedt, J., Richards, C., & Gerber, M. (2004). Effectiveness of explicit phonological-awareness instruction for at-risk English learners. *Learning Disabilities Research and Practice, 19,* 252–261.

Lecanuet, J.-P., Granier-Deferre, C., & Bushnel, M.-C. (1989). Differential fetal auditory reactiveness as a function of stimulus characteristics and state. *Seminars in Perinatology, 13,* 421–429.

Lee, H. B. (1999). Korean. In *Handbook of the International Phonetic Association* (pp. 120–122). Cambridge: Cambridge University Press.

Lee, L., Koenigsknecht, R., & Mulhern, S. (1975). *Interactive language development teaching.* Evanston, IL: Northwestern University Press.

Lehiste, I. (1970). *Suprasegmentals.* Cambridge: Massachusetts Institute of Technology.

Leinonen-Davis, E. (1988). Assessing the functional adequacy of children's phonological systems. *Clinical Linguistics and Phonetics, 2,* 257–270.

Leitao, S., Hogben, J., & Fletcher, J. (1997). Phonological processing skills in speech and language impaired children. *European Journal of Disorders of Communication, 32,* 73–93.

Leonard, L. (1988). Lexical development and processing in specific language impairment. In R. Schiefelbusch & L. Lloyd (Eds.), *Language perspectives: Acquisition, retardation, and intervention* (2nd ed.) (pp. 69–87). Austin, TX: PRO-ED.

Leonard, L. (1994). Some problems facing accounts of morphological deficits in children with specific language impairments. In R. Watkins & M. Rice (Eds.), *Specific language impairments in children* (pp. 91–106). Baltimore: Brookes.

Leonard, L., & Brown, B. (1984). Nature and boundaries of phonologic categories: A case study of an unusual phonologic pattern in a language-impaired child. *Journal of Speech and Hearing Disorders, 49,* 419–428.

Leonard, L., & Leonard, J. (1985). The contribution of phonetic context to an unusual phonological pattern: A case study. *Language, Speech, and Hearing Services in Schools, 16,* 110–118.

Leonard, L., & McGregor, K. (1991). Unusual phonological patterns and their underlying representations: A case study. *Journal of Child Language, 18,* 261–271.

Leonard, L., McGregor, K., & Allen, G. (1992). Grammatical morphology and speech perception in children with specific language impairment. *Journal of Speech and Hearing Research, 35,* 1076–1085.

Leonard, L., Newhoff, M., & Mesalam, L. (1980). Individual differences in early child phonology. *Applied Psycholinguistics, 1,* 7–30.

Leonard, L., Schwartz, R., Folger, M., Newhoff, M., & Wilcox, M. (1979). Children's imitations of lexical items. *Child Development, 50,* 19–27.

Leonard, L., Schwartz, R., Morris, B., & Chapman, K. (1981). Factors influencing early lexical acquisition: Lexical orientation and phonological composition. *Child Development, 52,* 882–887.

Leopold, W. F. (1947). *Speech development of a bilingual child: A linguist's record.* Evanston, IL: Northwestern University Press.

Lepschy, G. C. (1970). *A survey of structural linguistics.* London: Faber and Faber.

Levin, K. (1999). Babbling in infants with cerebral palsy, *Clinical Linguistics and Phonetics, 13,* 249–267.

Levitt, H., & Stromberg, H. (1983). Segmental characteristics of the speech of hearing-impaired children: Factors affecting intelligibility. In I. Hochberg, H. Levitt, & M. J. Osberger (Eds.), *Speech of the hearing impaired: Research, training, and personnel preparation* (pp. 53–73). Baltimore: University Park Press.

Lewis, B., Freebairn, L., Hansen, A., Taylor, H., Iyengar, S., & Shriberg, L. (2003). Family pedigrees of children with suspected childhood apraxia of speech. *Journal of Communication Disorders, 37,* 157–175.

Lewis, B., Freebairn, L., & Taylor, H. (2000). Correlates of spelling abilities in children with early speech sound disorders. *Reading and Writing: An Interdisciplinary Journal, 15,* 389–407.

Li, C., & Thompson, S. (1987). Chinese. In B. Comrie (Ed.), *The world's major languages* (pp. 811–833). New York: Oxford University Press.

Liberman, I. Y., & Shankweiler, D. (1985). Phonology and the problems of learning to read and write. *Topical Issues: Remedial and Special Education, 6,* 8–17.

Liberman, I. Y., Shankweiler, D., Fischer, W., & Carter, B. (1974). Reading and the awareness of linguistic segments. *Journal of Experimental Child Psychology, 18,* 201–212.

Liberman, I. Y., Shankweiler, D., Liberman, A. M., Fowler, C., & Fischer, F. W. (1977). Phonetic segmentation and recording in the beginning reader. In A. S. Reber & H. Scarborough (Eds.), *Toward a psychology of reading.* Hillsdale, NJ: Lawrence Erlbaum.

Liberman, M. (1975). *The intonational system of English.* Doctoral dissertation, Massachusetts Institute of Technology, Cambridge, MA.

Liberman, M., & Prince, A. (1977). On stress and linguistic rhythm. *Linguistic Inquiry, 8,* 249–336.

Ling, D. (1976). *Speech and the hearing-impaired child: Theory and practice.* Washington, DC: Alexander Graham Bell Association for the Deaf.

Lipke, B., Dickey, J., Selmer, J., & Soder, A. L. (1997). *PAT-3: Photo articulation test* (3rd ed.). Danville, IL: Interstate Press.

Lipsitt, L. (1966). Learning processes of human newborns. *Merrill-Palmer Quarterly, 12,* 45–71.

Lipski, J. (2000). The linguistic situation of Central Americans. In S. McKay & S. Wong (Eds.), *New immigrants in the United States* (pp. 189–215). Cambridge: Cambridge University Press.

Lloyd, L., & Fulton, R. (1972). Audiology's contribution to communications programming with the retarded. In J. McLean, D. Yoder, & R. Schiefelbusch (Eds.), *Language intervention with the retarded: Developmental strategies* (pp. 111–129). Baltimore: University Park Press.

Local, J. (1983). How many vowels in a vowel? *Journal of Child Language, 10,* 449–453.

Locke, J. L. (1980a). Mechanisms of phonological development in children: Maintenance, learning, and loss. *Papers from the Sixteenth Regional Meeting of the Chicago Linguistic Society.* Chicago: Chicago Linguistic Society.

Locke, J. L. (1980b). The inference of speech perception in the phonologically disordered child. Part I: A rationale, some criteria, the conventional tests. *Journal of Speech and Hearing Disorders, 45,* 431–434.

Locke, J. L. (1980c). The inference of speech perception in the phonologically disordered child. Part II: Some clinically novel procedures, their use, some findings. *Journal of Speech and Hearing Disorders, 45,* 435–468.

Locke, J. L. (1983). *Phonological acquisition and change.* New York: Academic Press.

Locke, J. L. (1990). Structure and stimulation in the ontogeny of spoken language. *Developmental Psychobiology, 23,* 621–643.

Locke, J. L., Bleile, K., Fey, M., & Folkins, J. (1996). *Does the distinction between articulation and phonology have clinical significance?* Paper presented at the national convention of the American Speech-Language-Hearing Association, Seattle, WA.

Lof, G. L. (2002). Two comments on this assessment series. *American Journal of Speech-Language Pathology, 11,* 255–256.

Lohr, F. E. (1978). The nonverbal apraxic child: Definition, evaluation, and therapy. *Western Michigan University Journal of Speech, Language, and Hearing, 12,* 71–82.

Long, S. H., & Long, S. T. (1994). Language and children with mental retardation. In V. R. Reed (Ed.), *An introduction to children with language disorders* (2nd ed.) (pp. 153–191). New York: Merrill.

Lonigan, C., Burgess, S., & Anthony, J. (2000). Development of emergent literacy and early reading skills in preschool children: Evidence from a latent-variable longitudinal study. *Developmental Psychology, 36,* 596–613.

Lonigan, C., Burgess, S., Anthony, J., & Berker, T. (1998). Development of phonological sensitivity in 2- to 5-year-old children. *Journal of Educational Psychology, 90,* 294–311.

Lorentz, J. P. (1976). An analysis of some deviant phonological rules of English. In D. M. Morehead & A. E. Morehead (Eds.), *Normal and deficient child language* (pp. 29–59). Baltimore: University Park Press.

Love, R. J. (2000). *Childhood motor speech disability.* (2nd ed.) Boston: Allyn & Bacon.

Love, R. J., & Fitzgerald, M. (1984). Is the diagnosis of developmental apraxia of speech valid? *Australian Journal of Human Communication Disorders, 12,* 71–82.

Lowe, R. J. (1986). *Assessment link between phonology and articulation: ALPHA.* Moline, IL: LinguiSystems.

Lowe, R. J. (1994). *Phonology: Assessment and intervention applications in speech pathology.* Baltimore: Williams & Wilkins.

Lowe, R. J. (1996). *Assessment link between phonology and articulation: ALPHA* (rev. ed.). Mifflinville, PA: Speech and Language Resources.

Lowe, R. J., Knutson, P., & Monson, M. (1985). Incidence of fronting in preschool children. *Language, Speech, and Hearing Services in Schools, 16,* 119–123.

Lowe, R. J., Mount-Weitz, J., & Schmidt, C. (1992). *Activities for the remediation of phonological disorders*. DeKalb, IL: Janelle.

Luchsinger, R., & Arnold, G. E. (1965). *Voice-speech-language. Clinical communicology: Its physiology and pathology*. Belmont, CA: Wadsworth.

Lund, N. J., & Duchan, J. F. (1993). *Assessing children's language in naturalistic contexts* (3rd ed.). Englewood Cliffs, NJ: Prentice-Hall.

Lundberg, I. (1988). Preschool prevention of reading failure: Does training in phonological awareness work? In R. L. Masland & M. W. Masland (Eds.), *Preschool prevention of reading failure* (pp. 163–176). Parkton, MD: York Press.

Lundberg, I., Olofsson, A., & Wall, S. (1980). Reading and spelling skills in the first school years predicted from phonemic awareness skills in kindergarten. *Scandinavian Journal of Psychology, 21*, 159–173.

Lundberg, I., Olofsson, A., & Wall, S. (1980). Reading and spelling skills in the first years predicted from phonemic awareness skills in kindergarten. *Scandinavian Journal of Psychology, 21*, 159–173.

Luria, A. R., & Hutton, J. T. (1977). A modern assessment of the basic forms of aphasia. *Brain and Language, 4*, 129–151.

Lynch, J. I. (1986). Langugage of cleft infants: Lessening the risk of delay through programming. In B. J. McWilliams (Ed.), Current methods of assessing and treating children with cleft palates. *Seminars in Speech and Language, 7*, 255–268.

Lyytinen, H., Ahonen, T., Eklund, K., Guttorm, T., Laakso, M., Leinonen, S., Leppanen, P., Lyytinen, P., Poikkeus, A., Puolakanaho, A., Richardson, U., & Viholainen, H. (2001). Developmental pathways of children with and without familial risk for dyslexia during the first years of life. *Developmental Neuropsychology, 20*, 535–554.

Mackay, I. (1987). *Phonetics: The science of speech production* (2nd ed.). Boston: Allyn & Bacon.

Maclean, M., Bryant, P., & Bradley, L. (1987). Rhymes, nursery rhymes and reading in early childhood. *Merrill-Palmer Quarterly, 33*, 255–282.

Mader, J. (1954). The relative frequency occurrence of English consonant sounds in words in the speech of children in grades one, two, and three. *Speech Monographs, 21*, 294–300.

Magnusson, E. (1983). The phonology of language disordered children: Production, perception and awareness. *Travaux de l'Institut de Linguistique de Lund XVIII*. Lund: CWK Gleerup.

Magnusson, E. (1991). Metalinguistic awareness in phonologically disordered children. In M. Yavaş (Ed.), *Phonological disorders in children: Theory, research and practice* (pp. 87–120). London: Routledge.

Magnusson, E., & Naucler, K. (1987). Language disordered and normally speaking children's development of spoken and written language: Preliminary results from a longitudinal study. *RUVL 16*, Uppsala University: Department of Linguistics.

Malikouti-Drachman, A., & Drachman, G. (1975). The acquisition of stress in Modern Greek. *Salzburger Beiträge zur Linguistik, 2*, 277–289.

Marcel, T. (1980). Surface dyslexia and beginning reading: A revised hypothesis of the pronunciation of print and its impairments. In M. Coltheart, K. Paterson, & J. Marshall (Eds.), *Deep dyslexia* (pp. 227–258). London: Routledge & Kegan Paul.

Marcos, H. (1987). Communicative function of pitch range and pitch direction in infants. *Journal of Child Language, 14*, 255–268.

Mareschal, D., & French, R. (2000). Mechanisms of categorization in infants. *Infancy, 1*, 59–76.

Marili, J., Andrianopoulos, K., Velleman, M., & Foreman, C. (2004*). Incidence of motor speech impairment in autism and Asperger's disorders*. Paper presented at the annual convention of the American Speech-Language-Hearing Association, Philadelphia.

Marion, M. J., Sussman, H. M., & Marquardt, T. P. (1993). The perception and production of rhyme in normal and developmentally apraxic children. *Journal of Communication Disorders, 26*, 129–160.

Markides, A. (1970). The speech of deaf and partially-hearing children with special reference to factors affecting intelligibility. *British Journal of Disorders of Communication, 5*, 126–140.

Marquardt, T. P. (1982). *Acquired neurogenic disorders*. Englewood Cliffs, NJ: Prentice-Hall.

Marquardt, T. P., Reinhart, J. B., & Peterson, H. A. (1979). Markedness analysis of phonemic substitution errors in apraxia of speech. *Journal of Communication Disorders, 12*, 481–494.

Marquardt, T. P., & Sussman, H. M. (1991). Developmental apraxia of speech: Theory and practice. In D. Vogel & M. P. Cannito (Eds.), *Treating disordered speech motor control* (pp. 341–390). Austin, TX: PRO-ED.

Marquardt, T. P., Sussman, H. M., Snow, T., & Jacks, A. (2002). The integrity of the syllable in developmental apraxia of speech. *Journal of Communication Disorders, 35*, 31–49.

Marsh, J. L., & Lehman, J. A. (1988). *Cleft care in 1986: An ACPA survey* [abstract]. American Cleft Palate–Craniofacial Annual Meeting, Williamsburg, VA.

Martin, A. D. (1974). Some objections to the term apraxia of speech. *Journal of Speech and Hearing Disorders, 39*, 53–64.

Martinet, A. (1960). *Elements de linguistique général I*. [Elements of general linguistics I]. Paris: Armand Colin.

Mase, D. (1946). Etiology of articulatory speech defects. *Teacher's College Contribution to Education, no. 921.* New York: Columbia University.

Masterson, J., Bernhardt, B., & Hofheinz, M. (2005). A comparison of single words and conversational speech in phonological evaluation. *American Journal of Speech-Language Pathology, 14,* 229–241.

Matheny, N., & Panagos, J. (1978). Comparing the effects of articulation and syntax programs on syntax and articulation improvement. *Language, Speech, and Hearing Services in Schools, 9,* 57–61.

Matisoff, J. (1991). Sino-Tibetan linguistics: Present state and future prospects. *Annual Review of Anthropology, 20,* 469–504.

Maye, J., & Gerken, L. (2000). *Learning phonemes without minimal pairs.* Proceeedings of the 24th Annual Boston University Conference on Language Development. Somerville, MA: Cascadia Press.

Maye, J., & Weiss, D. (2003). *Statistical cues facilitate infants' discrimination of difficult phonetic contrasts.* Proceedings of the 27th Boston University Conference on Language Development (pp. 508–518). Somerville, MA: Cascadilla Press.

Maye, J., Werker, J., & Gerken, L. (2002). Infant sensitivity to distributional information can affect phonetic discrimination, *Cognition, 82,* B101–B111.

McCabe, R. B., & Bradley, D. P. (1975). Systematic multiple phonemic approach to articulation therapy. *Acta Symbolica, 6,* 1–18.

McCarthren, R., Warren, S., & Yoder, P. (1996). Prelinguistic predictors of later language development. In K. Cole, P. Dale, & D. Thal (Eds.*), Assessment of communication and language* (pp. 57–75). Baltimore: Brookes.

McCarthy, J. (1988). Feature geometry and dependency: A review. *Phonetica, 43,* 84–108.

McCarthy, J., & Prince, A. (1993). *Prosodic morphology I: Constraint interaction and satisfaction.* Unpublished manuscript, University of Massachusetts, Amherst.

McCarthy, J. J., & Prince, A. S. (1995). Faithfulness and reduplicative identity. In *Papers in Optimality Theory: University of Massachusetts Occasional Papers in Linguistics 18* (pp. 249–384). Amherst, MA: Graduate Linguistics Student Association.

McCune, L., & Vihman, M. M. (2001). Early phonetic and lexical development: A productivity approach. *Journal of Speech, Language, and Hearing Research, 44,* 670–684.

McDonald, E. T. (1964). *A deep test of articulation—picture form.* Pittsburgh, PA: Stanwix.

McHenry, M. (2003). The effect of pacing strategies on the variability of speech movement sequences in dysarthria. *Journal of Speech, Language, and Hearing Research, 46,* 702–710.

McLeod, S. van Doorn, J., & Reed, V. (2001). Consonant cluster development in two-year-olds: General trends and individual difference. *Journal of Speech, Language, and Hearing Research, 44,* 1144–1171.

McMahon, K., Hodson, B., & Allen, E. (1983). Phonological analysis of cerebral palsied children's utterances. *Journal of Childhood Communication Disorders, 7,* 28–35.

McNeil, M. R., Rosenbek, J. C., & Aronson, A. E. (1984). *The dysarthrias: Physiology, acoustics, perception, management.* San Diego, CA: College-Hill Press.

McReynolds, L. V., & Bennett, S. (1972). Distinctive feature generalization in articulation training. *Journal of Speech and Hearing Disorders, 37,* 462–470.

McReynolds, L. V., & Elbert, M. (1981). Criteria for phonological process analysis. *Journal of Speech and Hearing Disorders, 46,* 197–204.

McReynolds, L. V., & Engmann, D. (1975). *Distinctive feature analysis of misarticulations.* Baltimore: University Park Press.

McReynolds, L. V., Engmann, D., & Dimmitt, K. (1974). Markedness theory and articulation errors. *Journal of Speech and Hearing Disorders, 39,* 93–103.

Meador, D. (1984). Effects of color on visual discrimination of geometric symbols by severely and profoundly mentally retarded individuals. *American Journal on Mental Deficiency, 89,* 275–286.

Mehler, J., Jusczyk, P., Lambertz, G., Halsted, N., Bertoncini, J., & Amiel-Tison, C. (1988). A precursor of language acquisition in young infants. *Cognition, 29,* 143–178.

Mehrabian, A. (1970). Measures of vocabulary and grammatical skills for children up to age six. *Developmental Psychology, 2,* 439–446.

Meitus, I. J., & Weinberg, B. (1983). *Diagnosis in speech-language pathology.* Baltimore: University Park Press.

Menn, L. (1971). Phonotactic rules in beginning speech. *Lingua, 26,* 225–251.

Menn, L. (1976). *Pattern, control and contrast in beginning speech: A case study in the development of word form and word function.* Unpublished doctoral dissertation, University of Illinois, Urbana–Champaign.

Menn, L. (1978). *Pattern, control and contrast in beginning speech: A case study in the development of word form and word function.* Bloomington, IN: Indiana University Linguistics Club.

Menyuk, P. (1980). The role of context in misarticulations. In G. Yeni-Komshian, J. Kavanagh, & C. Ferguson (Eds.), *Child phonology: Vol. 1. Production* (pp. 211–226). New York: Academic Press.

Menyuk, P., Liebergott, J., & Schultz, M. (1986). Predicting phonological development. In B. Lindblom & R. Zetterstrom (Eds.), *Precursors of early speech* (pp. 79–93). New York: Stockton Press.

Mercer, J. R. (1973). *Labeling the mentally retarded.* Berkeley: University of California Press.

Metter, E. J. (1985). *Speech disorders: Clinical evaluation and diagnosis.* Jamaica, NY: Spectrum Publications Medical & Scientific Books.

Miccio, A. W. (2002). Clinical problem solving: Assessment of phonological disorders. *American Journal of Speech-Language Pathology, 11,* 221–229.

Miccio, A. W., Elbert, M., & Forrest, K. (1999). The relationship between stimulability and phonological acquisition in children with normally developing and disordered phonologies. *American Journal of Speech-Language Pathology, 8,* 347–363.

Milisen, R. (1954). The disorder of articulation: A systematic clinical and experimental approach. *Journal of Speech and Hearing Disorders,* Monograph Supplement 4.

Miller, G., & Nicely, P. (1955). An analysis of perceptual confusions among some English consonants. *Journal of the Acoustical Society of America, 27,* 338–352.

Miller, J. F. (1988). Facilitating speech and language. In C. Tingey (Ed.), *Down syndrome. A resource book* (pp. 119–133). Boston: College-Hill Press.

Miller, J. F. (1992). Lexical development in young children with Down syndrome. In R. S. Chapman (Ed.), *Processes in language acquisition and disorder* (pp. 202–216). St. Louis, MO: Mosby Year Book.

Milloy, N. (1985). *The assessment and identification of developmental articulatory dyspraxia and its effect on phonological development.* Unpublished thesis, Leicester Polytechnic, Leicester, UK.

Milloy, N., & Morgan-Barry, R. (1990). Developmental neurological disorders. In P. Grunwell (Ed.), *Developmental speech disorders* (pp. 109–132). New York: Churchill Livingstone.

Mines, M., Hanson, B., & Shoup, J. (1978). Frequency of occurrence of phonemes in conversational English language and speech. *Language and Speech, 21,* 221–241.

Mitchell, P. R., & Kent, R. (1990). Phonetic variation in multisyllable babbling. *Journal of Child Language, 17,* 247–265.

Monnin, L. (1984). Speech sound discrimination testing and training: Why? Why not? In H. Winitz (Ed.), *Treating articulation disorders: For clinicians by clinicians* (pp. 1–20). Austin, TX: PRO-ED.

Monnin, L., & Huntington, D. (1974). Relationship of articulatory defects to speech-sound identification. *Journal of Speech and Hearing Research, 17,* 352–366.

Monsen, R. B. (1981). A usable test for the speech intelligibility of deaf talkers. *American Annals of the Deaf, 126,* 845–852.

Monsen, R. B., Moog, J. S., & Geers, A. E. (1988). *CID picture SPINE.* St. Louis, MO: Central Institute for the Deaf.

Moore, C., Yorkston, K., & Beukelman, D. R. (Eds.). (1991). *Dysarthria and apraxia of speech: Perspectives on management.* Baltimore: Paul H. Brooks.

Moore, W. M., Rosenbek, J. C., & LaPointe, L. L. (1976). Assessment of oral apraxia in brain-injured adults. In R. Brookshire (Ed.), *Clinical aphasiology: Proceedings of the conference* (pp. 64–79). Minneapolis, MN: BRK.

Moran, M., Money, S., & Leonard, L. (1984). Phonological process analysis of the speech of mentally retarded adults. *American Journal of Mental Deficiency, 89,* 304–306.

Morley, M. E. (1959). Defects of articulation. *Folia Phoniatrica, 11,* 65–124.

Morley, M. E. (1970). *Cleft palate and speech* (7th ed.). Baltimore: Williams & Wilkins.

Morley, M. E. (1972). Developmental articulatory apraxia. In M. E. Morley (Ed.), *The development and disorders of speech in childhood* (pp. 274–290). Baltimore: Williams & Wilkins.

Morley, M. E., Court, D., & Miller, H. (1954). Delayed speech and developmental aphasia. *British Medical Journal, 2,* 463–467.

Morley, M. E., & Fox, J. (1969). Disorders of articulation: Theory and therapy. *British Journal of Communication, 4,* 151–165.

Morris, H. L., Spriestersbach, D. C., & Darley, F. L. (1961). An articulation test for assessing competency of velopharyngeal closure. *Journal of Speech and Hearing Research, 4,* 48–55.

Morris, S. E. (1975). Pre-speech assessment. In S. E. Morris (Ed.), *Pre-speech and language programming for the young child with cerebral palsy.* Wauwatosa, WI: Curative Rehabilitation Center.

Morrisette, M., & Gierut, J. (2002). Lexical organization and phonological change in treatment. *Journal of Speech, Language, and Hearing Research, 45,* 143–159.

Morrison, J., & Shriberg, L. (1992). Articulation testing versus conversational speech sampling. *Journal of Speech and Hearing Research, 35,* 259–273.

Mortenson, D. (2004). *Preliminaries to Mong Leng (Hmong Njua) phonology.* Retrieved from ist-socrates.berkeley.edu/~dmort/mong_leng_phonology.pdf, May 2006.

Mosher, J. (1929). *The production of correct speech sounds.* Boston: Expression.

Moskowitz, A. (1971). *Acquisition of phonology.* Unpublished doctoral dissertation, University of California, Berkeley.

Munson, B., Edwards, J., & Beckman, M. (2005). Phonological knowledge in typical and atypical speech-sound development. *Topics in Language Disorders. Clinical Perspectives on Speech Sound Disorders, 25,* 190–206.

Murdoch, B. E., Porter, S., Younger, R., & Ozanne, A. (1984). Behaviors identified by South Australian clinicians as differentially diagnostic of developmental articulatory dyspraxia. *Australian Journal of Human Communication Disorders, 12,* 55–70.

Myers, F. L., & Myers, R. W. (1983). Perception of stress contrasts in semantic and non-semantic contexts by children. *Journal of Psycholinguistic Research, 12,* 327–338.

Myerson, R. F. (1978). Children's knowledge of selected aspects of sound pattern of English. In R. N. Campbell & P. T. Smith (Eds.), *Recent advances in the psychology of language* (Vol. III4) (pp. 377–402). New York: Plenum Press.

Mysak, E. D. (1959). A servomodel for speech therapy. *Journal of Speech and Hearing Disorders, 24,* 144–149.

Nakazima, S. A. (1962). A comparative study of the speech developments of Japanese and American English in childhood (1): A comparison of the developments of voices at the prelinguistic period. *Studia Phonologica, 2,* 27–46.

Nathani, S., Ertmer, D., & Stark, R. (2006). Assessing vocal development in infants and toddlers. *Clinical Linguistics and Phonetics, 20,* 351–369.

Neary, T. (1978). *Phonetic feature systems for vowels.* Doctoral dissertation, University of Connecticut. Reproduced by Indiana University Linguistic Club.

Nelson, K. (1973). Structure and strategy in learning to talk. *Monographs of the Society of Research in Child Development, 38*(149). Chicago: University of Chicago Press.

Nelson, N. W. (1998). *Childhood language disorders in context: Infancy through adolescence* (2nd ed.). Boston: Allyn & Bacon.

Nemoy, E. M. (1954). *Speech correction through story telling units.* Magnolia, MA: Expression.

Nemoy, E. M., & Davis, S. (1937). *The correction of defective consonant sounds.* Boston: Expression.

Newcomer, P., & Hammill, D. (1988). *Test of language development-2 primary.* Austin, TX: PRO-ED.

Newman, P. W., & Creaghead, N. A. (1989). Assessment of articulatory and phonological disorders. In N. A. Creaghead, P. W. Newman, & W. A. Secord (Eds.), *Assessment and remediation of articulatory and phonological disorders* (2nd ed.) (pp. 69–126). New York: Macmillan.

Nolan, M., McCartney, E., McArthur, K., & Rowson, V. (1980). A study of the hearing and receptive vocabulary of the trainees of an adult training centre. *Journal of Mental Deficiency Research, 24,* 271–286.

Noll, J. D. (1983). Diagnosis of speech and language disorders associated with acquired neuropathologies: Apraxia of speech and the dysarthrias. In I. J. Meitus & B. Weinberg (Eds.), *Diagnosis in speech-language pathology.* Baltimore: University Park Press.

Northern, J. L., & Downs, M. P. (1984). *Hearing in children* (3rd ed.). Baltimore: Williams & Wilkins.

Odell, K., McNeil, M. R., Rosenbek, J. C., & Hunter, L. (1990). Perceptual characteristics of consonant production by apraxic speakers. *Journal of Speech and Hearing Disorders, 55,* 345–359.

Oetting, J., & Horohov, J. (1997). Past tense marking by children with and without specific language impairment. *Journal of Speech and Hearing Research, 40,* 62–74.

Oetting, J., & Rice, M. (1993). Plural acquisition in children with specific language impairment. *Journal of Speech and Hearing Research, 36,* 1236–1248.

Office of English Language Acquisition. (2002). *Survey of the states' limited English proficient students and available educational programs and services: 2000–2001 summary report.* Washington, DC: National Clearinghouse for English Language Acquisition and Language Instruction Educational Programs.

Oller, D., Eilers, R., Neal, A., & Schwartz, G. (1999). Precursors to speech in infancy: The predication of speech and language disorders. *Journal of Communication Disorders, 32,* 223–245.

Oller, D. K. (1973). Regularities in abnormal child phonology. *Journal of Speech and Hearing Disorders, 38,* 36–47.

Oller, D. K. (1980). The emergence of the sounds of speech in infancy. In G. Yeni-Komshian, J. Kavanagh, & C. A. Ferguson (Eds.), *Child phonology: Vol. I. Production* (pp. 93–112). New York: Academic Press.

Oller, D. K., Jensen, H. T., & Lafayette, R. H. (1978). The relatedness of phonological processes of a hearing-impaired child. *Journal of Communication Disorders, 11,* 97–105.

Oller, D. K., Weiman, L. A., Doyle, W. J., & Ross, C. (1976). Infant babbling and speech. *Journal of Child Language, 3,* 1–11.

Olmsted, D. (1971). *Out of the mouth of babes: Earliest stages in language learning.* The Hague: Mouton.

Olofsson, A., & Neidersoe, J. (1999). Early language development and kindergarten phonological awareness as predictors of reading problems. *Journal of Learning Disabilities, 32,* 464–472.

Osberger, M. J. (1983). Development and evaluation of some speech training procedures for hearing-impaired children. In I. Hochberg, H. Levitt, & M. J. Osberger (Eds.), *Speech of the hearing impaired: Research, training, and personnel preparation* (pp. 333–348). Baltimore: University Park Press.

Osberger, M. J., & McGarr, N. (1982). Speech production characteristics of the hearing impaired. In N. Lass (Ed.), *Speech and language: Advances in basic science and research.* New York: Academic Press.

Otheguy, R., Garcia, O., & Roca, A. (2000). Speaking in Cuban: The language of Cuban Americans. In S. McKay & S. Wong (Eds.), *New immigrants in the United States* (pp. 165–188). Cambridge: Cambridge University Press.

Owens, R. E. (1992). *Language development: An introduction* (3rd ed.). New York: Macmillan.

Owens, R. E. (2002). Mental retardation: Difference and delay. In D. K. Bernstein & E. Tiegerman-Farber (Eds.), *Language and communication disorders in children* (5th ed.) (pp. 457–523). Boston: Allyn & Bacon.

Owens, R. E. (2008). *Language development: An introduction* (7th ed.). Boston: Allyn & Bacon.

Owens, R. E., & House, L. (1984). Decision-making processes in augmentative communication. *Journal of Speech and Hearing Disorders, 49,* 18–25.

Paavola, L., Kunnari, S., & Moilanen, I. (2005). Maternal responsiveness and infant intentional communication: Implications for the early communicative and linguistic development. *Child: Care, Health and Development, 31,* 727–735.

Pamplona, M., Ysunza, A., Gonzalez, M., Ramirez, E., & Patino, C. (2000). Linguistic development in cleft palate patients with and without compensatory articulation disorder. *International Journal of Pediatric Otorhinolaryngology, 54,* 81–91.

Pan, B., & Gleason, J. B. (2005). Semantic development: Learning the meanings of words. In J. Gleason (Ed.), *The development of language* (6th ed.) (pp. 125–161). Boston: Allyn & Bacon.

Panagos, J., & Prelock, P. (1982). Phonological constraints on the sentence production of language disordered children. *Journal of Speech and Hearing Research, 25,* 171–177.

Panagos, J., Quine, M., & Klich, R. (1979). Syntactic and phonological influences on children's articulation. *Journal of Speech and Hearing Research, 22,* 841–848.

Panconcelli-Calzia, G. (1924). *Experimental phonetik, Gehör und Lautwandel.* Tillägnat Hugo Pipping, Helsingfors, 429.

Parker, F. (1976). Distinctive features in speech pathology: Phonology or phonemics. *Journal of Speech and Hearing Disorders, 41,* 23–39.

Parker, F. (1994). Phonological theory. In R. Lowe (Ed.), *Phonology. Assessment and intervention applications in speech pathology* (pp. 17–34). Baltimore: Williams & Wilkins.

Parsons, C. L. (1984). A comparison of phonological processes used by developmentally verbal dyspraxic children and non-dyspraxic phonologically impaired children. *Australian Journal of Human Communication Disorders, 12,* 93–107.

Paschall, L. (1983). Development at 18 months. In J. V. Irwin & S. P. Wong (Eds.), *Phonological development in children: 18–72 months* (pp. 27–54). Carbondale, IL: Southern Illinois University Press.

Patel, R. (2002). Prosodic control in severe dysarthria. *Journal of Speech, Language, and Hearing Research, 45,* 858–870.

Paul, R. (1989). *Outcomes of specific expressive language delay.* Paper at Symposium for Research in Child Language Disorders, Madison, WI.

Paul, R. (1991). Profiles of toddlers with slow expressive language development. *Topics in Language Disorders, 11,* 1–13.

Paul, R. (1993). Patterns of development in late talkers: Preschool years. *Journal of Childhood Communication Disorders, 15,* 7–14.

Paul, R. (2001). *Language disorders from infancy through adolescence: Assessment and intervention.* (2nd ed.) St. Louis, MO: Mosby Year Book.

Paul, R., & Jennings, P. (1992). Phonological behavior in toddlers with slow expressive language development. *Journal of Speech and Hearing Research, 35,* 99–107.

Paul, R., Looney, S., & Dahm, P. (1991). Communication and socialization skills at ages 2 and 3 in "late talking" young children. *Journal of Speech and Hearing Research, 34,* 858–865.

Paul, R., & Shriberg, L. D. (1982). Associations between phonology and syntax in speech delayed children. *Journal of Speech and Hearing Research, 25,* 536–547.

Pena-Brooks, A., & Hegde, M. N. (2000). *Assessment and treatment of articulation and phonological disorders in children.* Austin: PRO-ED.

Penfield, J., & Ornstein-Galacia, J. (1985). *Chicano English: An ethnic dialect.* Philadelphia: John Benjamin.

Penney, G., Fee, E. J., & Dowdle, C. (1994). Vowel assessment and remediation: A case study, *Child Language Teaching and Therapy, 10,* 47–66.

Perez, E. (1994). Phonological differences among speakers of Spanish-influenced English. In J. Bernthal & N. Bankson (Eds.), *Child phonology: Characteristics, assessment, and intervention with special populations* (pp. 245–254). New York: Thieme.

Peterson, H. A., & Marquardt, T. P. (1990). *Appraisal and diagnosis of speech-language disorders* (2nd ed.). Englewood Cliffs, NJ: Prentice-Hall.

Pharoah, P. O. D., Cooke, T., Rosenbloom, I., & Cooke, R. W. I. (1987). Trends in birth prevalence of cerebral palsy. *Archives of Disease in Childhood, 62,* 379–384.

Pharr, A., Ratner, N., & Rescorla, L. (2000). Syllable structure development of toddlers with expressive specific language impairment. *Applied Psycholinguistics, 21,* 429–449.

Philips, B. J. W., & Bzoch, K. R. (1969). Reliability of judgements of articulation of cleft palate speakers. *Cleft Palate Journal, 6,* 24–34.

Piaget, J. (1952). *The origins of intelligence in children.* New York: International Universities Press.

Pierce, J. E., & Hanna, I. V. (1974). *The development of a phonological system in English speaking American children*. Portland: HaPi Press.

Pike, K. L. (1943). *Phonetics*. Ann Arbor, MI: University of Michigan Press.

Pollack, E., & Rees, N. (1972). Disorders of articulation: Some clinical applications of distinctive feature theory. *Journal of Speech and Hearing Disorders, 37*, 451–461.

Pollock, K. (1991). The identification of vowel errors using traditional articulation or phonological process test stimuli. *Language, Speech, and Hearing Services in Schools, 22*, 39–50.

Pollock, K. E. (2002). Identification of vowel errors: Methodological issues and preliminary data from the Memphis vowel project. In M. J. Ball & F. E. Gibbon (Eds.), *Vowel Disorders* (pp. 83–113). Boston: Butterworth-Heinemann.

Pollock, K., & Hall, P. K. (1991). An analysis of the vowel misarticulations of five children with developmental apraxia of speech. *Clinical Linguistics and Phonetics, 5*, 207–224.

Pollock, K., & Keiser, N. (1990). An examination of vowel errors in phonologically disordered children. *Clinical Linguistics and Phonetics, 4*, 161–178.

Pollock, K., & Schwartz, R. (1988). Structural aspects of phonological development: Case study of a disordered child. *Language, Speech, and Hearing Services in Schools, 19*, 5–16.

Pollock, K., & Swanson, L. (1986). *Analysis of vowel errors in a disordered child during training*. Paper presented at the annual convention of the American Speech-Language-Hearing Association, Detroit, MI.

Poole, I. (1934). Genetic development of articulation of consonant sounds in speech. *Elementary English Review, 11*, 159–161.

Powell, T. W., Elbert, M., & Dinnsen, D. A. (1991). Stimulability as a factor in the phonologic generalization of misarticulating preschool children. *Journal of Speech and Hearing Research, 34*, 1318–1328.

Powers, M. (1971). Clinical and educational procedures in functional disorders of articulation. In L. Travis (Ed.), *Handbook of speech pathology and audiology* (pp. 877–910). New York: Appleton-Century-Crofts.

Prather, E. M., Hedrick, D., & Kern, C. (1975). Articulation development in children aged two to four years. *Journal of Speech and Hearing Disorders, 40*, 179–191.

Pratt, C., & Grieve, R. (1983). The development of metalinguistic awareness: An introduction. In W. Tunmer, C. Pratt, & M. Herriman (Eds.), *Metalinguistic awareness in children: Theory, research and implications* (pp. 2–11). Berlin: Springer-Verlag.

Preisser, D. A., Hodson, B. W., & Paden, E. P. (1988). Developmental phonology: 18–29 months. *Journal of Speech and Hearing Disorders, 53*, 125–130.

President's Committee on Mental Retardation (PCMR). (1978). Washington, DC: PCMR Newsclipping Service.

Prince, A. S., & Smolensky, P. (1993). Optimality theory: Constraint interaction in generative grammar, *RUCCs Technical Report #2*, New Brunswick, NJ: Rutgers University Center for Cognitive Science, Rutgers University.

Prins, D. (1963). Relations among specific articulatory deviations and responses to a clinical measure of sound discrimination ability. *Journal of Speech and Hearing Disorders, 28*, 382–388.

Pulleyblank, D. (1986). Underspecification and low vowel harmony in Okpe2. *Studies in African Linguistics, 17*, 119–153.

Radziewicz, C., & Antonellis, S. (1997). Considerations and implications for habilitation of hearing impaired children. In D. K. Bernstein & E. Tiegerman (Eds.), *Language and communication disorders in children* (4th ed.) (pp. 574–603). Boston: Allyn & Bacon.

Raphael, L., & Bell-Berti, F. (1975). Tongue musculature and the feature of tension in English vowels. *Phonetica, 32*, 61–63.

Ratliff, M. (1992). *Meaningful tone: A study of tonal morphology in compounds, form classes, and expressive phrases in White Hmong*. Monograph Number 27, Southeast Asia. De Kalb, IL: Northern Illinois University Center for Southeast Asian Studies.

Ratner, N. B. (1994). Phonological analysis of child speech. In J. Sokolov & C. Snow (Eds.), *Handbook of Research in Language Development using CHILDES* (pp. 324–372). Northvale, NJ: Lawrence Erlbaum.

Read, C. (1978). Children's awareness of sounds, with emphasis on sound systems. In A. Sinclair, R. J. Jarvella, & W. J. Levelt (Eds.), *The child's conception of language* (pp. 65–82). Berlin: Springer Verlag.

Reed, V. (2005). *An introduction to children with language disorders* (3rd ed.). Boston: Allyn & Bacon.

Renfrew, C. (1966). Persistence of the open syllable in defective articulation. *Journal of Speech and Hearing Disorders, 31*, 370–373.

Rescorla, L. (1989). The Language Development Survey: A screening tool for delayed language in toddlers. *Journal of Speech and Hearing Disorders, 54*, 587–599.

Rescorla, L., Mirak, J., & Singh, L. (2000). Vocabulary growth in late talkers: Lexical development from 2;0 to 3;0. *Journal of Child Language, 27*, 293–311.

Rescorla, L., & Ratner, N. B. (1996). Phonetic profiles in toddlers with specific expressive language impairment (SLI-E). *Journal of Speech and Hearing Research, 39*, 153–165.

Rescorla, L., & Schwartz, E. (1990). Outcome of toddlers with expressive language delay. *Applied Psycholinguistics, 11*, 393–407.

Reynolds, J. (1987). *The development of the vowel system in phonologically disordered children*. Unpublished doctoral dissertation, University of Sheffield, UK.

Reynolds, J. (1990). Abnormal vowel patterns in phonologically disordered children: Some data and a hypothesis. *British Journal of Disorders of Communication, 25*, 115–148.

Reynolds, J. (2002). Recurring patterns and idiosyncratic systems in some English children with vowel disorders. In H. Ball & F. Gibbon (Eds.), *Vowel disorders* (pp. 115–143). Boston: Butterworth Heinemann.

Rice, M. (1991). Children with specific language impairment: Towards a model of teachability. In N. Krasnegor (Ed.), *Biological and behavioral determinants of language development* (pp. 447–480). Hillsdale, NJ: Lawrence Erlbaum.

Rice, M. (1994). Grammatical categories of children with specific language impairments. In R. Watkins & M. Rice (Eds.), *Specific language impairment in children* (pp. 69–90). Baltimore: Brookes.

Rice, M., & Bode, J. (1993). Gaps in the verb lexicons of children with specific language impairment. *First Language, 13*, 113–131.

Rice, M., & Oetting, J. (1993). Morphological deficits of children with SLI: Evaluation of number marking and agreement. *Journal of Speech and Hearing Research, 36*, 1249–1257.

Rice, M., Wexler, K., & Cleave, P. (1995). Specific language impairment as a period of extended optional infinitive. *Journal of Speech and Hearing Research, 38*, 850–863.

Richardson, U., Leppaenen, P., Leiwo, M., & Lyytinen, H. (2003). Speech perception of infants with high familial risk for dyslexia differ at the age of 6 months. *Developmental Neuropsychology, 23*, 385–397.

Robb, M., Bleile, K., & Yee, S. (1999). A phonetic analysis of vowel errors during the course of treatment. *Clinical Linguistics & Phonetics, 13*, 309–321.

Robb, M. P., & Saxman, J. H. (1990). Syllable durations of preword and early word vocalizations. *Journal of Speech and Hearing Research, 33*, 583–593.

Roberts, A. (1965). *A statistical linguistic analysis of American English*. The Hague: Mouton.

Roberts, J. E., Burchinal, M., & Footo, M. (1990). Phonological process decline from 2½ to 8 years. *Journal of Communication Disorders, 23*, 205–217.

Roberts, T. (2005). Articulation accuracy and vocabulary size contributions to phonemic awareness and word reading in English language learners. *Journal of Educational Psychology, 97*, 601–616.

Robin, D., Bean, C., & Folkins, J. (1989). Lip movement in apraxia of speech. *Journal of Speech and Hearing Research, 32*, 512–523.

Robin, D. A., Hall, P. K., & Jordan, L. S. (1987). *Prosodic impairment in developmental verbal apraxia*. Paper presented at the annual meeting of the American Speech-Language-Hearing Association, New Orleans, LA.

Robin, D. A., Hall, P. K., Jordan, L. S., & Gordan, A. J. (1991). *Developmentally apraxic speakers' stress production: Perceptual and acoustic analyses*. Paper presented at the annual meeting of the American Speech-Language-Hearing Association, Atlanta, GA.

Roe, K. V. (1975). Amount of infant vocalization as a function of age: Some cognitive implications. *Child Development, 46*, 936–941.

Roe, K. V. (1977). *Relationship between infant vocalizations and preschool cognitive functioning*. Paper presented at the Annual Meeting of the Washington Psychological Association, Seattle, WA.

Rosenbek, J. C. (1985). Treating apraxia of speech. In D. F. Johns (Ed.), *Clinical management of neurogenic communicative disorders* (pp. 267–312). Boston: Little, Brown.

Rosenbek, J. C., & LaPointe, L. L. (1985). The dysarthrias: Description, diagnosis and treatment. In D. F. Johns (Ed.), *Clinical management of neurogenic communicative disorders* (pp. 97–152). Boston: Little, Brown.

Rosenbek, J. C., & Wertz, R. T. (1972). A review of fifty cases of developmental apraxia of speech. *Language, Speech, and Hearing Services in Schools, 5*, 23–33.

Rosenbek, J. C., & Wertz, R. T. (1976). Workshop on speech motor disorders, Veterans Administration Hospital, Madison, WI.

Rosetti, A. (1959). *Sur la théorie de la syllable*. Gravenhage: Mouton.

Rothgaenger, H. (2003). Analysis of the sounds of the child in the first year of age and a comparison to the language. *Early Human Development, 75*, 55–69.

Ruhlen, M. (1976). *Guide to the languages of the world*. San Diego, CA: Los Amigos Research Associates.

Rvachew, S., & Nowak, M. (2001). The effect of target-selection strategy on phonological learning. *Journal of Speech, Language, and Hearing Research, 44*, 610–623.

Rvachew, S., Rafaat, S., & Martin, M. (1999). Stimulability, speech perception skills, and the treatment of phonological disorders. *American Journal of Speech-Language Pathology, 8*, 33–43.

Saben, C., & Ingham, J. (1991). The effects of minimal pairs treatment on the speech-sound production of two children with phonologic disorders. *Journal of Speech and Hearing Research, 34*, 1023–1040.

Sagey, E. (1986). *The representation of features and relations in non-linear phonology*. Unpublished doctoral dissertation, MIT, Cambridge, MA.

Sander, E. K. (1972). When are speech sounds learned? *Journal of Speech and Hearing Disorders, 37*, 55–63.

Sapir, E. (1921). *Language: An introduction to the study of speech*. New York: Harcourt, Brace and World.

Sapir, E. (1925). Sound patterns in language. *Language, 1,* 37–51.

Scarborough, H., & Dobrich, W. (1990). Development of children with early language delay. *Journal of Speech and Hearing Research, 33,* 70–83.

Schmauch, V., Panagos, J., & Klich, R. (1978). Syntax influences the accuracy of consonant production in language-disordered children. *Journal of Communication Disorders, 11,* 315–323.

Schonweiler, R., Schonweiler, B., Schmelzeisen, R., & Ptok, M. (1995). The language and speech skills in 417 children with cleft formations. *Fortschritte in der Kieferorthopadie, 56,* 1–6.

Schwartz, A., & Goldman, R. (1974). Variables influencing performance on speech discrimination tests. *Journal of Speech and Hearing Research, 17,* 25–32.

Schwartz, R. (1992a). Clinical applications of recent advances in phonological theory. *Language, Speech, and Hearing Services in Schools, 23,* 269–276.

Schwartz, R. (1992b). Nonlinear phonology as a framework for phonological acquisition. In R. Chapman (Ed.), *Processes in language acquisition and disorders* (pp. 108–124). St. Louis, MO: Mosby Year Book.

Schwartz, R., & Leonard, L. B. (1982). Do children pick and choose? An examination of phonological selection and avoidance in early lexical acquisition. *Journal of Child Language, 9,* 319–336.

Schwartz, R., Leonard, L., Folger, M., & Wilcox, M. (1980). Evidence for a synergistic view of linguistic disorders: Early phonological behavior in normal and language disordered children. *Journal of Speech and Hearing Disorders, 45,* 357–377.

Scripture, E. W. (1902). *Elements of experimental phonetics.* New York: Charles Scribner's Sons.

Scripture, E. W. (1927). Die Silbigkeit und die Silbe. *Archives fur das Studium der neueren Sprachen, CLII,* 74.

Scripture, M., & Jackson, E. (1919). *A manual of exercises for the correction of speech disorders.* Philadelphia: Davis.

Secord, W. (1981a). *C-PAC: Clinical probes of articulation consistency.* Sedona, AZ: Red Rock Education.

Secord, W. (1981b). *Eliciting sounds: Techniques for clinicians.* San Antonio, TX: Psychological Corporation.

Secord, W. (1989). The traditional approach to treatment. In N. A. Creaghead, P. W. Newman, & W. A. Secord (Eds.), *Assessment and remediation of articulatory and phonological disorders* (2nd ed.) (pp. 129–158). New York: Macmillan.

Seymour, H., Green, L., & Hundley, R. (1991). *Phonological patterns in the conversational speech of African American children.* Paper presented at the national convention of the American Speech-Language-Hearing Association, Atlanta, GA.

Seymour, H., & Miller-Jones, D. (1981). Language and cognitive assessment of Black children. *Speech Language: Advances in Basic Research and Practice, 6,* 203–255.

Shane, H., & Wilbur, R. (1980). Potential for expressive signing based on motor control. *Sign Language Studies, 29,* 331–347.

Shankweiler, D., & Harris, K. (1966). An experimental approach to the problem of articulation in aphasia. *Cortex, 2,* 277–292.

Share, D., Jorm, A., Maclean, R., & Matthews, R. (1984). Sources of individual differences in reading acquisition. *Journal of Educational Psychology, 76,* 1309–1324.

Shelton, I. K., & Graves, M. M. (1985). Use of visual techniques in therapy for developmental apraxia of speech. *Language, Speech, and Hearing Services in Schools, 16,* 129–131.

Shelton, R. (1993). Grand rounds for sound system disorder. Conclusion: What was learned. *Seminars in Speech and Language, 14,* 166–178.

Sherman, D., & Geith, A. (1967). Speech sound discrimination and articulation skill. *Journal of Speech and Hearing Disorders, 10,* 277–280.

Shibamoto, J., & Olmsted, D. (1978). Lexical and syllabic patterns in phonological acquistion. *Journal of Child Language, 5,* 417–456.

Shipley, K. G. (1997). *Interviewing and counseling in communicative disorders: Principles and procedures.* (2nd ed.). Boston: Allyn & Bacon.

Shipley, K. G., & McAfee, J. G. (1998). *Assessment in speech-language pathology: A resource manual* (2nd ed.). San Diego, CA: Singular Thomson Learning.

Shprintzen, R. J. (1995). *Cleft palate speech management. A multidisciplinary approach.* St. Louis, MO: Mosby Year Book.

Shprintzen, R. J., & Bardach, J. (Ed.). (1995). *Cleft palate speech management: A multidisciplinary approach.* St. Louis, MO: Mosby.

Shprintzen, R. J., Siegel-Sadewitz, V. L., Amato, J., & Goldberg, R. B. (1985). Anomalies associated with cleft lip, cleft palate, or both. *American Journal of Medical Genetics, 20,* 585–595.

Shriberg, L. D. (1975). A response evocation program for /ɝ/. *Journal of Speech and Hearing Disorders, 40,* 92–105.

Shriberg, L. D. (1980). An intervention procedure for children with persistent /r/ errors. *Language, Speech, and Hearing Services in Schools, 11,* 102–110.

Shriberg, L. D. (1991). Directions for research in developmental phonological disorders. In J. F. Miller (Ed.), *Research on child language disorders: A decade of progress* (pp. 267–276). Austin, TX: PRO-ED.

Shriberg, L. D., Aram, D. M., & Kwiatkowski, J. (1997a). Developmental apraxia of speech: I. Descriptive and theoretical perspectives. *Journal of Speech, Language, and Hearing Research, 40,* 273–285.

Shriberg, L. D., Aram, D. M., & Kwiatkowski, J. (1997b). Developmental apraxia of speech: II. Toward a diagnostic marker. *Journal of Speech, Language, and Hearing Research, 40,* 286–312.

Shriberg, L. D., Aram, D. M., & Kwiatkowski, J. (1997c). Developmental apraxia of speech: III. A subtype marked by inappropriate stress. *Journal of Speech, Language, and Hearing Research, 40,* 313–337.

Shriberg, L. D., Austin, D., Lewis, B., McSweeny, J. L., & Wilson, D. L. (1997). The percentage of consonants correct (PCC) metric: Extensions and reliability data. *Journal of Speech, Language, and Hearing Research, 40,* 708–722.

Shriberg, L. D., & Kent, R. D. (2003). *Clinical phonetics* (3rd ed.). Boston: Allyn & Bacon.

Shriberg, L. D., & Kwiatkowski, J. (1980). *Natural process analysis (NPA): A procedure for phonological analysis of continuous speech samples.* New York: John Wiley.

Shriberg, L. D., & Kwiatkowski, J. (1982a). Phonological disorders II: A conceptual framework for management. *Journal of Speech and Hearing Disorders, 47,* 242–256.

Shriberg, L. D., & Kwiatkowski, J. (1982b). Phonological disorders III: A procedure for assessing severity of involvement. *Journal of Speech and Hearing Disorders, 47,* 256–270.

Shriberg, L. D., & Kwiatkowski, J. (1983). Computer-assisted natural process analysis (NPA): Recent issues and data. *Seminars in Speech and Language, 4,* 389–406.

Shriberg, L. D., & Kwiatkowski, J. (1985). Continuous speech sampling for phonologic analyses of speech-delayed children. *Journal of Speech and Hearing Disorders, 50,* 323–334.

Shriberg, L. D., & Kwiatkowski, J. (1994). Developmental phonological disorders I: A clinical profile. *Journal of Speech and Hearing Research, 37,* 1100–1126.

Shriberg, L. D., Kwiatkowski, J., Best, S., Hengst, J., & Terselic-Weber, B. (1986). Characteristics of children with phonologic disorders of unknown origin. *Journal of Speech and Hearing Disorders, 51,* 140–161.

Shriberg, L. D., Kwiatkowski, J., & Rasmussen, C. (1990). *The prosody-voice screening profile.* Tucson, AZ: Communication Builders.

Shriberg, L. D., & Lof, G. L. (1991). Reliability studies in broad and narrow transcription. *Clinical Linguistics and Phonetics, 5,* 225–179.

Shriberg, L. D., Tomblin, J., & McSweeny, J. (1999). Prevalence of speech delay in 6-year-old children and comorbidity with language impairment. *Journal of Speech, Language, and Hearing Research, 42,* 1461–1481.

Shriberg, L. D., & Widder, C. J. (1990). Speech and prosody characteristics of adults with mental retardation. *Journal of Speech and Hearing Research, 33,* 627–653.

Shriner, T., Holloway, M., & Daniloff, R. (1969). The relationship between articulatory deficits and syntax in speech defective children. *Journal of Speech and Hearing Research, 12,* 319–325.

Shvachkin, N. K. (1973). The development of phonemic speech perception in early childhood. In C. A. Ferguson & D. I. Slobin (Eds.), *Studies of child language development* (pp. 91–127). New York: Holt, Rinehart and Winston.

Sievers, E. (1901). *Grundzüge der Phonetik: Zur Einführung in das Studium der indogermanischen Sprachen.* Leipzig: Breitkopf und Hartel.

Silverman, F. (1980). *Communication for the speechless.* Englewood Cliffs, NJ: Prentice-Hall.

Simon, C., & Fourcin, A. J. (1978). Cross language study of speech pattern learning. *Journal of the Acoustical Society of America, 63,* 925–935.

Singh, S. (1968). *Perceptual correlates of distinctive feature systems.* Washington, DC: Howard University Press.

Singh, S. (1976). *Distinctive features: Principles and practices.* Baltimore: University Park Press.

Singh, S., & Black, J. (1966). Study of twenty-six intervocalic consonants as spoken and recognized by four language groups. *Journal of the Acoustical Society of America, 39,* 372–387.

Singh, S., & Polen, S. (1972). Use of distinctive feature model in speech pathology. *Acta Symbolica, 3,* 17–25.

Sloat, C., Taylor, S., & Hoard, J. (1978). *Introduction to phonology.* Englewood Cliffs, NJ: Prentice-Hall.

Small, L. (2005). *Fundamentals of phonetics: A practical guide for students* (2nd ed.). Boston: Allyn & Bacon.

Smit, A. (1986). Ages of speech sound acquisition: Comparisons and critiques of several normative studies. *Language, Speech, and Hearing Services in Schools, 17,* 175–186.

Smit, A. B. (1993a). Phonologic error distributions in the Iowa-Nebraska Articulation Norms Project: Word-initial consonant clusters. *Journal of Speech and Hearing Research, 36,* 931–947.

Smit, A. B. (1993b). Phonologic error distributions in the Iowa-Nebraska Articulation Norms Project: Consonant singletons. *Journal of Speech and Hearing Research, 36,* 533–547.

Smit, A. B., & Bernthal, J. E. (1983). Voicing contrasts and their phonological implications in the speech of articulation-disordered children. *Journal of Speech and Hearing Research, 26,* 486–500.

Smit, A. B., Hand, L., Freilinger, J., Bernthal, J., & Bird, A. (1990). The Iowa Articulation Norms Project and its Nebraska replication. *Journal of Speech and Hearing Disorders, 55,* 779–798.

Smith, B., Marquardt, T. P., Cannito, M. P., & Davis, B. L. (1994). Vowel variability in developmental apraxia of speech. In J. A. Till, K. M. Yorkston, & D. R. Beukelman (Eds.), *Motor speech disorders* (pp. 81–89). Baltimore: Paul H. Brookes.

Smith, B. L. (1979). A phonetic analysis of consonant devoicing in children's speech. *Journal of Child Language, 6,* 19–28.

Smith, B. L., Brown-Sweeney, S., & Stoel-Gammon, C. (1989). A quantitative analysis of reduplicated and variegated babbling. *First Language, 9,* 175–189.

Smith, C. R. (1975). Residual hearing and speech production in deaf children. *Journal of Speech and Hearing Research, 18,* 795–811.

Smith, N. V. (1973). *The acquisition of phonology: A case study.* Cambridge: Cambridge University Press.

Smith, S., Simmons, D., & Kameenui, E. (1995). Synthesis of research on phonological awareness: Principles and implications for reading acquisition. *Technical Report No. 12.* Eugene, OR: National Center to Improve the Tools of Educators.

Snow, C., Burns, S., & Griffin, P. (1998). *Preventing reading difficulties in young children.* National Academy of Sciences—National Research Council. Washington, DC: Commission on Behavioral and Social Sciences and Education (BBB21833).

Snow, D. (2000). The emotional basis of linguistic and nonlinguistic intonation: Implications for hemispheric specialization. *Developmental Neuropsychology, 17,* 1–27.

Snow, D. (1998a). Children's imitations of intonation contours: Are rising tones more difficult than falling tones? *Journal of Speech, Language and Hearing Research, 41,* 576–587.

Snow, D. (1998b). A prominence account of syllable reduction in early speech development: The child's prosodic phonology of tiger and giraffe. *Journal of Speech, Language, and Hearing Research, 41,* 1171–1184.

Snowling, M., Bishop, D., & Stothard, S. (2000). Is preschool language impairment a risk factor for dyslexia? *Journal of Child Psychology and Psychiatry, 41,* 587–600.

Snowling, M., Goulandris, N., & Stackhouse, J. (1994). Phonological constraints on learning to read: Evidence from single case studies of reading difficulty. In C. Hulme & M. Snowling (Eds.), *Reading development and dyslexia* (pp. 86–104). London: Whurr.

So, L., & Dodd, B. (1994). Phonologically disordered Cantonese-speaking children. *Clinical Linguistics and Phonetics, 8,* 235–255.

Sommers, R. (1969). *Factors in the effectiveness of articulation with educable retarded children.* Final report of project 7–0432. Washington, DC: U.S. Department of Health, Education and Welfare.

Sommers, R., Patterson, J., & Wildgen, P. (1988). Phonology of Down syndrome speakers, ages 13–22. *Journal of Childhood Communication Disorders, 12,* 65–91.

Sonderman, J. (1971). *An experimental study of clinical relationships between auditory discrimination and articula-tion skills.* Paper presented at the national convention of the American Speech-Language-Hearing Association, San Francisco.

Sparks, R. W., Helm, N., & Albert, M. (1974). Aphasia rehabilitation resulting from Melodic Intonation Therapy. *Cortex, 10,* 303–316.

Square, P. A. (1999). Treatment of developmental apraxia of speech: Tactile-kinesthetic, rhythmic, and gestural approaches. In A. J. Caruso & E. A. Strand (Eds.), *Clinical management of motor speech disorders in children* (pp. 149–186). New York: Thieme.

Stackhouse, J. (1982). An investigation of reading and spelling performance in speech disordered children. *British Journal of Disorders of Communication, 17,* 53–60.

Stackhouse, J. (1985). Segmentation, speech and spelling difficulties. In M. Snowling (Ed.), *Children's written language difficulties: Assessment and management* (pp. 96–115). Windsor, UK: NFER Nelson.

Stackhouse, J. (1993). Phonological disorder and lexical development: Two case studies. *Child Language Teaching and Therapy, 9,* 230–241.

Stackhouse, J. (1997). Phonological awareness: Connecting speech and literacy problems. In B. W. Hodson & M. L. Edwards (Eds.), *Perspectives in applied phonology* (pp. 157–196). Gaithersburg, MD: Aspen.

Stackhouse, J., & Snowling, M. (1983). Segmentation and spelling in children with speech disorders. In M. Edwards (Ed.), *Proceedings of XIX congress of the international association of logopedics and phoniatrics* (pp. 282–287). London: College of Speech Therapists.

Stackhouse, J., & Snowling, M. (1996). Speech, spelling and reading: Who is at risk and why? In M. Snowling & J. Stackhouse (Eds.), *Dyslexia, speech and language: A practitioner's handbook* (pp. 12–30). San Diego, CA: Singular.

Stampe, D. (1969). The acquisition of phonetic representation. *Proceedings of the Fifth Regional Meeting of the Chicago Linguistic Circle,* 443–454.

Stampe, D. (1972). On the natural history of diphthongs. *Chicago Linguistic Society* (8th Regional Meeting), 578–590.

Stampe, D. (1973). *A dissertation on natural phonology.* Unpublished doctoral dissertation, University of Chicago.

Stampe, D. (1979). *A dissertation on natural phonology.* New York: Garland.

Stanovich, K. (2000). *Progress in understanding reading: Scientific foundations and new frontiers.* New York: Guilford.

Stark, R. (1980). Stages of speech development in the first year of life. In G. Yeni-Komshian, J. Kavanagh, & C. A. Ferguson (Eds.), *Child phonology: Vol. I. Production* (pp. 73–92). New York: Academic Press.

Stark, R. (1986). Prespeech segmental feature development. In P. Fletcher & M. Garman (Eds.), *Language acquisition. Studies in first language development* (pp. 149–173). Cambridge: Cambridge University Press.

Starr, C. D. (1993). Behavioral approaches to treating velopharyngeal closure and nasality. In K. T. Moller & C. D. Starr (Eds.), *Cleft palate: Interdisciplinary issues and treatment* (pp. 337–356). Austin, TX: PRO-ED.

Stathopoulos, E. T., & Sapienza, C. (1993). Respiratory and laryngeal measures of children during vocal intensity variation. *Journal of the Acoustical Society of America, 94,* 2531–2543.

Stemberger, J. P., & Bernhardt, B. (1997). Optimality theory. In M. Ball & R. Kent (Eds.), *The new phonologies* (pp. 211–245). San Diego, CA: Singular.

Stern, D., & Wasserman, G. (1979). *Maternal language to infants.* Paper presented at a meeting of the Society for Research in Child Development.

Stern, H. (1927). Zur Pathogenese des Sigmatismus nasalis. *Zeitschrift fur Hals-, Nasen-, Ohrenheilkunde, 18,* 585ff.

Stetson, R. H. (1936). The relation of the phoneme and the syllable. *Proceedings of the Second International Congress of Phonetic Sciences,* 245–254.

Stetson, R. H. (1951). *Motor phonetics: A study of speech movements in action.* Amsterdam: North-Holland.

Stockman, I. (1996). Phonological development and disorders in African American children. In A. Kamhi, K. Pollock, & J. Harris (Eds.), *Communication development and disorders in African American children: Research, assessment, and intervention* (pp. 117–154). Baltimore: P. H. Brookes.

Stockman, I. (1996). The promises and pitfalls of language sample analysis as an assessment tool for linguistic minority children. *Language, Speech, and Hearing Services in Schools, 27,* 355–366.

Stockman, I. J., Woods, D. R., & Tishman, A. (1981). Listener agreement on phonetic segments in early infant vocalizations. *Journal of Psycholinguistic Research, 10,* 593–617.

Stoel-Gammon, C. (1985). Phonetic inventories, 15–24 months: A longitudinal study. *Journal of Speech and Hearing Research, 28,* 505–512.

Stoel-Gammon, C. (1987). Phonological skills of two-year-olds. *Language, Speech, and Hearing Services in Schools, 18,* 323–329.

Stoel-Gammon, C. (1989). Prespeech and early speech development of two late talkers. *First Language, 9,* 207–223.

Stoel-Gammon, C. (1998). Phonological development in Down syndrome. *Mental Retardation and Developmental Disabilities Research Reviews, 3,* 300–306.

Stoel-Gammon, C., & Cooper, J. A. (1984). Patterns of early lexical and phonological development. *Journal of Child Language, 11,* 247–271.

Stoel-Gammon, C., & Dunn, C. (1985). *Normal and disordered phonology in children.* Baltimore: University Park Press.

Stoel-Gammon, C., & Herrington, P. (1990). Vowel systems of normally developing and phonologically disordered children. *Clinical Linguistics and Phonetics, 4,* 145–160.

Stoel-Gammon, C., & Menn, L. (1997). Phonological development: Learning sounds and sound patterns. In J. Berko Gleason (Ed.), *The development of language* (4th ed.) (pp. 69–121). Boston: Allyn & Bacon.

Stoel-Gammon, C., & Otomo, K. (1986). Babbling development of hearing-impaired and normally hearing subjects. *Journal of Speech and Hearing Disorders, 51,* 33–41.

Storkel, H. (2001). Learning new words: Phonotactic probability in language development. *Journal of Speech, Language, and Hearing Research, 44,* 1321–1337.

Storkel, H. (2003). Learning new words II: Phonotactic probability in verb learning. *Journal of Speech, Language, and Hearing Research, 46,* 1312–1323.

Storkel, H. (2004). The emerging lexicon of children with phonological delays: Phonotactic constraints and probability in acquisition. *Journal of Speech, Language, and Hearing Research, 47,* 1194–1212.

Storkel, H. L., & Morrisette, M. L. (2002). The lexicon and phonology: Interactions in language acquisition. *Language, Speech, and Hearing Services in Schools, 33,* 24–37.

Storkel, H. L., & Rogers, M. A. (2000). The effect of probabilistic phonotactics on lexical acquisition. *Clinical Linguistics and Phonetics, 14,* 407–425.

Strand, E. A., & Skinder, A. (1999). Treatment of developmental apraxia of speech: Integral stimulation methods. In. A. J. Caruso & E. A. Strand (Eds.), *Clinical management of motor speech disorders in children* (pp. 109–148). New York: Thieme.

Subtelny, J. D. (1980). *Speech assessment and speech improvement for the hearing impaired.* Washington, DC: Alexander Graham Bell Association for the Deaf.

Swank, L. (1997). Linguistic influences on the emergence of written word decoding in first grade. *American Journal of Speech-Language Pathology, 6,* 62–66.

Sweet, H. (1877). *A handbook of phonetics.* Oxford: Clarendon Press.

Sweet, H. (1890). *Primer of phonetics.* Oxford: Oxford University Press.

Swift, E., & Rosin, P. (1990). A remediation sequence to improve speech intelligibility for students with Down syndrome. *Language, Speech, and Hearing Services in Schools, 21,* 140–146.

Tallal, P., Stark., R. E., Kallman, C., & Mellits, D. (1980). Perceptual constancy for phonemic categories: A developmental study with normal and language-impaired children. *Applied Psycholinguistics, 1,* 49–64.

Tarjan, G., Wright, S. W., Eyman, R. K., & Keeran, D. V. (1973). Natural history of mental retardation: Some aspects of epidemiology. *American Journal of Mental Deficiency, 77,* 369–379.

Tatham, M., & Morton, K. (1997). Recording and displaying speech. In M. J. Ball & C. Code (Eds.), *Instrumental clinical phonetics* (pp. 1–21). San Diego, CA: Singular.

Templin, M. (1957). *Certain language skills in children: Their development and interrelationships.* Institute of Child Welfare, Monograph 26. Minneapolis, MN: University of Minnesota Press.

Terrell, S., & Terrell, F. (1993). African American cultures. In D. Battle (Ed.), *Communication disorders in multicultural populations* (pp. 3–37). Boston: Andover Medical Publishers.

Thiele, G. (1980). *Handlexikon der Medizin.* Munchen: Urban & Schwarzenberg.

Thompson, L. C. (1965). *A Vietnamese grammar.* Seattle: University of Washington Press.

Thurlbeck, W. (1982). Postnatal human lung growth, *Thorax, 37,* 465–571.

Tillmann, H. G. (1964). *Das phonetische Silbenproblem.* Unpublished doctoral dissertation, University of Bonn, Germany.

Toombs, M. S., Singh, S., & Hayden, M. E. (1981). Markedness of features in the articulatory substitutions of children. *Journal of Speech and Hearing Disorders, 46,* 184–191.

Toppelberg, C., Shapiro, M., & Theodore, M. (2000). Language disorders: A 10-year research update review. *Journal of the American Academy of Child and Adolescent Psychiatry, 39,* 143–152.

Torgesen, J. (2000). Individual differences in response to early interventions in reading: The lingering problem of treatment resisters. *Learning Disabilities Research and Practice, 15,* 55–64.

Torgesen, J., Wagner, R., & Rashotte, C. (1994). Longitudinal studies of phonological processing and reading. *Journal of Learning Disabilities, 27,* 276–286.

Torgesen, J., Wagner, R., Rashotte, C., Burgess, S., & Hecht, S. (1997). Contributions of phonological awareness and rapid automatic naming ability to the growth of word-reading skills in second- to fifth-grade children. *Scientific Studies of Reading, 1,* 161–185.

Torgesen, J., Wagner, R., Simmons, K., & Laughon, P. (1990). Identifying phonological coding problems in disabled readers: Naming counting, or span measures? *Learning Disability Quarterly, 13,* 236–243.

Torneus, M. (1984). Phonological awareness and reading: A chicken and egg problem? *Journal of Educational Psychology, 76,* 1346–1358.

Travis, L., & Rasmus, B. (1931). The speech sound discrimination ability of cases with functional disorders of articulation. *Quarterly Journal of Speech, 17,* 217–226.

Trehub, S. E. (1976). The discrimination of foreign speech contrasts by infants and adults. *Child Development, 47,* 466–472.

Trost, J. E. (1981). Articulatory additions to the classical description of the speech of persons with cleft palate. *Cleft Palate Journal, 18,* 193–203.

Trost-Cardamone, J. E. (1990a). The development of speech: Assessing cleft palate misarticulations. In D. A. Kernahan & S. W. Rosenstein (Eds.), *Cleft lip and palate: A system of managment* (pp. 227–235). Baltimore: Williams & Wilkins.

Trost-Cardamone, J. E. (1990b). Speech: Anatomy, physiology, and pathology. In D. A. Kernahan & S. W. Rosenstein (Eds.), *Cleft lip and palate: A system of management* (pp. 91–103). Baltimore: Williams & Wilkins.

Trost-Cardamone, J. E., & Bernthal, J. E. (1993). Articulation assessment procedures and treatment decisions. In K. T. Moller & C. D. Starr (Eds.), *Cleft palate. Interdisciplinary issues and treatment* (p. 307 ff.). Austin, TX: PRO-ED.

Trubetzkoy, N. S. (1931). Gedanken über Morphophonologie. *Travaux du Cercle Linguistique de Prague, 4,* 160 ff.

Trubetzkoy, N. S. (1939). *Grundzüge der Phonologie.* Prague: TCLP, 4.

Trubetzkoy, N. S. (1969). *Principles of phonology.* Berkeley: University of California Press. (Original work published 1939)

Tsao, F.-M., Liu, H.-M., & Kuhl, P. (2004). Speech perception in infancy predicts language development in the 2nd year of life: A longitudinal study. *Child Development, 75,* 1067–1084.

Turk, A., Jusczyk, P., & Gerken, L. (1995). Do English-learning infants use syllable weight to determine stress? *Language and Speech, 38,* 143–158.

Tyler, A., & Langsdale, T. (1996). Consonant–vowel interactions in early phonological development. *First Language, 16,* 159–191.

Tyler, A., & Tolbert, L. (2002). Speech-language assessment in the clinical setting. *American Journal of Speech-Language Pathology, 11,* 215–220.

Tyler, A., & Watterson, K. (1991). Effects of phonological versus language intervention in preschoolers with both phonological and language impairment. *Child Language Teaching and Therapy, 7,* 141–160.

United States Bureau of the Census. (1990). *Statistical abstract of the United States: 1990. The national data book* (110th ed.). Washington, DC: U.S. Department of Commerce.

United States Census Bureau. (2000). United States Department of Commerce. Washington, D.C.

Van Demark, D. R., & Hardin, M. A. (1990). Speech therapy for the child with cleft lip and palate. In J. Bardach & H. L. Morris (Eds.), *Multidisciplinary man-*

agement of cleft lip and palate. Philadelphia: W. B. Saunders.

Van Keulen, J. E., Weddington, G. T., & DeBose, C. E. (1998). *Speech, language, learning, and the African American child.* Boston: Allyn & Bacon.

Van Riper, C. (1939a). Ear training in the treatment of articulation disorders. *Journal of Speech Disorders, IV,* 141–142.

Van Riper, C. (1939b). *Speech correction: Principles and methods.* Englewood Cliffs, NJ: Prentice-Hall.

Van Riper, C. (1963). *Speech correction: Principles and methods* (4th ed.). Englewood Cliffs, NJ: Prentice-Hall.

Van Riper, C. (1978). *Speech correction: Principles and methods* (6th ed.). Englewood Cliffs, NJ: Prentice-Hall.

Van Riper, C., & Emerick, L. (1984). *Speech correction: An introduction to speech pathology and audiology* (7th ed.). Englewood Cliffs, NJ: Prentice-Hall.

Van Riper, C., & Irwin, J. (1958). *Voice and articulation.* Englewood Cliffs, NJ: Prentice-Hall.

Velleman, S. (2003). *Childhood apraxia of speech resource guide.* Cliften Park, NY: Thomson Delmar Learning.

Velleman, S., & Shriberg, L. (1999). Metrical analysis of the speech of children with suspected developmental apraxia of speech. *Journal of Speech, Language, and Hearing Research, 42,* 1158–1170.

Velleman, S. L., & Strand, K. (1994). Developmental verbal dyspraxia. In J. E. Bernthal & N. W. Bankson (Eds.), *Child phonology: Characteristics, assessment, and intervention with special populations* (pp. 110–139). New York: Thieme.

Velleman, S., & Strand, K. (1998). *Dynamic remediation strategies for children with developmental verbal dyspraxia.* Videoteleconference available from the American Speech-Language-Hearing Association.

Velleman, S., & Vihman, M. (2002). Whole-word phonology and templates: Trap, bootstrap, or some of each? *Language, Speech, and Hearing Services in Schools, 33,* 9–23.

Velten, H. (1943). The growth of phonemic and lexical patterns in infant language. *Language, 19,* 281–292.

Vihman, M. M. (1984). *Individual differences in phonological development: Age one and age three.* Unpublished manuscript.

Vihman, M. M. (1992). Early syllables and the construction of phonology. In C. A. Ferguson, L. Menn, & C. Stoel-Gammon (Eds.), *Phonological development: Models, research, implications* (pp. 393–422). Timonium, MD: York Press.

Vihman, M. M. (2004). Early phonological development. In J. E. Bernthal & N. W. Bankson (Eds.), *Articulation and phonological disorders* (5th ed.) (pp. 63–112). Boston: Allyn & Bacon.

Vihman, M. M., Ferguson, C. A., & Elbert, M. (1986). Phonological development from babbling to speech: Common tendencies and individual differences. *Applied Psycholinguistics, 7,* 3–40.

Vihman, M. M., & Greenlee, M. (1987). Individual differences in phonological development: Ages one through three years. *Journal of Speech and Hearing Research, 30,* 503–521.

Vihman, M. M., Macken, M. A., Miller, R., Simmons, H., & Miller, J. (1985). From babbling to speech: A reassessment of the continuity issue. *Language, 61,* 397–445.

Voiers, W. D. (1967). *Performance evaluation of speech processing devices: Vol. 3. Diagnostic evaluation of speech intelligibility.* Bedford, MA: Air Force Research Laboratories.

Von Bremen, V. (1990). *A nonlinear phonological approach to intervention with severely phonologically disordered twins.* Unpublished master's thesis, University of British Columbia.

von Essen, O. (1979). *Allgemeine und angewandte Phonetik* (5th ed.). Berlin: Akademie-Verlag.

Waengler, H.-H. (1981). *Atlas deutscher Sprachlaute* (7th ed.). Berlin: Akademie-Verlag.

Waengler, H.-H. (1983). *Grundriss einer Phonetik des Deutschen* (4th ed.). Marburg: Elwert Verlag.

Waengler, H.-H., & Bauman-Waengler, J. A. (1980). Lautdauerverhältnisse im Sprechen von Patienten mit zentral-nervalen Störungen. In W. Kühlwein & A. Rasch (Eds.), *Sprache und Verstehen, Bd. II. Kongressberichte der 10. Jahrestagung der Gesellschaft für Angewandte Linguistik* (p. 134ff). Tübingen: Gunter Narr Verlag.

Waengler, H.-H., & Bauman-Waengler, J. A. (1984). *Phonetische Logopädie, Lieferung 2: S-Lautbildungen und ihre Störungen.* Berlin: Marhold Verlag.

Waengler, H.-H., & Bauman-Waengler, J. A. (1985). *Phonetische Logopädie, Lieferung 4.* Berlin: Marhold Verlag.

Waengler, H.-H., & Bauman-Waengler, J. A. (1987a). *Phonetische Logopädie. Die Behandlung von Kommunikationstörungen auf phonetischer Grundlage. 2.4 Dysarthrien* (p. 562ff). Berlin: Marhold Verlag.

Waengler, H.-H., & Bauman-Waengler, J. A. (1987b). *Phonetische Logopädie. Die Behandlung von Kommunikationstörungen auf phonetischer Grundlage. 2.3.8. LKG-Spalten* (pp. 503ff). Berlin: Marhold Verlag.

Waengler, H.-H., & Bauman-Waengler, J. A. (1989). *Phonological development of normal and speech/language disordered 4-year-olds.* Paper presented at the national convention of the American Speech-Language-Hearing Association, St. Louis.

Wagner, R., & Torgesen, J. (1987). The nature of phonological processing and its causal role in the acquisition of reading skills. *Psychological Bulletin, 101,* 192–212.

Walsh, H. (1974). On certain practical inadequacies of distinctive feature systems. *Journal of Speech and Hearing Disorders, 39,* 32–43.

Wambaugh, J., Martinez, A., McNeil, M., & Rogers, M. (1999). Sound production treatment for apraxia of speech: Overgeneralization and maintenance effects. *Aphasiology, 13,* 821–837.

Wang, W. (1990). Theoretical issues in studying Chinese dialects. *Journal of the Chinese Language Teachers Association, 25,* 1–34.

Ward, I. (1923). *Defects of speech.* New York: E. P. Dutton.

Warren, S. (1979). PERCI: A method for rating palatal efficiency. *Cleft Palate Journal, 16,* 279–285.

Washington, J. (1998). *African American English research: A review and future directions.* Retrieved from www.rcgd.isr.umich.edu/prba/perspectives/spring1998/jwashington.pdf, May 2006.

Washington, J. A., & Craig, H. K. (1994). Dialectal forms during discourse of poor, urban, African American preschoolers. *Journal of Speech and Hearing Research, 37,* 816–823.

Watkins, R., Rice, M., & Moltz, C. (1993). Verb use by language-impaired and normally developing children. *First Language, 13,* 133–143.

Webb, J. C., & Duckett, B. (1990). *The RULES phonological evaluation.* Vero Beach, FL: The Speech Bin.

Webster, P. E., & Plante, A. S. (1992). Effects of phonological impairment on word, syllable, and phoneme segmentation and reading. *Language, Speech, and Hearing Services in Schools, 23,* 176–182.

Webster, P. E., Plante, A. S., & Couvillion, L. (1997). Phonologic impairment and prereading: Update on a longitudinal study. *Journal of Learning Disabilities, 30,* 365–375.

Webster, R., Majnemer, A., Platt, R., & Shevell, M. (2005). Motorfunction at school age in children with a preschool diagnosis of developmental language impairment. *Journal of Pediatrics, 146,* 80–85.

Weiner, F. (1979). *Phonological process analysis.* Baltimore: University Park Press.

Weiner, F. (1981). Treatment of phonological disability using the method of meaningful minimal contrast: Two case studies. *Journal of Speech and Hearing Disorders, 46,* 97–103.

Weiner, F., & Bankson, N. (1978). Teaching features. *Language, Speech, and Hearing Services in Schools, 9,* 29–34.

Weiner, F., & Ostrowski, A. (1979). Effects of listener uncertainty on articulatory inconsistency. *Journal of Speech and Hearing Disorders, 44,* 487–493.

Weiner, P. (1967). Auditory discrimination and articulation. *Journal of Speech and Hearing Disorders, 32,* 19–28.

Weinert, H. (1974). *Die Bekämpfung von Sprechfehlern.* Berlin: VEB Verlag Volk und Gesundheit.

Weismer, G. (1984). Acoustic analysis strategies for the refinement of phonological analysis. In M. Elbert, D. Dinnsen, & G. Weismer (Eds.), *Phonological theory and the misarticulating child. ASHA Monographs, 22,* 30–52. Rockville, MD: ASHA.

Weismer, G., Dinnsen, D., & Elbert, M. (1981). A study of the voicing distinction associated with omitted, word-final stops. *Journal of Speech and Hearing Disorders, 46,* 320–328.

Weiss, C. (1980). *Weiss comprehensive articulation test.* Allen, TX: DLM Teaching Resources.

Weiss, C. E. (1982). *Weiss intelligibility test.* Tigard, OR: C. C. Publicatons.

Weiss, C. E., Gordon, M. E., & Lillywhite, H. S. (1987). *Clinical management of articulatory and phonologic disorders* (2nd ed.). Boston: Williams & Wilkins.

Weiss, C. E., & Lillywhite, H. E. (1981). *Communication disorders* (2nd ed.). St. Louis, MO: C. V. Mosby.

Wellman, B. L., Case, I. M., Mengert, I. G., & Bradbury, D. E. (1931). Speech sounds of young children. *University of Iowa Studies in Child Welfare, 5.* Iowa City, IA: University of Iowa Press.

Wells, B., Peppé, S., & Goulandris, N. (2004). Intonation development from five to thirteen. *Journal of Child Language, 31,* 749–778.

Wells, B., Stackhouse, J., & Vance, M. (1996). A specific deficit in onset-rhyme assembly in a 9-year-old child with speech and literacy difficulties. In T. W. Powell (Ed.), *Pathologies of speech and language: Contributions of clinical phonetics and linguistics.* New Orleans, LA: International Clinical Phonetics and Linguistics Association.

Wepman, J. (1973). *Wepman auditory discrimination test.* Chicago: Language Research Association.

Werker, J., & Fennell, C. (2004). Listening to sounds versus listening to words: Early steps in word learning. In D. Hall & S. Waxman (Eds.), *Weaving a Lexicon* (pp. 79–110). Cambridge, MA: MIT Press.

Werker, J., & Tees, R. (2005). Speech perception as a window for understanding plasticity and commitment in language systems of the brain. *Developmental Psychobiology, 46,* 233–251.

Werker, J. F., & Tees, R. C. (1983). Developmental changes across childhood in the perception of non-native speech sounds. *Canadian Journal of Psychology, 37,* 278–286.

Wertz, R. T. (1985). Neuropathologies of speech and language. In D. F. Johns (Ed.), *Clinical management of neurogenic communicative disorders* (pp. 1–96). Boston: Little, Brown.

Wertz, R. T., LaPointe, L. L., & Rosenbek, J. C. (1984). *Apraxia of speech in adults: The disorder and its management.* Orlando, FL: Grune and Stratton.

Wesseling, R., & Reitsma, P. (2000). The transcient role of explicit phonological recoding for reading acquisition. *Journal of Reading and Writing, 13,* 313–336.

West, R., & Ansberry, M. (1968). *The rehabilitation of speech* (4th ed.). New York: Harper & Row.

West, R., Kennedy, L., & Carr, A. (1937). *The rehabilitation of speech*. New York: Harpers.

Westlake, H., & Rutherford, D. (1961). *Speech therapy for the cerebral palsied*. Chicago: National Society for Crippled Children and Adults.

Whalen, D. H., Levitt, A. G., & Wang, Q. (1991). Intonational differences between reduplicative babbling of French- and English-learning infants. *Journal of Child Language, 18,* 501–516.

Whitehill, T., Francis, A., & Ching, C. (2003). Perception of place of articulation by children with cleft palate and posterior placement. *Journal of Speech, Language, and Hearing Research, 46,* 451–461.

Whitehurst, G., Fischel, J., Lonigan, C., Valdez-Menchaca, M., Arnold, D., & Smith, M. (1991). Treatment of early expressive language delay: If, when, and how. *Topics in Language Disorders, 11,* 55–68.

Whitehurst, G., Smith, M., Fischel, J., Arnold, D., & Lonigan, C. (1991). The continuity of babble and speech in children with specific expressive language delay. *Journal of Speech and Hearing Research, 34,* 1121–1129.

Wickelgren, W. (1966). Distinctive features and errors in short-term memory for English consonants. *Journal of the Acoustic Society of America, 39,* 388–398.

Wilcox, K. A., Schooling, T. L., & Morris, S. R. (1991). *The preschool intelligibility measure (P-SIM)*. Paper presented at the annual convention of the American Speech-Language-Hearing Association, Atlanta, GA.

Wilkins, J. (1668). *An essay towards a real character and a philosophical language*. London: S. Gellibrand.

Williams, A. L. (1992). *Multiple oppositions: An alternative contrastive therapy approach*. Paper presented at the annual convention of the American Speech-Language-Hearing Association, San Antonio, TX.

Williams, A. L. (2000a). Multiple oppositions: Theoretical foundations for an alternative contrastive intervention approach. *American Journal of Speech-Language Pathology, 9,* 282–288.

Williams, A. L. (2000b). Multiple oppositions: Case studies of variables in phonological intervention. *American Journal of Speech-Language Pathology, 9,* 289–299.

Williams, A. L., Epperly, R., Rodgers, J. R., & Feltes, L. (1999). *Treatment efficacy in phonological intervention: Clinical case studies*. Poster session presented at the annual convention of the American Speech-Language-Hearing Association, San Francisco, CA.

Williams, F., Cairns, H. S., Cairns, C. E., & Blosser, D. F. (1970). *Analysis of production errors in the phonetic performance of school-age standard English-speaking children*. Austin, TX: University of Texas.

Williams, G., & McReynolds, L. (1975). The relationship between discrimination and articulation training in children with misarticulations. *Journal of Speech and Hearing Research, 18,* 401–412.

Williams, R. L., & Wolfram, W. (1977). Social dialects: Differences versus disorders. In K. Jeter (Ed.), *Bilingual language learning system*. Rockville, MD: American Speech-Language-Hearing Association.

Winitz, H. (1969). *Articulation acquisition and behavior*. New York: Appleton-Century-Crofts.

Winitz, H. (1975). *From syllable to conversation*. Baltimore: University Park Press.

Winitz, H. (1984). Auditory considerations in articulation training. In H. Winitz (Ed.), *Treating articulation disorders: For clinicians by clinicians*. Baltimore: University Park Press.

Winitz, H. (1989). Auditory considerations in treatment. In N. Creaghead, P. Newman, & W. Secord (Eds.), *Assessment and remediation of articulatory and phonological disorders* (2nd ed.) (pp. 243–264). New York: Macmillan.

Winitz, H., & Irwin, O. C. (1958). Syllabic and phonetic structure of infants' early words. *Journal of Speech and Hearing Research, 1,* 250–256.

Winitz, H., Sanders, R., & Kort, J. (1981). Comprehension and production of the /əz/ plural allomorph. *Journal of Psycholinguistic Research, 10,* 259–271.

Winteler, J. (1876). *Die Kerenzer Mundart des Kantons Glarus in ihren Grundzügen dargestellt*. Leipzig: C. F. Winter'sche Verlagsbuchhandlung.

Wise, C. M. (1958). *Introduction to phonetics*. Englewood Cliffs, NJ: Prentice-Hall.

Witzel, M. A. (1995). Communicative impairment associated with clefting. In R. J. Schprintzen & J. Bardach (Eds.), *Cleft palate speech management: A multidisciplinary approach*. St. Louis, MO: Mosby.

Wolfram, W. (1986). Language variation in the United States. In O. Taylor (Ed.), *Treatment of communication disorders in culturally and linguistically diverse populations* (pp. 73–116). San Diego, CA: College-Hill Press.

Wolfram, W. (1994). The phonology of a sociocultural variety: The case of African American Vernacular English. In J. Bernthal & N. Bankson (Eds.), *Child phonology: Characteristics, assessment, and intervention with special populations* (pp. 227–244). New York: Thieme.

Wolfram, W., & Schilling-Estes, N. (2006). *American English: Dialects and variation* (2nd ed.). Malden/Oxford: Blackwell.

Wolk, L. (1986). Markedness analysis of consonant error productions in apraxia of speech. *Journal of Communication Disorders, 19,* 133–160.

Wolk, L., & Meisler, A. (1998). Phonological assessment: A systematic comparison of conversation and picture naming. *Journal of Communication Disorders, 31,* 291–313.

Yavaş, M. (1998). *Phonology development and disorders*. San Diego, CA: Singular.

Yearbook of immigration statistics. (2003). U.S. Department of Commerce. Springfield, VA: National Technical Information Service.

Yeni-Komshian, G., Flege, J., & Liu, S. (2000). Pronunciation proficiency in the first and second languages of Korean-English bilinguals. Bilingualism: Language. *Cognition, 3,* 131–150.

Yorkston, K. (1996). Treatment efficacy: Dysarthria. *Journal of Speech and Hearing Research, 39,* S42–S57.

Yorkston, K. M., & Beukelman, D. R. (1981). Communication efficiency of dysarthric speakers as measured by sentence intelligibility and speaking rate. *Journal of Speech and Hearing Disorders, 46,* 296–301.

Yorkston, K. M., & Beukelman, D. R. (Eds.). (1988). *Recent advances in clinical dysarthria.* Boston: Little, Brown.

Yorkston, K. M., Beukelman, D. R., & Bell, K. R. (1988). *Clinical management of dysarthric speakers.* Boston: College-Hill Press.

Yoss, K. A., & Darley, F. L. (1974a). Developmental apraxia of speech in children with defective articulation. *Journal of Speech and Hearing Research, 17,* 399–416.

Yoss, K. A., & Darley, F. L. (1974b). Therapy in developmental apraxia of speech. *Language, Speech, and Hearing Services in Schools, 5,* 23–31.

Young, E. H., & Hawk, S. S. (1955). *Moto-kinesthetic speech training.* Palo Alto, CA: Stanford University Press.

Zeltner, T., Caduff, J., Gehr, P., Pfenninger, J., & Burri, P. (1987). The postnatal growth and development of the human lung I. *Morphometry Respiratory Physiology, 67,* 247–267.

Zemlin, W. R. (1998). *Speech and hearing science: Anatomy and physiology* (4th ed.). Englewood Cliffs, NJ: Prentice-Hall.

Zentella, A. (2000). Puerto Ricans in the United States: Confronting the linguistic repercussions of colonialism. In S. McKay & S. Wong (Eds.), *New immigrants in the United States* (pp. 137–164). Cambridge: Cambridge University Press.

Author Index

Subject Index

substitution processes, 77, 78
syllable structure processes, 77–78, 132–133
systematic sound preference, 230
therapy, 321–323, 324–325
unusual processes, 230–231
variable use of processes, 231
Place-manner-voice analysis, 224–228
Prelinguistic behavior. *See* Prelinguistic stages
Prelinguistic stages, 114–116, 118, 119–120
canonical babbling, 115–116
contoids, 116
cooing and laughter stage, 115
first words, distinctions from, 114
jargon stage, 116
and language development, 114, 118
nonreduplicated babbling, 115
reflexive crying and vegetative sounds, 114–115
and transition to first words, 119–120
variegated babbling, 115
vocal play stage, 115
vocoids, 116
Productive phonological knowledge, 232–236
breadth of distribution, 233–234
distribution by morpheme, 234
distribution of sounds, 233, 234
levels, 236
phonemic inventory, 233
phonological rules, static, 234
dynamic rules, 234
neutralization rules, 235
Prosodic features, 119, 126–127, 137, 145–146
as contrastive stress, 137
defined, 119
development in infants, 119
in first fifty words, 126–127
in preschool children, 137
in school-age children, 145–146
tone unit, 137
Protowords, 120

Quasi-words, 120

Regression, 132
Resonatory system, development of structures in infants, 109–111
Respiration, development of structures in infants, 109
Rhotics, 25–26. *See also* Misarticulations

Salience factor, 126
Screening, 152–153
Semivowels, 364
Sensory-perceptual training, 248–249
Severity measures, 238–239
percentage of consonants correct, 238–239
procedures for analysis, 239
severity divisions, 239

Sibilants, 23, 314, 367
Sonorants, 17, 67, 68, 69
Sonority, 16
Spanish American English, 188–191
clinical application, 190
consonant inventory, 189
Cuban American English, 190
Nicaraguan American English, 188
Puerto Rican American English, 191
vowel inventory, 188
Speech, 1
Speech disorders, 1
Speech mechanism, 162–165
assessment form, 203–207
evaluation of, 162–165, 172–173
Speech sound, 60–61, 107–150, 210–215
analysis forms, 211–215
form, 60–61
definition, 107
development, 107–150. *See also* Phonological development
distribution, 210–211
inventory, 209
Speech sound development. *See* Phonological development
Stimulability testing, 159–160
Suprasegmentals. *See* Prosodic features
Syllabic, 17, 18, 31, 43, 45
Syllable, 31–33, 117, 222–224
analysis, 223–224
closed (checked), 32
constraints, 223
open (unchecked), 32
parts of, 31–32
shapes in early development, 117
structure, 31–33

Theories, phonological, 57–96. *See individual theories*
Therapy, phonetic approach. *See* Phonetic therapy approach
Tongue thrust, 258, 260
Traditional approach. *See* Phonetic approach

Unintelligible child, 176–177
characteristics of, 176
problems during evaluation, 176–177

Vietnamese American English, 191–193
clinical application, 192–193
consonants in inventory, 192
vowels in inventory, 192
Vocables, 120
Vowel therapy, 338–342
limited vowel inventory, 341–342
multiple vowel errors, 338–340
vowel substitutions, 342